BIOPSY INTERPRETATION SERIES

BIOPSY INTERPRETATION OF THE LUNG

BIOPSY INTERPRETATION SERIES

Series Editor: Jonathan I. Epstein, M.D.

Biopsy Interpretation of the Gastrointestinal Tract Mucosa: Neoplastic, 2/e (Vol. 2)
Elizabeth A. Montgomery and Lysandra Voltaggio, 2012

Biopsy Interpretation of the Upper Aerodigestive Tract and Ear, 2/e
Edward B. Stelow and Stacey E. Mills, 2012

Biopsy Interpretation of the Breast, 2/e
Stuart J. Schnitt and Laura C. Collins, 2013

Biopsy Interpretation of the Lung
Saul Suster and Cesar A. Moran, 2013

Biopsy Interpretation of the Gastrointestinal Tract Mucosa: Non-Neoplastic, 2/e (Vol. 1)
Elizabeth A. Montgomery and Lysandra Voltaggio, 2011

Biopsy Interpretation of the Central Nervous System
Matthew J. Schniederjan, Daniel J. Brat, 2011

Biopsy Interpretation of the Bladder, 2/e
Jonathan I. Epstein, Mahul B. Amin, and Victor E. Reuter, 2010

Biopsy Interpretation of Soft Tissue Tumors
Cyril Fisher, Elizabeth A. Montgomery, and Khin Thway, 2010

Biopsy Interpretation of the Thyroid
Scott L. Boerner and Sylvia L. Asa, 2009

Biopsy Interpretation of the Skin
A. Neil Crowson, Cynthia M. Magro, and Martin C. Mihm, 2009

Biopsy Interpretation: The Frozen Section
Jerome B. Taxy, Aliya N. Husain, and Anthony G. Montag, 2009

Biopsy Interpretation of the Uterine Cervix and Corpus
Anais Malpica, Michael T. Deavers and Elizabeth D. Euscher, 2009

Biopsy Interpretation of the Liver, 2/e
Stephen A. Geller and Lydia M. Petrovic, 2009

Biopsy Interpretation of the Prostate, 4/e
Jonathan I. Epstein and George Netto, 2007

BIOPSY INTERPRETATION SERIES

BIOPSY INTERPRETATION OF THE LUNG

Saul Suster, M.D.
Professor and Chairman
Department of Pathology
Medical College of Wisconsin
Milwaukee, Wisconsin

Cesar A. Moran, M.D.
Professor of Pathology
Director of Thoracic Pathology
The University of Texas M.D. Anderson Cancer Center
Houston, Texas

Wolters Kluwer | Lippincott Williams & Wilkins
Health
Philadelphia · Baltimore · New York · London
Buenos Aires · Hong Kong · Sydney · Tokyo

Senior Executive Editor: Jonathan W. Pine, Jr.
Product Director: Julia Seto
Vendor Manager: Alicia Jackson
Senior Manufacturing Manager: Benjamin Rivera
Creative Director: Doug Smock
Production Service: S4Carlisle

Two Commerce Square
2001 Market Street
Philadelphia, PA 19103

Printed in the People's Republic of China

Library of Congress Cataloging-in-Publication Data

Suster, Saul.
Biopsy interpretation of the lung / Saul Suster, Cesar A. Moran.—1st ed.
p. ; cm.—(Biopsy interpretation series)
Includes bibliographical references and index.
ISBN 978-0-7817-8467-2—ISBN 0-7817-8467-0
I. Moran, Cesar. II. Title. III. Series: Biopsy interpretation series.
[DNLM: 1. Lung Diseases—pathology. 2. Biopsy—methods. WF 600]

616.2'40758—dc23

2012013175

10 9 8 7 6 5 4 3 2 1

RRS1207

To my wife, Jenny, and to our children,
David and Dana, for their endless support

S.S.

With love to my wife, Susan, and my
children Kate and Eliza

C.A.M.

PREFACE

Lung biopsies represent some of the most common types of specimens seen by pathologists during routine daily practice. The introduction of flexible bronchoscopy has allowed pulmonologists and clinicians ready access to the lungs in patients suffering from pulmonary disease. The small size of the biopsies and frequent artifactual changes induced by the procedure, however, can create serious challenges for the pathologist. The level of expectation by clinicians regarding the diagnostic yield of such biopsies can sometimes be at odds with the realities imposed by the limitations of this biopsy modality. Close communication with the pneumonologist and radiologist is of the highest importance in this setting for adequate interpretation and for educating the clinician regarding the limitations of the technique. Despite all of its limitations, small lung biopsy specimens can provide valuable information that will be of importance for the clinician in patient management and treatment. Computer tomographic scans prior to the biopsy are useful for selecting appropriate patients to undergo the biopsy procedure and in elaborating an appropriate differential diagnosis.

This book addresses the various aspects of lung biopsy interpretation. Although there are numerous excellent textbooks of pulmonary pathology in print, most are based on the pathology of resected specimens and very few address the particular challenges and special limitations of small lung biopsies. The book is organized by traditional disease groups and covers the major clinical aspects of the various disease processes, plus histopathologic features and use of ancillary diagnostic techniques such as special stains, immunohistochemistry, electron microscopy, and molecular pathology. The differential diagnosis in the context of small biopsies and the particular limitations imposed by the procedure are also highlighted when pertinent. Numerous tables summarize the main features of the processes described, and ample illustrations are provided to highlight the most salient and distinctive features of the various conditions discussed. The indications for the various types of biopsies (i.e., endoscopic versus core needle versus open/wedge biopsy) are discussed in the context of the various lesions.

The content of this book represents the result of the personal experience of the authors plus a thoughtful review of the published literature. The authors apologize for any omissions in the text, particularly when dealing with esoteric and extremely rare conditions, of for the natural personal bias all pathologists have when dealing with controversial concepts or poorly defined entities. We have tried to achieve balance in our exposition of controversial subjects and hope that this volume will be of assistance for general pathologist confronted with the task of interpreting lung biopsies.

Saul Suster, M.D.
Cesar A. Moran, M.D.

CONTENTS

1

METHODS FOR OBTAINING LUNG BIOPSIES

Lung biopsies represent an important and oftentimes definitive method for establishing a diagnosis in patients afflicted with pulmonary disorders. Three basic methods are currently routinely employed for the evaluation of lung tissue: endoscopic biopsies, transthoracic (percutaneous) core needle biopsies, and video-assisted thoracoscopic surgery (VATS) lung biopsy. The older method of open lung biopsy via thoracotomy was associated with significant morbidity and has been largely abandoned in favor of VATS. Techniques based on the cytologic examinations of specimens obtained through fine needle aspiration (FNA) or bronchial brushings and washings also play a role in the evaluation of patients with lung disorders but will not be a subject of discussion in this book. The selection of the biopsy method employed will be dictated by the clinical circumstances and the level of experience and skill of the thoracic surgeon, pneumonologist, or interventional radiologist. Obviously, the diagnostic yield for a focalized endobronchial lesion will be much higher on endobronchial biopsy than for a diffuse or peripheral lung processes. Diffuse lung diseases with predominant peribronchial distribution such as sarcoidosis are particularly amenable to diagnosis on transbronchial biopsy. Conditions in which diagnostic features depend on demonstration of temporal heterogeneity and variations in the histopathologic features from site to site, such as the idiopathic interstitial pneumonias, will require a VATS approach and will yield only extremely limited results on endoscopic biopsies. Correlation of the clinical information and radiographic findings will be indispensable for a correct interpretation of the findings. It is important that the pathologist be provided with a full clinical history, results of imaging studies, and other clinical test results, as well as a provisional or suspected differential diagnosis by the surgeon or clinician at the time the biopsy specimen is submitted.

BRONCHIAL ENDOSCOPIC BIOPSY

Endoscopic bronchial or transbronchial biopsy constitutes a technique whereby biopsy material is generally obtained through a flexible tube that is inserted into the airways (fiberoptic bronchoscopy). It is the most commonly used invasive technique currently available for obtaining lung tissue biopsies. Although rigid bronchoscopes were used for obtaining biopsy material as far back as the 1940s,[1,2] it was not until the development of fiberoptic technology that this technique truly came of age. The first flexible fiberoptic bronchoscope was developed and introduced into clinical practice by Ikeda[3] in 1970. Since then, further refinements and additional experience with this instrument have firmly established this modality as a highly valuable technique for obtaining lung tissue biopsies for diagnosis. The development of videobronchoscopy has further refined our capabilities for diagnosis and currently permits capturing digital images using a video chip that transmits them to a digital monitor. The latter technique provides the advantage of capturing images and storing them in various formats for teaching and research in addition to procuring the biopsy samples.

Rigid bronchoscopy is more limited in terms of the depth of airways examination and is usually used for evaluation of proximal lesions in the upper airways and for the extraction of foreign bodies or the management of hemoptysis. It is limited by the inability to properly visualize terminal bronchi and the need for general anesthesia.

Bronchoscopy is generally carried out with light sedation and topical anesthesia in an outpatient setting. The bronchoscope can be introduced by either a transnasal or transoral approach. The field of vision is usually 80° with the angle of deflection usually 160° to 180°. The scope is equipped with a light source, camera, suction and irrigation ports, and biopsy tools. The size and width of the instrument will depend on the number of fiberoptic bundles; the larger the number of fiberoptic bundles, the greater the light transmitted by the scope. Most scopes have the ability to permit examination of segmental and subsegmental bronchi up to sixth-order bronchi.[4] Diagnostic yield can be enhanced in certain settings when the results of bronchial biopsy are combined with the findings of bronchial washings, brushings, and alveolar lavage.[5,6]

There are very few contraindications for fiberoptic bronchoscopy. They mostly involve coagulopathy, recent myocardial ischemia or high-risk patients with increased intracranial pressure. The main risk of bronchoscopy is compromising the patient's airway, particularly in cases of tracheal stenosis or tumor. Rare complications include bradycardia, hypotension, syncope, and arrythmias. Morbidity in most large studies has varied from 0.05% to 1%, and mortality is around 0.01%.[7] The biopsy samples can be either endobronchial, comprising only the superficial mucosal surface (Figs. 1.1 and 1.2; eFig. 1.1), or transbronchial for deeper lesions within the parenchyma of the lung or lesions lying beneath the bronchial surface (Fig. 1.3). Biopsy of the bronchial mucosa is accomplished using a cupped forceps that is introduced through the flexible shaft of the bronchoscope. This allows visualization of the mucosa, lamina propria, muscle layer, and peribronchial lymphovascular network. The transbronchial technique uses a different kind of forceps that is generally advanced into a distal airway

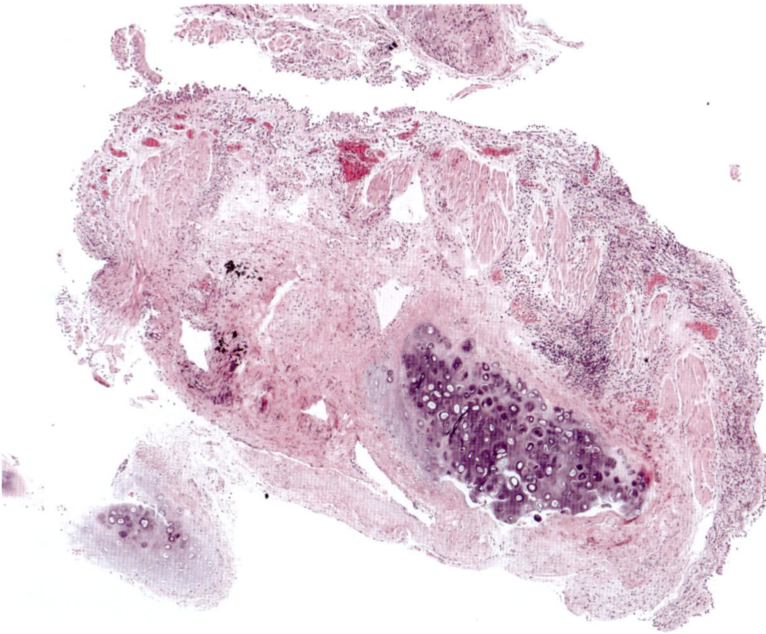

FIGURE 1.1 Endobronchial biopsy showing normal bronchial mucosa. Notice surface mucosa overlying hyaline bronchial cartilage and smooth muscle in the lamina propria.

and forces the bronchiolar wall and peribronchial lung parenchyma into the mouth of the device. The material sampled usually comprises lung parenchyma beyond the cartilaginous plate and includes alveolar spaces.

Although bronchial biopsies can be highly effective for the diagnosis of certain lung conditions, they may have serious limitations in many instances (Table 1.1).

The most useful role for bronchial biopsies is in the diagnosis of lung tumors involving the bronchial tree. Tumors most commonly accessible to the bronchoscope in the major airways include bronchogenic squamous cell carcinoma, small cell carcinoma, well-differentiated neuroendocrine carcinoma ("carcinoid" tumor), and certain salivary gland-type tumors such as mucoepidermoid carcinoma and adenoid cystic carcinoma (Fig. 1.4). Adenocarcinomas, particularly those in peripheral locations or not involving the bronchial tree, may not be easily detected by endobronchial or transbronchial biopsies.

Bronchoscopy has become increasingly used for the diagnosis and staging of lung cancer in recent years.[8] Endoscopic evaluation of early stage squamous cell carcinoma can provide a basis for the determination of therapeutic strategies depending on the gross configuration of the tumor (i.e., polypoid, diffuse).[9] Ultrasound-guided transbronchial endoscopic biopsies have also increased the yield of positive diagnosis

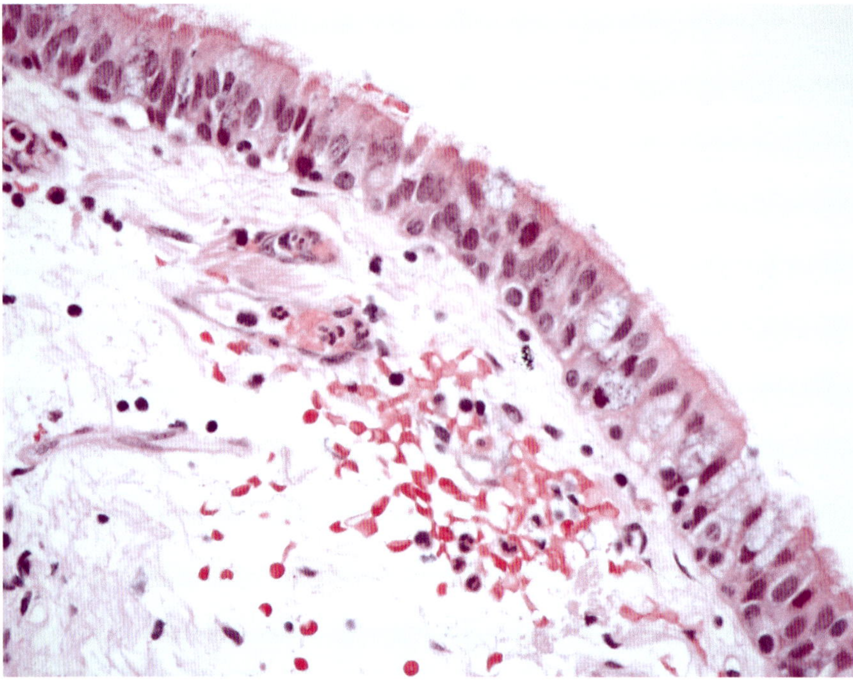

FIGURE 1.2 Higher magnification of endobronchial biopsy showing normal columnar ciliated surface epithelium.

for solitary pulmonary nodules less than 3 cm in diameter that cannot be normally visualized under conventional fluoroscopy.[10] Diagnosis of endobronchial metastases can also be successfully accomplished in many instances by bronchoscopic biopsy techniques.[11] Clinical correlation and a thorough patient history, however, are required in most instances to distinguish these tumors from primary cancers.

Another indication for endoscopic biopsy is for the diagnosis of opportunistic infections, including *Pneumocystis carinii*, fungal and viral infections, and cytomegalovirus. Bronchial biopsy is also very useful for the evaluation of lung transplant patients, particularly in the diagnosis of acute allograft rejection. Diagnostic yield for opportunistic infections in AIDS patients can be as high as 90% when cytologic and biopsy methods are combined.[12,13]

Conditions in which transbronchial lung biopsies may yield diagnostic information in certain circumstances include diffuse alveolar hemorrhage with necrotizing capillaritis in patients with Wegener granulomatosis and other antineutrophil cytoplasmic antibody-related conditions. Bronchial biopsy may also yield diagnostic tissue in cases of pulmonary alveolar proteinosis or lymphangioleiomyomatosis, particularly when there is extensive disease. The same applies to cases of sarcoidosis in which transbronchial biopsy may yield well-formed epithelioid granulomas, although

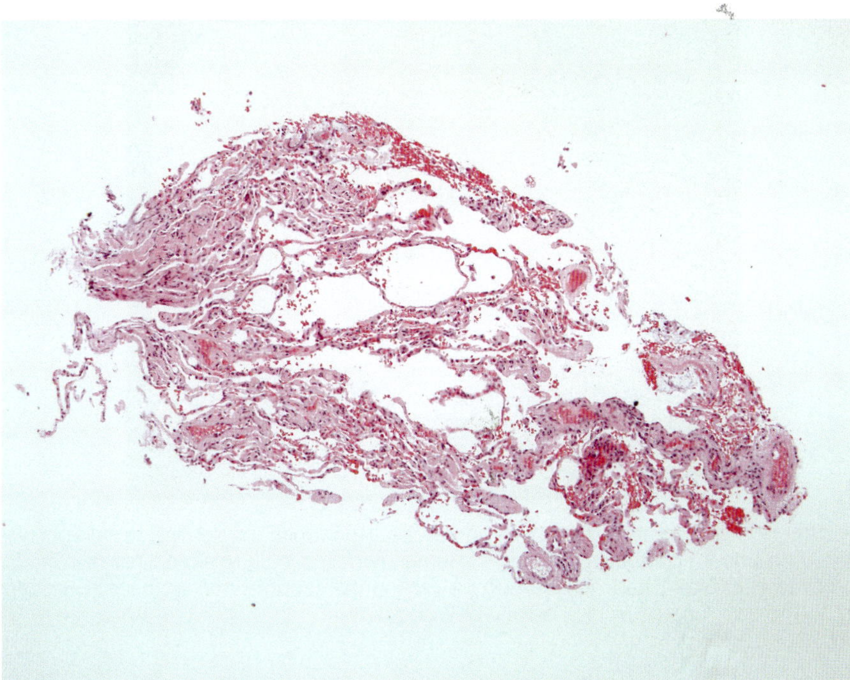

FIGURE 1.3 Transbronchial biopsy showing normal lung parenchyma with preserved alveolar spaces. Notice the dilated capillaries within the interstitium in the alveolar walls.

TABLE 1.1 Limitations and Indications of Bronchial Endoscopic Biopsies

High Diagnostic Yield	Moderate Diagnostic Yield	Poor Diagnostic Yield
Squamous cell carcinoma	Alveolar hemorrhagic syndromes	Adenocarcinoma
Carcinoid tumor	Capillaritis	Metastatic tumors
Small cell carcinoma	Collagen vascular diseases	Sarcomas
Mucoepidermoid carcinoma	Alveolar proteinosis	Other unusual tumors
Adenoid cystic carcinoma	Lymphangioleiomyo matosis	Interstitial lung diseases
Opportunistic infections	Sarcoidosis	Acute pneumonias
Lung transplant patients	Lymphoproliferative disorders	Wegener granulomatosis

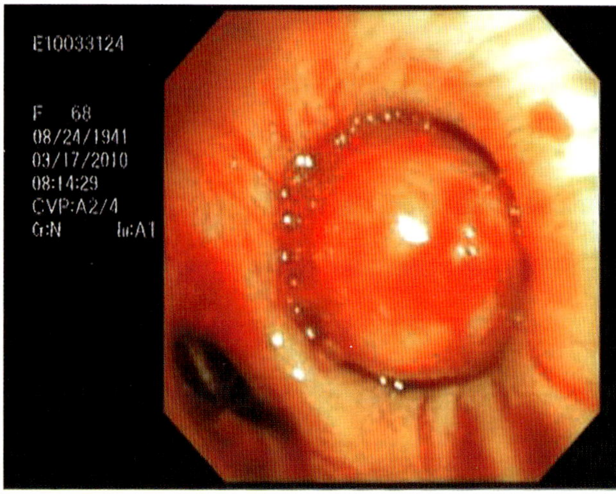

FIGURE 1.4 Bronchoscopic examination reveals a polypoid, intraluminal endobronchial mass with smooth contours occluding the lumen corresponding to a bronchial "carcinoid" tumor (well-differentiated neuroendocrine carcinoma). (Courtesy of Dr. George Haasler, Ph.D., Thoracic Surgery, Medical college of Wisconsin.)

the latter remains strictly a diagnosis of exclusion and requires clinical correlation. Diagnostic information can also be obtained from limited bronchial biopsy material containing dense lymphoid infiltrates, particularly when utilizing modern molecular techniques for the study of clonal gene rearrangements, specific translocations, and detection of light chain restriction using paraffin-embedded tissue biopsies with polymerase chain reaction, fluorescence in situ hybridization, or other techniques.

Transbronchial biopsies may be of very limited or no value in the evaluation of various lung conditions, including peripheral tumors that are not accessible via the fiberoptic bronchoscope, metastatic tumors that do not involve the major airways, and sarcomas and other rare tumors in which a limited sample may not supply the necessary information for a definitive diagnosis. In acute pneumonias, the findings will be so nonspecific that anything beyond a generic diagnosis of diffuse alveolar damage may not be possible. The size and number of tissue fragments obtained for evaluation may also influence the diagnostic yield of the procedure; the smaller the size of the biopsy and the fewer the tissue samples obtained, the lower the yield (Fig. 1.5).[14,15]

One of the most abused uses of endoscopic lung biopsies is for the evaluation of interstitial lung disease.[16] Criteria for the diagnosis of these conditions are currently based on the examination of open lung biopsies.[17] Because the diagnosis of interstitial lung disease is heavily dependent on the temporal and spatial relationship of the changes requiring comparison from various areas of the lung (often from separate lobes), results obtained from transbronchial biopsies will be of extremely

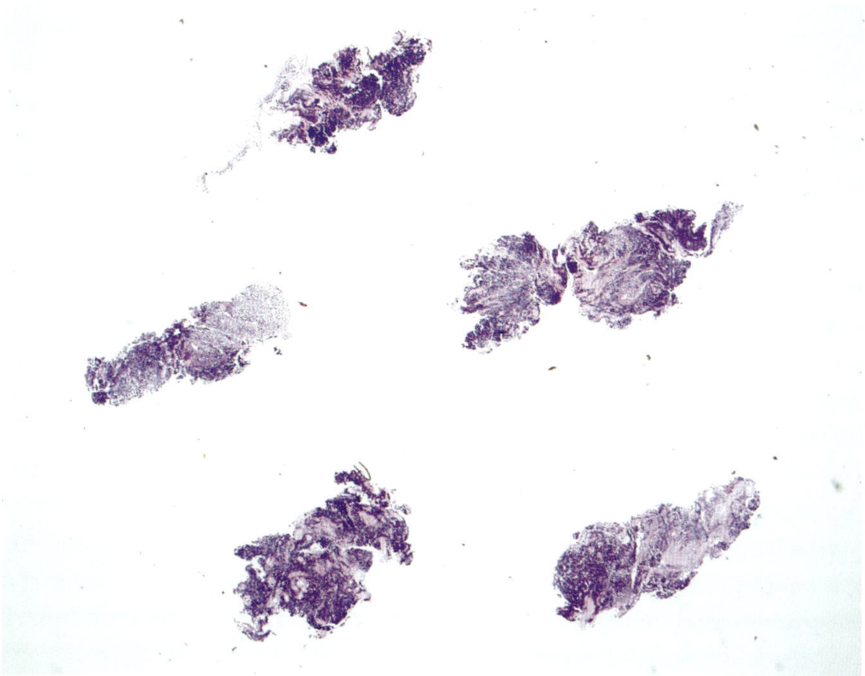

FIGURE 1.5 Multiple small transbronchial biopsies dramatically improve the chances for a definitive diagnosis than a single, small biopsy.

limited value for the diagnosis of usual interstitial pneumonia, desquamative interstitial pneumonia, respiratory bronchiolitis-associated interstitial lung disease, nonspecific interstitial pneumonia, hypersensitivity pneumonitis, and others. Attempting to establish a definitive diagnosis of a specific interstitial lung disease on a transbronchial biopsy may often be misleading and nearly impossible in most cases. The bulk of the literature has demonstrated that the diagnostic yield and accuracy of endoscopic bronchial biopsy for the diagnosis of diffuse interstitial lung disease is much less than that of other techniques such as open biopsy and VATS.[18,19] In recent years, video-assisted thoracoscopic biopsies have become increasingly favored over open lung biopsy for the diagnosis of interstitial lung disorders owing to the decreased morbidity and hospital stay associated with the former.[20–22]

Use of transbronchial biopsy in patients with interstitial lung disease to rule out certain conditions that present with a similar clinical and radiographic picture, such as sarcoidosis and lymphangitis carcinomatosa, may be justified and indicated in selected instances. The appropriate approach by the endoscopist who submits a biopsy in such instances would be to provide the pathologist with a pertinent clinical history, provide information regarding the existence of interstitial lung infiltrates in the requisition form, state the differential diagnosis and request that alternative conditions such as sarcoidosis, lymphangitis carcinomatosa, or others be ruled out.

Endoscopic biopsy procedures of the bronchial tree are often complicated by artifacts and nonspecific changes that can obscure the underlying process and create pitfalls for diagnosis. These include tissue compression with crushing artifact or collapse of the lung parenchyma and bleeding. Compression of lung parenchyma may superficially simulate interstitial fibrosis on scanning magnification owing to the apposition of alveolar walls against one another. Closer examination will demonstrate that the alveolar septa are of normal thickness and that only their close proximity creates an illusion of fibrosis (Fig. 1.6). Tangential sectioning of medium and large caliber vessel walls may also contribute to the impression of interstitial fibrosis in endoscopic biopsies. Crushing of lymphocytes may create a picture suggestive of small cell bronchogenic carcinoma (Fig. 1.7; eFig. 1.2); use of immunostains may be warranted under such circumstances to identify CD45-positive cells versus keratin-positive cells in these areas (Fig. 1.8). Bleeding is a common complication of the biopsy procedure and may be confused for pathologic hemorrhage. In most instances of pathologic pulmonary

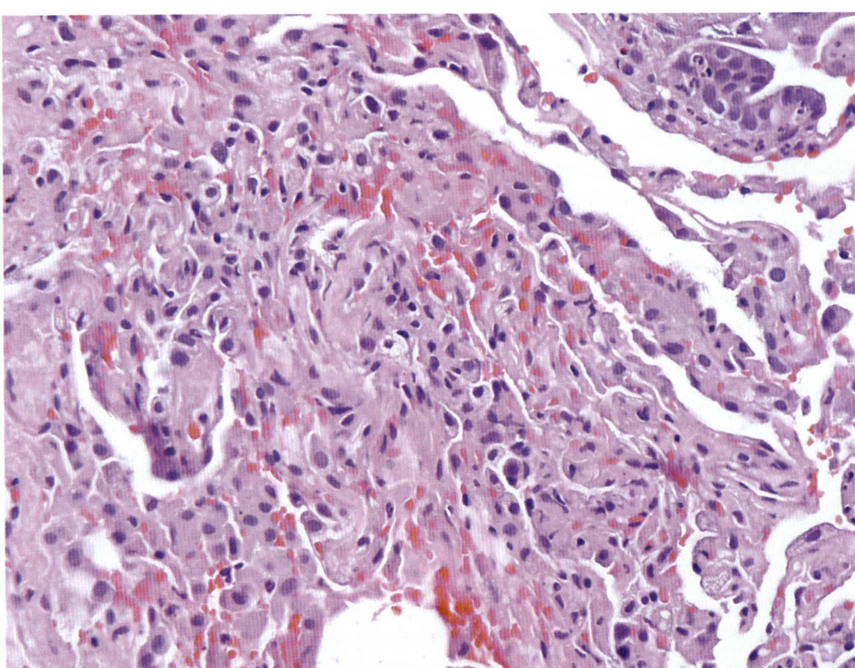

FIGURE 1.6 Collapse of alveolar walls with close apposition of alveolar septa may give an initial impression of interstitial fibrosis; closer examination shows that alveolar septa are of normal thickness.

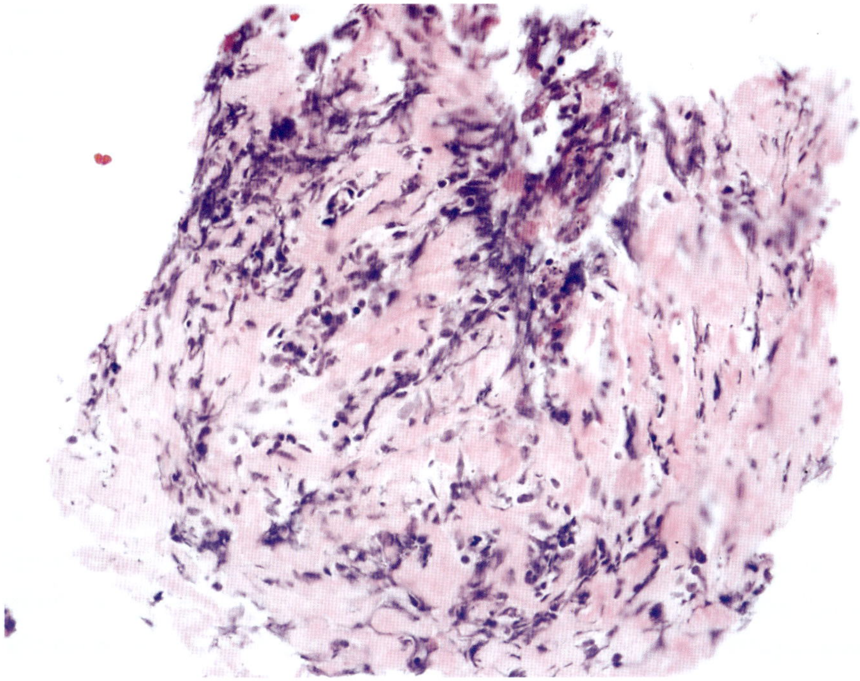

FIGURE 1.7 Transbronchial biopsy with extensive crushing of lymphocytes may suggest the possibility of small cell carcinoma.

bleeding, however, the lung parenchyma will also contain fibrin and hemosiderin-laden macrophages (Fig. 1.9) (eFig. 1.3).

TRANSTHORACIC PERCUTANEOUS CORE NEEDLE BIOPSY

Transthoracic percutaneous biopsies under computerized tomography (CT)-guidance or using ultrasound techniques have been employed during the past two decades with great success for the evaluation of pulmonary pathology. The technique is typically employed in the radiology department because it requires advanced radiologic equipment and expertise. This approach is particularly well suited to the evaluation of peripheral lung lesions, in particular pleural-based tumors.[23] Ultrasound-guided percutaneous biopsies offer the advantage of real-time visualization of the path of the needle, thus allowing a more rapid examination than that possible under CT guidance.[24] Recent advances in CT scan technology, however, are now also allowing real-time visualization of the procedure using continuous CT fluoroscopy.[25] A fairly recent survey of transthoracic needle biopsies of lung masses disclosed that approximately 70% of participating medical centers in the United States and Canada performed the procedure under CT guidance, 8% under fluoroscopy, and 22% used a

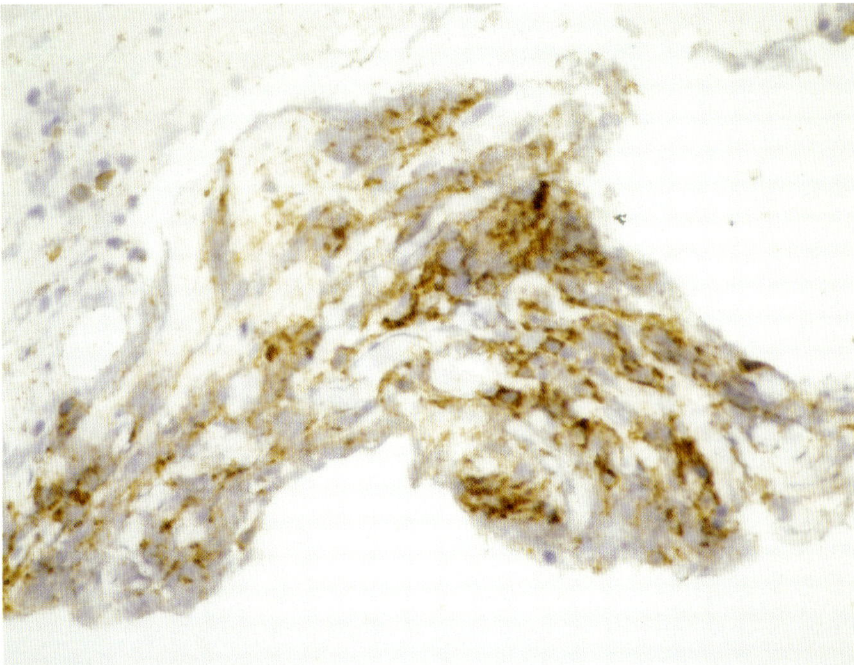

FIGURE 1.8 Immunohistochemical stain for CD45 (leukocyte common antigen) shows a positive reaction, indicating that the crushed cells correspond to lymphoid cells.

combination of CT and fluoroscopy. FNA was the procedure of choice in 73% of centers, while 14% preferred core biopsies, and 13% employed a combination of both techniques.[26] Core biopsies have had wider acceptance in the United Kingdom than in the United States, where more than 30% of centers utilize it as their sole technique.[27] The combined use of FNA and core biopsy, however, appears to yield the best results.[28,29] There may be specific indications, advantages, and disadvantages to both techniques. The role of FNA in the evaluation of pulmonary processes is beyond the scope of this book and will not be dealt with here. The reader is referred to the various specialized texts addressing this issue in the literature.

The main indications for transthoracic core needle biopsy are listed in Table 1.2. These include evaluation of a patient with a new or enlarging solitary pulmonary nodule, especially in peripheral locations; a patient with a hilar mass in whom bronchoscopy was negative; for the staging of patients with intrathoracic malignancy; in patients with consolidation of lung parenchyma in whom an infectious organism has not been isolated; and in patients with pleural thickening suspicious for malignancy (Fig. 1.10; eFig. 1.4). Although there are no absolute contraindications to transthoracic needle biopsy, a few relative contraindications do exist, including patients with bleeding diathesis, on mechanical ventilation, with

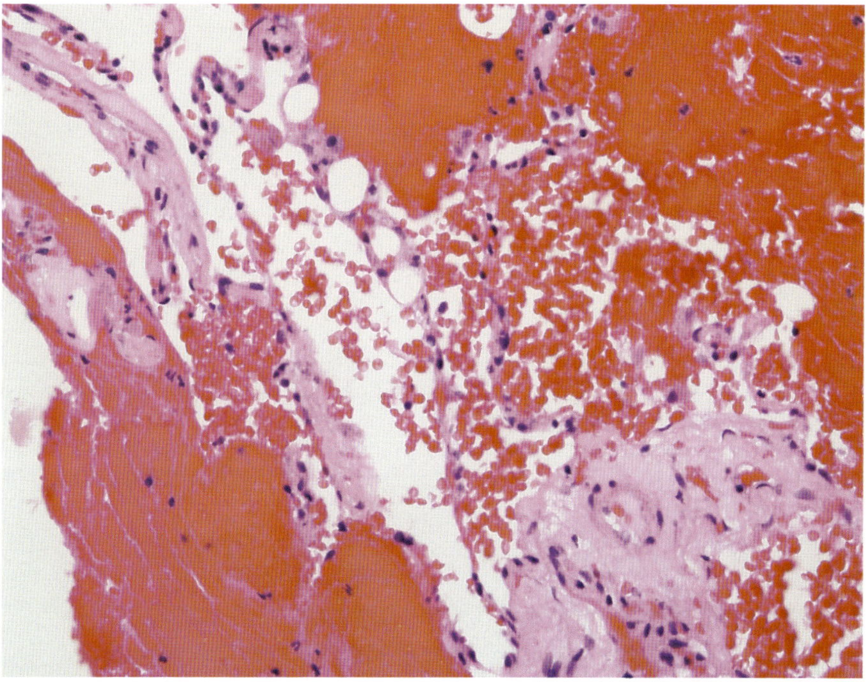

FIGURE 1.9 Bleeding caused by the biopsy procedure in transbronchial lung biopsy. Notice the absence of hemosiderin-laden macrophages and fibrin; this should not be confused for actual pathologic bleeding caused by bleeding disorders.

TABLE 1.2 Indications for Percutaneous Core Biopsy

Indications
Patient with a peripheral pulmonary nodule
Patient with a hilar mass with negative bronchoscopy
Staging of intrathoracic malignancies
Patient with suspected lung infection in whom other techniques failed to identify the organism
Patient with pleural thickening suspicious for malignancy
Relative contraindications
Bleeding disorders
Obstructive lung disease/mechanical ventilation
Pulmonary hypertension
Patients on mechanical ventilation
Patients with subpleural bulla, vascular lesions, or possible echinococcal cyst

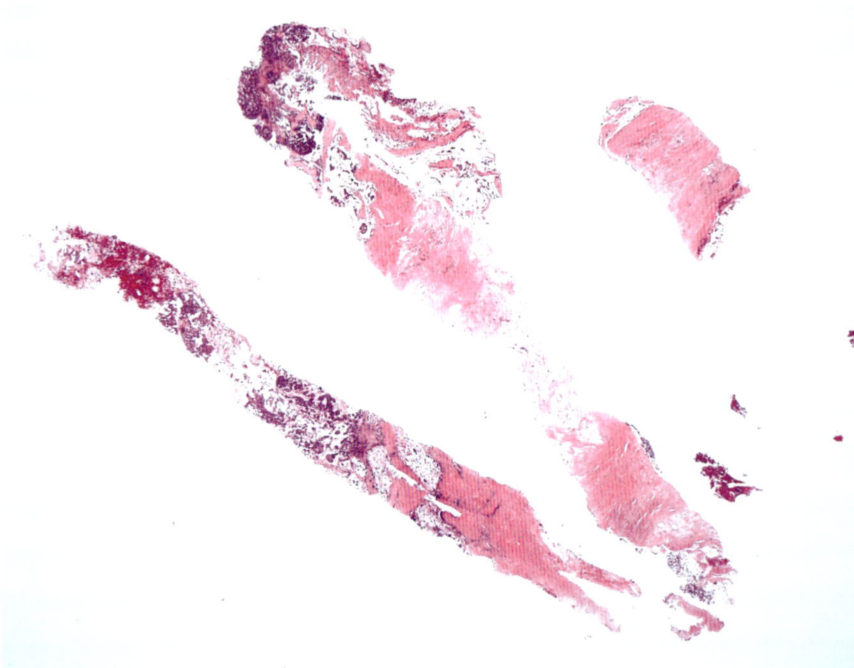

FIGURE 1.10 Percutaneous needle core biopsy of peripheral lung nodule demonstrating tumor identifiable as an adenocarcinoma.

moderate or severe obstructive lung disease, pulmonary hypertension, or patients with a history of contralateral pneumonectomy. Also, patients with a history of or clinical circumstances suspicious for subpleural bulla, vascular lesions, or echinococcal cyst should be approached with great caution to avoid unnecessary complications. All patients undergoing the transthoracic core biopsy should have a blood coagulation profile prior to the procedure, including platelet count and prothrombin time. Patients with central lesions in whom intravenous contrast is required for CT-guided biopsy should have renal function tests done prior to the procedure.

Percutaneous core biopsy is performed under local anesthesia and involves the introduction of a large-bore cutting needle through the pleura into the chest cavity. Obviously, the patients need to have the ability to cooperate with the procedure; patients who cannot maintain a prone or decubitus position, who cannot hold their breath, or who cannot lie still are poor candidates for this procedure. The main complication is the development of pneumothorax, the majority of which can usually be detected immediately following the procedure. The second most common complication is hemorrhage, with or without hemoptysis. Hemorrhage from transthoracic biopsies, however, is usually self-limited. Widely used guidelines for percutaneous core biopsy have been developed.[30] The majority of published studies demonstrate that the technique is safe with a low incidence of complications, morbidity, and mortality. Trucut (14G) and Surecut (15G or 16G, modified Menghini) needles are the types most commonly used.[31,32]

The use of large-bore cutting needles has been found to be superior to FNA sampling in terms of providing more specific diagnoses, particularly for the characterization of neoplastic processes.[31] FNA, although yielding a high rate of positive diagnosis of malignancy, has been found to have a limited capability for accurately identifying the cell type in up to one-third of cases, thus limiting management options for the treatment of the tumors.[33] Moreover, diagnosis of benign lesions is made more difficult on FNA material than with core biopsies.[31,34] CT-guided core needle biopsy has also been found to be associated with a higher diagnostic accuracy for the evaluation of pneumonia and its mimics than FNA.[35] In a study from the United Kingdom,[36] significantly more core biopsies than fine needle aspirates were diagnostic (93% vs. 78%; $P < .005$). No differences were found in the frequency of complications between the two groups.

VIDEO-ASSISTED THORACOSCOPIC LUNG BIOPSY

VATS offers the opportunity for obtaining multiple, relatively large tissue samples from lesions of the lung using a minimally invasive approach that involves the use of small incisions without spreading the ribs. This approach reduces the morbidity and mortality and allows a quicker return to normal activities with minimal hospitalization. The technique involves the use of trochars and a thoracoscope that is usually inserted through a 2-cm incision in about the sixth or seventh intercostal space along the midclavicular line. Two additional 2-cm incisions are made in about the fifth intercostal space, one anteriorly and the other posteriorly, creating a triangular configuration that facilitates access to various parts of the chest. VATS is generally performed under general anesthesia, although relatively limited procedures such as pleural biopsies can also be performed under local anesthesia. The procedure is accomplished by ventilating the opposite lung through a double-lumen endotracheal tube and allowing the affected lung to collapse. Following insertion of the thoracoscope the lung collapses and quickly separates from the chest wall, allowing clear visualization of all the major structures in the chest cavity.

A large number of thoracic operations can now be performed with VATS, including wedge resection and lobectomy. Lung biopsy is the most common procedure performed by VATS (eFig. 1.5).[37] The morbidity and mortality are very low, and patients are usually discharged on the first or second postoperative day. The procedure can even be performed on an outpatient basis.

VATS is particularly well suited to the evaluation of diffuse interstitial lung disease. The technique allows for generous sampling of multiple sites without the need for an open thoracotomy incision and permits

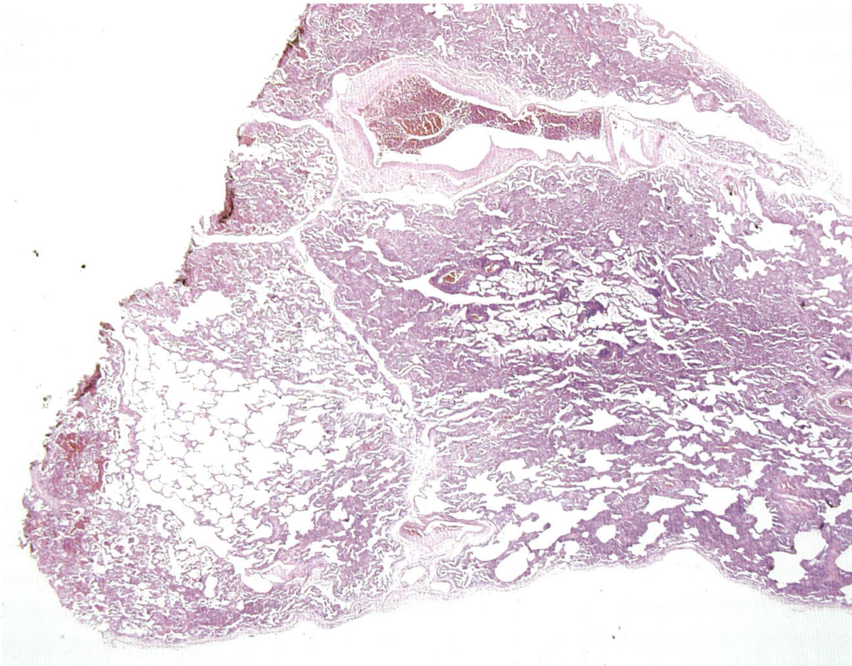

FIGURE 1.11 VATS biopsy for evaluation of interstitial lung disease. Notice wedge-shaped contour of the biopsy with the apex opposite to the pleural surface.

adequate evaluation of lung tissues (Fig. 1.11). VATS has been shown to be as effective as open lung biopsy for the diagnosis of interstitial lung disease, resulting in shorter hospital stays and fewer complications.[38] The procedure is considered safe in most patients; however, a recent study found a 4.4% mortality rate (3 of 68 patients) in a retrospective study of patients undergoing VATS biopsy for interstitial lung disease.[39]

VATS is also useful for the evaluation of peripheral lung lesions, in particular, indeterminate solitary pulmonary nodules.[40,41] This technique is particularly valuable for those cases in which endoscopic biopsy or core needle biopsy yield equivocal results. It has been shown that as many as 29% of patients whose condition was not diagnosed as malignant on transthoracic needle biopsy are ultimately found to have carcinoma.[42] VATS is not suitable for centrally located lesions because they generally cannot be reached by a thoracoscopic approach. Also, new lesions larger than 3 cm in greatest diameter are more likely to be malignant and may require thoracotomy.

The only absolute contraindication to VATS lung biopsy is a patient's inability to tolerate a general anesthetic with single-lung ventilation. This situation, however, is extremely unusual, except among mechanically ventilated patients with severe respiratory failure. VATS is also not feasible in patients who have previously undergone a pneumonectomy and thus do not have an opposite lung to ventilate. Prior thoracotomy with the development of adhesions can also make VATS difficult; however, in most instances the adhesions can be lysed under direct vision, allowing the procedure to be carried out safely.

HANDLING AND PROCESSING OF THE LUNG BIOPSY

Lung biopsy samples should be placed immediately into fixative or sterile transport medium. If transport medium is not available, the material may be placed on a sterile non stick dressing and immediately transported fresh to the laboratory for processing. Placing of a biopsy on saline-soaked gauze or mesh pads is discouraged as the biopsy material may become entrapped in the mesh, making extraction difficult with ensuing tissue damage. Exposure to air should be minimized to avoid air-drying artifacts. Procuring tissue for special techniques such as microbiologic cultures, cytogenetics, flow cytometry, electron microscopy (EM) or immunofluorescence always needs to be coordinated in advance with the pathology department. Tissues for microbial cultures should be sampled under sterile conditions in the operating room and submitted directly to the microbiology laboratory in a sterile container. Once the tissue has been transported to surgical pathology, the chance of contamination is great, thus compromising the results of microbiologic culture studies. If direct immunofluorescence is to be performed, a tissue sample must be frozen. Freezing to –20° C is usually sufficient for the initial handling of the specimen. If the specimen is to be retained longer than a few weeks, freezing at –70° C will be required. Tissues for EM need to be sampled fresh, carefully diced into 1-mm^3 cubes, and placed in a solution of 2% to 3% glutaraldehyde or other EM fixative. The vials containing the tissue must be carefully labeled, stored at 4° C and transferred to the EM facility. Tissues for cytogenetics or flow cytometry must be placed in an appropriate transport solution and transferred immediately to the appropriate facility for proper processing. Tissues intended for routine histopathologic examination are best placed in 10% neutral buffered formalin using a tissue to volume ratio of approximately 1:10. Alternative nonformalin fixatives such as alcohol and others may also be used, depending on the local usage at any given laboratory.

Specimens obtained through video-assisted thoracoscopy or thoracotomy may require different handling techniques than small endoscopic or core biopsy samples. In many instances, such specimens are subjected to intraoperative consultation with frozen section examination at the time of surgery. This is best accomplished by sectioning the specimen fresh with a sharp new blade avoiding unnecessary compression and distortion of the tissue. After frozen section consultation is complete, the remainder of the specimen can be routinely fixed in neutral buffered formalin or carefully injected with formalin using a 21G to 23G needle and syringe. Frozen section consultation is obtained in some instances to determine whether the sample is representative for the evaluation of interstitial lung disease;

however, the frozen section must be followed by an additional sample, preferably from the same site, because the frozen tissues will become distorted by the freezing artifact, rendering them useless for proper evaluation on permanent sections. Frozen section examination is not an optimal modality for evaluating interstitial lung disease and should be discouraged, unless there is a proper indication for it and additional, properly fixed tissue will be subsequently submitted for definitive evaluation.

REFERENCES

1. Edell ES, Sanderson DR. History of bronchoscopy. In: Prakash UBS, ed. *Bronchoscopy*. New York, NY: Raven Press; 1994:7–11.
2. Herbut PA, Clerf LH. Bronchogenic carcinoma: diagnosis by cytological study of bronchoscopically removed secretions. *JAMA*. 1946;130:1006.
3. Ikeda S. Flexible bronchofiberscope. *Ann Otol Rhinol Laryngol*. 1970;79:916–923.
4. Kovnat DM, Rath GS, Anderson WM, et al. Maximal extent of visualization of bronchial tree by flexible fiberoptic bronchoscopy. *Am Rev Respir Dis*. 1974;110:88–90.
5. Lauver GI, Hasan FM, Morgan RB, et al. The usefulness of fiberoptic bronchoscopy in evaluating new pulmonary lesions in the compromised host. *Am J Med*. 1979;66:580–587.
6. Poletti V, Patelli M, Poggi S, et al. Transbronchial lung biopsy and bronchoalveolar lavage in diagnosis of diffuse infiltrative lung diseases. *Respiration*. 1988;54(suppl):66–79.
7. Pue CA, Pacht ER. Complications of fiberoptic bronchoscopy at a university hospital. *Chest*. 1995;107:430–432.
8. Savage C, Morrison RJ, Zwischenberger JB. Bronchoscopic diagnosis and staging of lung cancer. *Chest Surg Clin N Am*. 2001;11:701–721.
9. Konaka C, Hirano T, Kato H, et al. Comparison of endoscopic features of early-stage squamous cell lung cancer and histological findings. *Br J Cancer*. 1999;80:1435–1439.
10. Herth FJF, Eberhardt R, Becker HD, et al. Endobronchial ultrasound-guided transbronchial lung biopsy in fluoroscopically invisible solitary pulmonary nodules: a prospective trial. *Chest*. 2006;129:147–150.
11. Dursun AB, Demirag F, Bayiz H, et al. Endobronchial metastases: a clinicopathological analysis. *Respirology*. 2005;10:510–514.
12. Poe RH, Utell MJ, Israel RH, et al. Sensitivity and specificity of the nonspecific transbronchial lung biopsy. *Am Rev Respir Dis*. 1979;119:25–32.
13. House AJS. Biopsy techniques in the investigation of diseases of the lung, mediastinum, and chest wall. *Radiol Clin North Am*. 1979;17:393–412.
14. Fraire AE, Cooper SP, Greenberg SD, et al. Transbronchial lung biopsy. Histopathologic and morphometric assessment of diagnostic utility. *Chest*. 1992;102:748–753.
15. Shure D. Transbronchial biopsy and needle aspiration. *Chest*. 1989;95:1130–1138.
16. Gal AA. Use and abuse of lung biopsy. *Adv Anat Pathol*. 2005;12:195–202.
17. Travis WD, King TE Jr, Bateman ED, et al. American Thoracic Society/European Respiratory Society international multidisciplinary consensus classification of the idiopathic interstitial pneumonias. *Am J Respir Crit Care Med*. 2002;165:277–304.
18. Wall CP, Gaensler EA, Carrington CB, et al. Comparison of transbronchial and open biopsies in chronic infiltrative lung diseases. *Am Rev Respir Dis*. 1981;123:280–285.
19. Katzenstein A-LA, Askin FB. Interpretation and significance of pathologic findings in transbronchial lung biopsy. *Am J Surg Pathol*. 1980;4:223–234.
20. Ferson PF, Landreneau RJ. Thoracoscopic lung biopsy or open lung biopsy for interstitial lung disease. *Chest Surg Clin N Am*. 1998;8:749–762.

21. Tiitto L, Heiskanen U, Bloigu R, et al. Thoracoscopic lung biopsy is a safe procedure in diagnosing usual interstitial pneumonia. *Chest.* 2005;128:2375–2380.

22. Riley DJ, Costanzo EJ. Surgical biopsy: its appropriateness in diagnosing interstitial lung disease. *Curr Opin Pulm Med.* 2006;12:331–336.

23. Clore F, Virapongse C, Saterfiel J. Low-risk large-needle biopsy of chest lesions. *Chest.* 1989;96:538–541.

24. Yang PC, Chang DB, Yu CJ, et al. Ultrasound-guided core biopsy of thoracic tumors. *Am Rev Respir Dis.* 1992;146:763–767.

25. Tsushima K, Sone S, Hanaoka T, et al. Comparison of bronchoscopic diagnosis for peripheral pulmonary nodule under fluoroscopic guidance with CT guidance. *Respir Med.* 2006;100:737–745.

26. Aviram G, Schwartz DS, Meirsdorf S, et al. Transthoracic needle biopsy of lung masses: a survey of techniques. *Clin Radiol.* 2005;60:370–374.

27. Richardson CM, Pointon KS, Manhire AR, et al. Percutaneous lung biopsies: a survey of UK practice based on 5444 biopsies. *Br J Radiol.* 2002;75:731–735.

28. Yamagami T, Iida S, Kato T, et al. Combining fine-needle aspiration and core biopsy under CT fluoroscopy guidance: a better way to treat patients with lung nodules? *AJR Am J Roentgenol.* 2003;180:811–815.

29. Kim HK, Shin BK, Cho SJ, et al. Transthoracic fine needle aspiration and core biopsy of pulmonary lesions. A study of 296 patients. *Acta Cytol.* 2002;46:1061–1068.

30. Manhire A, Charig M, Clelland C, et al. Guidelines for radiologically guided lung biopsy. *Thorax.* 2003;58:920–936.

31. Pang JA, Tsang V, Hom BL, et al. Ultrasound-guided tissue-core biopsy of thoracic lesions with Trucut and Surecut needles. *Chest.* 1987;91:823–828.

32. Yamagami T, Iida S, Kato T, et al. Usefulness of new automated cutting needle for tissue-core biopsy of lung nodules under CT fluoroscopic guidance. *Chest.* 2003;124:147–154.

33. Zavala DC, Schoell JE. Ultrathin needle aspiration of the lung in infectious and malignant disease. *Am Rev Respir Dis.* 1981;123:125–131.

34. Greif J, Marmor S, Schwarz Y, et al. Percutaneous core needle biopsy vs. fine needle aspiration in diagnosing benign lung lesions. *Acta Cytol.* 1999;43:756–760.

35. Thanos L, Galani P, Mylona S, et al. Percutaneous CT-guided core needle biopsy versus fine needle aspiration in diagnosing pneumonia and mimics of pneumonia. *Cardiovasc Intervent Radiol.* 2004;27:329–334.

36. Anderson JM, Murchison J, Patel D. CT-guided lung biopsy: factors influencing diagnostic yield and complication rate. *Clin Radiol.* 2003;58:791–797.

37. Ayed AK. Video-assisted thoracoscopic lung biopsy in the diagnosis of diffuse interstitial lung disease. A prospective study. *J Cardiovasc Surg (Torino).* 2003;44:115–118.

38. Ferson PF, Landreneau RJ, Dowling RD, et al. Comparison of open versus thoracoscopic lung biopsy for diffuse infiltrative pulmonary disease. *J Thorac Cardiovasc Surg.* 1993;106:194–199.

39. Kreider ME, Hansen-Flaschen J, Ahmad NN, et al. Complications of video-assisted thoracoscopic lung biopsy in patients with interstitial lung disease. *Ann Thorac Surg.* 2007;83:1140–1145.

40. Mack MJ, Hazelrigg SR, Landreneau RJ, et al. Thoracoscopy for the diagnosis of the indeterminate solitary pulmonary nodule. *Ann Thorac Surg.* 1993;56:825–830.

41. Santambrogio L, Nosotti M, Bellaviti N, et al. Videothoracoscopy versus thoracotomy for the diagnosis of the indeterminate solitary pulmonary nodule. *Ann Thorac Surg.* 1995;59:868–870.

42. Calhoun P, Feldman PS, Armstrong P, et al. The clinical outcome of needle aspirations of the lung when cancer is not diagnosed. *Ann Thorac Surg.* 1986;41:592–596.

2

INFLAMMATORY LUNG CONDITIONS

Lung injury can result from various inflammatory conditions. The changes affecting the lung parenchyma may be relatively nonspecific, and a detailed clinical history and results of imaging studies and ancillary tests will be required to arrive at a definitive or more specific diagnosis. Inflammatory conditions may lead to diverse changes ranging from acute inflammation, to subacute and chronic inflammation, to reparative changes characterized by fibrous scarring of lung parenchyma. It is important to understand that such changes do not constitute specific diagnoses or discrete clinicopathologic entities but merely represent patterns of tissue response to injury that are nonspecific and that may be observed in a wide variety of conditions (Table 2.1).

ACUTE LUNG INJURY

Several conditions can result in acute lung inflammation. The acute inflammatory reaction may affect any component of the lung parenchyma, including the alveolus, the bronchial tree and mucosa, and the bronchial vasculature.

The most common form of acute lung injury involves the alveolus and is characterized histologically by diffuse alveolar damage (DAD). The clinical counterpart of DAD has been designated over the years by different terms, including "shock lung," "postperfusion lung," and "acute respiratory distress syndrome" (ARDS). The term ARDS was introduced in 1967 by Ashbaugh et al.[1] for patients characterized by severe respiratory distress of acute onset following different insults, with dyspnea, reduction in lung diffusing capacity, radiographic changes, and hypoxemia refractory to oxygen administration. ARDS follows a rapidly progressing clinical course and is associated with a high-mortality rate, with approximately more than half of patients dying of respiratory insufficiency within days to weeks.[2,3]

Because the lung reacts to various types of injuries in a similar fashion regardless of the etiology, the changes observed in acute lung injury are nonspecific and have been generically designated as "DAD." Causes

TABLE 2.1 Nonspecific Patterns of Tissue Response to Injury in Lung Parenchyma
DAD with hyaline membranes
Organizing bronchopneumonia
Bronchiolitis obliterans (peribronchial fibrosis)
Interstitial pneumonitis
Interstitial fibrosis
Hyperplasia of alveolar type II pneumocytes
Bronchiolar and squamous metaplasia
Respiratory bronchiolitis
Vasculitis/capillaritis
Granulomatous inflammation

of DAD in patients with the ARDS include infections, drugs, radiation, ingestion or inhalation of poisons and chemicals, oxygen toxicity, shock, sepsis, collagen-vascular diseases, and others (Table 2.2).

The histologic picture in DAD can be quite variable, depending on the stage of the process. The initial phase is characterized by acute endothelial and mucosal injury with resulting exudation of fluid and cells (so-called exudative phase) (Fig. 2.1) (eFig. 2.1). The alveolar walls are characterized by interstitial and intra-alveolar edema with varying amounts of hemorrhage and fibrin deposition (eFig. 2.2). Interstitial inflammatory infiltrates comprise small lymphocytes, and histiocytes with small fibrin thrombi within the pulmonary microvasculature are also present. The morphologic hallmark of the exudative phase is the formation of so-called hyaline membranes characterized by deposition of acellular eosinophilic proteinaceous exudates on the surface of the alveolar walls (Fig. 2.2) (eFig. 2.3). Another change that occurs toward the end of the exudative phase is hyperplasia of type II pneumocytes. The reactive

TABLE 2.2 Causes of Acute Lung Injury
Infection
Drugs
Poisons, toxins
Inhalants (smoke, toxic gases, etc.)
Oxygen toxicity
Shock/sepsis
Radiation
Collagen-vascular/autoimmune diseases
Surgery, trauma

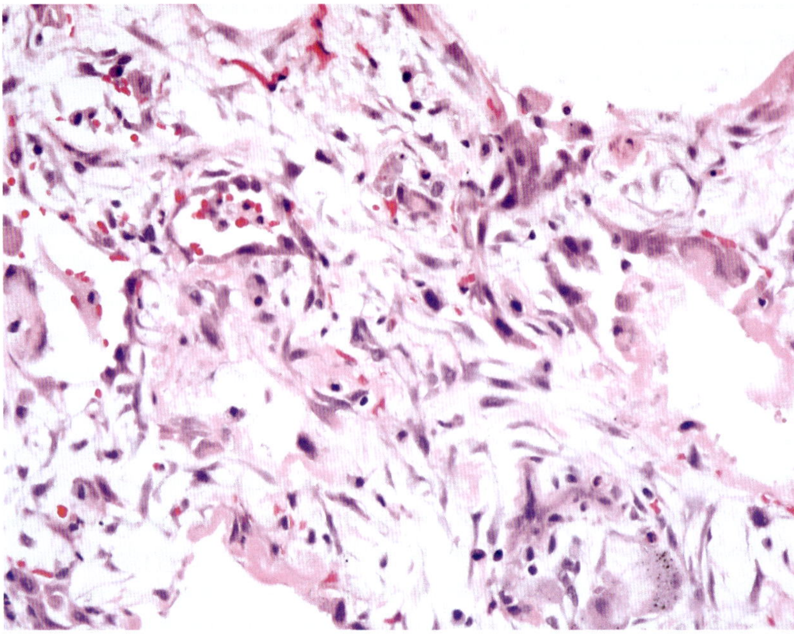

FIGURE 2.1 Exudative phase of DAD. Notice acute endothelial and mucosal damage with abundant edema fluid in the interstitium and alveolar lumens and abundant fibrin deposition.

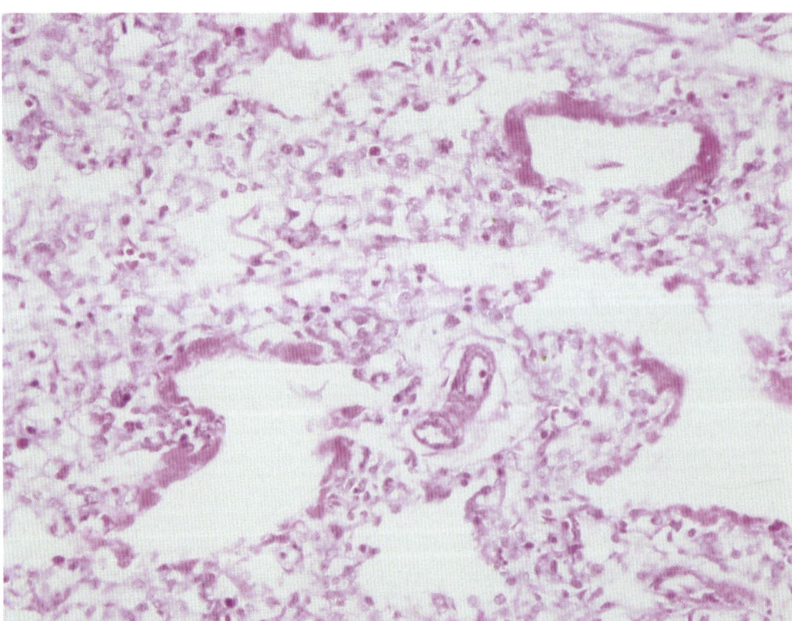

FIGURE 2.2 Exudative phase of DAD showing formation of hyaline membranes characterized by acellular eosinophilic proteinaceous material lining the surface of alveolar walls.

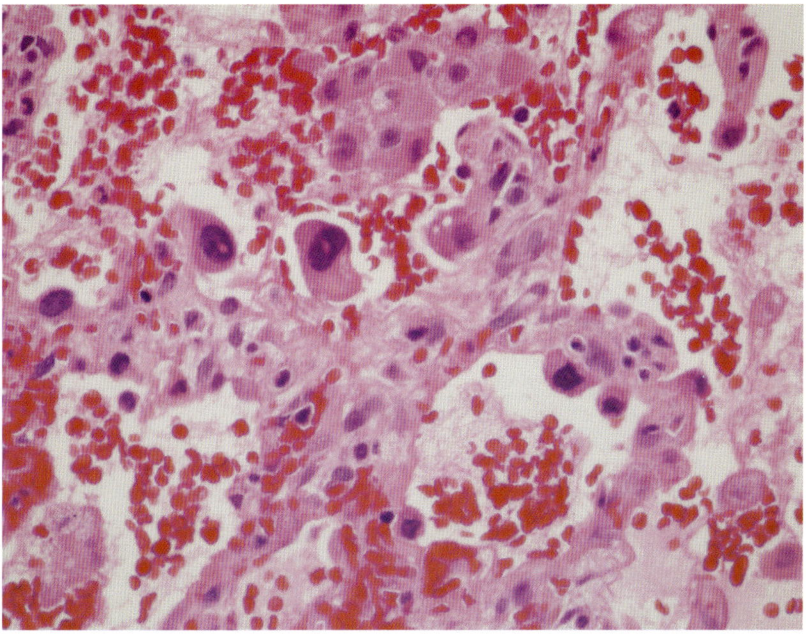

FIGURE 2.3 Exudative phase of DAD showing hyperplasia of type II alveolar pneumocytes. Notice enlarged, atypical nuclei protruding from the alveolar walls.

type II pneumocytes may display marked cytologic atypia with enlarged, hyperchromatic nuclei and mitotic figures (Fig. 2.3). The exudative phase generally lasts from 3 to 7 days and is followed by a proliferative phase characterized by active fibroblastic proliferation mainly involving the interstitium and eventually extending to the alveolar spaces (Fig. 2.4). The fibroblastic plugs usually comprise loose aggregates of fibroblasts against a myxoid stroma admixed with scattered inflammatory cells and are devoid of significant collagen deposition (Fig. 2.5) (eFig. 2.4). Hyperplasia of type II pneumocytes persists during this stage and may be accompanied by immature squamous metaplasia with atypia (Fig. 2.6). Hyaline membranes are usually reabsorbed by the end of the exudative stage but may persist into the proliferative phase. The natural evolution of the process at this stage may be followed by complete resolution with little residual change and complete regeneration of the alveolar lining, or it may progress to a fibrotic stage, characterized by extensive collagen deposition in and around alveolar septa, eventually resulting in extensive remodeling and honeycombing of lung parenchyma (Fig. 2.7). It should be noted that DAD in any given patient may be the result of repeated injury over a period, in which case the lung biopsy may show superimposed features of acute early exudative damage along with reparative and proliferative changes in the same biopsy specimen (eFig. 2.5). DAD will usually regress if the inciting stimulus is removed.

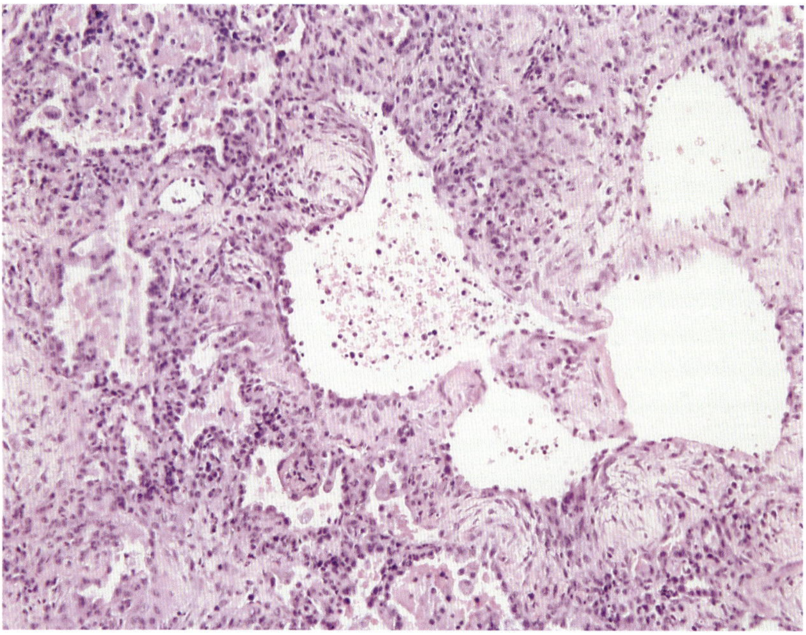

FIGURE 2.4 Proliferative phase of DAD characterized by active fibroblastic proliferation involving the interstitium of the alveolar walls and extending into alveolar spaces.

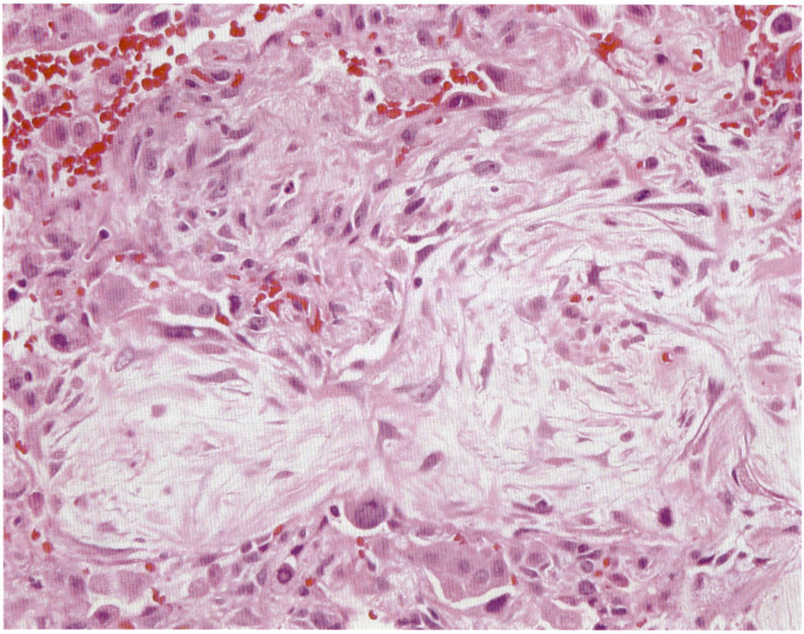

FIGURE 2.5 Proliferative phase of DAD showing fibroblastic plugs within the alveolar lumens comprising aggregates of spindle fibroblasts embedded in loose myxoid matrix.

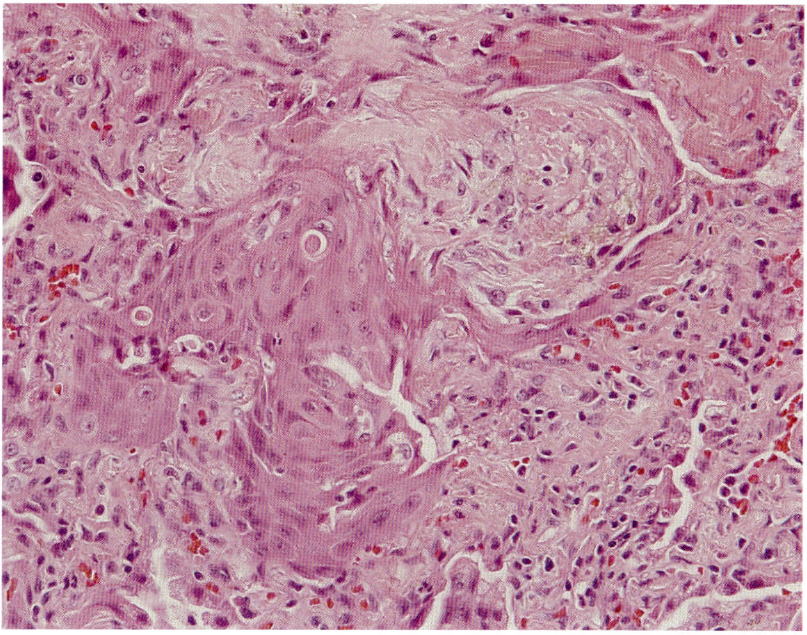

FIGURE 2.6 Proliferative stage of DAD with hyperplasia of type II pneumocytes and squamous metaplasia of alveolar lining.

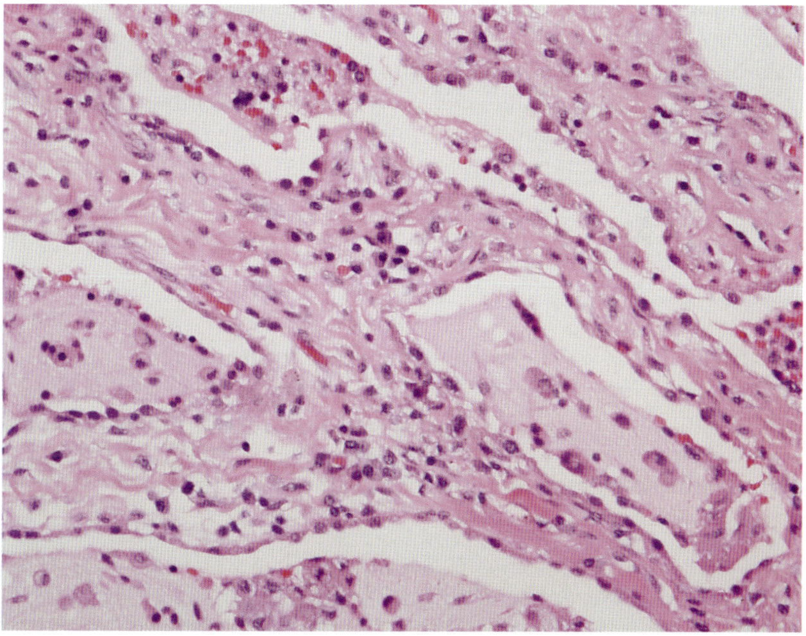

FIGURE 2.7 Fibrotic stage of DAD showing extensive collagen deposition in and around alveolar septa with remodeling of lung parenchyma.

SPECIFIC CAUSES OF ACUTE LUNG INFLAMMATION

There may be several specific etiologic causes of acute lung inflammation. Most of them result in a similar nonspecific histopathologic picture; however, in some instances some specific features may point to a specific diagnosis, or a more specific diagnosis can be achieved with the aid of a good clinical history or results of additional clinical tests. In the absence of corroborating history or laboratory tests supporting a specific etiology for the changes observed in the lung biopsy, the pathologist's role is limited to making a detailed reporting of the findings of acute injury and making a generic diagnosis of DAD.

Acute Interstitial Pneumonia (Hamman–Rich Syndrome)

Acute interstitial pneumonia (AIP), also known as the Hamman–Rich syndrome, represents a fulminant and rapidly progressive lung condition of unknown etiology mostly affecting previously healthy young adults. It is characterized clinically by sudden onset of fever, cough, and shortness of breath with diffuse bilateral pulmonary infiltrates on chest X-rays.[4,5] Patients usually develop respiratory failure with a high-mortality rate—usually within a few days to weeks.

Histologically, AIP is characterized by changes indistinguishable from DAD as seen in the adult respiratory distress syndrome (ARDS). Unlike ARDS in which DAD can be traced to a well-defined inciting stimulus such as infection, drugs, shock, radiation, trauma, oxygen toxicity, and noxious inhalants, the term AIP is reserved for cases where the etiology is unknown.[3] A thorough clinical history, serologic tests, and microbiologic studies are indicated to rule out specific causes of acute lung injury in these patients. The early changes resemble the exudative phase of DAD, with inflammation and edema of alveolar walls and formation of hyaline membranes (Fig. 2.8). This is followed by an organizing phase with acute interstitial and intra-alveolar fibrosis accompanied by hyperplasia of type II pneumocytes. If the patient survives, residual scarring with severe interstitial fibrosis will ensue.

Collagen-Vascular Diseases

Lung involvement is a frequent manifestation of collagen-vascular diseases. There may be several specific etiologic causes of acute lung inflammation. The majority of them result in a similar nonspecific histopathologic picture; however, in the setting of a well-defined clinical picture and with the support of appropriate laboratory tests, a more specific diagnosis may be rendered.

SYSTEMIC LUPUS ERYTHEMATOSUS. Patients with systemic lupus erythematosus (SLE) may present with diffuse acute or chronic inflammation of the lungs or with changes affecting primarily the pulmonary vasculature (vasculitis and thromboembolic phenomena). Acute lupus pneumonitis is a form of the disease associated with highly aggressive evolution and

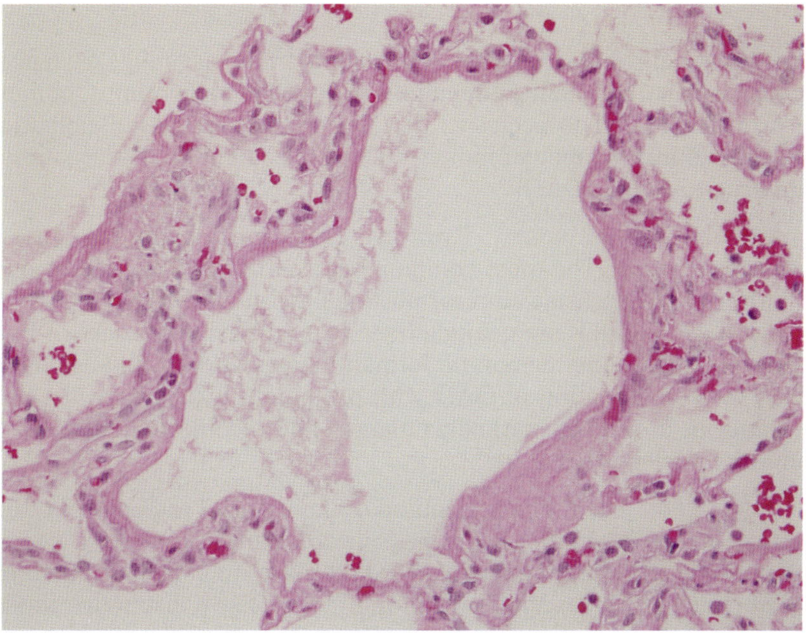

FIGURE 2.8 Formation of hyaline membrane lining the alveolar wall is seen in patient with AIP.

a high-mortality rate.[6] This condition is characterized by dyspnea, tachypnea, fever, and hypoxemia. The histopathologic changes are primarily those of DAD, although acute alveolar hemorrhage with capillaritis and small vessel vasculitis can also be observed.[7,8] Diffuse fibrosis with changes indistinguishable from those of usual interstitial pneumonia (UIP) will develop in 1% to 5% of patients with SLE.[9] Vascular changes are also a common manifestation of lung involvement by SLE. Capillaritis with diffuse alveolar hemorrhage, small vessel vasculitis, and pulmonary hypertension are a major cause of morbidity and mortality in patients with SLE.[10,11] Immune complex deposition, including IgG, IgM, IgA, and C3, can be demonstrated by immunofluorescence in the alveolar interstitium and vessel walls.[12,13]

RHEUMATOID ARTHRITIS. Pulmonary manifestations of rheumatoid arthritis (RA) can vary from acute lung injury to the characteristic rheumatoid nodule. Acute lung injury in patients with RA takes the form of DAD, and the findings are indistinguishable from those seen in adult respiratory distress syndrome (ARDS).[14,15] Correlation with serologic tests and a good clinical history are indispensable for diagnosis.

POLYMYOSITIS AND DERMATOMYOSITIS. These conditions can also be associated with pulmonary manifestations, which can range from acute respiratory distress with DAD-like changes, to organizing pneumonia, to organizing fibrosis.[16,17]

Drug Toxicity

Many drugs can result in damage to the airways that may range from acute alveolar damage, organizing pneumonia, interstitial pneumonitis, obliterative bronchiolitis, veno-occlusive disease, granulomatous inflammation, and diffuse fibrosing pneumonitis.[18,19] The most common manifestation of acute drug toxicity is DAD.[18]

CHEMOTHERAPEUTIC AGENTS. Cytotoxic drugs are a common cause of acute lung damage. The most common agents are busulfan and bleomycin, although methotrexate and carmustine have also been implicated.[18–21] The histologic findings are characterized by nonspecific changes of DAD with extensive hyaline membrane formation. Busulfan toxicity is characterized by a combination of DAD with prominent hyperplasia of type II pneumocytes displaying markedly enlarged and pleomorphic nuclei with prominent nucleoli (Fig. 2.9).[22]

AMIODARONE. The ß-blocker, amiodarone, used for the control of cardiac arrythmias, is another well-recognized cause of pulmonary toxicity. The pathologic findings comprise DAD, chronic interstitial pneumonitis with fibrosis, and organizing pneumonia.[23–25] A fairly distinctive finding in amiodarone toxicity is the presence of fine cytoplasmic vacuolation of intra-alveolar macrophages and type II pneumocytes (Fig. 2.10).

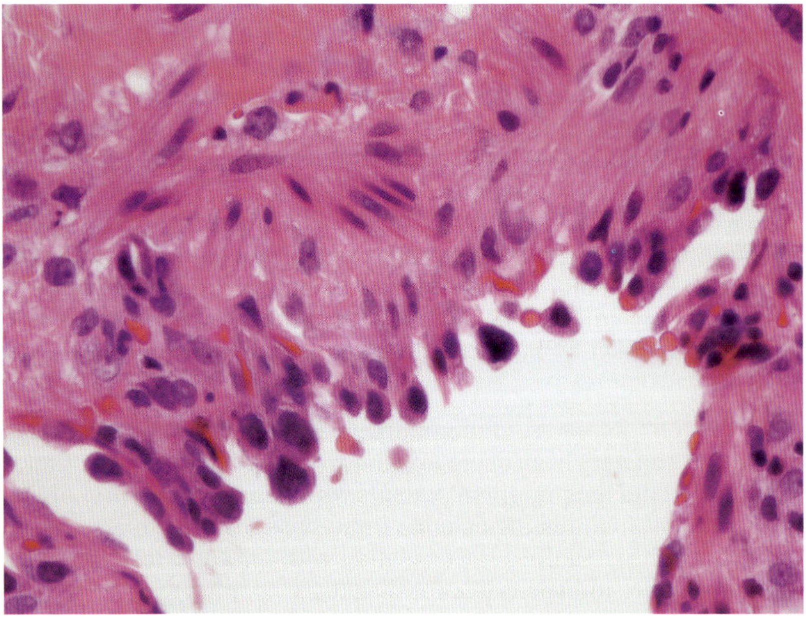

FIGURE 2.9 Acute lung injury in patient with drug toxicity secondary to busulfan. Notice alveolar type II pneumocytes displaying markedly enlarged and pleomorphic nuclei with prominent nucleoli.

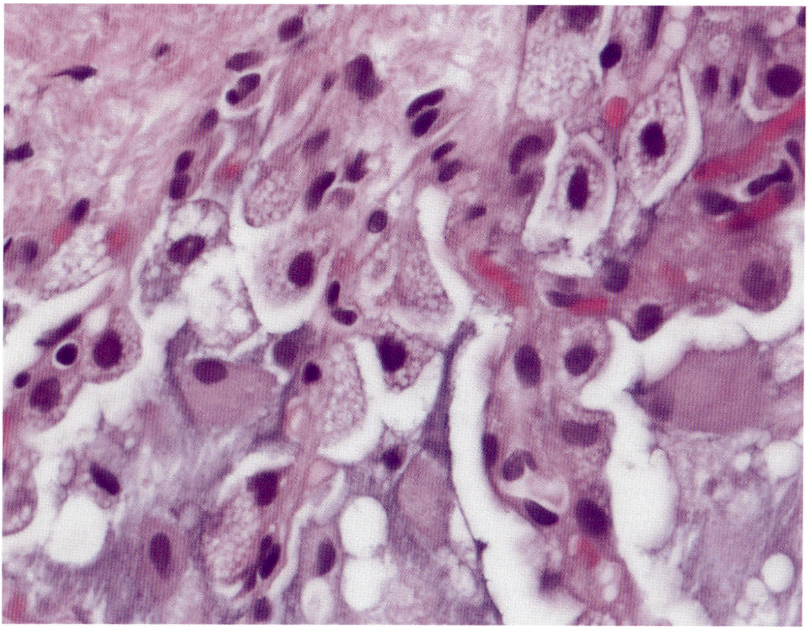

FIGURE 2.10 Acute lung injury in amiodarone toxicity characterized by prominent fine cytoplasmic vacuoles in intra-alveolar macrophages and type II alveolar pneumocytes.

Acute Eosinophilic Pneumonia

Acute eosinophilic pneumonia is a condition of unknown etiology that presents clinically as acute respiratory distress without any identifiable underlying cause.[26] Patients present with symptoms of acute respiratory distress with or without peripheral eosinophilia. It is histologically characterized by alveolar septal edema admixed with macrophages and reactive atypia of alveolar type II macrophages. The distinctive feature of the process is the presence of eosinophils in varying numbers within the alveolar lumens. Hyaline membranes and intra-alveolar fibrin deposition may also be seen. It is important to recognize the eosinophils because patients respond favorably to treatment with corticosteroids.

CHRONIC LUNG INJURY

Chronic lung inflammation results from long-standing lung injury that may affect alveolar walls, bronchioles, segmental bronchi, and the interstitium. The findings in subacute and chronic inflammation of pulmonary parenchyma range from bronchiolitis obliterans with organizing pneumonia (BOOP) to extensive interstitial fibrosis with remodeling of lung parenchyma. The patterns of BOOP as well as interstitial fibrosis are quite nonspecific and represent a common tissue response to various injuries and stimuli. In the majority of instances, correlation with the clinical history and radiographic and laboratory test results is required for a more specific diagnosis.

The term idiopathic BOOP is of historical interest and was used in the past to refer to a form of idiopathic interstitial lung disease characterized by abundance of intra-alveolar fibroblastic polyps in the terminal airways and surrounding alveoli.[27] This process is currently referred to as cryptogenic organizing pneumonia (COP). The term "bronchiolitis obliterans" is also currently employed to refer to the airway injury in chronic lung transplant rejection (so-called bronchiolitis obliterans syndrome).[28,29] "BOOP" should no longer be used to define a specific "entity" and the more descriptive term of organizing pneumonia or airspace organization should be employed, as this pattern may be observed in a large number of conditions (Table 2.3).

The organizing pneumonia pattern is characterized by plugs of granulation tissue that are located within the lumen of small airways and extend into the alveolar ducts and alveoli (Fig. 2.11) (eFig. 2.6). These plugs comprise inflammatory cells (neutrophils, macrophages, lymphocytes, and plasma cells) that may be admixed with small vessels and occasional fibroblasts and are embedded in a loose myxoid matrix (Fig. 2.12). The plugs may appear as polypoid masses that penetrate through the walls of the alveoli into adjacent spaces (so-called Masson bodies) or may completely fill the alveoli obliterating their lumen (Fig. 2.13). The fibrous plugs may also completely fill the alveolar ducts, adopting a branching configuration (Fig. 2.14) (eFigs. 2.7 and 2.8).

TABLE 2.3 Conditions Associated with Organizing Pneumonia Pattern

In advanced stages of DAD
As a complication of aspiration pneumonia
As a response to drug reactions or inhalation of toxic gases
In systemic connective tissue disorders
In the vicinity of malignant neoplasms or distal to obstructed bronchi
In association with idiopathic interstitial pneumonia (UIP)
In hypersensitivity pneumonitis
In association with other inflammatory lung diseases such as abscess, infarcts, and infections
In association with chronic obstructive bronchiolitis
In chronic lung transplant rejection
As an idiopathic process associated with mild interstitial pneumonia (COP)

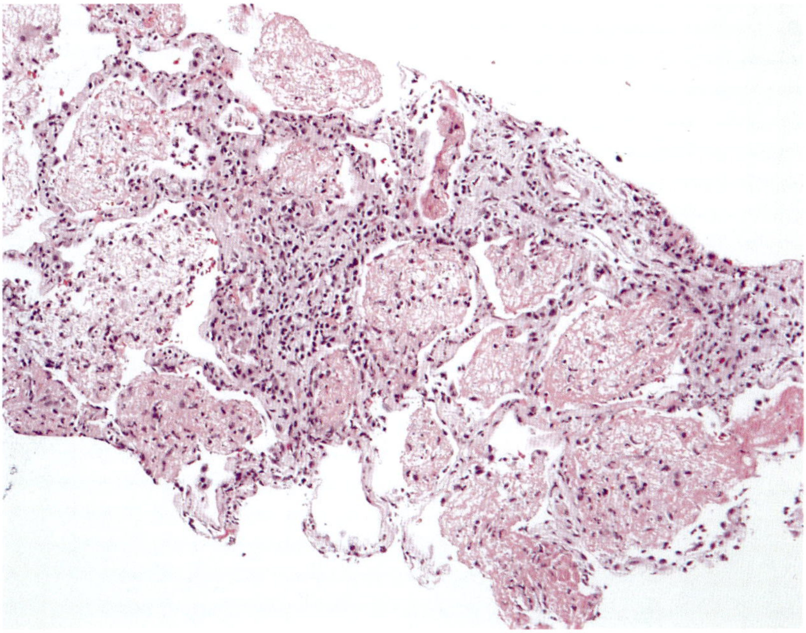

FIGURE 2.11 Chronic lung injury tissue response pattern characterized by organizing pneumonia (formerly known as BOOP). Notice the plugs of granulation tissue located within the lumen of the small airways and extending into alveolar ducts and alveoli.

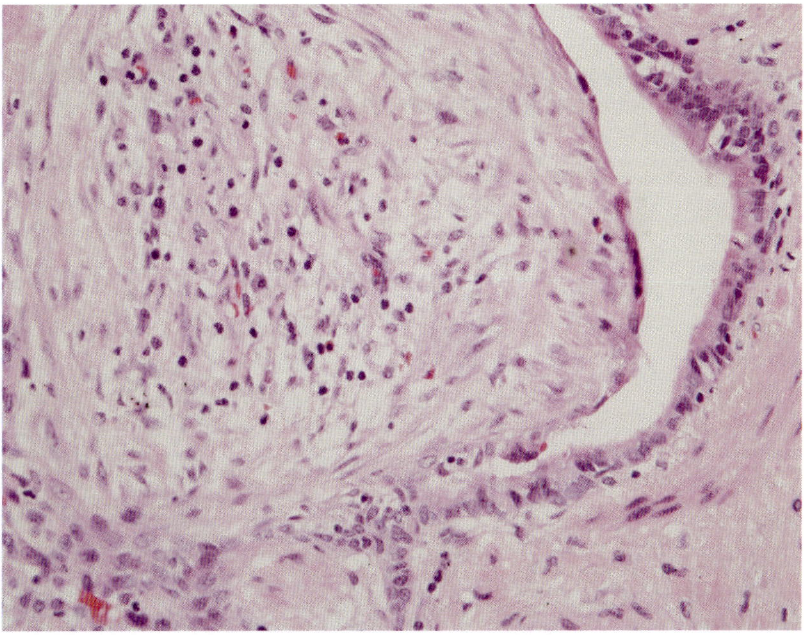

FIGURE 2.12 Organizing pneumonia pattern showing admixture of inflammatory cells (neutrophils, plasma cells, small lymphocytes, and macrophages) with small vessels and spindled fibroblasts; notice abundant fibrin in alveolar lumens due to acute exacerbation.

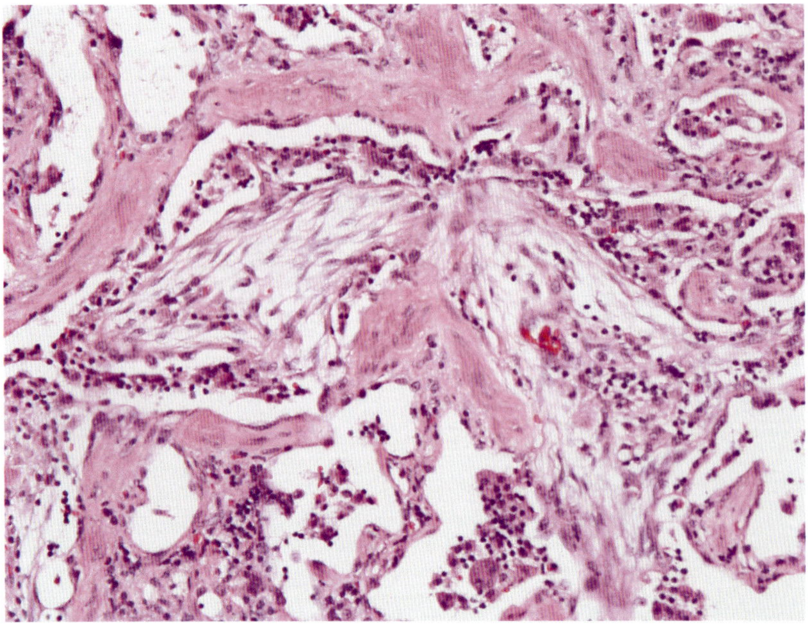

FIGURE 2.13 Polypoid masses comprising fibroblastic proliferation with loose myxoid matrix are seen filling the lumen of alveolar spaces and penetrating through pores of Kohn into the adjacent alveoli.

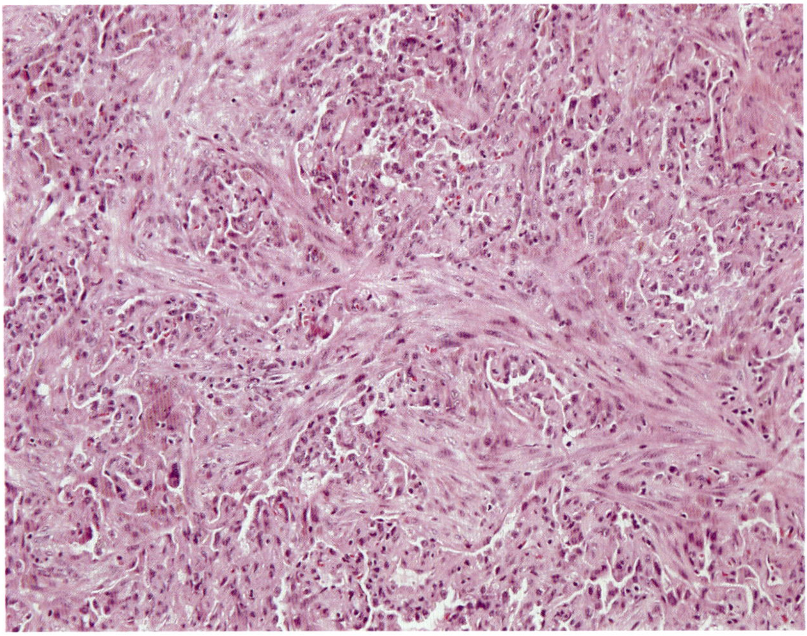

FIGURE 2.14 Branching configuration of fibroblastic plugs extending along alveolar ducts in advanced organizing pneumonia.

Another pattern of chronic inflammation that must be distinguished from the organizing pneumonia pattern is constrictive bronchiolitis (bronchiolitis obliterans). The latter comprise mucosal, submucosal, and peribronchiolar inflammatory infiltrates that eventually progress to peribronchiolar fibrosis and collagenization, leading to partial or total obstruction of the bronchiole (Fig. 2.15). This pattern may be observed in association with pulmonary infections such as mycoplasma or viruses, exposure to dusts, drug reactions, toxic gases, and collagen-vascular disorders such as RA. It can also be seen as a nonspecific response complicating DAD and other injuries to lung parenchyma.

Another nonspecific pattern that may result from long-standing chronic inflammation is interstitial fibrosis. This must be distinguished from the idiopathic interstitial fibrosing pneumonitides that will be dealt with in another chapter. Interstitial fibrosis is characterized by narrowing and obliteration of alveolar spaces by interstitial collagen deposition (Fig. 2.16) (eFig. 2.9). When the process is advanced, it leads to honeycombing of lung parenchyma. Interstitial fibrosis may be associated with various metaplastic processes, including bronchiolar metaplasia and squamous metaplasia. The former is characterized by replacement of the alveolar lining by columnar, ciliated bronchiolar epithelium (Fig. 2.17). It has been hypothesized that the metaplastic epithelium derives from the

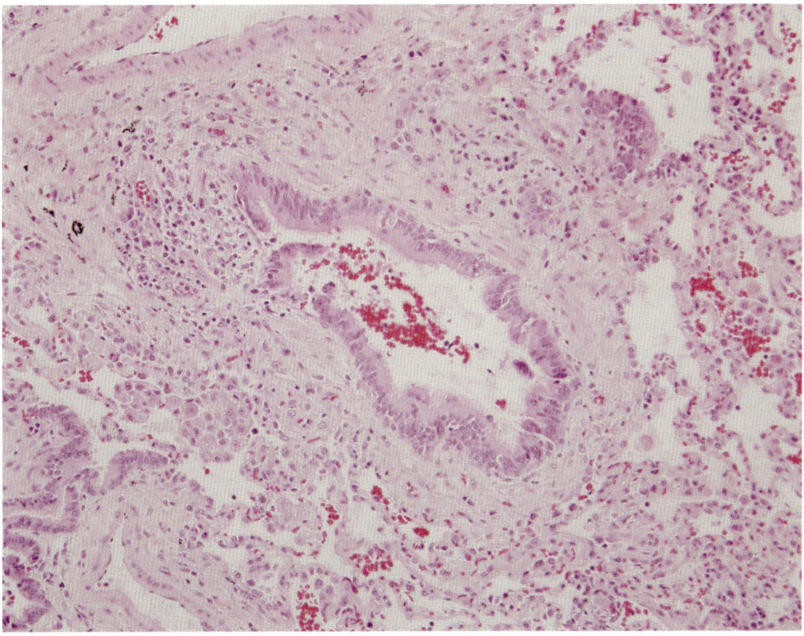

FIGURE 2.15 Response to chronic inflammation characterized by bronchiolitis obliterans showing constrictive pattern of fibrosis and inflammation around the lumen of a small bronchiole.

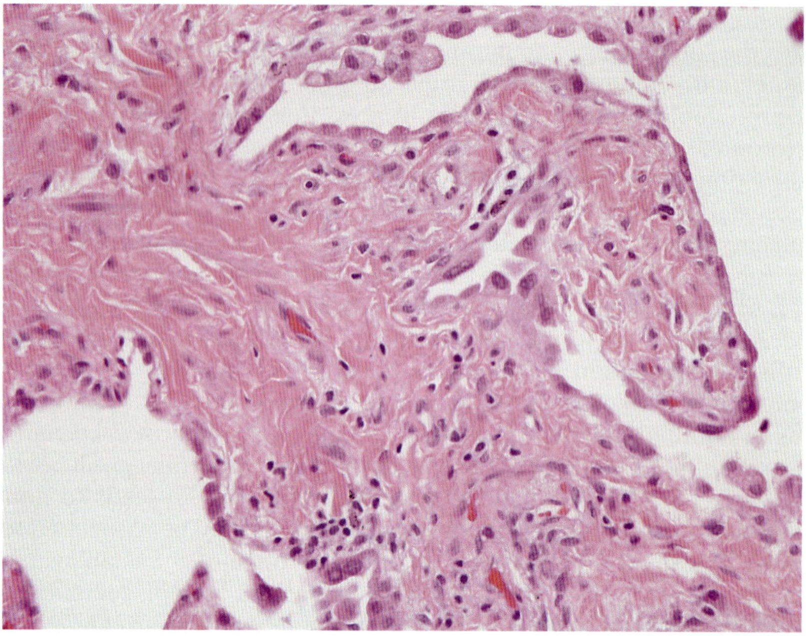

FIGURE 2.16 Interstitial fibrosis resulting from chronic lung injury. Notice thickening of alveolar walls by interstitial collagen deposition.

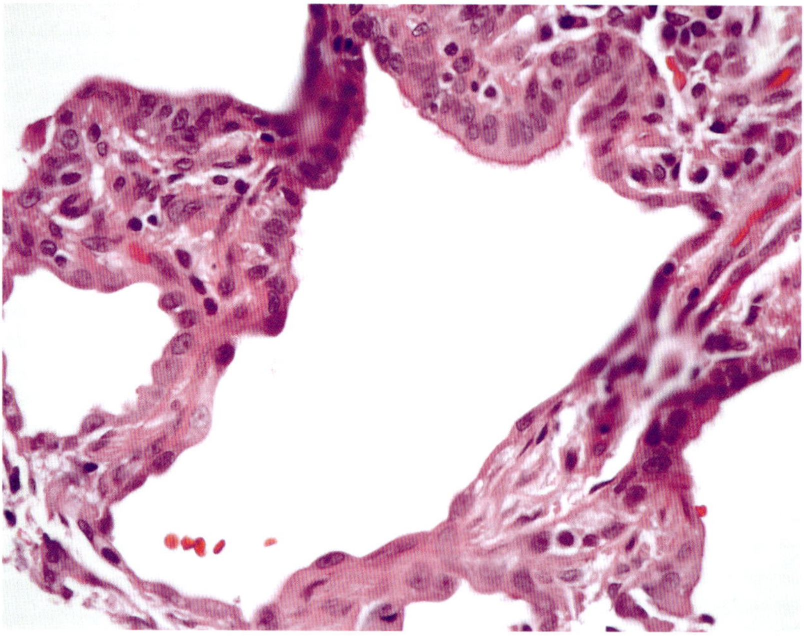

FIGURE 2.17 Bronchiolar metaplasia ("lambertosis") in chronic lung injury characterized by replacement of the alveolar lining by columnar, ciliated bronchiolar epithelium.

canals of Lambert that normally connect the bronchioles with the alveoli, hence the alternate designation of "lambertosis" for this phenomenon. Squamous metaplasia can also be observed under a wide range of circumstances and can be most striking in advanced stages of interstitial fibrosis. Another phenomenon that can be commonly observed in advanced stages of interstitial fibrosis is bronchiolar smooth muscle hyperplasia, which in advanced stages may lead to a distinctive macroscopic appearance that has been termed in the British literature "pulmonary cirrhosis" (eFig. 2.10).

Finally, another manifestation of chronic inflammation is the presence of granulomatous pneumonitis, which will be discussed separately in more detail.

SPECIFIC CAUSES OF CHRONIC LUNG INFLAMMATION

There may be several specific etiologic causes of chronic lung inflammation. Most of them result in a similar nonspecific histopathologic picture; however, in some instances some specific features may point to a specific diagnosis, or a more specific diagnosis can be achieved with the aid of a good clinical history or results of additional clinical tests.

Collagen-Vascular Diseases

Collagen-vascular diseases affecting the lungs are principally characterized by a chronic inflammatory response of pulmonary parenchyma. The majority of them result in a similiar nonspecific histopathologic picture. Result, of laboratory tests and a detailed clinical history are required for arriving at a more specific diagnosis.

RHEUMATOID ARTHRITIS. It has been estimated that about 14% of patients who meet the criteria for the diagnosis of RA by the American Rheumatism Association develop significant lung disease.[30] A distinctive, but not unique, feature of lung involvement by RA is the development of multiple discrete lymphoid follicles with germinal centers. When these lymphoid follicles aggregate around the terminal airways, the pattern is designated as "follicular bronchiolitis." A variable cellular chronic interstitial infiltrate rich in plasma cells and small lymphocytes is usually present in the vicinity of the lymphoid nodules. Another common finding is the combination of subacute and chronic inflammation manifested by hyperplasia of type II pneumocytes and interstitial pneumonia that may progress to diffuse interstitial fibrosis. The end-stage of the fibrotic process will lead to the formation of the typical rheumatoid nodules, which must be distinguished from the nodules in Wegener granulomatosis and of various infectious processes. It cannot be overemphasized that a specific diagnosis of RA cannot be rendered solely on the basis of biopsy material and requires strict correlation and confirmation from the clinical findings.

SYSTEMIC LUPUS ERYTHEMATOSUS. SLE is a chronic systemic autoimmune disease that may often affect the lungs and can range from acute lupus pneumonitis to advanced fibrosis. Acute lung injury and pulmonary hemorrhage and vasculitis are more commonly associated with SLE than with other connective tissue disorders and are the more common pulmonary manifestation of the disease.[11] However, a significant number of patients will present in advanced stages with cellular interstitial pneumonia and variable degrees of interstitial fibrosis. This latter presentation is associated with a more favorable prognosis than acute lupus pneumonitis. The subacute and chronic manifestations of lupus pneumonitis manifest with a nonspecific interstitial pneumonia (NSIP) pattern, which is characterized by a cellular interstitial pneumonia with variable interstitial fibrosis (Fig. 2.18). More rarely, the process will progress to a more advanced pattern of interstitial fibrosis that may be indistinguishable from UIP (Fig. 2.19). Clinical correlation and laboratory findings are indispensable for correct diagnosis. Other less common chronic pulmonary manifestations of SLE include bronchiolitis obliterans and lymphocytic interstitial pneumonia.[31]

SCLERODERMA (PROGRESSIVE SYSTEMIC SCLEROSIS). Diffuse lung involvement represents the fourth most common manifestation of progressive systemic sclerosis (PSS) after skin, peripheral vascular, and esophageal involvement.[32] Patients with pulmonary involvement in scleroderma are

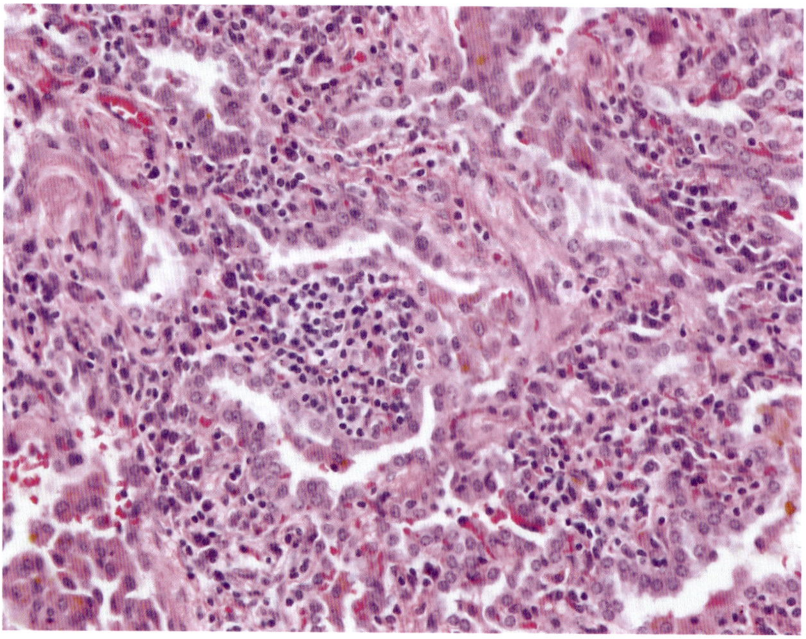

FIGURE 2.18 Cellular interstitial pneumonia in patient with lupus erythematosus. Notice the dense interstitial lymphoid infiltrate expanding the alveolar walls.

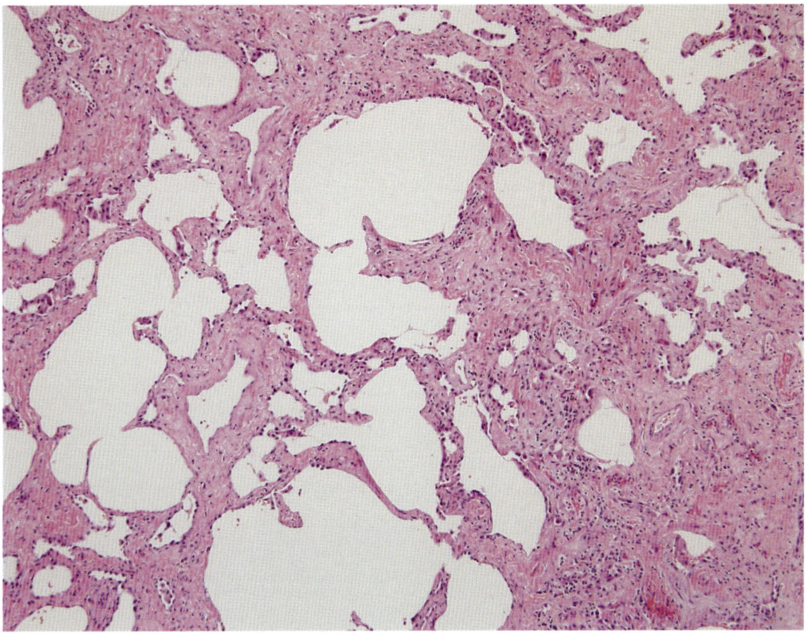

FIGURE 2.19 Advanced stage of lupus pneumonitis showing severe interstitial fibrosis with extensive remodeling of lung parenchyma. This picture is morphologically indistinguishable from idiopathic UIP and a diagnosis of lupus cannot be rendered in the absence of a clinical history.

associated with increased morbidity and mortality. A rare complication of pulmonary involvement in PSS is the development of lung carcinoma from areas of fibrosis. Lung involvement in PSS is usually characterized by diffuse interstitial fibrosis. The interstitial fibrosis is characterized by a paucicellular collagenization of the interstitium with preservation of the underlying lung architecture; however, in more advanced stages it may closely resemble that seen in UIP (Fig. 2.20). The absence of "temporal heterogeneity" of the lesions, a distinctive feature of UIP, is helpful to differentiate PSS from the latter.[33] Vascular changes secondary to pulmonary hypertension are another feature seen in the lungs of patients with PSS and represent a major cause of mortality in such patients.[34]

POLYMYOSITIS AND DERMATOMYOSITIS. Pulmonary involvement in polymyositis (PM) and dermatomyositis (DM) occurs with much less frequency than in other systemic diseases and usually manifests late in the course of the process. However, in occasional cases, they may precede the clinical and serologic diagnoses of the disease.[17] The most common manifestation of PM/DM in the lungs is an interstitial pneumonitis with a pattern very similar to NSIP. The interstitium shows a cellular interstitial pneumonia with temporal heterogeneity (i.e., all lesions are in the same stage of

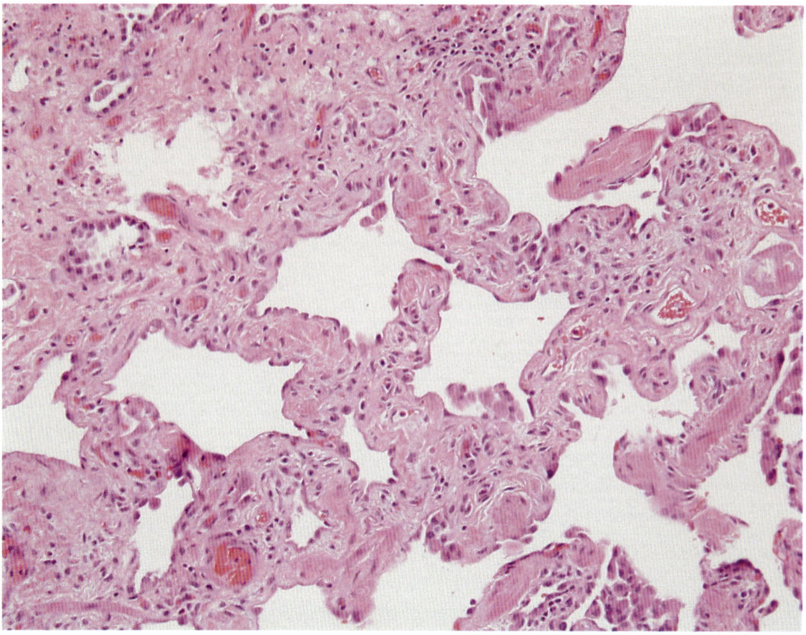

FIGURE 2.20 Interstitial fibrosis in PSS. This pattern of fibrosis is nonspecific and can be observed in various other disorders. Clinical correlation is required to establish the cause of the sclerosing process.

development). There is a variable degree of fibrosis and the changes may resemble those seen in the cellular or fibrotic forms of NSIP. In more advanced stages, the fibrosis associated with PM/DM may be indistinguishable from that of idiopathic UIP. Clinical correlation and a good history will be essential for correct interpretation. In limited biopsy samples, it may be impossible to establish a definitive diagnosis.

SJOGREN SYNDROME. Sjogren syndrome (SS) is an autoimmune disease characterized by dense lymphocytic infiltration of the salivary glands resulting in the clinical manifestations of dry mouth and dry eyes. Lung involvement often occurs in SS and is characterized by a lymphocytic interstitial pneumonitis principally distributed around the airways. When the infiltrates form lymphoid follicles, they can result in a pattern of follicular bronchiolitis. The most common pattern is that of lymphoid interstitial pneumonia (LIP) that may closely resemble a low-grade lymphoproliferative disorder. A common finding is the presence of small, nonnecrotizing interstitial granulomas admixed with the lymphoid cell population. It should be kept in mind that patients with SS are at increased risk for developing lymphoproliferative disorders, and proper evaluation of dense lymphoid infiltrates in SS patients with lung involvement to rule out lymphoma should always be considered.

Drug Toxicity

Many drugs, including amiodarone, bleomycin, carmustine, and methotrexate, can result in lung damage leading to chronic inflammation and fibrosis. Most of the chronic inflammatory changes induced by drugs are nonspecific and can resemble other causes of diffuse lung injury, such as cellular interstitial pneumonia, bronchiolitis obliterans, and diffuse interstitial fibrosis.[35,36] Clinical correlation, with adequate information regarding specific types of drugs, and timing of administration in relation to the onset of symptoms are important for specific diagnosis. Cessation of symptoms or their improvement following discontinuation of the drug is also a helpful clue to verify the etiology of the pathologic findings. Chronic lung inflammation caused by drugs may manifest as diffuse interstitial fibrosis that can resemble UIP, sometimes leading to honeycombing of lung parenchyma. Tissue eosinophilia can be seen in some cases, and some drugs may be associated with the formation of small interstitial granulomas, in particular, methotrexate.[21] Clinical correlation is necessary for adequate interpretation of the pathologic findings.

CHRONIC EOSINOPHILIC PNEUMONIA

CEP is a condition of unknown etiology characterized by a typical clinical syndrome and radiographic appearance that includes fever, weight loss, cough and dyspnea with or without peripheral blood eosinophilia,

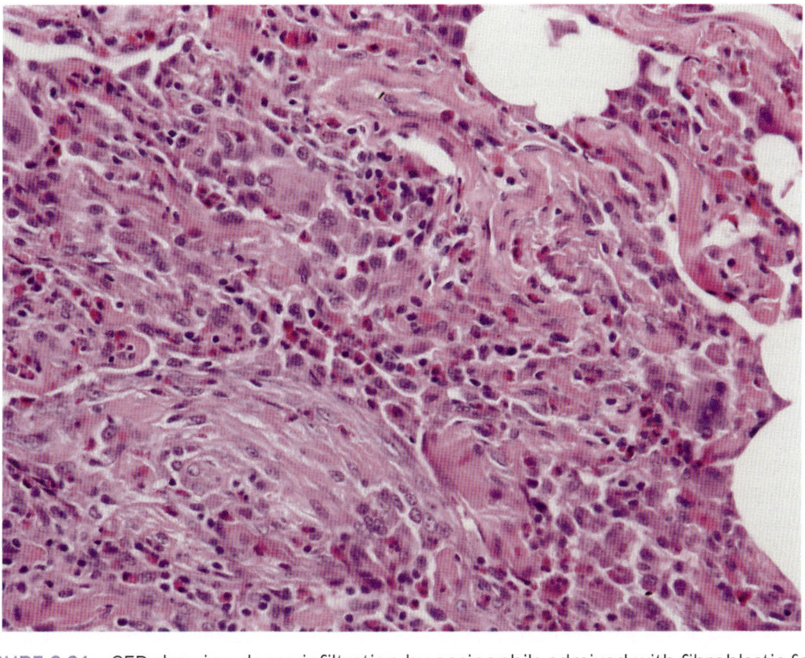

FIGURE 2.21 CEP showing dense infiltration by eosinophils admixed with fibroblastic foci.

and bilateral subpleural infiltrates with poorly defined margins that may disappear spontaneously only to recur later at the same sites ("migratory" infiltrates). The radiologic appearance has been likened to the photographic negative of pulmonary edema.[37] The disease occurs most often in middle-aged women and can be accompanied by asthma or nasal symptoms.[38] The histologic features are very similar to those of the acute form of the disease, and the distinction is made based on the constellation of clinical findings. Usually, there is mild interstitial pneumonia with hyperplasia of type II pneumocytes and accumulation of fibrin within alveolar spaces. Macrophages are also seen within the lumen of alveolar spaces. The cytologic atypia of the type II pneumocyte hyperplasia can be quite striking, sometimes simulating viral cytopathic effect. The most distinctive feature of the process, however, is the dense accumulation of eosinophils admixed with the macrophages within the alveolar lumens (Fig. 2.21). Discrete eosinophilic microabscesses may also be present. The differential diagnosis for the condition is with the Churg–Strauss syndrome, from which it is distinguished histologically by the absence of vasculitis. The condition responds well to treatment with corticosteroids.

REFERENCES

1. Ashbaugh D, Bigelow D, Petty T, et al. Acute respiratory distress in adults. *Lancet*. 1967;2:319–323.
2. Tomashefsky J Jr. Pulmonary pathology of acute respiratory distress syndrome. *Clin Chest Med*. 2000;21:435–466.
3. Katzenstein A, Bloor C, Liebow A. Diffuse alveolar damage—the role of oxygen, shock and related factors. *Am J Pathol*. 1976;85:209–228.
4. Hamman L, Rich A. Acute diffuse interstitial fibrosis of the lungs. *Bull Johns Hopkins Hosp*. 1944;74:177–212.
5. Katzenstein A-L, Myers J, Mazur M. Acute interstitial pneumonia. A clinicopathologic, ultrastructural and cell kinetic study. *Am J Surg Pathol*. 1986;10:256–267.
6. Matthay R, Schwanz M, Petty T, et al. Pulmonary manifestations of systemic lupus erythematosus: review of twelve cases of acute lupus pneumonia. *Medicine*. 1974;54:392–409.
7. Colby T. Pulmonary pathology in patients with systemic autoimmune disease. *Clin Chest Med*. 1998;19:587–612.
8. Quismorio F Jr, Cheema G. Interstitial lung disease in systemic lupus erythematosus. *Curr Opin Pulm Med*. 2000;6:424–429.
9. Eisenberg H. The interstitial lung diseases associated with collagen-vascular disorders. *Clin Chest Med*. 1982;3:565–573.
10. Haupt HM, Moore GW, Hutchins GM. The lung in systemic lupus erythematosus: analysis of the pathologic changes in 120 patients. *Am J Med*. 1981;71:791–813.
11. Myers JL, Katzenstein AA. Microangitis in lupus-induced pulmonary hemorrhage. *Am J Clin Pathol*. 1986;85:552–556.
12. Pertschuk LP, Moccia LF, Rosen Y, et al. Acute pulmonary complications in systemic lupus erythematosus. Immunofluorescence and light microscopic study. *Am J Clin Pathol*. 1977;68:553–559.
13. Eagen JW, Roberts H, Schwartz MM, et al. The composition of pulmonary immune deposits in systemic lupus erythematosus. *Clin Immunol Immunopathol*. 1979;12:204–212.

14. Yousem S, Colby T, Carrington C. Lung biopsy in rheumatoid arthritis. *Am Rev Respir Dis*. 1985;131:770–777.
15. Hakala M, Paakko P, Huhti E, et al. Open lung biopsy of patients with rheumatoid arthritis. *Clin Rheumatol*. 1990;9:452–460.
16. Lakhanpal S, Lie J, Conn D, et al. Pulmonary disease in polymiositis/dermatomyositis: a clinicopathologic analysis of 65 autopsy cases. *Ann Rheum Dis*. 1987;46:23–29.
17. Tazelaar HD, Viggiano RW, Pickersgill J, et al. Interstitial lung disease in polymiositis and dermatomyositis. Clinical features and prognosis as correlated with histologic findings. *Am Rev Respir Dis*. 1990;141:727–733.
18. Rossi S, Erasmus J, McAdams H, et al. Pulmonary drug toxicity: radiologic and pathologic manifestations. *Radiographics*. 2000;20:1245–1259.
19. Cooper JA Jr. Drug-induced lung disease. *Adv Intern Med*. 1997;42:231–268.
20. Ozkan M, Dweik RA, Ahmad M. Drug-induced lung disease. *Cleve Clin J Med*. 2001;68:782–785.
21. Imokawa S, Colby TV, Leslie KO, et al. Methotrexate pneumonitis: review of the literature and histopathological findings in nine patients. *Eur Respir J*. 2000;15:373–381.
22. Littler W, Kay J, Haselton P, et al. Busulphan lung. *Thorax*. 1969;24:639–655.
23. Myers JL, Kennedy JI, Plumb VJ, et al. Amiodarone pulmonary toxicity: clinical, radiologic and pathologic correlation. *Arch Intern Med*. 1987;147:50–55.
24. Dean P, Groshart K, Potterfield JG, et al. Amiodarone-associated pulmonary toxicity: a clinical and pathological study of eleven cases. *Am J Clin Pathol*. 1987;87:7–13.
25. Myers JL, Kennedy JI, Plumb VJ. Amiodarone lung: pathologic findings in clinically toxic patients. *Hum Pathol*. 1987;18:349–354.
26. Tazelaar H, Linz L, Colby TV, et al. Acute eosinophilic pneumonia: histopathologic findings in nine patients. *Am J Respir Crit Care Med*. 1997;155:296–302.
27. Epler GR, Colby TV, McLoud TC, et al. Bronchiolitis obliterans organizing pneumonia. *N Engl J Med*. 1985;312:152–158.
28. Paradis I, Yousem S, Griffith B. Airway obstruction and bronchiolitis obliterans after lung transplantation. *Clin Chest Med*. 1993;14:751–763.
29. Estenne M, Maurer JR, Boehler A, et al. Bronchiolitis obliterans syndrome 2001: an update of the diagnostic criteria. *J Heart Lung Transplant*. 2002;21:297–310.
30. Gabbay E, Tarala R, Will R, et al. Interstitial lung disease in recent onset rheumatoid arthritis. *Am J Respir Crit Care Med*. 1997;156:528–535.
31. Kinney WW, Angelillo VA. Bronchiolitis in systemic lupus erythematosus. *Chest*. 1982;82:646–648; Mum MN, Ziegler JR, Walker PD, et al. Pseudolymphoma of the lung in a patient with systemic lupus erythematosus. *Am J Med*. 1979;66:172–175.
32. Cheema GS, Quismorio FP Jr. Interstitial lung disease in systemic sclerosis. *Curr Opin Pulm Med*. 2001;7:283–290.
33. Bouros D, Wells AU, Nicholson AG, et al. Histopathologic subsets of fibrosing alveolitis in patients with systemic sclerosis and their relationship to outcome. *Am J Respir Crit Care Med*. 2002;165:1581–1586.
34. Yamane K, Ihn H, Asano Y, et al. Clinical and laboratory features of scleroderma patients with pulmonary hypertension. *Rheumatology (Oxford)*. 2000;39:1269–1271.
35. Kreisman H, Wolcove N. Pulmonary toxicity of antineoplastic therapy. *Semin Oncol*. 1992;19:508–520.
36. Zitnik RJ, Matthay RA. Drug-induced lung disease. In: Schwartz MI, King TE, eds. *Interstitial Lung Disease*. London, UK: BC Decker; 1998:423–449.
37. Gaensler E, Carrington C. Peripheral opacities in chronic eosinophilic pneumonia. The photographic negative of pulmonary edema. *AJR Am J Roentgenol*. 1977;128:1–13.
38. Liebow A, Carrington C. The eosinophilic pneumonias. *Medicine (Baltimore)*. 1969;48:251–285.

3

PULMONARY NONINFECTIOUS GRANULOMAS

Granulomas can occur in the lung under different circumstances, including infectious and noninfectious processes. For the most part, granulomatous pneumonitis is a relatively nonspecific reaction pattern that requires strict clinicopathologic correlation for proper interpretation. Granulomas are frequent findings in endoscopic lung biopsies; a specific diagnosis is often not attainable in most circumstances from the review of the biopsy material alone.

The most frequent cause of pulmonary granulomas is infectious diseases, and these will be discussed separately in other chapters. This chapter will deal with noninfectious granulomas and their possible etiology (Table 3.1).

SARCOIDOSIS

Sarcoidosis is a systemic disease of unknown etiology. Pulmonary involvement is a common feature of the disease.[1,2] Pulmonary involvement by sarcoidosis is usually accompanied by cough and shortness of breath. As many as two-thirds of patients may be asymptomatic. The disease has a predilection for young adults and for African Americans. Serum angiotensin-converting enzyme can be detected in 30% to 80% of patients and may be helpful for diagnosis; however, the test is not specific and elevated levels can be observed in other conditions also including infectious granulomas, lymphomas, hepatitis, and diabetes. The Kveim test, which employs an injected antigenic serum derived from human sarcoid granuloma extracts, is relatively specific but has largely been abandoned for the use of endoscopic lung biopsy to confirm the presence of the granulomas.[2] On chest X-rays, the disease tends to preferentially occupy the upper lobes and is characterized by reticulonodular infiltrates with a lymphatic distribution.

The histopathologic hallmark of sarcoidosis is the formation of nonnecrotizing ("productive") epithelioid granulomas (Fig. 3.1) (eFig. 3.1). The granulomas show a tendency to be surrounded by a rim of collagenous stroma (Fig. 3.2). They are usually small but tend to coalesce to form larger granulomas. Scattered small lymphocytes are often present in the

TABLE 3.1 Causes of Noninfectious Granulomas in the Lung
Sarcoidosis
Berylliosis
Necrotizing sarcoid granulomatosis
Wegener granulomatosis
Bronchocentric granulomatosis
Hypersensitivity pneumonitis
Aspiration pneumonia
Less common causes of granulomas:
– Hard metal pneumoconiosis
– Autoimmune disorder (Sjogren syndrome)
– Drug reaction (methotrexate)
– Hematologic malignancies (Hodgkin lymphoma, lymphomatoid granulomatosis)
– Intravenous drug abuse
– Exogenous lipid pneumonia

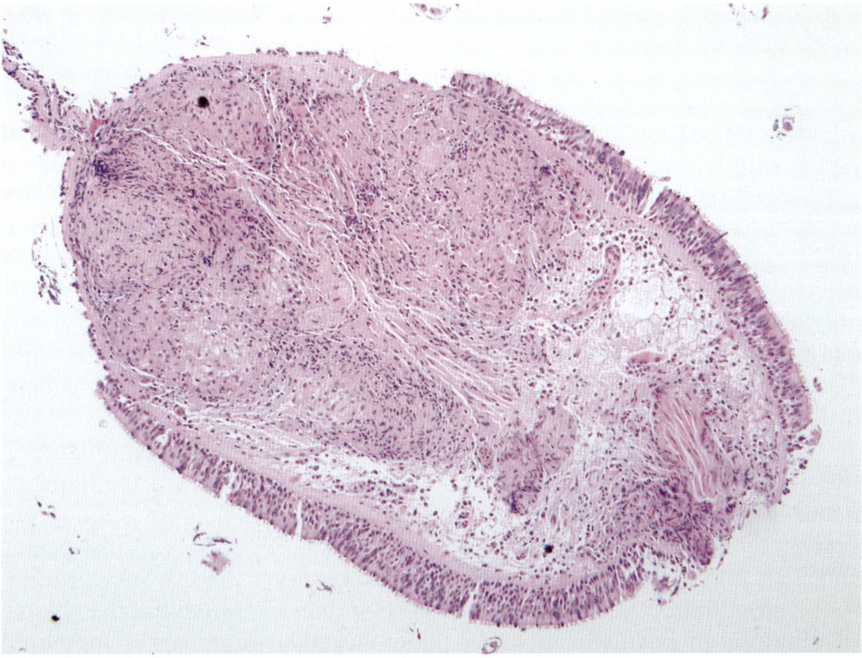

FIGURE 3.1 Endobronchial biopsy showing multiple small, confluent epithelioid granulomas in the subepithelial lamina propria in patient with sarcoidosis.

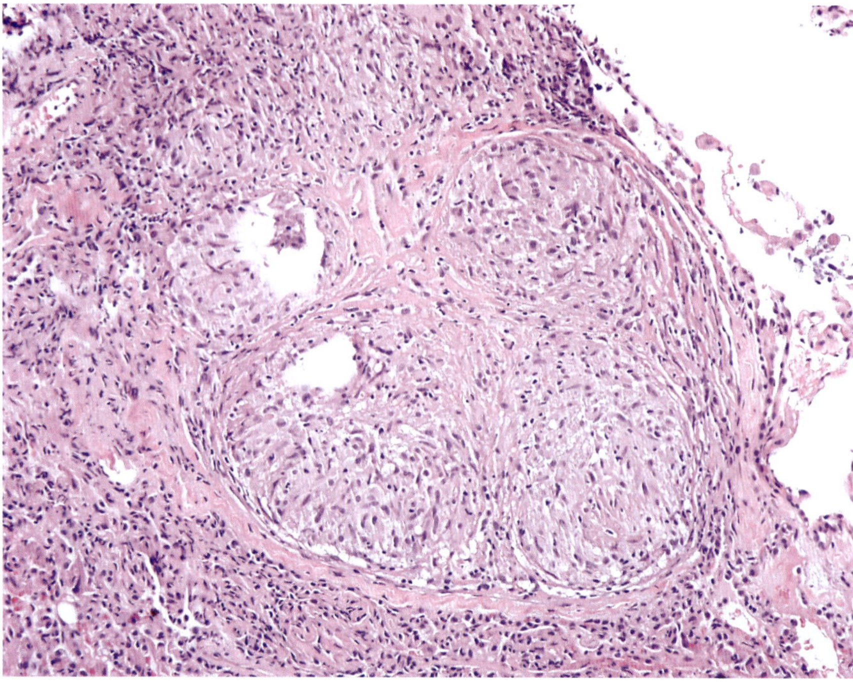

FIGURE 3.2 Typical sarcoid granuloma characterized by nodular aggregate of epithelioid histiocytes. Notice that the granuloma is surrounded by a thin rim of collagenous stroma that separates it from the surrounding tissues. Small scattered lymphocytes are seen in the vicinity of the granuloma.

vicinity of the granulomas. The granulomas are characteristically distributed along lymphatics and bronchovascular bundles and can often adopt a perivascular distribution (Figs. 3.3 and 3.4). The granulomas comprise collections of epithelioid histiocytes that contain abundant lightly eosinophilic cytoplasm (Fig. 3.5) (eFigs. 3.2 and 3.3). The histiocytes are devoid of cytologic atypia or mitotic activity (Fig. 3.6). Multinucleated giant cells are characteristically seen within the granulomas and may contain various cytoplasmic inclusions such as Schaumman bodies and asteroid bodies. The latter are nonspecific and can be seen in various granulomatous conditions other than sarcoidosis.

Transbronchial biopsies are the preferred method for demonstrating the granulomas in sarcoidosis. The granulomas will show a tendency to occur in submucosal distribution and may sometimes be quite subtle, presenting as discrete subepithelial accumulations of epithelioid histiocytes (Figs. 3.7 and 3.8). The positive yield of the biopsy is directly proportional to the amount of tissue biopsied. It has been demonstrated that the chance of obtaining a positive biopsy in patients with sarcoidosis is increased when four biopsy specimens are obtained rather than a single biopsy.[3]

The diagnosis of sarcoidosis is a diagnosis of exclusion. The pathology report on transbronchial biopsies should read only "nonnecrotizing

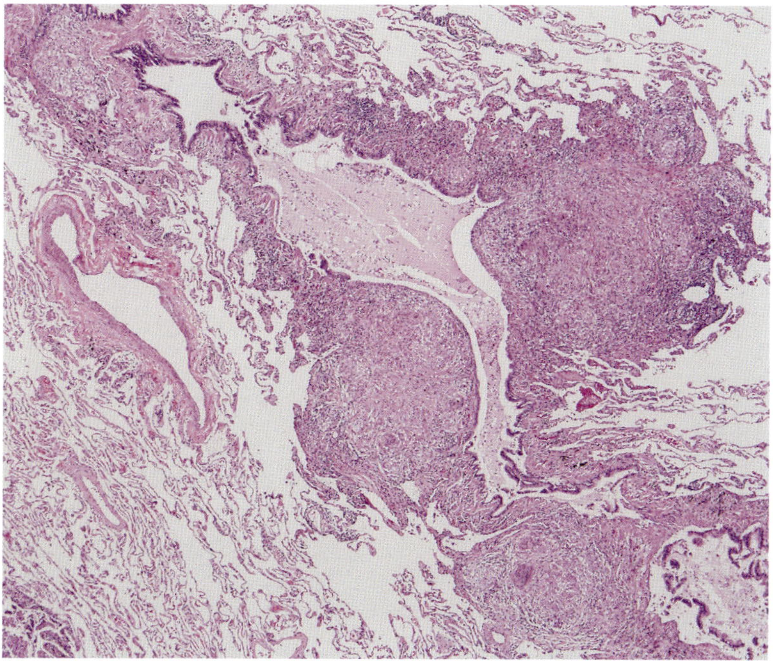

FIGURE 3.3 Characteristic distribution of sarcoid granulomas along lymphatics and bronchovascular bundles.

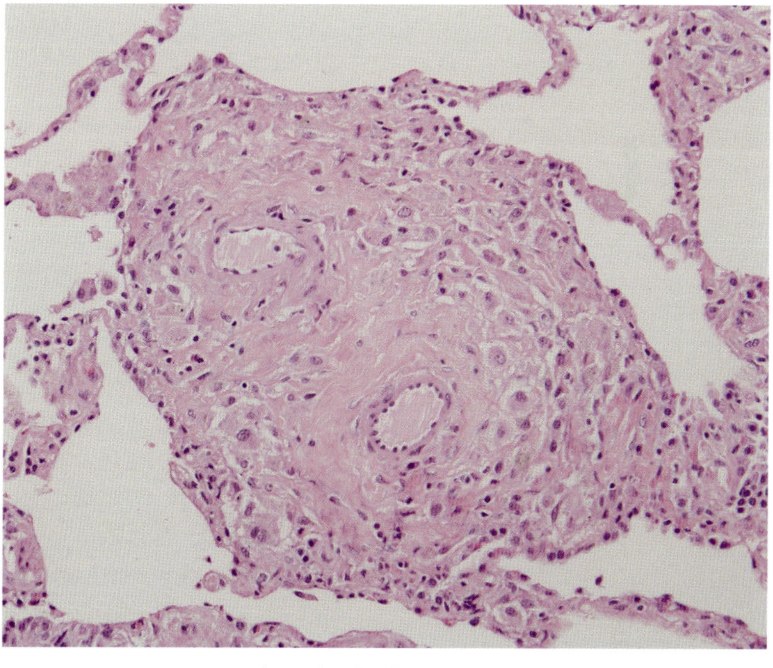

FIGURE 3.4 Perivascular distribution in sarcoid granuloma.

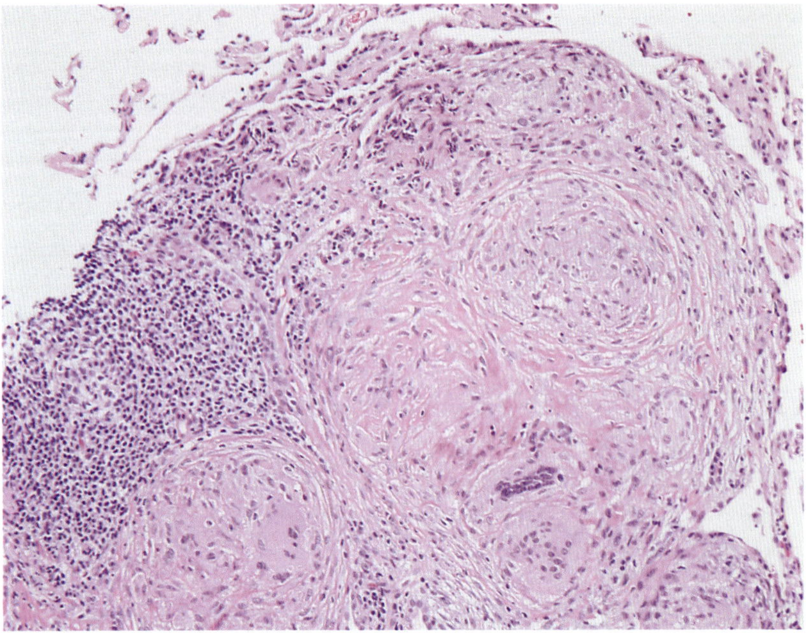

FIGURE 3.5 Sarcoid granulomas comprising collections of epithelioid histiocytes surrounded by dense collections of small lymphocytes.

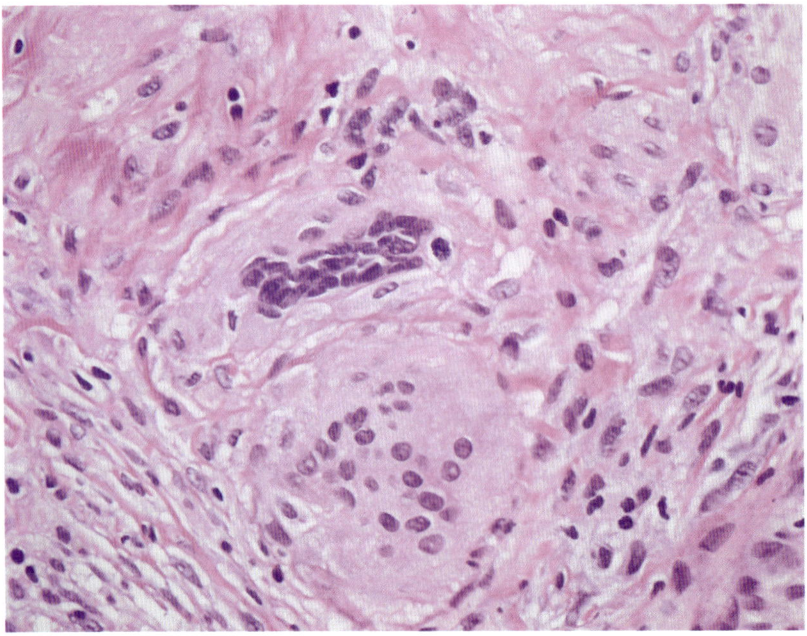

FIGURE 3.6 High magnification of sarcoid granuloma showing epithelioid histiocytes and multinuclear giant cells.

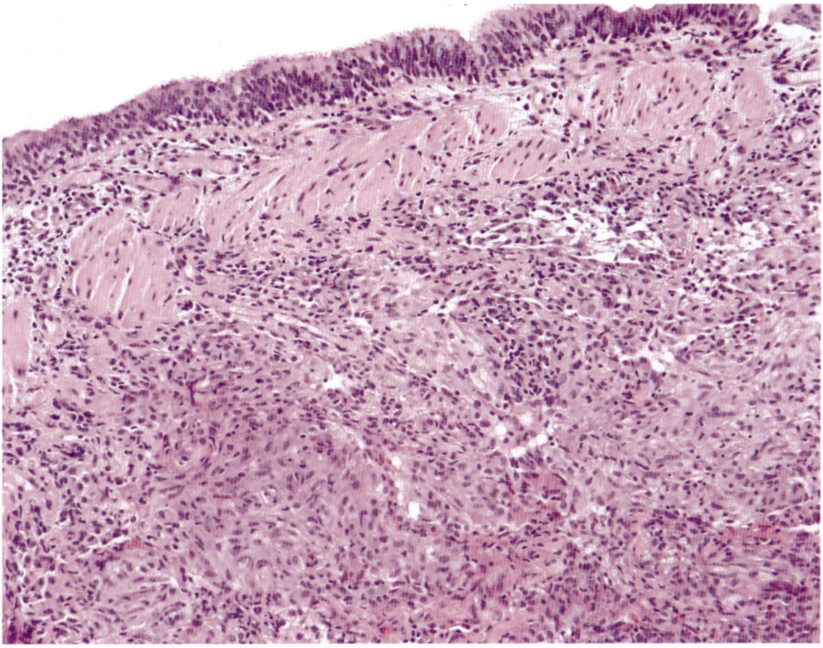

FIGURE 3.7 Discrete submucosal granulomas in bronchial biopsy in patient with sarcoidosis.

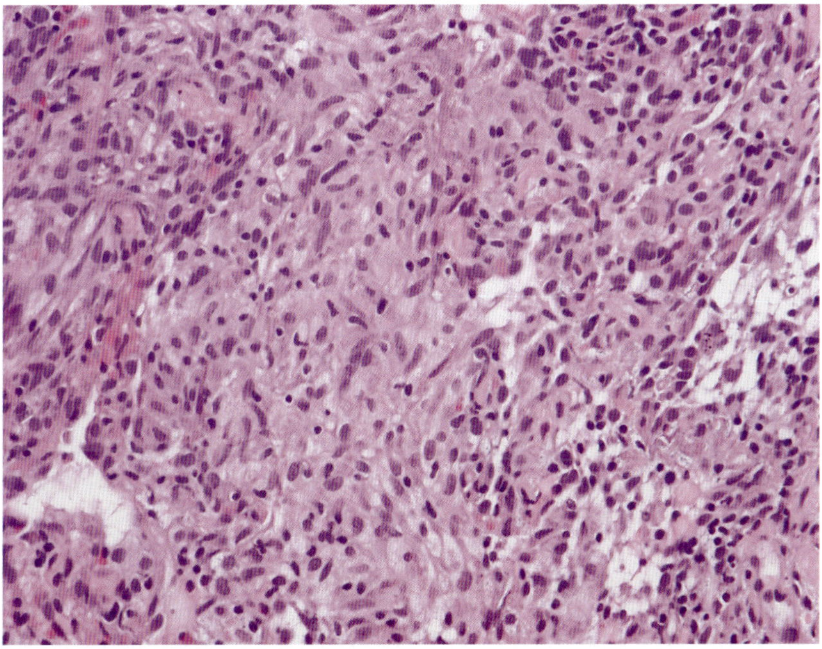

FIGURE 3.8 Higher magnification showing discrete clusters of epithelioid histiocytes gradually merging with the surrounding tissues.

epithelioid granulomas present" or "nonnecrotizing granulomatous pneumonitis." The pathologist can then state in a note that the findings are consistent with sarcoidosis if the clinical information provided was suggestive of the disease but should also suggest that alternate diagnostic possibilities must be first ruled out clinically. It is always a sound practice to routinely order special stains for microorganisms in cases of pulmonary granulomas to exclude infection, even in the absence of necrosis. We recommend routinely ordering acid-fast and silver stains. Submitting tissue for microbiologic cultures on cases in which clinical and radiographic findings are not highly suspicious for sarcoidosis is recommended because one study documented positive microbiologic cultures in up to 11% of biopsies of granulomas that were negative for microorganisms on special stains.[4]

BERYLLIOSIS

Berylliosis is a chronic occupational lung disease caused by inhalation of beryllium or its salts.[5,6] Because chronic berylliosis can develop in patients at relatively low levels of exposure and in a minority of individuals at risk, it has been postulated that the mechanism of disease may be the result of a hypersensitivity reaction, whereby beryllium will function as a hapten binding to some large carrier molecules to form an antigen.[7] The histopathologic findings in chronic berylliosis are essentially indistinguishable from those of sarcoidosis and are characterized by multiple nonnecrotizing epithelioid granulomas with giant cells associated with variable degrees of fibrosis. In advanced stages, the granulomas may coalesce to form large, centrally hyalinized masses that can resemble old lesions of histoplasmosis. There is also an acute form of the disease characterized by a chemical pneumonitis with diffuse alveolar damage that develops rapidly following short-term, massive exposure to soluble beryllium salts. This form of the disease has now disappeared owing to the air quality standards imposed in 1949 following the first cases of acute beryllium exposure reported in this country.[8]

The diagnosis of berylliosis is dependent on the demonstration of a history of beryllium exposure and can be confirmed by demonstration of beryllium in lung tissue by wet chemical spectrometry techniques. Electron energy loss spectrometry and laser microprobe or ion microprobe mass spectrometry have also been utilized to demonstrate beryllium in tissue sections.[9] In the past, beryllium was an important component of fluorescent lights, but it is now mainly used in the aerospace industry and computer manufacturing.[10] Exposure can also occur during mining and extraction of beryllium ores.

NECROTIZING SARCOID GRANULOMATOSIS

Necrotizing sarcoid granulomatosis (NSG) is a rare condition of unknown etiology characterized by nodular masses of necrotizing epithelioid granulomas involving the lung parenchyma. It is still not clear whether this condition represents a variant of sarcoidosis or whether it belongs in the family of pulmonary vasculitides. The condition affects mostly adults older than 50 years but can also occur in adolescents or in elderly patients. There is an increased incidence in women (approximately 1:2 male/female ratio). The disease is usually confined to the lungs and presents with cough, fever, weight loss, and chest pain. Up to 25% of patients may be asymptomatic. There has been no evidence found of systemic vasculitis, multiorgan involvement, or positive antineutrophil cytoplasmic antibodies (ANCA) in these patients.[11,12] NSG presents radiologically as bilateral, multifocal nodular opacities involving lung parenchyma following a bronchovascular and subpleural distribution. Solitary lesions have also been reported.

Histologically the lesions are characterized by confluent epithelioid granulomas with large areas of necrosis (Fig. 3.9). Foci of vasculitis may be present involving the media and subintimal region of small pulmonary arteries and veins. The granulomas may also circumferentially surround large arteries impinging on the adventitia. Scattered giant cells may be seen in the areas of vasculitis. The viable portions of the granulomas, however, are indistinguishable from those seen in sarcoidosis and comprise epithelioid histiocytes admixed with multinucleated giant cells. The granulomas may vary considerably in size and usually coalesce to form larger granulomas. They follow a similar lymphangitic distribution as in sarcoidosis

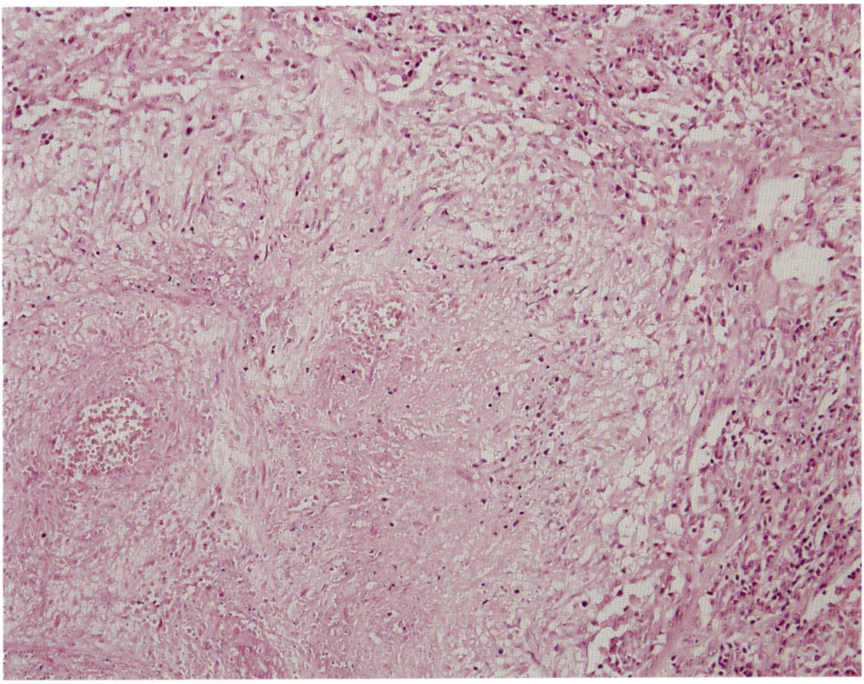

FIGURE 3.9 NSG showing confluence of epithelioid granulomas with central areas of necrosis.

and differ only because of the prominent areas of necrosis and the foci of vasculitis.[11–13] NSG may be very difficult to diagnose in transbronchial biopsies and may require video-assisted thoracoscopic surgery (VATS) or wedge resection for adequate evaluation. Special stains for organisms are mandatory to rule out the possibility of infectious granulomas.

The differential diagnosis of NSG includes infectious granulomas, sarcoidosis, and Wegener granulomatosis (WG). Infectious granulomas may be the most difficult to exclude because they too can produce vasculitis and sarcoid-like epithelioid necrotizing granulomas. Special stains for organisms and microbiologic culture studies are the only reliable means for making this distinction. Separation from WG may be problematic in some cases but can be accomplished by identifying the palisaded necrotizing granulomas with deeply basophilic areas of necrosis in WG as opposed to the nonpalisading epithelioid granulomas of NSG and by the absence of cytoplasmic ANCA (C-ANCA) reactivity in the latter.

The prognosis for NSG is generally excellent. Most patients respond to systemic corticosteroids. A small percentage of patients will develop a relapse or have persistent disease. Death is rare and is usually the result of opportunistic infections.[11–14]

WEGENER GRANULOMATOSIS

WG is a rare disease of unknown etiology. It primarily affects the upper and lower respiratory tract and the kidneys. The granulomas in WG resemble more closely infectious granulomas than the granulomas of sarcoidosis owing to extensive central necrosis with peripheral palisading of macrophages (Fig. 3.10) (eFig. 3.4). WG occurs in adults with a mean age of 50. Clinically, it presents with various symptoms that may involve the head and neck, eyes, lungs, and kidney, including sinusitis, nasal ulceration, otitis media, ear pain, oral lesions, cough, hemoptysis, pleuritic pain, conjunctivitis, eye pain, corneal ulcers, iritis, renal manifestations, and systemic manifestations including arthritis, weight loss, fever, and peripheral neuropathy.[15,16] The most important laboratory diagnostic test for WG is the determination of serum ANCA. Two immunofluorescent patterns have been demonstrated; cytoplasmic or classical type (C-ANCA) and the perinuclear pattern (P-ANCA). The C-ANCA pattern is the one most closely associated with WG and is present in most patients with generalized disease.[17,18] The basic histopathologic finding in WG is a necrotizing vasculitis affecting small arteries and veins (Fig. 3.11) (eFig. 3.5). The vasculitis is often centered in areas of necrosis and may display granulomas involving the media and the adventitia of the vessel (Figs. 3.12 and 3.13). Small neutrophilic microabscesses are also a distinctive feature of WG (Fig. 3.14) (eFig. 3.6). They are seen within connective tissue and may contain a central area of necrosis surrounded by variable numbers of lymphocytes, plasma cells, histiocytes, and fibroblasts (Fig. 3.15). The areas of necrosis in WG are often large and irregular with "geographic" contours.

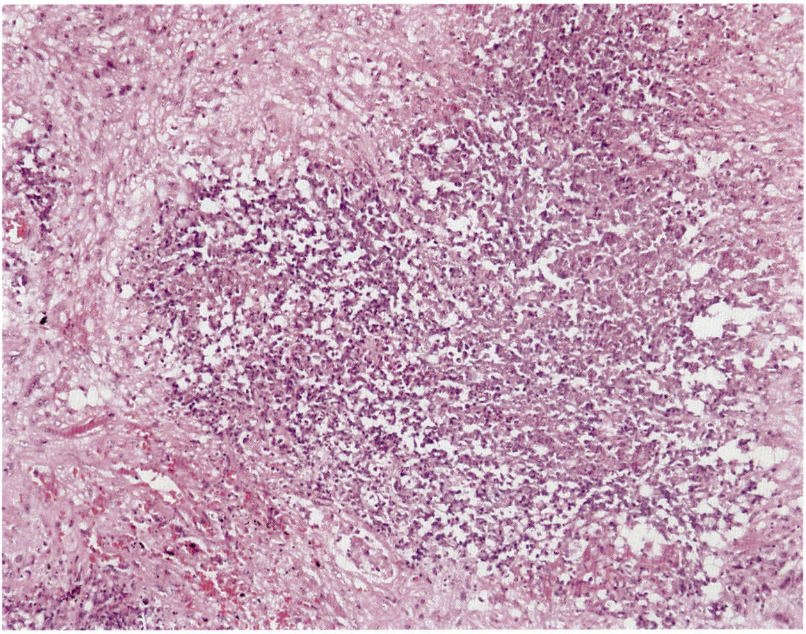

FIGURE 3.10 WG showing granuloma with characteristic area of geographic necrosis with deep basophilic appearance owing to abundant nuclear debris, surrounded by a palisaded rim of histiocytes.

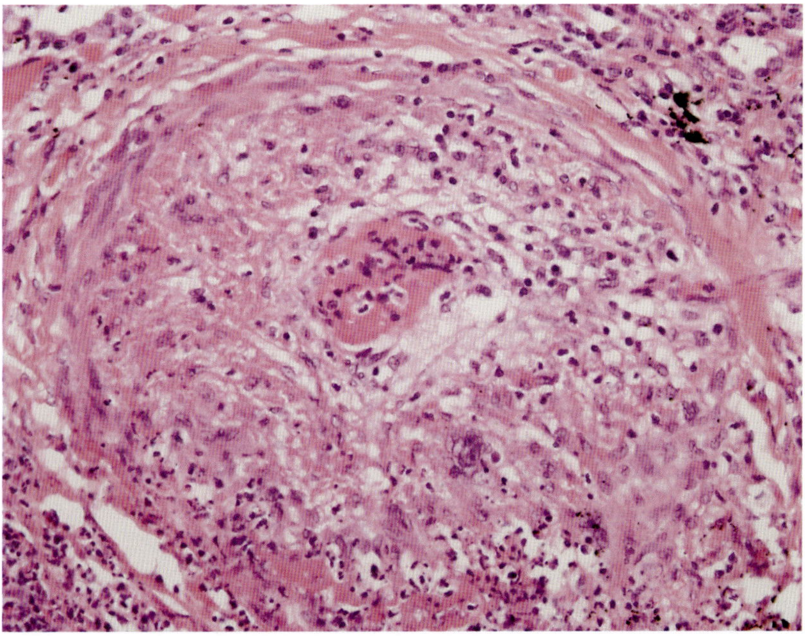

FIGURE 3.11 WG showing necrotizing vasculitis involving a small artery with small areas of necrosis in the media and adventitia of the vessels.

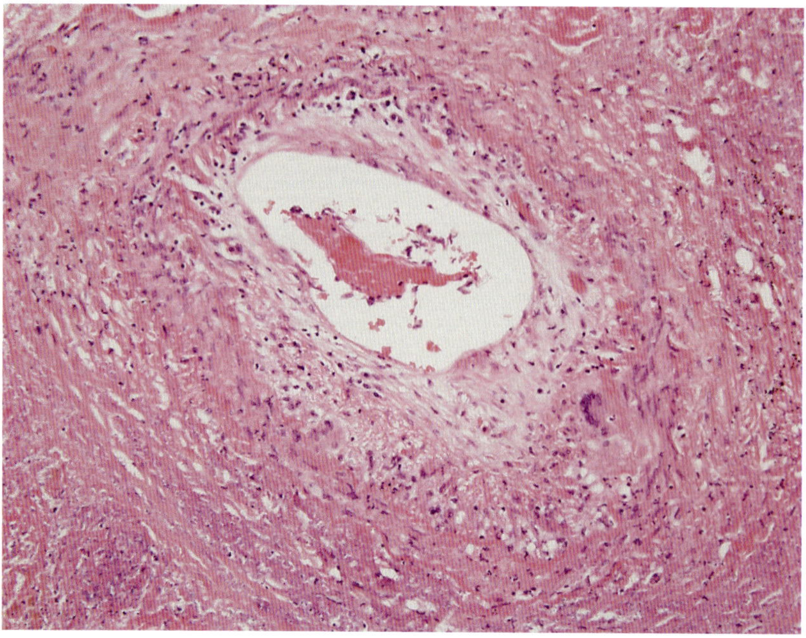

FIGURE 3.12 Medium-sized vessel in WG showing involvement of the media by granulomatous inflammation.

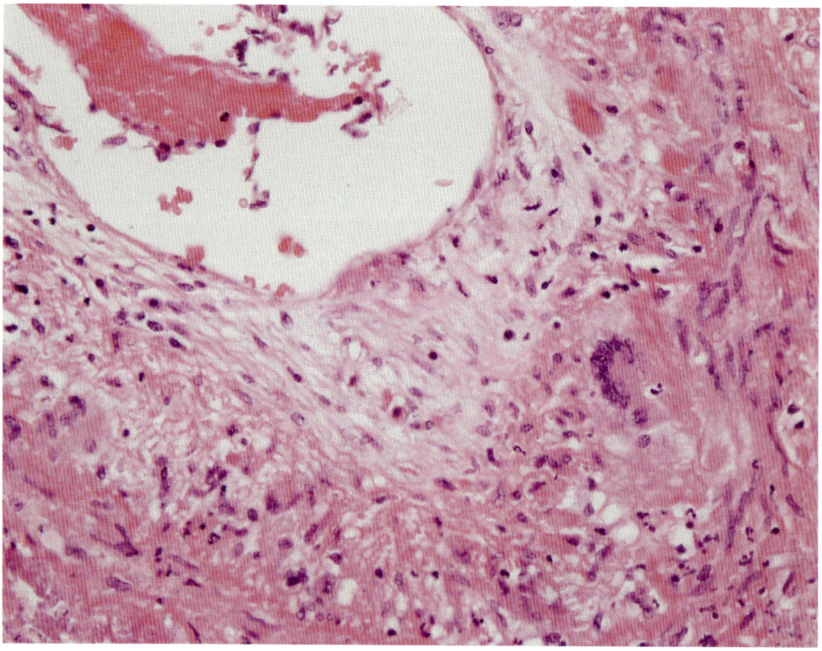

FIGURE 3.13 Higher magnification of vasculitis in WG showing multinucleated giant cells and mononuclear cells within the wall of the vessel.

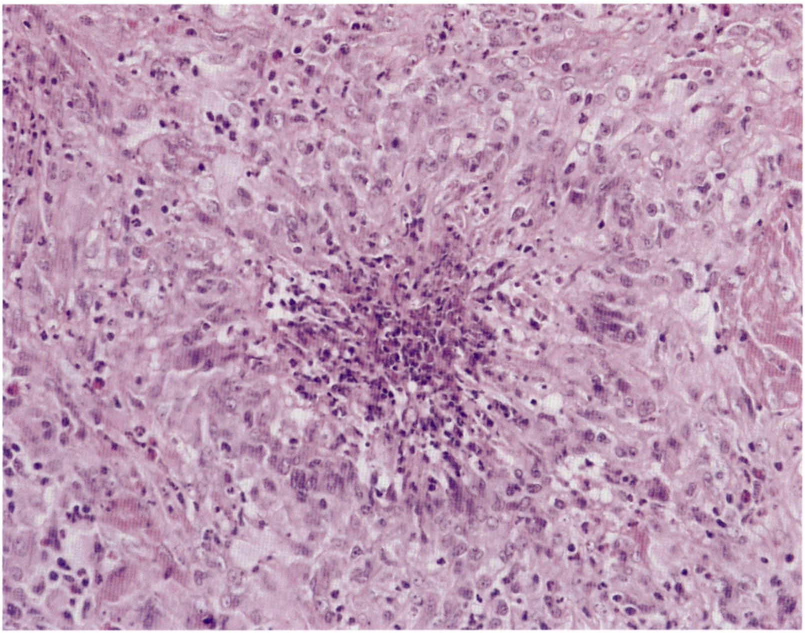

FIGURE 3.14 Small neutrophilic microabscesses in WG with central area of suppuration and necrosis and numerous scattered eosinophils in the periphery of the granuloma.

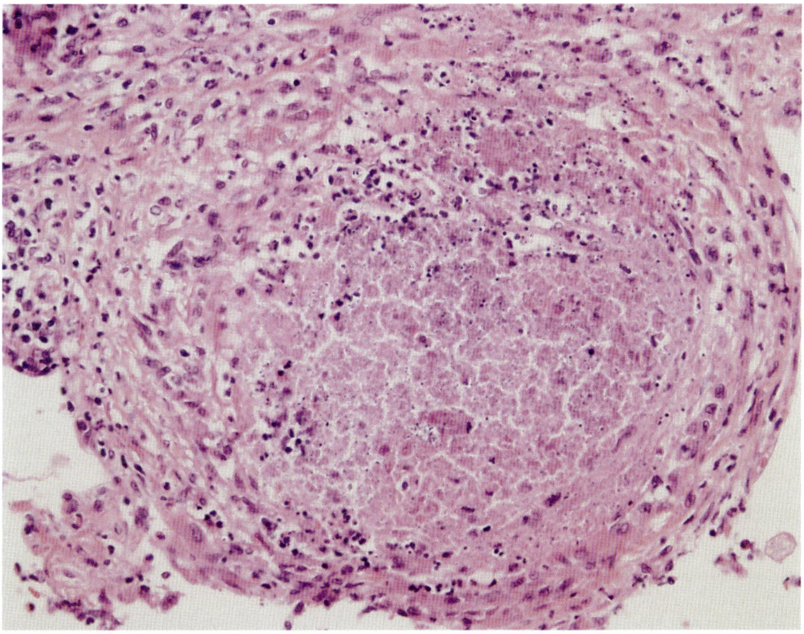

FIGURE 3.15 Another example of a small necrotizing microabscess in WG showing extensive central area of necrosis surrounded by neutrophils and nuclear debris and bounded by a peripheral rim of histiocytes.

Unlike infectious granulomas, the areas of necrosis tend to display a deeply basophilic appearance owing to the accumulation of abundant nuclear debris rather than the pink (eosinophilic) areas of necrosis seen in infectious granulomas. The areas of necrosis are characteristically surrounded by a rim of palisaded histiocytes. Multinucleated giant cells can be seen randomly scattered singly or forming small aggregates at the edges of the areas of necrosis. Well-formed, nonnecrotizing epithelioid granulomas are not a feature of WG and should suggest an alternative diagnosis. Central cavitation with necrotic centers can often be seen in large granulomas. Extensive degeneration of collagen may also be appreciated surrounding the areas of necrosis. The lesions are often multiple and nodular with skip areas of uninvolved normal parenchyma. Secondary nonspecific changes that can be seen in association with WG include an organizing pneumonia pattern, alveolar hemorrhage, interstitial fibrosis, lipid pneumonia, lymphoid hyperplasia, and acute bronchiolitis. WG may be very difficult to diagnose on small transbronchial biopsies, but the diagnosis can be suggested when the characteristic granulomatous vasculitis is identified. VATS biopsy is usually required for proper histopathologic evaluation. Clinical correlation and serologic testing are required for making a definitive diagnosis.

BRONCHOCENTRIC GRANULOMATOSIS

Bronchocentric granulomatosis (BG) is a condition characterized by necrotizing granulomatous inflammation that surrounds and replaces the bronchial wall and mucosa. The process involves the bronchi and the more distal bronchioles. The term BG is purely a descriptive diagnosis rather than a specific pathologic entity and may be the result of infectious and noninfectious conditions, including allergic bronchopulmonary fungal disease, bacterial or parasitic infection, rheumatoid arthritis, WG, and necrotizing sarcoidosis. Between one-third and one-half of all cases occur in the setting of allergic bronchopulmonary aspergillosis in patients with asthma. Serum precipitin titers to aspergillus or candida species are elevated in about 50% of patients.[19] Cultures will grow the fungus in 20% to 50% of cases.[20] In asthmatic patients, the condition usually presents with progressive wheezing, cough, and fever with mucoid impaction. The lesions usually present as localized areas of consolidation or nodular parenchymal lesions on chest radiographs. Cavitation may be present in some of the nodules. The prognosis for patients with this condition is generally good. Asthmatic patients usually respond to corticosteroid treatment. Isolated lesions can be cured by simple surgical excision. Approximately half of the cases of BG are of noninfectious nature and may be owing to a specific etiology, such as rheumatoid arthritis or WG, or of unknown etiology.

Histologically, the hallmark of the process is the destruction of the airway lumen by necrotizing palisaded granulomas (Fig. 3.16) (eFig. 3.7). In some cases, the bronchial or bronchiolar wall may be partially preserved,

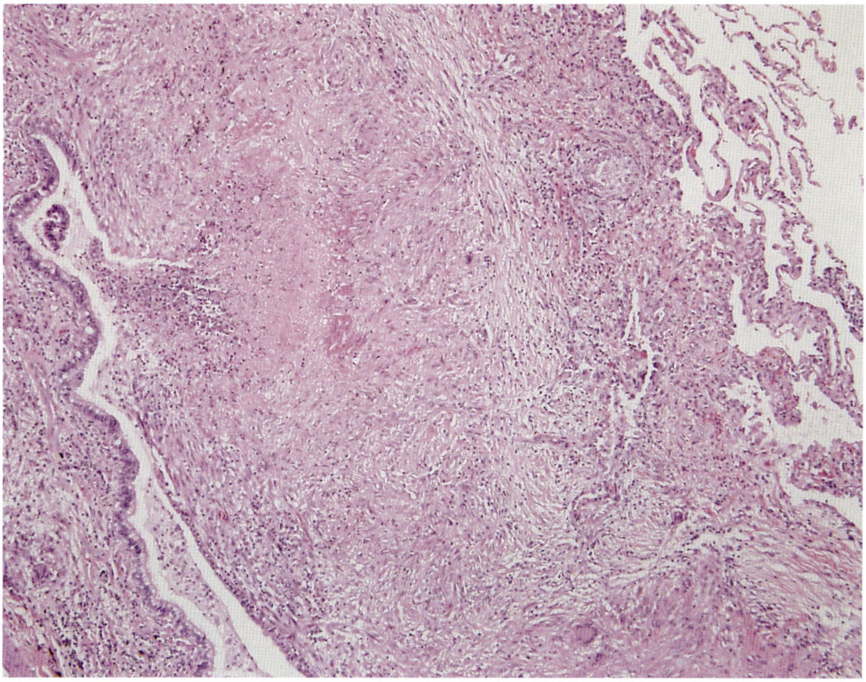

FIGURE 3.16 Necrotizing palisaded granulomas are seen causing destruction of the airway lumen in BG.

and there will be only partial obliteration of the airway by the necrotizing granulomatous process. In cases where there is complete obliteration of the bronchial wall, identification of residual bronchial epithelium or identification of adjacent pulmonary arteries will help to confirm the bronchocentric nature of the process. In equivocal cases, elastic stains may help to identify the residual elastica of the airway or to highlight the proximity to a pulmonary artery. The centers of the granulomas may contain abundant eosinophils, particularly in asthmatic patients. A foreign body giant cell reaction to the necrotic debris can also be observed in some cases. Fungal hyphae can be found in 20% to 90% of samples of patients with allergic bronchopulmonary aspergillosis.[19–21] The hyphae are often distorted and fragmented and are noninvasive. They are more frequently present within proximal bronchial plugs rather than in the necrotizing granulomas. Special stains for organisms should always be routinely ordered in cases of BG. Some cases of BG do not display any eosinophilia but are characterized instead by intense neutrophilia and total absence of organisms on special stains. Such cases may represent a manifestation of rheumatoid arthritis or WG. Clinical correlation with serologic tests and identification of the other features distinctive for these conditions are necessary for correct interpretation. BG can also occur in patients with tuberculosis, blastomycosis, and histoplasmosis.[22,23] Transbronchial biopsies may yield limited information in cases of BG, and an open lung biopsy may be preferable for more definitive interpretation. However, destruction of bronchial walls by necrotizing granulomas, especially when containing prominent eosinophils, should raise the suspicion of this condition and prompt further clinical studies and special stains to rule out organisms.

HYPERSENSITIVITY PNEUMONITIS

Hypersensitivity pneumonitis, also known as extrinsic allergic alveolitis (EAA), represents an allergic response of the small airways and lung parenchyma to various inhaled organic antigens. The most well-known examples are farmer's lung, caused by sensitivity to thermophilic actinomycetes, and pigeon breeder or "bird fancier" lung, caused by inhalation of avian antigens. Although a similar effect can be observed with some ingested antigens, EAA generally refers to disease occurring as a result of inhalation exposure. These antigens include thermophilic bacteria such as actinomyces, other bacteria or bacterial products (humidifier lung, bissinosis), molds, amoeba, and chemicals (such as toluene diisocyanate used in plastics manufacture, or pyromellitic dianhydride used in epoxy resin).

The disease can occur as an acute or chronic process. The acute form occurs within hours of exposure to the inhaled antigen. The symptoms resemble an acute viral infection, with fever, chills, malaise, shortness of breath, and dry cough. The chronic form of the disease may be initially more subtle but will lead to progressive symptoms of shortness of breath.[24,25] Some cases can progress to end-stage diffuse interstitial fibrosis leading to death resulting from respiratory compromise. Radiologic studies show diffuse ground glass infiltrates, sometimes accompanied by reticulonodular densities. The findings mostly involve the upper half of the lung fields and generally spare the apices and bases.

The pathologic features of EAA are mainly characterized by a chronic interstitial pneumonitis associated with bronchiolitis and small, poorly formed epithelioid granulomas (Fig. 3.17). The granulomas are characteristically nonnecrotizing and located in the interstitium. The granulomas are usually poorly formed and small; they can be sometimes difficult to identify and will blend imperceptibly with the surrounding inflammatory cells in the alveolar septa (Fig. 3.18). The chronic interstitial pneumonia is usually mild and causes only slight widening of the alveolar septa by small lymphocytes and occasional plasma cells. The inflammatory infiltrate is often present around the walls of terminal bronchioles. The interstitial granulomas in EAA can be very subtle and often only recognizable on higher magnification (eFig. 3.8), although we have seen examples of "hot tub" pneumonitis in which well-formed epithelioid granulomas were prominent. Scattered isolated multinucleated giant cells may also be seen in the interstitium unassociated with the granulomas. Refractile oxalate crystals may be present within the giant cells and can lead to confusion with aspiration pneumonia or pneumoconiosis. Patchy airspace

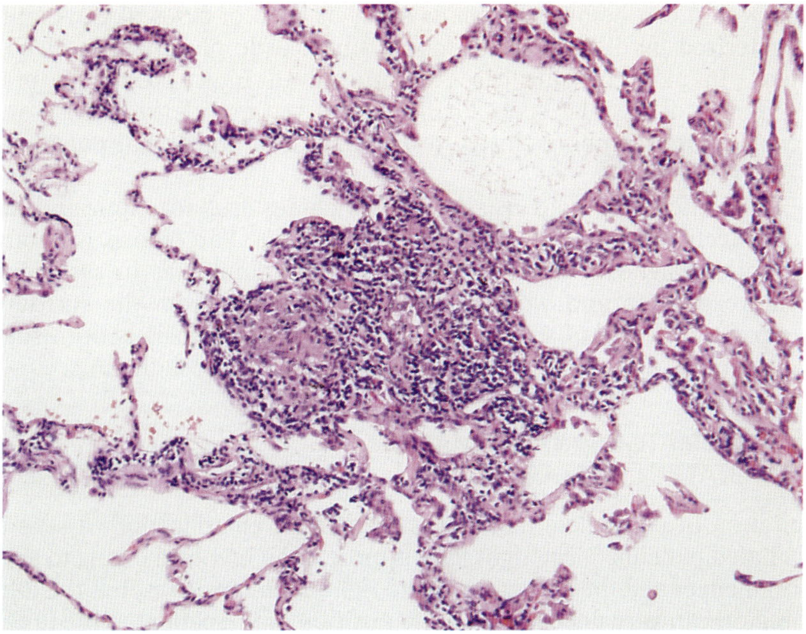

FIGURE 3.17 Chronic interstitial pneumonia in patient with EAA (hypersensitivity pneumonitis) showing interstitial lymphoid infiltrates within alveolar walls and scattered small epithelioid granulomas.

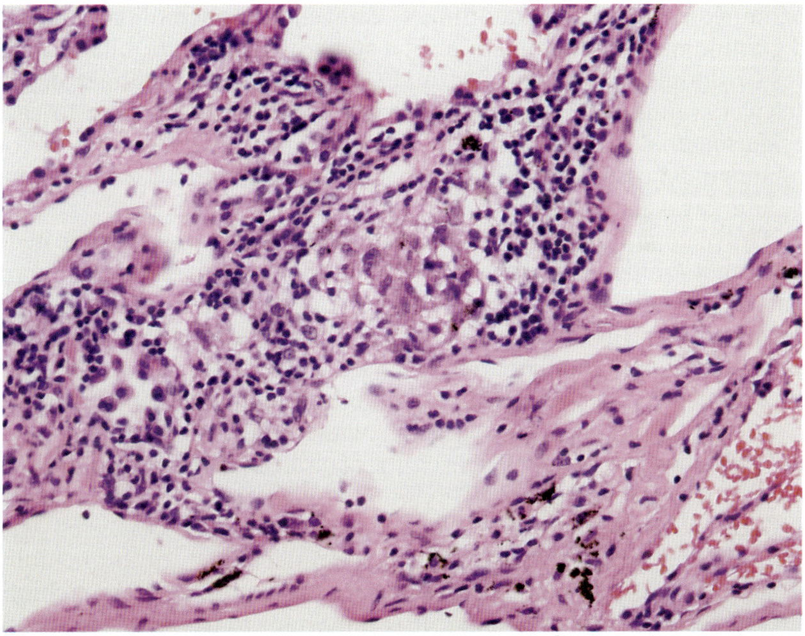

FIGURE 3.18 Higher magnification of EAA (hypersensitivity pneumonitis) showing ill-defined, poorly formed small epithelioid granulomas characteristic of this condition.

organization can be observed in as many as 60% of cases of EAA and is characterized by discrete small foci of fibroblastic plugs within alveolar lumens. In more chronic cases of unresolved EAA, prominent bronchiolization of alveolar spaces can be observed and dense fibrosis with extensive honeycombing closely resembling usual interstitial pneumonia (UIP) will develop.

The differential diagnosis for EAA includes drug reactions and low-grade infections caused by atypical mycobacteria. Sarcoidosis is another differential diagnostic consideration, but the granulomas in sarcoidosis are more discrete and well defined and separated from the surrounding stroma by a rim of sclerosis. Furthermore, sarcoidosis is not usually accompanied by marked interstitial inflammation as seen in EAA.

GRANULOMATOUS INFLAMMATION IN ASPIRATION PNEUMONIA

Aspiration of particulate material is a common complication of severely debilitated patients.[26] The right lung is more often involved owing to gravitational effect and the trajectory of the right main bronchus, but the affected region can vary depending on the position of the patient at the time of aspiration. Most aspirated materials are foods and other organic materials, including seeds, meat particles, vegetable peels and pits, chicken bones, candy, and gum.[27] Complications of aspiration of particulate material can include lung abscess formation, bronchial stenosis, bronchiectasis, bronchocutaneous fistula, pneumothorax, empyema, bronchiolitis obliterans, and granulomatous inflammation. In a study of 59 patients, bilateral infiltrates or nodules were identified in 17 cases, unilateral nodules or infiltrates were found in 17 cases, and solitary nodules were seen in 13 cases. Foreign material was identified in all cases, including vegetable or food remnants in 54 cases, talc or microcrystalline cellulose in 7, crospovidone in 4, and kayaxelate in 2 patients.[28]

The histopathologic features of aspiration pneumonia include necrotizing pneumonitis with abscess formation, acute necrotizing and granulomatous bronchiolitis, and necrotizing suppurative granulomas with foreign body-type giant cell reaction to the aspirated material (Fig. 3.19). An organizing pneumonia pattern is often found distal to the obstructed bronchus or bronchioles. Hyaline membranes can develop within 48 to 72 hours and may lead to confusion with diffuse alveolar damage on endoscopic biopsies. Careful search for aspirated foreign material is necessary for a correct diagnosis. The foreign material is usually surrounded by multinucleated giant cells. The diagnosis must be suspected when multinucleated giant cells, acute bronchopneumonia or bronchiolitis, and suppurative granulomas are seen in a background of bronchiolitis obliterans organizing pneumonia. It is important to examine the sections always under polarized microscopy to identify birefringent foreign particles. Polarized microscopy may help identify crystalline material within

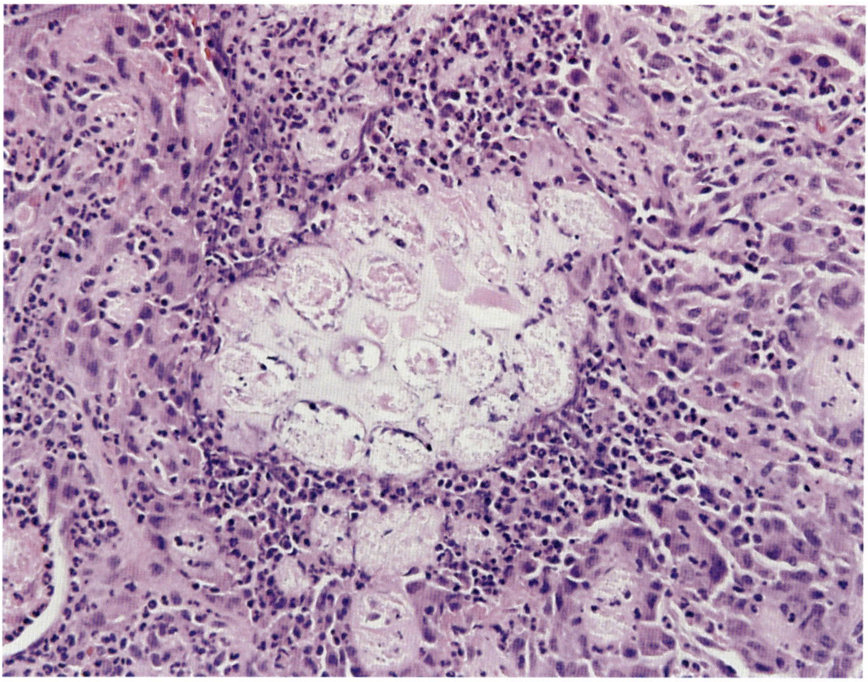

FIGURE 3.19 Necrotizing suppurative granulomas are seen in aspiration pneumonia. Notice the foreign body type giant cell reaction surrounding the aspirated material.

macrophages and multinucleated giant cells. Care must be taken, however, not to misinterpret the presence of conchoidal calcifications or calcium oxalate crystals for evidence of aspiration, as these can occur in various inflammatory granulomatous reactions unrelated to aspiration.

Less Frequent Causes of Pulmonary Granulomatous Inflammation

Less frequent causes of pulmonary granulomatous inflammation can be seen in patients with hard metal pneumoconiosis, autoimmune disorders, particularly Sjogren syndrome (SS), drug reactions (particularly with methotrexate), and in certain hematolymphoid neoplasms, particularly Hodgkin disease and lymphomatoid granulomatosis (LYG).

HARD METAL PNEUMOCONIOSIS. Hard metal lung disease occurs as the consequence of the inhalation of hard metal dusts. Exposure can occur during the manufacture of products containing hard metals or during their use.[29] The two most frequent agents involved in hard metal pneumoconiosis are tungsten carbide used in the manufacture of cutting tools and drilling equipment and cobalt. Patients usually present with insidious onset of dyspnea and restrictive changes on pulmonary function tests. Radiologic studies show diffuse interstitial infiltrates. The fact that a very low percentage

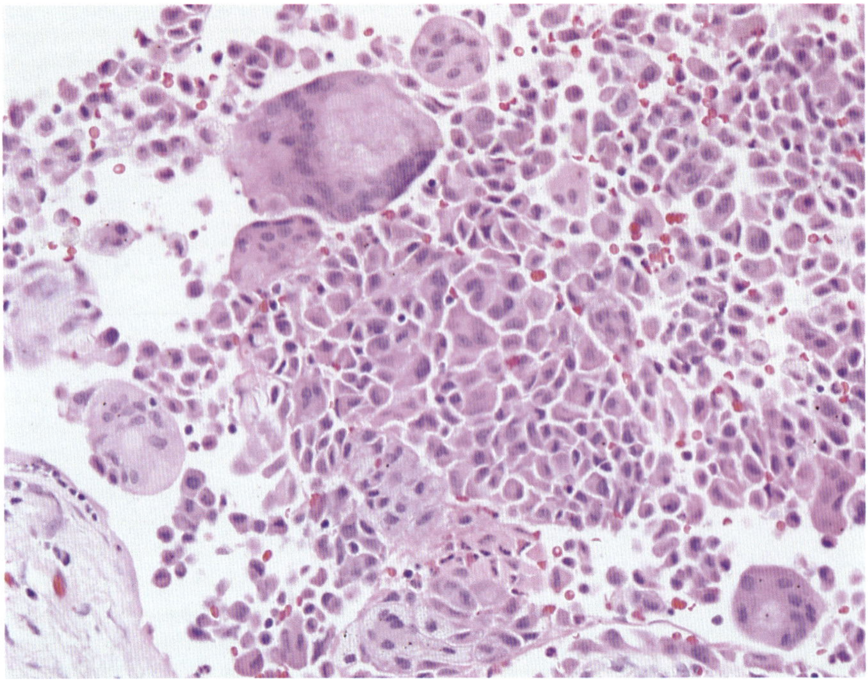

FIGURE 3.20 Hard metal pneumoconiosis showing multinucleated giant cells admixed with macrophages within alveolar spaces and lining the alveolar septa.

(<1%) of exposed workers develop the disease suggests that the underlying pathogenetic mechanism may be related to a hypersensitivity reaction.

The histopathologic hallmark of hard metal lung disease is the presence of abundant multinucleated giant cells within the alveolar spaces and lining the alveolar septa (Fig. 3.20) (eFig. 3.9). In fact, a term applied in the past to this condition was giant cell interstitial pneumonia, which was believed to represent one of the idiopathic interstitial pneumonias.[30] The alveolar septa are usually thickened and fibrotic and lined by hyperplastic type II pneumocytes. The alveolar lumens are filled with abundant macrophages in a pattern reminiscent of desquamative interstitial pneumonia. In advanced cases, interstitial fibrosis may be very striking leading to honeycombing of lung parenchyma and extensive bronchiolar metaplasia similar to that observed in the advanced stages of UIP. Discrete or well-formed epithelioid granulomas are *not* a feature of the disease. The metal particles can be visualized using analytical electron microscopy.[31]

SJOGREN SYNDROME. SS is an autoimmune disease characterized by a dense lymphocytic infiltration of the salivary glands resulting in the clinical manifestations of dry mouth and dry eyes. The principal morphologic manifestation of SS is a lymphocytic interstitial pneumonitis principally distributed around the airways. However, a common finding is the presence of small, nonnecrotizing interstitial granulomas admixed with the

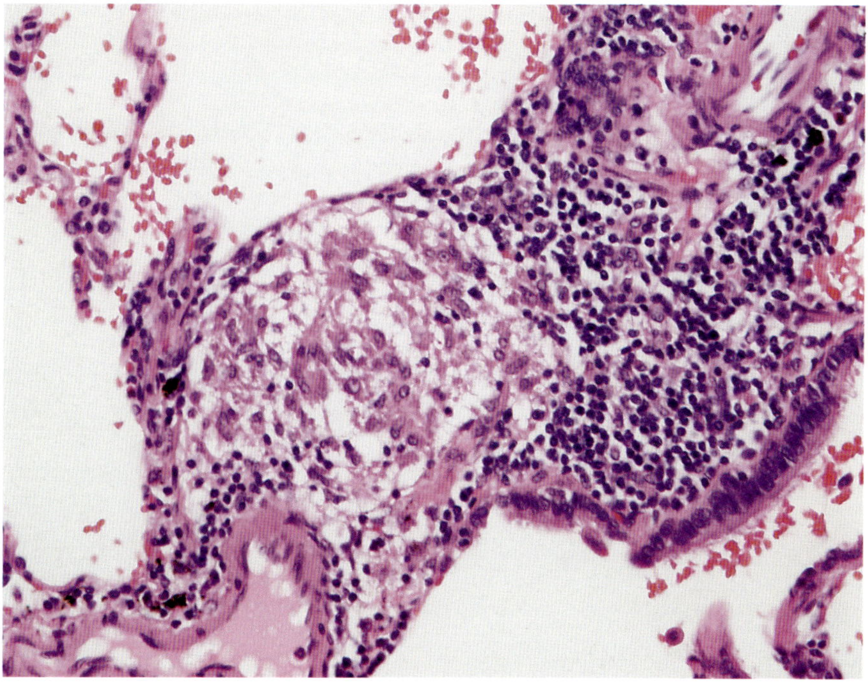

FIGURE 3.21 Small granulomas can be seen in SS admixed with dense lymphoid cell infiltrates.

lymphoid cell population.[32] For the most part, the granulomas are small and poorly formed, somewhat reminiscent of those seen in allergic extrinsic alveolitis, and are commonly admixed with the dense lymphoid interstitial infiltrate along with scattered multinucleated giant cells (Fig. 3.21). However, in some instances, the granulomas may become more numerous and diffuse, raising the possibility of an infectious process or aspiration pneumonia in the differential diagnosis.

METHOTREXATE TOXICITY. Methotrexate, a drug used in the treatment of various disorders, including rheumatoid arthritis and cancer, may cause interstitial inflammation with airspace organization and fibrosis. Hyperplasia of type II pneumocytes and tissue eosinophilia can be seen in some cases. The findings are nonspecific, except for the presence of giant cells and small nonnecrotizing granulomas (Fig. 3.22), which are the only relatively specific features for this drug in comparison with other drugs causing lung toxicity.[33]

HEMATOLYMPHOID NEOPLASMS. Hematolymphoid neoplasms involving the lung may occasionally be accompanied by granulomas. These include Hodgkin lymphoma and LYG. Both will be discussed in more detail under hematolymphoid malignancies (chapter 11).

INFLAMMATORY BOWEL DISEASE. Pulmonary manifestations in inflammatory bowel disease have been well documented.[34,35] These include bronchitis,

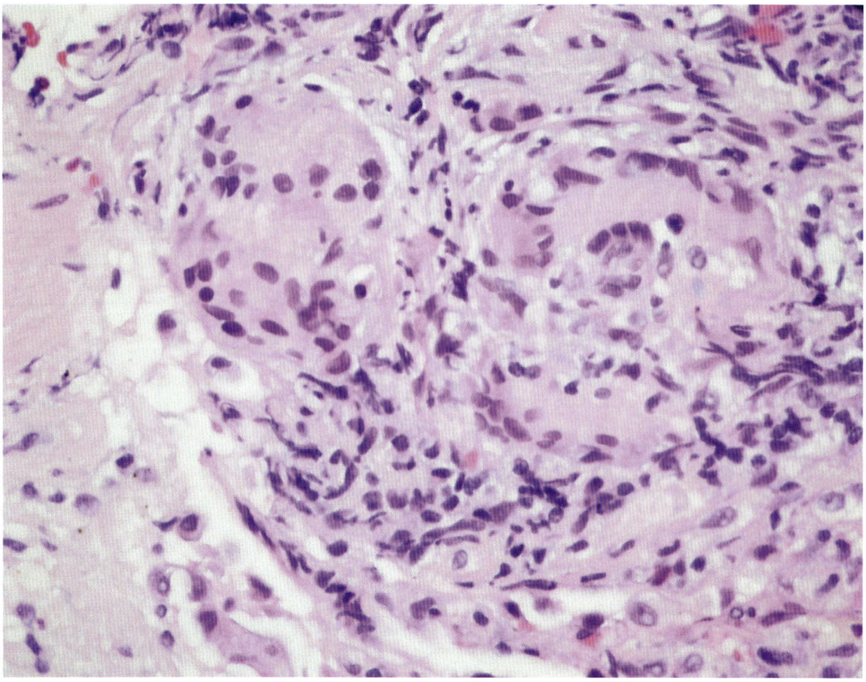

FIGURE 3.22 Small, poorly formed epithelioid granulomas similar to those observed in EAA can be seen in methotrexate toxicity.

bronchiectasis, bronchiolitis obliterans, organizing pneumonia, vasculitis, and granulomatous inflammation. Granulomatous pneumonitis can be observed in patients with Crohn disease and has also been reported in patients with ulcerative colitis under treatment with azathioprine.[36] In patients with Crohn disease, small, nonnecrotizing epithelioid granulomas with multinucleated giant cells tend to involve the interstitium and surrounding bronchioles. Special stains for organisms are indicated to rule out infectious agents. Clinical correlation is indispensable for correct interpretation.

INTRAVENOUS DRUG ABUSE. Intravenous injection of drugs that are normally intended for oral administration elicits a foreign body granulomatous reaction in the lung parenchyma secondary to the deposition of "filler" substances such as talc, starch, cellulose, and others within capillaries, arterioles, or small vessels. Talc used for "cutting" or diluting illicit drugs such as heroin can also deposit in the lung microvasculature in intravenous drug abusers. The granulomatous reaction can take place within the vasculature or may occur in the interstitium (Fig. 3.23). Multinucleated giant cells will usually contain polarizable crystalline foreign material. The most common types of foreign material include cornstarch, which shows a characteristic "maltese cross" pattern of polarization, or talc which assumes the shape of elongated plate-like crystalline material (Fig. 3.24).

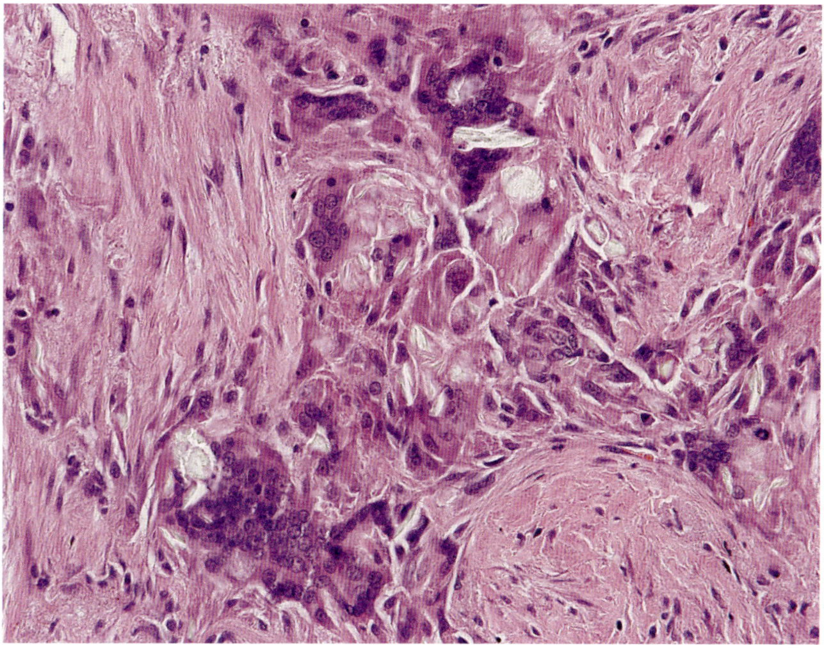

FIGURE 3.23 Small plate-like crystalline particles are seen surrounded by foreign body type multinucleated giant cells in intravenous drug abuser.

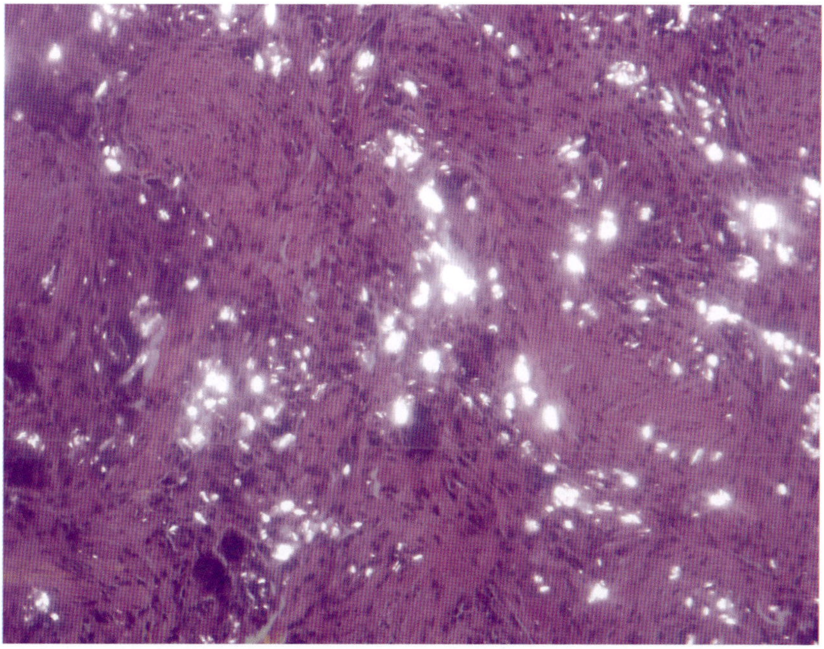

FIGURE 3.24 Intense birefringence is observed under polarized light in the foreign particles in intravenous drug abuse.

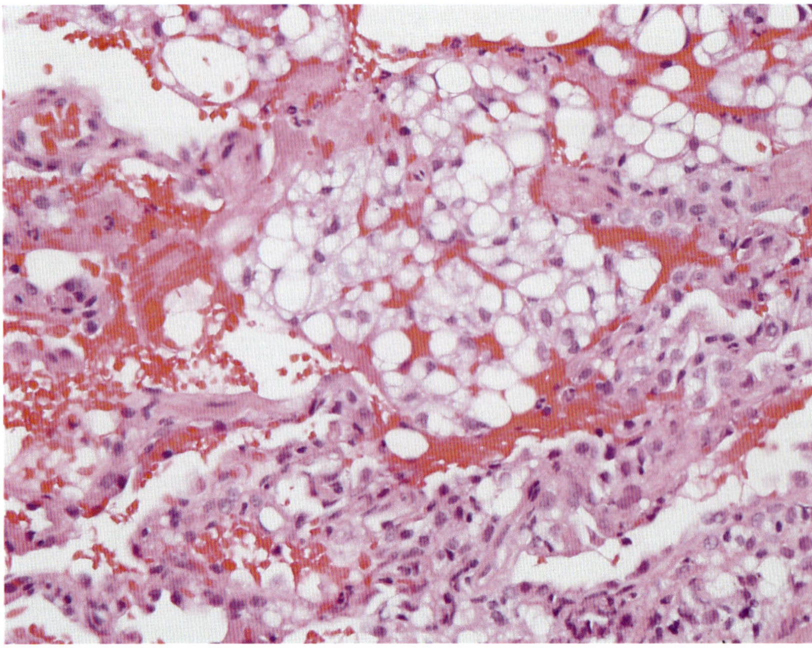

FIGURE 3.25 Transbronchial biopsy showing vacuolated histiocytes filling the alveolar lumens in lipid pneumonia.

LIPID PNEUMONIA. Lipid pneumonia may result from exogenous airway aspiration of mineral oils or by endogenous causes owing to breakdown of cells and release of their lipid constituents. The alveoli in exogenous lipid pneumonia become filled with lipid-rich histiocytes containing abundant vacuolated cytoplasm (Fig. 3.25) (eFig. 3.10). The vacuoles are filled with the engulfed mineral oil particles. Lipid stains, such as oil red-O, can be of help in identifying the lipid content of the vacuoles. With organization of the process, fibroblastic proliferation ensues leading to the formation of a tumor mass (paraffinoma).

REFERENCES

1. Lynch JP III, Kazerooni EA, Gay SE. Pulmonary sarcoidosis. *Clin Chest Med.* 1997; 18:755–785.
2. Hunninghake GW, Costabel U, Ando M, et al. ATS/ERS/WASOG statement on sarcoidosis. American Thoracic Society/European Respiratory Society/Word Association of Sarcoidosis and other Granulomatous Disorders. *Sarcoidosis Vasc Diffuse Lung Dis.* 1999;16:149–173.
3. Gilman MJ, Wang KP. Transbronchial lung biopsy in sarcoidosis. An approach to determine the optimal number of biopsies. *Am Rev Respir Dis.* 1980;122:721–724.
4. Hsu RM, Connors AF Jr, Tomashefski JF Jr. Histologic, microbiologic and clinical correlates of the diagnosis of sarcoidosis by transbronchial biopsy. *Arch Pathol Lab Med.* 1996;120:364–368.

5. Kriebel D, Brain JD, Sprince NL, et al. The pulmonary toxicity of beryllium. *Am Rev Respir Dis.* 1988;137:464–473.
6. Freiman D, Hardy H. Beryllium disease: the relation of pulmonary pathology to clinical course and prognosis based on a study of 130 cases from the U.S. Beryllium Case Registry. *Hum Pathol.* 1970;1:25–44.
7. Newman LS, Kreiss K, King TE Jr, et al. Pathologic and immunologic alterations in early stages of beryllium disease: re-examination of disease definition and natural history. *Am Rev Respir Dis.* 1989;139:1479–1487.
8. Eisenbud M. Origins of the standards for control of beryllium disease (1947–1949). *Environ Res.* 1982;27:79–85.
9. Ingram P, Shelburne JD, Roggli VL, eds. *Microprobe Analysis in Medicine.* New York, NY: Hemisphere; 1989.
10. Kriebel D, Sprince NL, Eisen EA, et al. Beryllium exposure and pulmonary function: a cross-sectional study of beryllium workers. *Br J Ind Med.* 1988;45:167–173.
11. Churg A, Carrington C, Gupta R. Necrotizing sarcoid granulomatosis. *Chest.* 1979; 76:406–413.
12. Koss M, Hochholzer L, Feigin D, et al. Necrotizing sarcoid-like granulomatosis: clinical, pathologic and immunopathologic findings. *Hum Pathol.* 1980;11(S):510–519.
13. Singh H, Cole S, Krause P, et al. Necrotizing sarcoid granulomatosis with extrapulmonary involvement. Clinical, pathologic, ultrastructural and immunologic features. *Am Rev Respir Dis.* 1981;124:189–192.
14. Spiteri M, Gledhill A, Campbell D, et al. Necrotizing sarcoid granulomatosis. *Br J Dis Chest.* 1987;81:70–75.
15. Hoffman G, Kerr G, Leavitt R, et al. Wegener's granulomatosis: an analysis of 158 patients. *Ann Int Med.* 1992;116:488–498.
16. Cotch M, Hoffman G, Yerg D, et al. The epidemiology of Wegener's granulomatosis. Estimates of the five-year period prevalence, annual mortality, and geographic disease distribution from population-based data sources. *Arthritis Rheum.* 1996;39:87–92.
17. Gross W, Csernok E. Immunodiagnostic and pathophysiologic aspects of antineutrophil cytoplasmic antibodies in vasculitis. *Curr Opin Rheumatol.* 1995;7:11–19.
18. Nolle B, Specks U, Ludemann J, et al. Anticytoplasmic autoantibodies: their immunodiagnostic value in Wegener's granulomatosis. *Ann Intern Med.* 1989;111:28–40.
19. Katzenstein A-L, Liebow A, Friedman P. Bronchocentric granulomatosis, mucoid impaction, and hypersensitivity reactions to fungi. *Am Rev Respir Dis.* 1975;111: 497–509.
20. Koss M, Robinson R, Hochholzer L. Bronchocentric granulomatosis. *Hum Pathol.* 1981;12:632–639.
21. Bosken CH, Myers JL, Greenberger PA, et al. Pathologic features of allergic bronchopulmonary aspergillosis. *Am J Surg Pathol.* 1988;12:216–220.
22. Maguire G, Lee M, Rosen Y, et al. Pulmonary tuberculosis and bronchocentric granulomatosis. *Chest.* 1986;89:606–609.
23. Myers J, Katzenstein A-L. Granulomatous infection mimicking bronchocentric granulomatosis. *Am J Surg Pathol.* 1986;10:317–320.
24. Bourke SJ, Dalphin JC, Boyd G, et al. Hypersensitivity pneumonitis: current concepts. *Eur Respir J Suppl.* 2001;32:81s–92s.
25. Patel AM, Ryu JH, Reed CE. Hypersensitivity pneumonitis: current concepts and future questions. *J Allergy Clin Immunol.* 2001;108:661–670.
26. Shigemitsu H, Ashfar K. Aspiration pneumonias: under-diagnosed and under-trated. *Curr Opin Pulm Med.* 2007;13:192–198.
27. Kollef MR, Winn RE. Occult coiled drinking straw aspiration. *Heart Lung.* 1990;19:24–28.

28. Mukhopadhyay S, Katzenstein A-L. Pulmonary disease due to aspiration of food and other particulate matter: a clinicopathologic study of 59 cases diagnosed on biopsy or resection specimens. *Am J Surg Pathol.* 2007;31:752–759.
29. Sprincc NL, Oliver LC, Eisen EA, et al. Cobalt exposure and lung disease in tungsten carbide production: a cross-sectional study of current workers. *Am Rev Respir Dis.* 1988;138:1220–1226.
30. Ohori NP, Sciuba FC, Owens GR, et al. Giant cell interstitial pneumonia and hard-metal pneumoconiosis: a clinicopathologic study of four cases and review of the literature. *Am J Surg Pathol.* 1989;13:581–587.
31. Stettler LE, Groth DH, Platek SF. Automated characterization of particles extracted from human lungs: three cases of tungsten carbide exposure. *Scanning Electron Microsc.* 1983;1:439–448.
32. Deheinzelin D, Capelozzi VL, Kairalla RA, et al. Interstitial lung disease in primary Sjogren's syndrome. Clinical–pathological evaluation and response to treatment. *Am J Respir Crit Care Med.* 1996;154:794–799.
33. Imokawa S, Colby TV, Leslie KO, et al. Methotrexate pneumonitis: review of the literature and histopathological findings in nine patients. *Eur Respir J.* 2000;15:373–381.
34. Black H, Mendoza M, Murin S. Thoracic manifestations of inflammatory bowel disease. *Chest.* 2007;131:524–532.
35. Casey MB, Tazelaar HD, Myers JL, et al. Noninfectious lung pathology in patients with Crohn's disease. *Am J Surg Pathol.* 2003;27:213–219.
36. Nagy F, Molnar T, Makula E, et al. A case of interstitial pneumonitis in a patient with ulcerative colitis treated with azathioprine. *World Gastroenterol.* 2007;13:316–319.
37. Leslie KO, Gruden JF, Parish JM, et al. Transbronchial biopsy interpretation in the patient with diffuse parenchymal lung disease. *Arch Pathol Lab Med.* 2007;131:407–423.

4

LUNG VASCULITIS AND HEMORRHAGIC DISORDERS

The involvement of blood vessels and hemorrhage as the primary pathologic findings can affect the lung parenchyma under many conditions. Vasculitis can be the result of autoimmune-mediated disease or can be secondary to infections and other types of inflammation. Although rare, vasculitic processes in the lung can be the source of major morbidity. A diagnosis of vasculitis has serious implications as it generally requires immediate therapeutic intervention. Clinical correlation and, in many instances, ancillary serologic testing are required for a specific and definitive diagnosis.

For ease and convenience of presentation, lung vasculitis can be categorized into conditions where vasculitis is the main or major manifestation of the disease and those where it is a secondary phenomenon (Table 4.1).

The majority of vasculitic syndromes affecting the lung belong to the category of idiopathic vasculitides. The most common ones affecting the lungs are Wegener granulomatosis (WG) and microscopic polyangiitis (MP). Other idiopathic vasculitides that affect the lung parenchyma more rarely include the Churg–Strauss syndrome (CSS), polyarteritis nodosa, small vessel vasculitis, Takayasu syndrome, Henoch–Schoenlein purpura, Behcet syndrome, cryoglobulinemia, and giant cell arteritis. The diagnosis of these conditions is often fraught with difficulties and relies heavily on a good clinical history and correlation with the radiology and the results of specialized laboratory tests.

WEGENER GRANULOMATOSIS

This condition, formerly classified by Liebow under the category of "pulmonary angiitis and granulomatosis,"[1] primarily represents a vasculitic process with predominant involvement of the lungs and an often prominent granulomatous component. The disease can occur at all extremes of age but is most common in middle-aged adults. The classic presentation of the disease is the triad of upper respiratory tract, lung involvement, and glomerulonephritis. Other organs, including skin, eyes, joints, and nervous system, can also be affected. Less than 20% of patients present

TABLE 4.1 Conditions in Which Pulmonary Vasculitis Is the Principal Manifestation and Those in Which It Represents a Secondary Manifestation of the Disease

Principal Manifestation	Secondary Manifestation
Wegener granulomatosis	Necrotizing sarcoid granulomatosis
Microscopic polyangiitis	Classical sarcoid
Churg–Strauss syndrome	Collagen-vascular disease
Polyarteritis nodosa	Inflammatory bowel disease
Small vessel vasculitis (capillaritis)	Malignancy
Takayasu syndrome	Pulmonary infection
Henoch–Schoenlein purpura	Bronchocentric granulomatosis
Behcet syndrome	Sequestration
Cryoglobulinemia	Drug or toxic substances
Giant cell arteritis	Transplantation
	Radiation
	Malignant lymphoma

initially with renal disease but at least 75% eventually develop a focal segmental necrotizing glomerulonephritis. However, the disease can be limited to the lungs (i.e., limited or localized form of WG); such patients are usually associated with a better prognosis.[2,3] The main clinical symptoms of WG include cough, chest pain, hemoptysis, nasal ulceration, sinus pain, fever, malaise, and weight loss. Other symptoms include hematuria, renal failure, otitis, arthralgia, myalgia, neurologic abnormalities, and skin lesions. It is interesting to note that some patients may be relatively asymptomatic despite having numerous necrotic nodules involving the lungs. As indicated previously, the most diagnostic laboratory abnormality is the presence of antineutrophil cytoplasmic antibodies (ANCA) in serum.[4,5] ANCA are autoantibodies to components of neutrophil and monocyte granules that can be detected by indirect immunofluorescence or by enzyme-linked immunoabsorbent assay techniques. Of the two immunofluorescent patterns observed (cytoplasmic ANCA or C-ANCA and perinuclear ANCA or P-ANCA), the one characterized by diffuse cytoplasmic immunofluorescence staining (C-ANCA) appears to be highly specific for WG and can be found in more than 90% of systemic cases and in about 60% of localized cases. False-positive results, however, can also be observed under various circumstances. Lung biopsies are usually indicated for definitive diagnosis.

The granulomatous features of WG have been explained in detail in the chapter 3 on "Lung granulomas." In this chapter, we will detail the vascular changes that characterize the disease. The vascular changes in WG can be of various types, including small vessel vasculitis (capillaritis), acute necrotizing vasculitis affecting small arteries and veins, and granulomatous vasculitis. *Capillaritis* is a distinctive feature of WG and normally involves alveolar septal capillaries and venules. It is frequently present within the parenchyma surrounding areas of necrosis. Transbronchial lung biopsy can be highly useful in identifying capillaritis in WG. The process is characterized by acute neutrophilic inflammation that expands and destroys alveolar septa (Figs. 4.1 and 4.2) (eFigs. 4.1 and 4.2). When extensive destruction of alveolar walls ensues, the capillaritis can only be inferred from the alveolar septal distribution of the acute inflammation (Fig. 4.3) (eFig. 4.3). A histologic variant of WG is characterized by the absence of granulomas and necrosis and by prominent alveolar hemorrhage and capillaritis. Clinically such patients usually present with hemoptysis and diffuse pulmonary infiltrates and follow a fulminant clinical course. The biopsy shows extensive intra-alveolar hemorrhage and capillaritis characterized by focal expansion of alveolar septa by neutrophils admixed with nuclear debris. The involved vessel walls may show features of fibrinoid necrosis. *Necrotizing vasculitis* is a constant feature of most cases of WG characterized by infiltration and destruction of vessel walls by a neutrophilic infiltrate, sometimes accompanied by fibrinoid necrosis (Fig. 4.4). The vasculitis can be seen involving only a

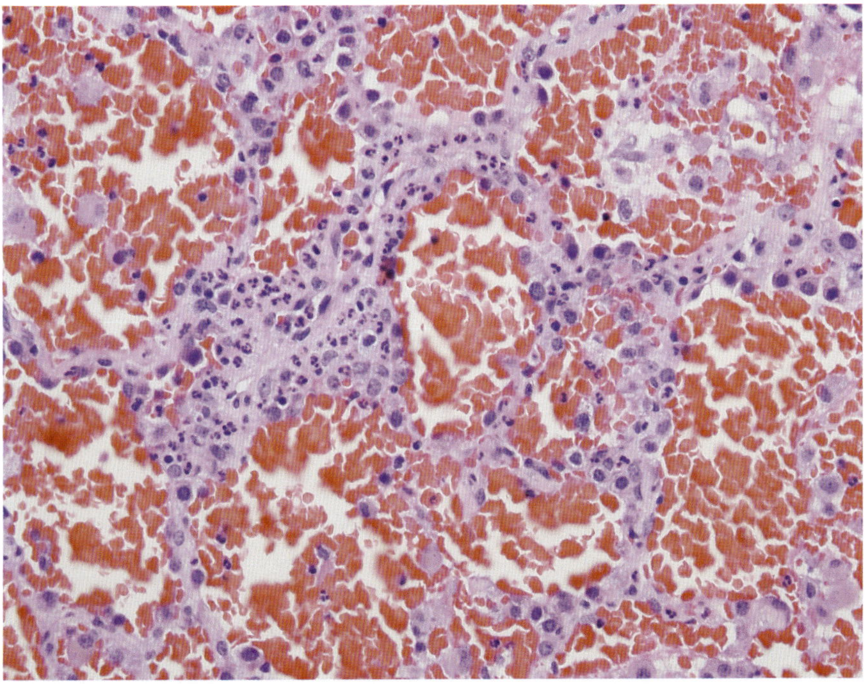

FIGURE 4.1 Capillaritis in WG characterized by acute neutrophilic infiltration that expands the alveolar septa.

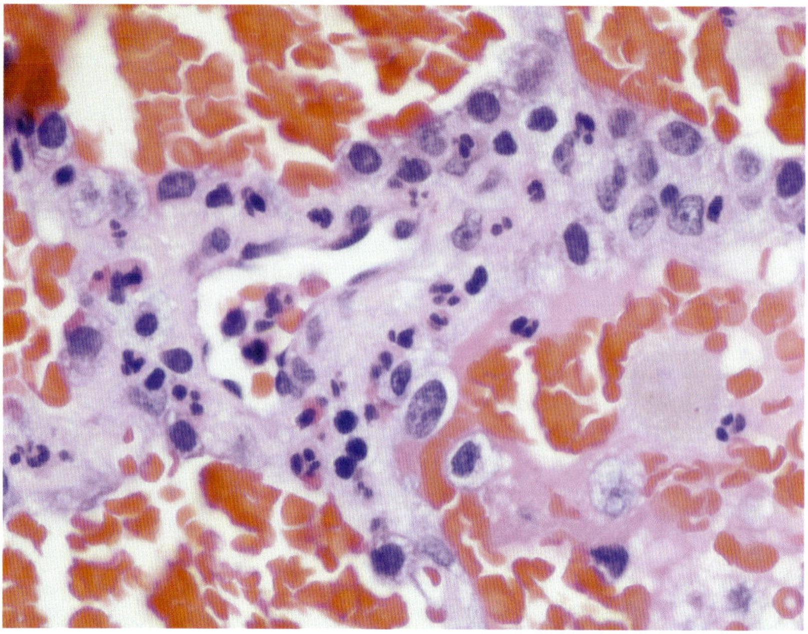

FIGURE 4.2 Higher magnification of capillaritis in WG. Notice the expansion of the alveolar septa by abundant neutrophils admixed with nuclear debris and fibrinous exudate.

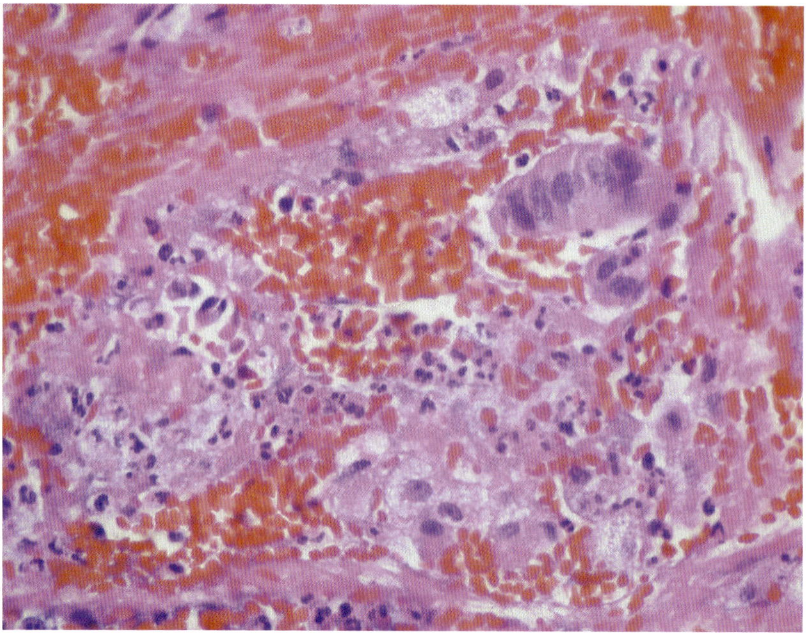

FIGURE 4.3 Necrotizing capillaritis in WG. The process has already destroyed the alveolar septa and only their outline can be discerned by tracing the neutrophils.

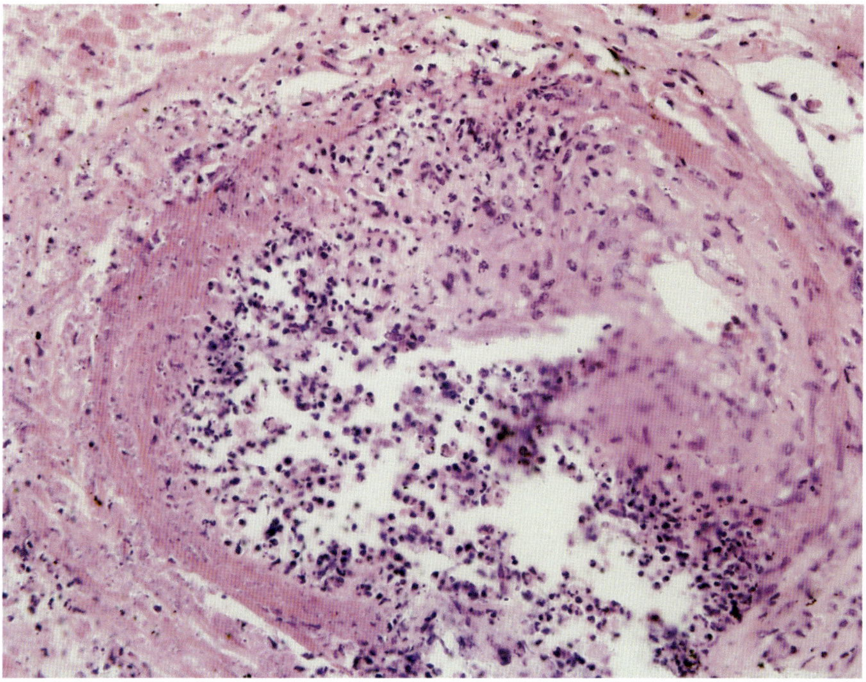

FIGURE 4.4 Necrotizing vasculitis in WG shows destruction of vessel walls by neutrophilic infiltrate admixed with fibrinoid exudates.

portion of the vessel wall leading to an "eccentric" or partial distribution. Circumferential and transmural involvement by acute and chronic inflammatory infiltrate, accompanied by necrosis and destruction of the vessel wall, however, is the more common manifestation. Elastic tissue stains will help to demonstrate the destruction of the internal elastic lamina (Fig. 4.5). The necrotizing vasculitis may lead to complete destruction of the vessel walls (Fig. 4.6). *Granulomatous vasculitis* was covered in detail in the chapter 3 on granulomatous pneumonitis and is characterized by necrotizing granulomas and multinucleated giant cells involving the adventitia and media of small and middle-sized vessels (Fig. 4.7) (eFigs. 4.4 to 4.6).

The histologic features of WG can be quite distinctive in fully developed lesions that are sampled on open lung or VATS biopsies but may be more difficult to appreciate on endoscopic biopsies. A descriptive diagnosis should be rendered by the pathologist under such circumstances. In some instances, when both the clinical and histopathologic findings are highly consistent with WG, the diagnosis can be made even in the absence of C-ANCA positivity.[6] A definitive diagnosis, however, should be rendered only after a strict correlation is done of the histopathologic findings with the clinical picture and serologic studies for C-ANCA.

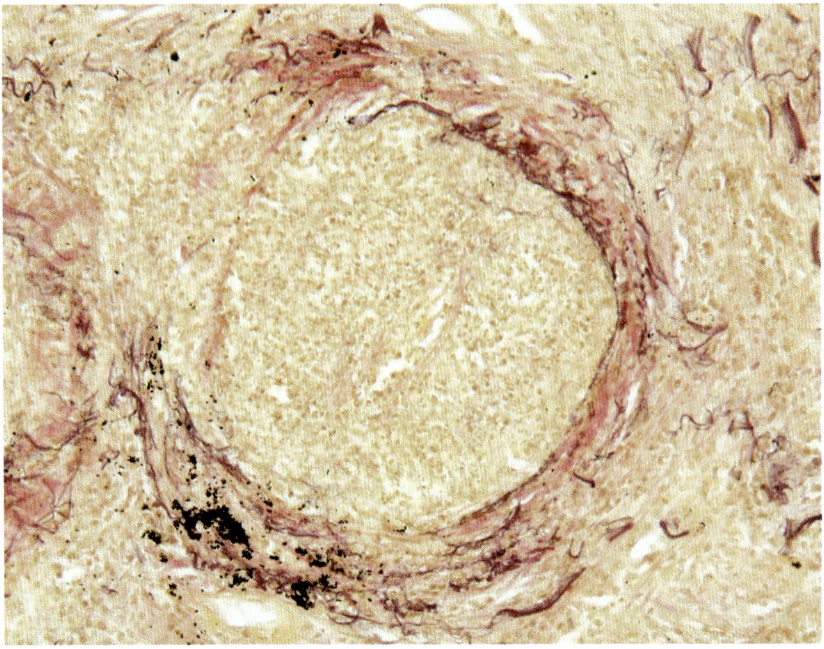

FIGURE 4.5 Elastic Van Gieson stain in Wegener vasculitis shows almost complete destruction of internal elastic lamina.

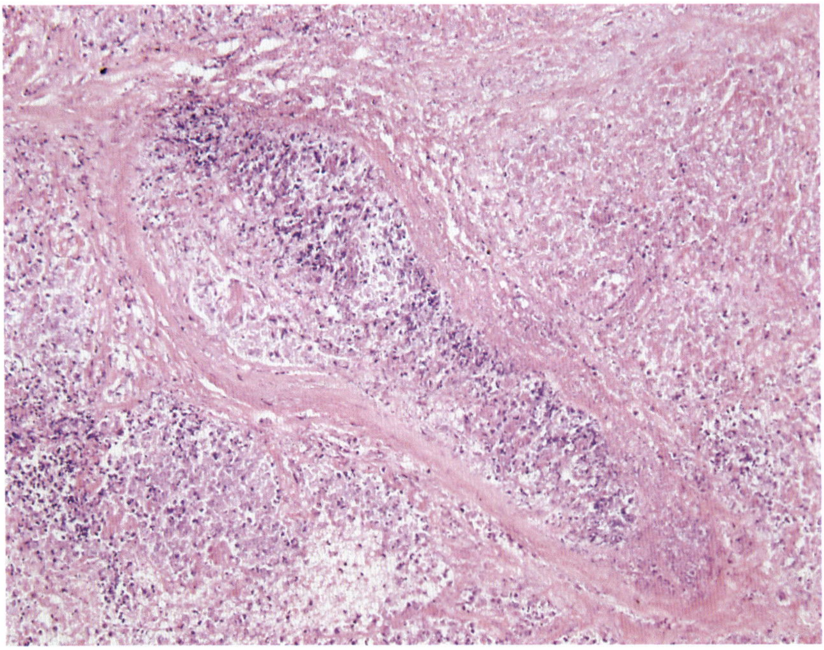

FIGURE 4.6 Necrotizing vasculitis in WG showing complete destruction of vessel wall with extensive fibrinoid necrosis.

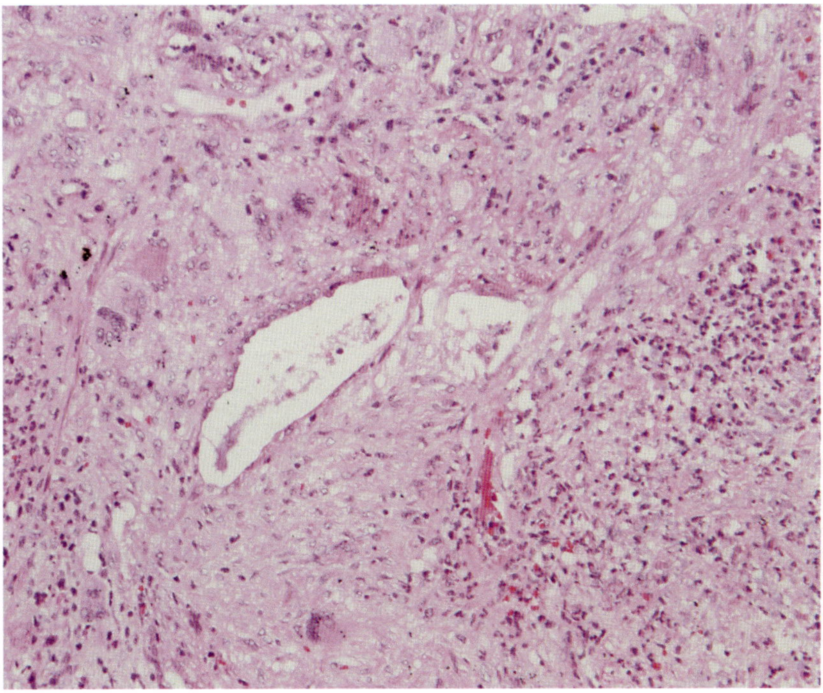

FIGURE 4.7 Granulomatous vasculitis in WG shows necrotizing granulomas and multinucleated giant cells involving the adventitia and the media of a mid-sized artery.

MICROSCOPIC POLYANGIITIS

MP is a term that encompasses conditions that were termed in the past as leukocytoclastic vasculitis, systemic necrotizing vasculitis, and hypersensitivity vasculitis.[7] A recent International Consensus Conference has defined MP as a vasculitis restricted to arterioles, venules, and capillaries.[8] MP is a systemic disease that involves the lungs in approximately 50% of cases. Other symptoms include necrotizing glomerulonephritis, fever, myalgia, arthralgia, otitis, rhinitis, and skin involvement.[9] More than 80% of patients have positive ANCA, especially P-ANCA.[9] The typical presentation of the disease is with pulmonary hemorrhage. Bilateral lung infiltrates are present in chest X-rays, and CT scans will usually demonstrate ground-glass attenuation, involving in particular the lower zones of the lungs. The treatment of choice is immunosuppressive agents, although supportive treatment with steroids, plasmapheresis, dialysis, and mechanical ventilation may also be needed.[10] The disease has a high-mortality rate, although complete recovery was observed in up to 69% of patients in one study.[10]

The principal histologic manifestation of MP is alveolar hemorrhage with capillaritis (Fig. 4.8). The capillaritis may appear on cursory examination as

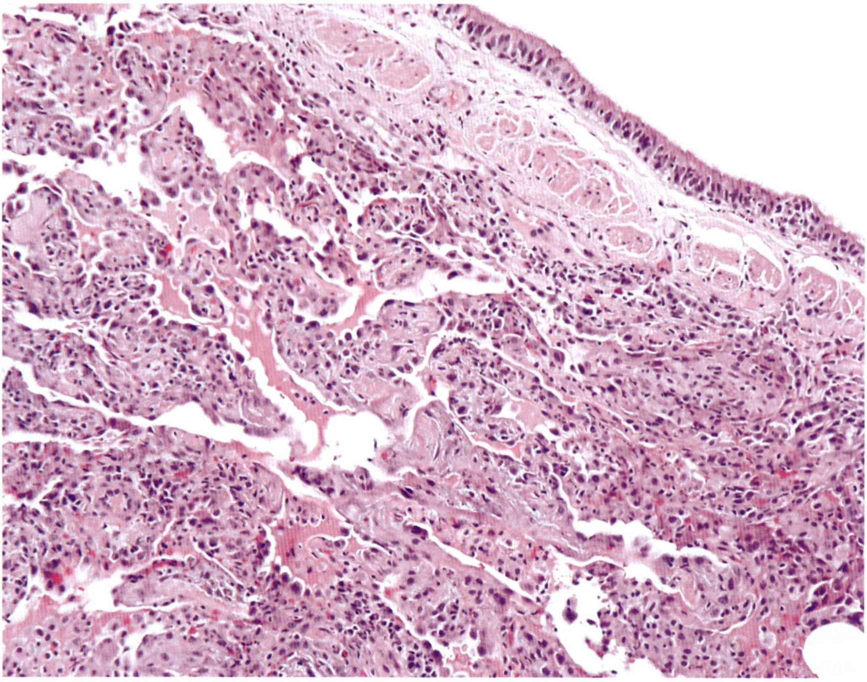

FIGURE 4.8 Transbronchial biopsy in patient with MP showing widening of alveolar septa by cellular infiltrate.

foci of increased alveolar wall cellularity against a background of alveolar hemorrhage, but on higher magnification the alveolar walls will show neutrophilic infiltration, which sometimes spills out onto the alveolar lumens simulating acute bronchopneumonia (Fig. 4.9). The intra-alveolar hemorrhage is often admixed with fibrin and hemosiderin-laden macrophages. In the healing phase, the alveolar hemorrhage can become organized resulting in a bronchiolitis obliterans with organizing pneumonia- or BOOP-like pattern.

The differential diagnosis includes infections, WG, Goodpasture syndrome, and other small vessel vasculitides (eFig. 4.7). The histologic variant of WG characterized by alveolar hemorrhage and capillaritis in the absence of granulomas and necrosis may be impossible to distinguish from MP on histologic grounds.

CHURG–STRAUSS SYNDROME

CSS is a condition of unknown etiology that affects mainly the respiratory tract and is characterized by the association of vasculitis with eosinophilia. The classical triad in CSS is asthma, peripheral blood eosinophilia, and vasculitis.[11,12] Other manifestations include neuropathy, sinus abnormalities, pulmonary infiltrates, arthritis, arthralgias, serositis, skin manifestations

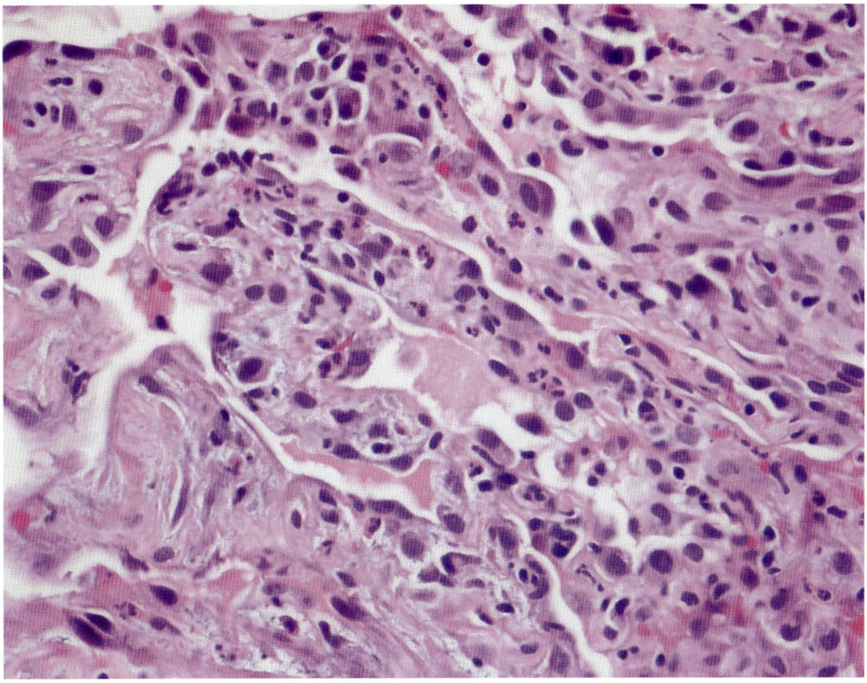

FIGURE 4.9 Higher magnification of capillaritis in patient with MP. Notice the neutrophilic infiltration of alveolar walls.

(urticaria), central nervous system abnormalities, gastrointestinal bleeding, and renal failure.[13] CSS is currently regarded as a clinical syndrome that requires meeting certain criteria for diagnosis as established by the American College of Rheumatology.[14] The diagnosis is no longer predicated on the results of lung biopsy but on the fulfillment of the clinical criteria. The traditional approach is based on the identification of six main criteria, including asthma, greater than 10% eosinophilia in peripheral blood, mono- or polyneuropathy, nonfixed radiographic pulmonary infiltrates, paranasal sinus abnormalities, and a biopsy containing a blood vessel with extravascular eosinophils. A fairly specific diagnosis can generally be established when four of the six criteria are met.[14] An alternate method for reaching the diagnosis involves identifying three major criteria: asthma, eosinophilia greater than 10%, and a history of allergy, although patients without asthma but with history of allergic disease can also develop CSS. The latter method is more sensitive but les specific.[14]

The process can affect patients at any age but shows a predilection for adults between 30 and 50 years of age. CSS can involve the upper respiratory tract, lungs, skin, peripheral nerves, heart, and kidneys. The disease generally progresses through three stages: the prodromal phase is characterized by asthma, rhinitis, and peripheral eosinophilia. The asthma may be present over a period of years before the onset of vasculitis.[11,15,16]

This is followed by the vasculitic phase during which the patients develop signs and symptoms of vasculitis and will test positive for P-ANCA. The damage sustained during this phase is usually permanent. Approximately half of the patients with CSS develop cardiac disease, including pericarditis, hypertension, acute myocardial infarction, and heart failure.[11,17] Other common manifestations include peripheral neuritis, cutaneous leukocytoclastic vasculitis, and sinonasal compromise. Renal, gastrointestinal, and central nervous system manifestations owing to vasculitis may also occur but are rarer. The final phase, or postvasculitic phase, is characterized by persistent asthma and allergic rhinitis as well as neuropathy and hypertension.[13] There are no specific laboratory tests for CSS. The most characteristic finding is peripheral blood eosinophilia. Bronchoalveolar lavage will also demonstrate increased eosinophilia. The radiographic abnormalities include multifocal lung infiltrates that are nonfixed (i.e., they change in location and distribution over time). High-resolution computerized tomography scans will usually show parenchymal opacifications or ground-glass attenuation. The treatment of choice consists of systemic corticosteroids. Immunosuppressive agents, interferon, and high doses of immune globulin have also been used in patients with severe or fulminant symptoms. Patient most often die of cardiac complications, including congestive heart failure and acute myocardial infarct.

The pathologic findings of CSS on lung biopsy in patients with the full-blown syndrome include vasculitis, eosinophilic pneumonia, and granulomas. The lesion may extend along the pleura and interlobular septa. The most consistent finding is eosinophilic pneumonia, characterized by accumulation of eosinophils in the airspaces as well as within the interstitium. The vasculitis can affect arteries, veins, or capillaries and is comprised mainly of neutrophils admixed with eosinophils, small lymphocytes and, sometimes, multinucleated giant cells (Figs. 4.10 and 4.11) (eFig. 4.8). Vasculitis can also manifest as capillaritis with diffuse pulmonary hemorrhage.[18] The granulomas in CSS are usually small, with central fibrinoid necrosis and peripheral palisading of histiocytes. They can contain multinucleated giant cells.

UNCOMMON FORMS OF LUNG VASCULITIS

Various uncommon forms of vasculitis, including giant cell (temporal) arteritis, polyarteritis nodosa, Takayasu arteritis (TA), Bechet syndrome, Henoch–Schonlein purpura, and the vasculitis associated with necrotizing sarcoid granulomatosis, may affect the lung.

Giant Cell (Temporal) Arteritis

Temporal arteritis is a disorder that involves primarily the temporal arteries in older adults. The disease is associated with upper respiratory tract symptoms and lower respiratory tract involvement only in a minority of

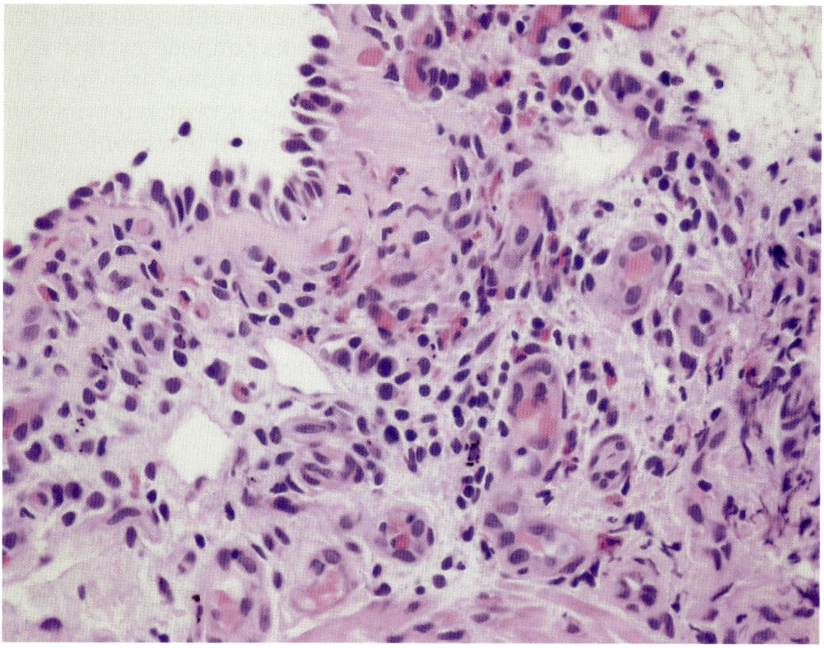

FIGURE 4.10 Endobronchial biopsy in patient with CSS shows dense lymphoid infiltrates admixed with eosinophils surrounding the vessel walls in the submucosa.

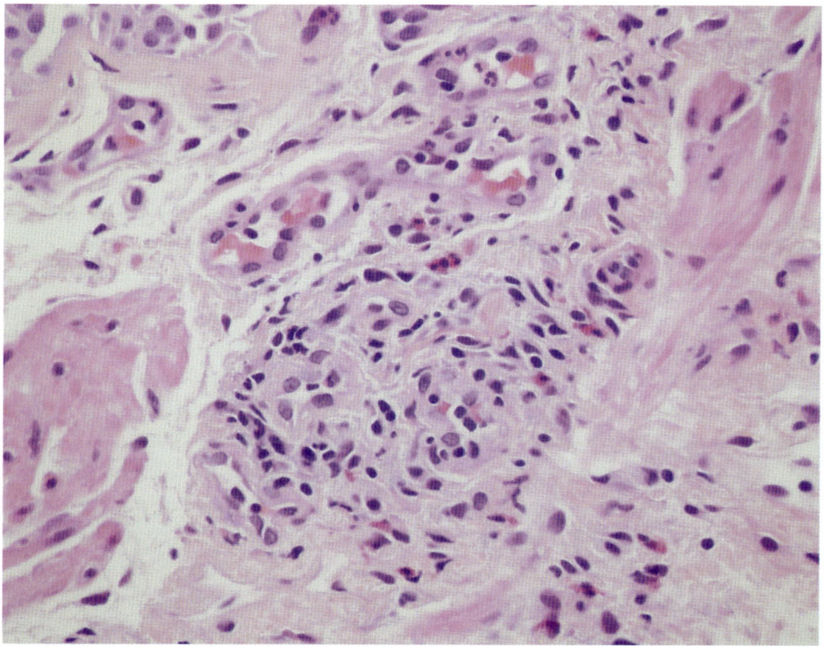

FIGURE 4.11 Higher magnification of vasculitis in CSS shows infiltration of vessel walls by neutrophils admixed with eosinophils.

cases.[19] Pulmonary involvement is usually bilateral resulting in interstitial opacities or small nodules.[20,21] Giant cell arteritis confined exclusively to the lungs has also been described.[22] The disease involves principally the large and medium pulmonary arteries. The damage is centered principally in the elastic lamina of the vessel, which is destroyed by chronic inflammation admixed with multinucleated giant cells. On bronchoscopic biopsies, the main finding is the destruction of the media of pulmonary arteries by granulomatous inflammation with fragmented elastic fibers.[23] Unlike other types of granulomatous vasculitis, such as WG, giant cell temporal arteritis is distinguished by the lesions being confined to the vessel wall without involvement of the surrounding lung parenchyma. Temporal arteritis is distinguished from WG by the younger age of the patients and by the involvement of temporal arteries. TA is a vasculitis that principally affects the aorta in women under the age of 40.[24] Pulmonary arteries are commonly involved and may rarely be the initial manifestation of the disease. The vessels show transmural infiltration of their walls by lymphocytes, histiocytes, and giant cells. Owing to the multisystem compromise and primary involvement of large caliber arteries such as the aorta and pulmonary artery, the diagnosis is generally established by angiography in the correct clinical setting.

Behcet Syndrome

Behcet syndrome is a systemic inflammatory disorder of unknown etiology that involves the skin, eyes (uveitis), mouth, and genitalia (aphtous ulcers). The disease has a marked geographic distribution and predominantly affects young or middle-aged individuals of Middle Eastern, Japanese, and Mediterranean origin.[25,26] The most common clinical feature of the disease is recurrent and painful oral or genital ulcers. Symptoms of pulmonary involvement include cough, chest pain, dyspnea, and hemoptysis.[26,27] The lesions are characterized by a necrotizing vasculitis that involves arteries, veins, and capillaries (Fig. 4.12). The inflammatory infiltrate involving the vessel walls in Behcet syndrome comprises small lymphocytes. Resolving lesions may show recanalized thrombi and perivascular adventitial fibrosis. Hemorrhage with severe hemoptysis may result as a complication of the necrotizing vasculitis. Other secondary complications resulting from the vasculitis include pulmonary artery aneurysms, arterial and venous thrombosis, and pulmonary infarcts.[28,29] The diagnosis is made by fulfilling the clinical requirements, including oral aphtous ulcers occurring more than three times in 1 year and at least two of the following clinical manifestations: recurrent genital aphtous ulcers, uveitis, synovitis, cutaneous vasculitis, and meningoencephalitis. In addition, there should be absence of inflammatory bowel disease or other collagen-vascular disorder. Circulating immune complexes have been demonstrated in patients with active pulmonary disease, suggesting that they may play a role in the pathogenesis of the process.[27,30]

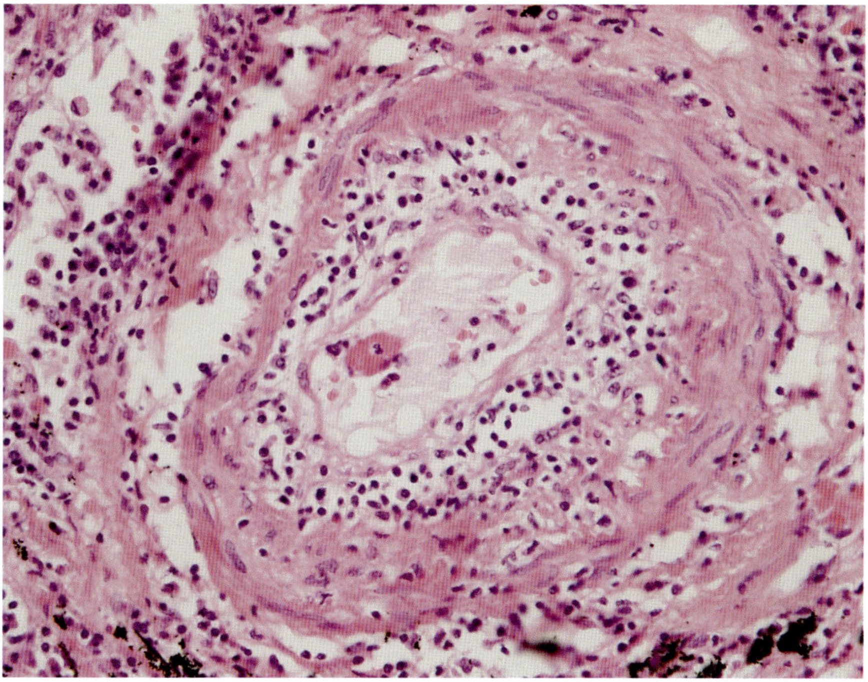

FIGURE 4.12 Necrotizing vasculitis in Behcet disease. The lesions are characterized by infiltration of small vessel walls by small lymphocytes.

Henoch–Schonlein Purpura

Henoch–Schonlein purpura is a rare form of pulmonary hemorrhagic vasculitis that most often affects children. Pulmonary manifestations are quite rare and the disease most often affects the skin, kidneys, and joints. The pathologic findings in the lung are characterized by intra-alveolar hemorrhage and neutrophilic capillaritis (Fig. 4.13). The capillaritis may be subtle and masked by the capillary congestion (Fig. 4.14) (eFig. 4.9). The findings are nonspecific and must be correlated with the clinical history and laboratory studies.

Necrotizing Sarcoid Granulomatosis

Systemic vasculitis is seldom observed in patients with sarcoidosis. The pathologic findings comprise sarcoid-like granulomas involving pulmonary vessels, sometimes showing foci of necrosis. The granulomatous necrotizing vasculitis may be systemic and also involve the skin, lymph nodes, bone, synovium, liver, trachea, and bone marrow.[31] In rare instances, classical sarcoid may also show a nonnecrotizing granulomatous vasculitis as an incidental finding in lung biopsies. The lesions will display typical nonnecrotizing epithelioid granulomas with giant cells involving the walls of blood vessels.[32]

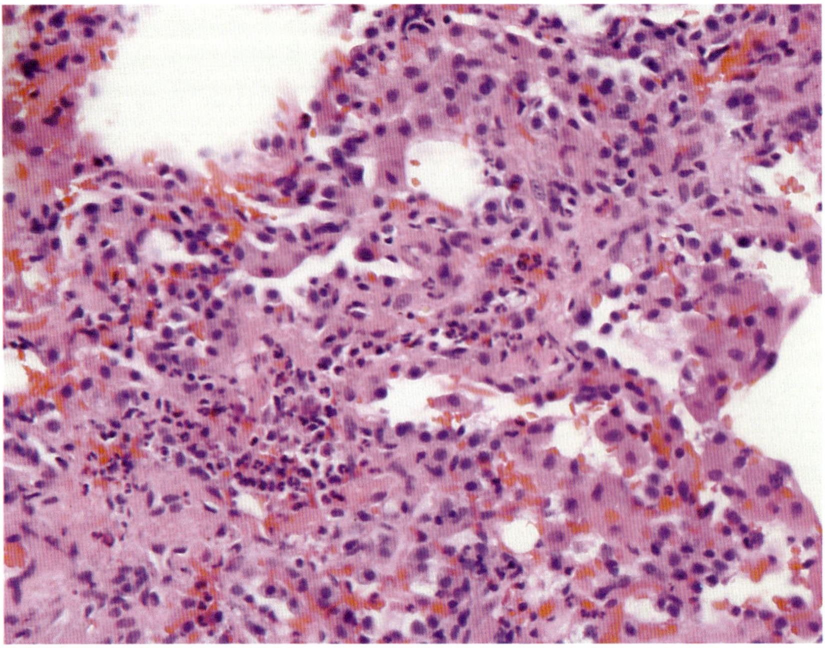

FIGURE 4.13 Intra-alveolar hemorrhage and capillaritis in patient with Henoch–Schonlein purpura. Notice thickening of alveolar septa by cellular infiltrate.

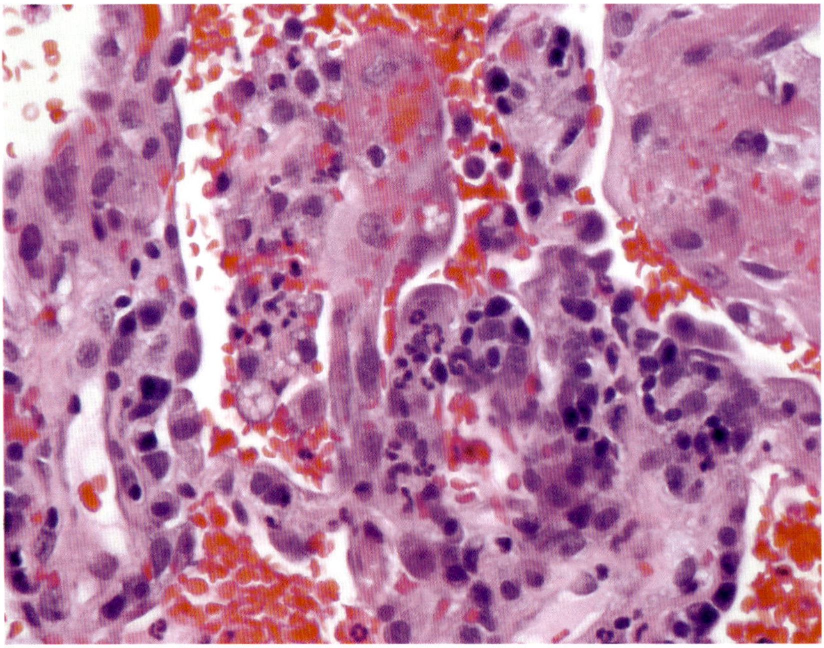

FIGURE 4.14 Higher magnification of capillaritis in Henoch–Schonlein purpura shows congestion of alveolar wall capillaries admixed with neutrophilic infiltrates.

PULMONARY HEMORRHAGE

Pulmonary hemorrhage can be caused by various mechanisms. The main clinical symptom is hemoptysis, followed by cough, fever, and dyspnea. The cause could be a localized event, such as thromboembolus, hemorrhage secondary to bleeding from tumor, abscess, or bronchiectasis; otherwise it may be diffuse, such as in Goodpasture syndrome, vasculitis, and collagen-vascular disease (eFig. 4.10). The former presents clinically and radiologically as a localized airspace infiltrate. Bronchoscopy in such instances can localize the source of the bleeding and determine the underlying cause. The latter is characterized clinically by diffuse and often bilateral airspace infiltrates on chest X-ray and computerized tomography scans. Hemoptysis may be absent at the time of initial presentation in one-third of the patients with pulmonary hemorrhage. The radiologic features of diffuse alveolar hemorrhage comprise patchy or diffuse bilateral areas of lung consolidation, particularly in the lower lobes and perihilar regions.

Transbronchial biopsy is, in general, of very limited value in confirming a specific diagnosis. It may serve to confirm only the clinical impression of intra-alveolar hemorrhage or help to rule out other conditions. The histopathologic evaluation of intra-alveolar hemorrhage should take into consideration the clinical context for adequate interpretation.[33] Some degree of extravasation of red blood cells can be observed in routine lung biopsies as a result of trauma caused by the biopsy procedure itself. The presence of fresh blood in the lumen of the alveoli per se is not an indication that the patient is suffering from clinically significant intra-alveolar hemorrhage. In such instances, the presence of red blood cells in the absence of fibrin, hemosiderin-laden macrophages, or reactive changes in the surrounding alveolar walls should suggest the possibility of artefactual hemorrhage rather than pathologic hemorrhage. When hemorrhage is accompanied by fibrin deposition, coarse granules of hemosiderin within macrophages, and the correlation with the radiologic images demonstrate a diffuse alveolar infiltrate, the process corresponds to one of the diffuse alveolar hemorrhage syndromes (Figs. 4.15 and 4.16). Intra-alveolar hemorrhage should also be distinguished on small endoscopic biopsies from hemosiderin-laden macrophages seen in smoker's lungs. In the latter, the macrophages filling the alveolar lumens and within the bronchioles contain very fine, dusty hemosiderin pigment, as opposed to the darkly staining, heavily pigmented macrophages seen in hemorrhagic syndromes, in which the hemosiderin granules are more coarse and abundant. The causes of diffuse alveolar hemorrhage are listed in Table 4.2.

A specific diagnosis of diffuse alveolar hemorrhage cannot be rendered in the absence of adequate clinical and laboratory data. Most causes of diffuse alveolar hemorrhage are immunologically mediated.[34] Some of these conditions display specific patterns of immunoglobulin deposition that can be demonstrated by immunofluorescence on adequately prepared tissue sections from the lung biopsy. Coordination between the clinician

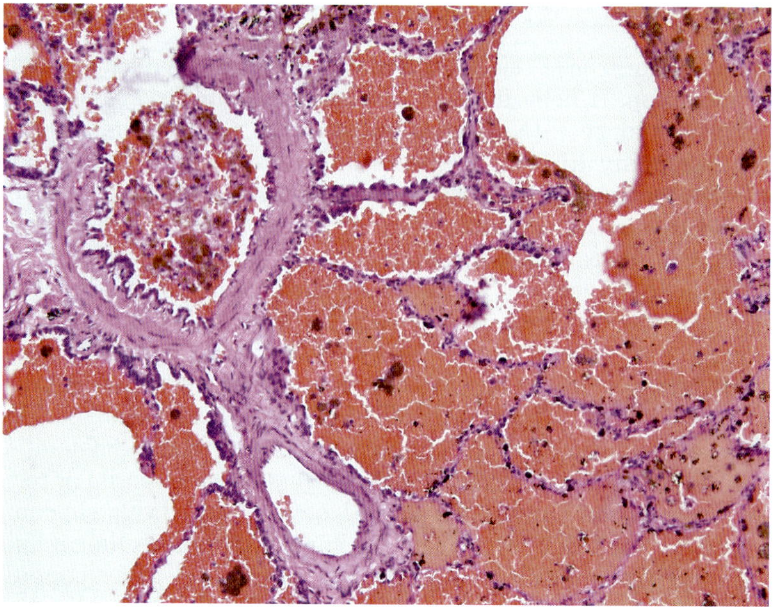

FIGURE 4.15 Diffuse alveolar hemorrhage in a patient with Goodpasture syndrome. The diagnosis cannot be rendered based on the biopsy findings alone. Correlation with clinical and laboratory findings and immunofluorescence studies are necessary for arriving at a definitive diagnosis.

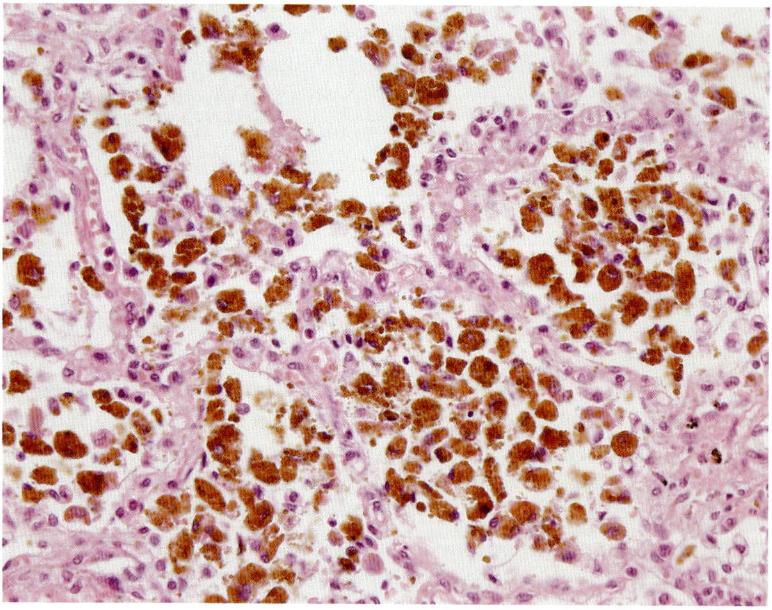

FIGURE 4.16 Alveolar hemorrhage in idiopathic pulmonary hemosiderosis. Notice the abundance of hemosiderin-laden macrophages admixed with the red blood cells, characteristic of this disorder.

TABLE 4.2 Causes of Diffuse Alveolar Hemorrhage

Immunologic Conditions	Infectious Diseases
– Wegener granulomatosis – Churg–Strauss syndrome – Systemic lupus erythematosus – Microscopic polyangiitis – Goodpasture syndrome – Henoch–Schonlein purpura – Connective tissue diseases	– Bacterial (lung abscess, tuberculosis, bacterial pneumonia, etc.) – Viral – Fungal – Parasites (paragonimus Westermani, leptospirosis)
Drugs and Toxins	**Neoplasia**
– Anticoagulants – Streptokinase – Cocaine – Solvents – Amiodarone	– Lung cancer – Carcinoid tumor – Kaposi sarcoma/angiosarcoma – Metastasis to the lung/bronchus
Bleeding Disorders	**Cardiac Causes**
– Coagulopathies – Thrombocytopenia	– Pulmonary thromboembolism – Left ventricular failure – Mitral stenosis – Aneurysms
Trauma	**Other Causes**
– Ruptured bronchus (bronchoscopy, Swan Ganz catheter, lung biopsy, Hickman catheter) – Lung contusion – Aortic tear, others	– Idiopathic pulmonary hemosiderosis – Aspiration of foreign body – Intralobar sequestration – Endometriosis – Broncholithiasis – Lymphangioleiomyomatosis

and the pathologist before the biopsy is carried out is therefore critical to obtain adequately processed samples for immunofluorescence microscopy if a hemorrhagic pulmonary disorder is suspected clinically. A more convenient substitute for immunofluorescent studies currently is the use of serologic tests that are widely available and reasonably specific for the various subtypes of diffuse alveolar hemorrhage.

TABLE 4.3 Causes of Diffuse Alveolar Hemorrhage Associated or Not Associated with Capillaritis

Alveolar Hemorrhage with Capillaritis	Alveolar Hemorrhage without Capillaritis
Wegener granulomatosis	Idiopathic pulmonary hemosiderosis
Microscopic polyangiitis	Systemic lupus erythematosus
Goodpasture syndrome	Goodpasture syndrome
Henoch–Schoenlein purpura	Diffuse alveolar damage
Mixed cryoglobulinemia	Coagulation disorders
Behcet syndrome	Pulmonary veno-occlusive disease
Connective tissue diseases	Mitral stenosis
Drug-induced	Neoplasms

Diffuse alveolar hemorrhage can present histologically in association with capillaritis or may not show evidence of capillaritis. This particular histologic finding is of importance because specific entities are associated with capillaritis while others are not (Table 4.3).

Correlation of the pathologic findings with clinical and laboratory findings is of importance for arriving at a more specific diagnosis (Table 4.4), as the histopathologic findings are generally nonspecific in the majority of cases of diffuse alveolar hemorrhage.

TABLE 4.4 Clinical and Pathologic Findings in Main Causes of Diffuse Alveolar Hemorrhage

Condition	Pathologic Findings	Laboratory Findings	Clinical Findings
Goodpasture syndrome	Nonspecific, can be associated with mild capillaritis and hyaline membranes	Antiglomerular basement membrane antibody +	Young male smokers Also involves kidneys
Wegener granulomatosis	Diffuse alveolar hemorrhage with prominent capillaritis with eosinophilia	C-ANCA +	Multiorgan involvement, including kidneys, nasal passage and others

TABLE 4.4 *(Continued)*

Condition	Pathologic Findings	Laboratory Findings	Clinical Findings
Idiopathic pulmonary hemosiderosis	Alveolar hemorrhage unassociated with capillaritis, with abundant hemosiderin-laden macrophages	No immunologic mechanism identified	Children with recurrent bouts of hemorptysis and anemia
Microscopic polyangiitis	Diffuse alveolar hemorrhage with prominent capillaritis	P-ANCA +	Frequent multiorgan involvement
Systemic lupus erythematosus	Diffuse alveolar hemorrhage with prominent capillaritis	Antinuclear antibodies +	Shows all the typical features of the disease. Patients with lupus nephritis are at increased risk for developing alveolar hemorrhage

REFERENCES

1. Liebow AA. The J. Burns Amberson lecture: pulmonary angiitis and granulomatosis. *Am Rev Respir Dis*. 1973;108:1–18.
2. Katzenstein AL, Locke WK. Solitary lung lesions in Wegener's granulomatosis. Pathologic findings and clinical significance in 25 cases. *Am J Surg Pathol*. 1995;19:545–552.
3. Carrington C, Liebow A. Limited forms of angiitis and granulomatosis of Wegener's type. *Am J Med*. 1966;41:497–527.
4. Gal AA, Salinas FF, Staton GW Jr. The clinical and pathological spectrum of antineutrophil cytoplasmic autoantibody-related pulmonary disease. A comparison between perinuclear and cytoplasmic antineutrophil cytoplasmic autoantibodies. *Arch Pathol Lab Med*. 1994;118:1209–1214.
5. Rao JK, Weinberger M, Oddone EZ, et al. The role of antineutrophil cytoplasmic antibody (c-ANCA) testing in the diagnosis of Wegener granulomatosis. A literature review and meta-analysis. *Ann Intern Med*. 1995;123:925–932.
6. Jennings CR, Jones NS, Dugar J, et al. Wegener's granulomatosis—a review of diagnosis and treatment in 53 subjects. *Rhinology*. 1998;36:188–191.

7. Churg J. Nomenclature of vasculitic syndromes: a historical perspective. *Am J Kidney Dis*. 1991;18:148–153.
8. Jennette JC, Falk RJ, Andrassy K, et al. Nomenclature of systemic vasculitides. Proposal of an international consensus conference. *Arthritis Rheum*. 1994;37:187–192.
9. Jennette JC, Falk RJ. Small-vessel vasculitis. *N Engl J Med*. 1997;337:1512–1523.
10. Lauque D, Cadranel J, Lazor R, et al. Microscopic polyangiitis with alveolar hemorrhage. A study of 29 cases and review of the literature. *Medicine (Baltimore)*. 2000;79:222–233.
11. Lanham JG, Elkon KB, Pusey CD, et al. Systemic vasculitis with asthma and eosinophilia: a clinical approach to the Churg–Strauss syndrome. *Medicine (Baltimore)*. 1984;63:65–81.
12. Guillevin L, Cohen P, Gayraud M, et al. Churg-Strauss syndrome. Clinical study and long-term follow-up of 96 patients. *Medicine (Baltimore)*. 1999;78:26–37.
13. Lanham JG, Churg J. Churg–Strauss syndrome. In: Churg A, Churg J, eds. *Systemic Vasculitides*. New York, NY: Igaku-Shoin; 1991:101–120.
14. Masi A, Hunder GG, Lie JT, et al. The American College of Rheumatology 1990 criteria for the classification of Churg–Strauss syndrome (allergic granulomatosis and angiitis). *Arthritis Rheum*. 1990;33:1094–1100.
15. Chumbley LC, Harrison EG Jr, DeRemee R. Allergic granulomatosis and angiitis (Churg–Strauss syndrome). Report and analysis of 30 cases. *Mayo Clin Proc*. 1977;52:477–484.
16. Specks U, DeRemee RA. Granulomatous vasculitis. Wegener's granulomatosis and Churg–Strauss syndrome. *Rheum Dis Clin North Am*. 1990;16:377–397.
17. Churg J, Strauss L. Allergic granulomatosis, allergic angiitis, and periarteritis nodosa. *Am J Pathol*. 1951;27:277–301.
18. Lai RS, Lin SL, Lai NS, et al. Churg–Strauss syndrome presenting with pulmonary capillaritis and diffuse alveolar damage. *Scand J Rheumatol*. 1998;27:230–232.
19. Larson TS, Hall S, Hepper NG, et al. Respiratory tract symptoms as a clue to giant cell arteritis. *Ann Intern Med*. 1984;101:594–597.
20. Bradley JD, Pinals RS, Blumenfeld HB, et al. Giant cell arteritis with pulmonary nodules. *Am J Med*. 1984;77:135–140.
21. Karam GH, Fulmer JD. Giant cell arteritis presenting as interstitial lung disease. *Chest*. 1982;82:781–784.
22. Wagenaar SS, van den Bosch JM, Westermann CJ, et al. Isolated granulomatous giant cell vasculitis of the pulmonary elastic arteries. *Arch Pathol Lab Med*. 1986;110:962–964.
23. Ladanyi M, Fraser RS. Pulmonary involvement in giant cell arteritis. *Arch Pathol Lab Med*. 1987;111:1178–1180.
24. Arend WP, Michel BA, Bloch DA, et al. The American College of Rheumatology 1990 criteria for the classification of Takayasu arteritis. *Arthritis Rheum*. 1990;33:1129–1134.
25. Fairley C, Wilson JW, Barraclough D. Pulmonary involvement in Behcet's syndrome. *Chest*. 1989;96:1428–1429.
26. Raz I, Okon E, Chajek-Shaul T. Pulmonary manifestations in Behcet's syndrome. *Chest*. 1989;95:585–589.
27. Efthimiou J, Johnston C, Spiro SG, et al. Pulmonary disease in Behcet's syndrome. *Q J Med*. 1986;58:259–280.
28. Slavin RE, de Groot WJ. Pathology of the lung in Behcet's disease. Case report and review of the literature. *Am J Surg Pathol*. 1981;5:779–788.
29. Lakhanpal S, Tani K, Lie JT, et al. Pathologic features of Behcet's syndrome: a review of Japanese autopsy registry data. *Hum Pathol*. 1985;16:790–795.
30. Gamble CN, Wiesner KB, Shapiro RF, et al. The immune complex pathogenesis of glomerulonephritis and pulmonary vasculitis in Behcet's disease. *Am J Med*. 1979;66: 1031–1039.

31. Fernandes SR, Singsen BH, Hoffman GS. Sarcoidosis and systemic vasculitis. *Semin Arthritis Rheum*. 2000;30:33–46.

32. Takemura T, Matsui Y, Saiki S, et al. Pulmonary vascular involvement in sarcoidosis: a report of 40 autopsy cases. *Hum Pathol*. 1992;23:1216–1223.

33. Colby TV, Fukuoka J, Ewaskow SP, et al. Pathologic approach to pulmonary hemorrhage. *Ann Diagn Pathol*. 2001;5:309–319.

34. Lynch J, Leatherman J. Alveolar hemorrhage syndromes. In: Fishman A, ed. *Fishman's Pulmonary Diseases and Disorders*. New York, NY: McGraw-Hill; 1998:1193–1210.

5

BACTERIAL LUNG INFECTIONS

Bacterial infections are a common cause of lung morbidity and mortality. Transbronchial biopsies are often used as an effective means for making a specific diagnosis, particularly in immunosuppressed patients. Various clinical settings besides immunosuppression can be associated with bacterial pneumonia, including alcoholism, aspiration, intravenous drug abuse, various immune deficiency syndromes, and chronic obstructive pulmonary disease.

Common bacterial pneumonias are found in various clinical settings, both nosocomial and community acquired. Two major types are recognized: lobar pneumonia, in which consolidation of an entire lobe of lung results from diffuse and uniform inflammation of the pulmonary parenchyma, and patchy bronchopneumonia, in which multiple foci of inflammation are present involving the terminal airways.[1] The most common causative organisms are gram-positive cocci, including *Staphylococcus aureus* and *Streptococcus pneumonia*, and gram-negative rods, including *Klebsiella pneumonia*, *Haemphilus influenza*, *Escherichia coli*, and *Pseudomonas aeruginosa* (eFigs. 5.1 and 5.2). These types of pneumonia are generally diagnosed by cultures of sputum or other respiratory secretions and do not generally require a biopsy unless specific culture and sensitivity assays are unsuccessful on sputum samples.[2] The histologic hallmark of the process is the presence of acute inflammatory exudate filling the alveolar spaces admixed with fibrin and often with necrosis of alveolar walls (Fig. 5.1). Tissue Gram stains will usually highlight the organisms.

UNCOMMON BACTERIAL PNEUMONIAS

Several uncommon bacterial pneumonias are seen in clinical practice that may be amenable to specific diagnosis by transbronchial biopsy, including legionella pneumonia, botryomycosis, nocardia, actinomyces, tularemia, malakoplakia, bacillary angiomatosis, mycobacterial pneumonias, and others (Table 5.1).

Legionella Pneumonia

Legionella pneumonia is a pulmonary infection caused by gram-negative bacteria, *Legionella pneumophila*. The organism is not normally

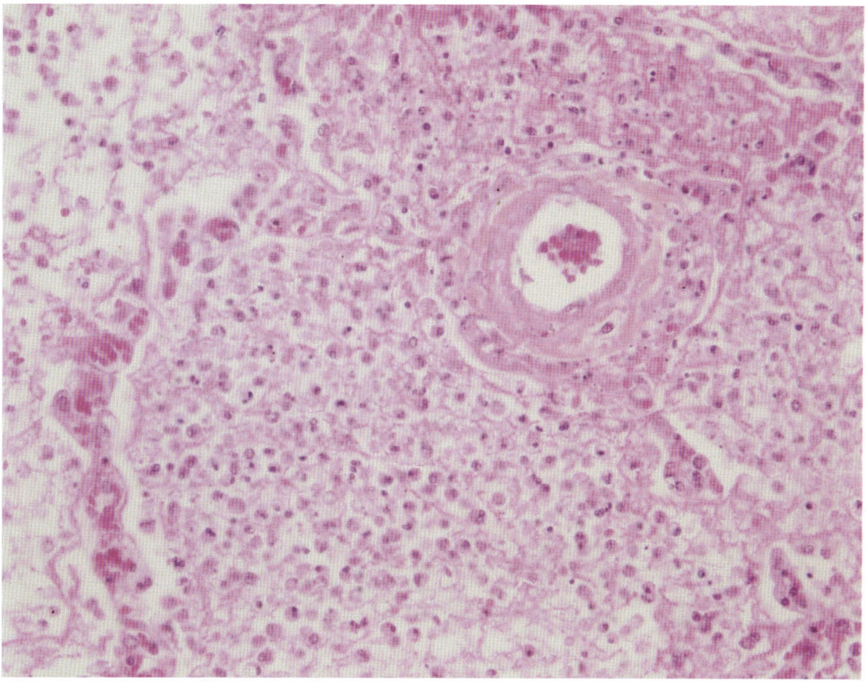

FIGURE 5.1 Acute bronchopneumonia owing to Klebsiella pneumonia shows filling of alveolar spaces with abundant neutrophils.

transmitted by direct contact; human infection results from inhalation of aerosolized droplets from contaminated air-handling equipment, such as evaporator pans, air conditioners, humidifiers, respiratory therapy equipment, and so on. This microorganism can cause nosocomial outbreaks as well as sporadic infection.[3] Patients present with constitutional symptoms including headache, fever, and myalgia. Cough, shortness of breath, and pleuritic pain are present in about half of patients, and one-third may present with hemoptysis. Chest radiographs show patchy peripheral areas of consolidation that may rapidly progress to extensive lobar involvement. The organism may be difficult to culture and microbiological studies have yielded only up to 60% sensitivity.[4] Histologically, transbronchial biopsies will show extensive neutrophilic infiltration of alveolar spaces admixed with fibrin (Fig. 5.2) (eFig. 5.3). In one-third of patients, the infiltrate may comprise monocytes and macrophages, or an admixture of neutrophils and monocytic cells. Often, there is abundant nuclear debris owing to karyorrhexis of neutrophils imparting the biopsy with a distinctive "dusty" appearance. Diffuse alveolar damage and organizing pneumonia may be seen in adjacent areas (Fig. 5.3), and secondary vasculitis can also be observed in some cases. In more advanced stages, the lung biopsy may show a desquamative interstitial pneumonia-like pattern (Fig. 5.4). The organisms can be visualized within macrophages by

TABLE 5.1 Uncommon Bacterial Pneumonias

Infection	Organisms	Histology	Stains	Clinical Features
Legionella	*Legionella pneumophila* (gram-negative bacteria)	Neutrophilic pneumonia admixed with fibrin and nuclear debris	Silver stains (Dieterle, Whartin–Starry, Steiner) Immunofluorescence staining, DNA-in-situ, PCR	Inhalation of aerosolized droplets in air-handling equipment
Nocardia	*Nocardia asteroides* (gram-positive, long beaded and branching filamentous bacteria)	Necrotizing neutrophilic pneumonia	GMS, B&B, and Fite–Faraco stain (weakly acid-fast)	Adult men, immunocompromised
Actinomyces	*Actinomyces israelii* (anaerobic, thin filamentous bacteria)	Suppurative inflammation with abscess formation and "sulfur granules"	GMS and B&B (filamentous branching bacteria) Negative acid-fast	Secondary to aspiration in debilitated patients
Tularemia	*Franciscella tularensis* (gram-negative coccobacillus)	Acute fibrinous and necrotizing pneumonia	Immunofluorescent antibody testing	Zoonosis—bite of deer tick or deer fly
Yersinia	*Yersinia pestis* (gram-negative rod)	Necrotizing and hemorrhagic pneumonia with abundant organisms	Silver stains (Whartin–Starry, Dieterle, Steiner) Direct immunofluorescence	Zoonosis—bite of rodent tick
Melioidosis	*Burkholderia pseudomallei* (gram-negative bacteria)	Acute necrotizing bronchopneumonia with abscess formation	Bacteria, cultures	Endemic in tropic regions in Southeast Asia

Malakoplakia	*Rhodococcus equi* (gram-positive coccobacillus)	Dense histiocytic infiltrate with scattered concentric calcifications (Michaelis–Guttman bodies)	Bacteria stain with B&B, Fite–Faraco Michaelis–Gutmann bodies stain with Von Kossa and Alizarin red stains	Organism found in soil and feces of animal, especially horses
Whipple disease	*Tropheryma whippelii*	Sheets of macrophages with abundant clear, PAS-positive foamy cytoplasm	GMS, Whartin–Starry	Multisystem disorder associated with malabsorption, diarrhea, weight loss, and lymphadenopathy
Bacillary angiomatosis	*Bartonella henselae* (small coccobacillus)	Vascular proliferation lined by large epithelioid endothelial cells with acute inflammatory infiltrates	Modified Whartin–Starry at pH 3.2 Immunohistochemistry and PCR	Immunocompromised patients; transmitted through cats by fleas
Botriomycosis	*S. aureus* and other bacteria	Neutrophilic pneumonia with "sulfur granules"	B&B ("grape-like" cultures composed on non filamentous, non branching bacteria)	Immunosuppressed patients

PCR, polymerase chain reaction; GMS, Gomori methenamine silver; B&B, Brown and Brenn.

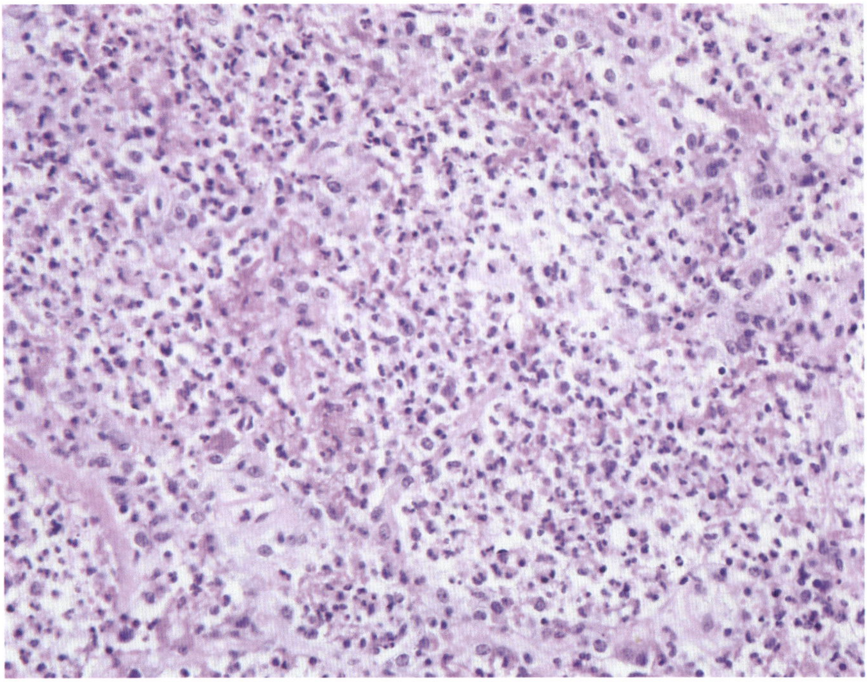

FIGURE 5.2 Transbronchial biopsy in patient with Legionnaire disease showing massive neutrophilic infiltration of alveolar spaces admixed with fibrin and nuclear debris imparting the biopsy with a characteristic "dusty" appearance.

use of special stains.[5] The best stains for *Legionella* are the silver stains, including Steiner, Whartin–Starry, and Dieterle. The organisms will present as small, short singly scattered bacilli (Fig. 5.5). Immunoperoxidase and immunofluorescent staining can also be used with specific antibodies on deparaffinized, formalin-fixed tissue samples.[6] The use of molecular techniques such as DNA-in-situ hybridization and PCR to detect these agents has recently been reported as a more sensitive and rapid method for diagnosis.[7]

Nocardia

Nocardia is a filamentous, gram-positive bacteria with a characteristically beaded histology. Pulmonary infection occurs from inhalation of saprophytic organisms in the soil or in decaying vegetable matter.[1] There are multiple species of *Nocardia* but lung infection most often is caused by *N. asteroides*. The process most often affects adult men, particularly among immunocompromised patients. Cavitation is a common complication of nocardosis, and pleural effusions, fistulas, and empyema can also supervene. Histologically, nocardia is characterized by a necrotizing pneumonia with extensive acute inflammation and large areas of necrosis (Fig. 5.6). The organisms display long, thin,

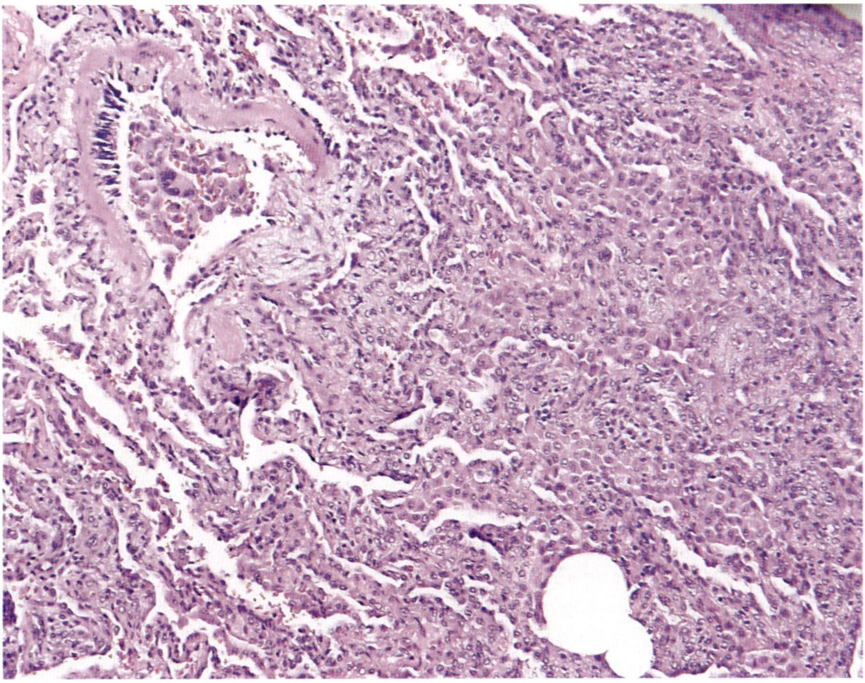

FIGURE 5.3 Legionella pneumonia showing a focal organizing pneumonia pattern.

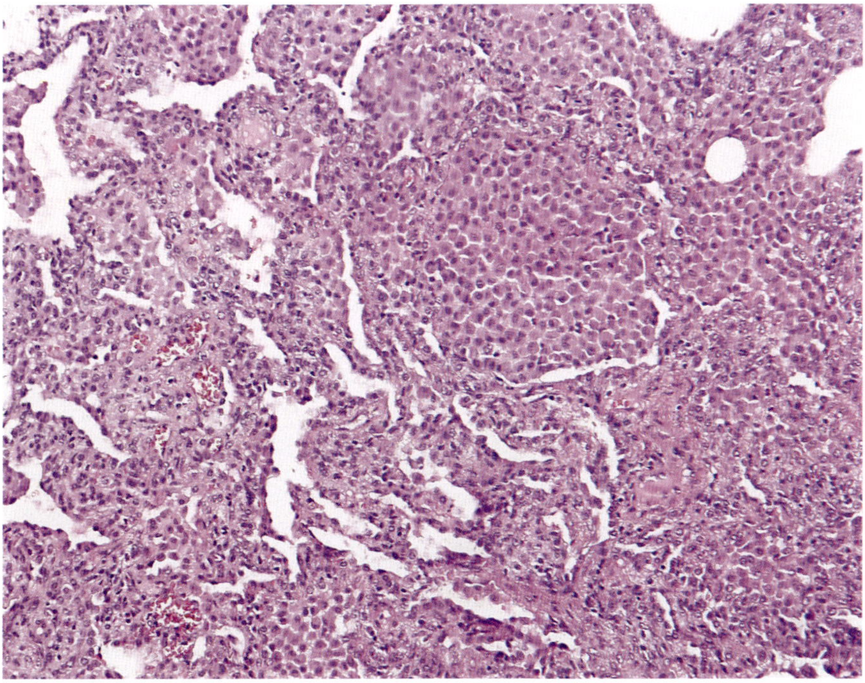

FIGURE 5.4 Desquamative interstitial pneumonia pattern in Legionella pneumonia.

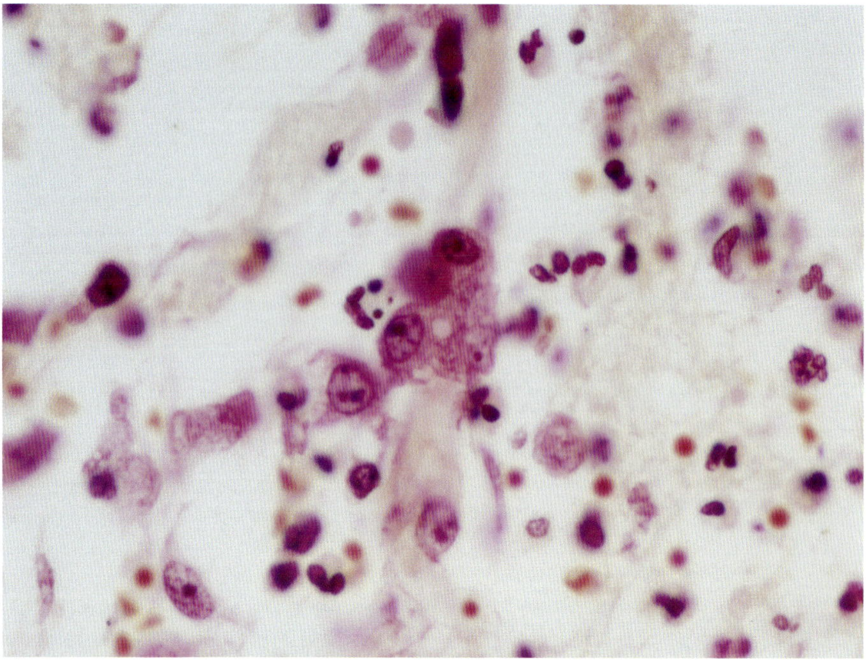

FIGURE 5.5 Steiner silver stain showing *Legionella* organisms within alveolar macrophages.

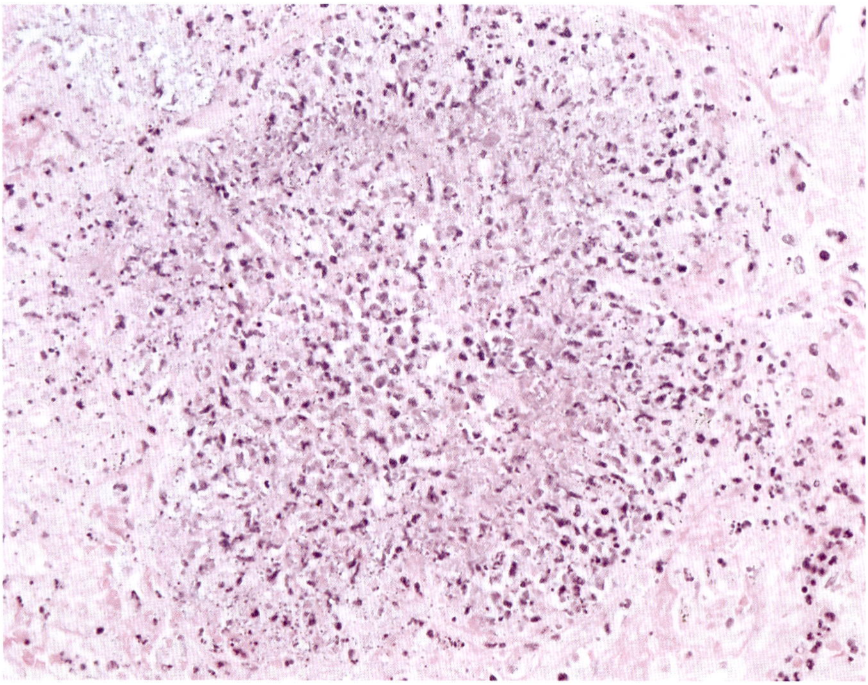

FIGURE 5.6 Lung biopsy showing focus of necrosis owing to *Nocardia*. The organisms are not easily visualized on routine hematoxylin and eosin (H&E) stains.

beaded filamentous bacteria that branch at right angles. They are not easily visualized on routine H&E tissue sections, and special stains are required for their identification. *Nocardia* stains with GMS, and with tissue Gram stains such as Brown and Brenn, and Brown and Hopps (Fig. 5.7). *Nocardia* is also weakly acid-fast and will be positive for the Fite–Faraco stain. However, the organisms can be difficult to detect and may be easily overlooked unless one pays attention to the peculiar complex branching appearance of the filamentous bacteria. Periodic acid–Schiff (PAS) stain for the fungus is usually negative. Definitive diagnosis is established by culture of lung biopsy tissue or bronchioloalveolar lavage fluid. Because cultures usually require 1 to 2 weeks, a more rapid diagnosis may be obtained from a transbronchial biopsy. Identification of *Nocardia* species requires a high degree of suspicion and use of the appropriate special stains such as the Brown and Brenn, GMS, or Fite–Faraco acid-fast stain. The filamentous branching bacteria of *Nocardia* can be easily overlooked on routine special stains. *Nocardia* is distinguished from *Actinomyces* by its weak acid-fast positivity.

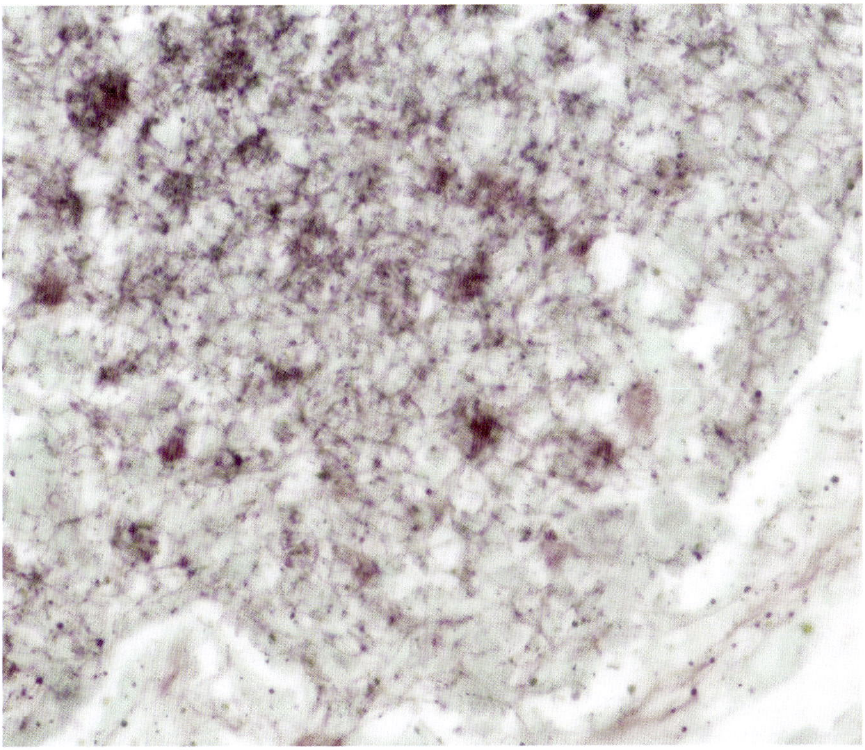

FIGURE 5.7 Thin, beaded filamentous bacteria that branch at right angles characteristic for *Nocardia* (GMS stain).

Actinomyces

Actinomyces is an anaerobic filamentous bacteria that commonly inhabits the mouth and nasal passages. There are several species but the most common pathogen in the lungs is *Actinomyces israelii.* Lung infection is usually the result of aspiration of oropharyngeal contents. Chest X-rays usually show unilateral patchy lower lobe areas of consolidation that may cause multifocal and nodular opacities. The process may extend to the pleura and chest wall and produce sinus tracts with broncho-pleural and cutaneous fistulas. Actinomycosis is characterized by suppurative inflammation, abscess formation, and the formation of so-called sulfur granules (eFig. 5.4).[8] The latter correspond to focalized masses of organisms that seem to radiate from the center of the structure. When these structures develop an eosinophilic, amorphous layer around the periphery of the granules, the process is referred to as the "Splendore–Hoeppli" phenomenon (Fig. 5.8). The lesions often tend to cavitate and form abscesses that may be surrounded by a prominent histiocytic reaction. The organisms are thin, gram-positive, beaded filamentous bacteria that show branching at right angles. At the periphery of the sulfur granules, the organisms often show a radial orientation with club-shaped swellings at the periphery. The

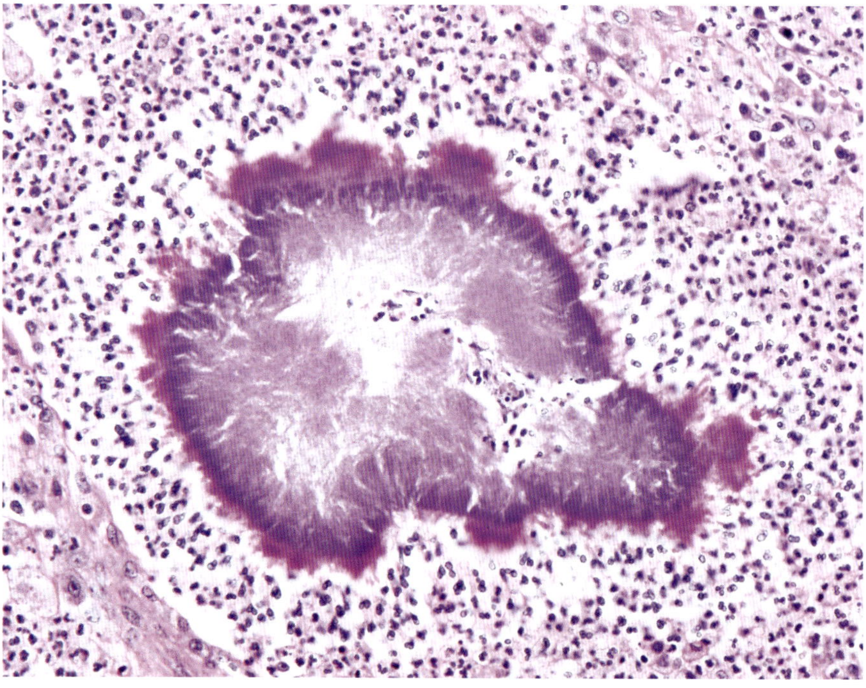

FIGURE 5.8 "Sulfur granules" in actinomycosis showing filamentous structures that radiate from the center toward the periphery and show an amorphous peripheral eosinophilic layer of proteinaceous material (so-called Splendore–Hoeppli phenomenon).

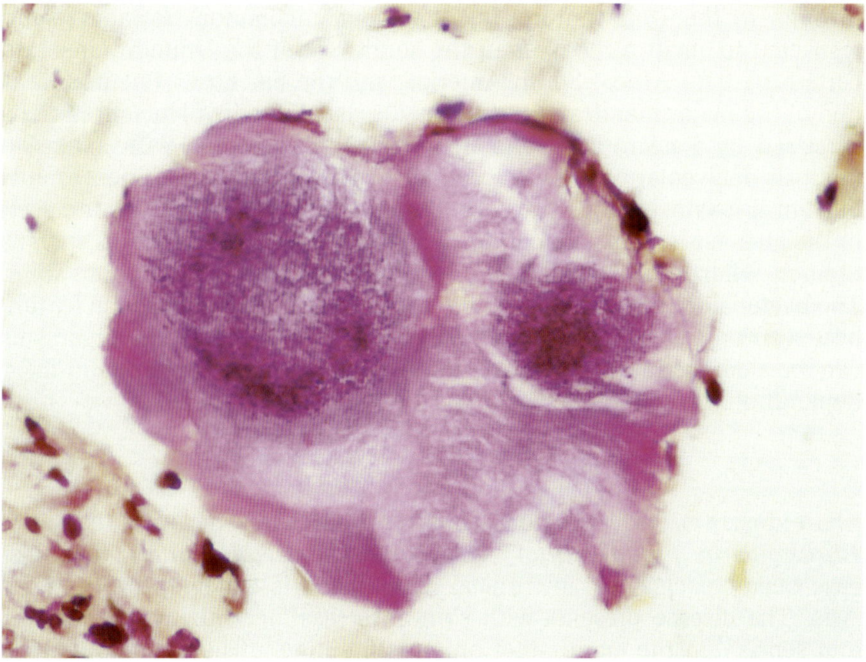

FIGURE 5.9 Positive staining of *Actinomyces* with tissue Gram stain (Brown and Brenn).

organisms are positive for GMS and the Brown and Brenn tissue Gram stain (Fig. 5.9). The differential diagnosis includes other organisms that can form sulfur granules with the Splendore–Hoeppli phenomenon, such as botryomycosis. *Nocardia* can closely resemble actinomycosis but is weakly acid-fast positive with the Fite–Faraco and other acid-fast stains, and it does not form sulfur granules.

Tularemia

Tularemic pneumonia is caused by a small, gram-negative cocobacillus, *Franciscella tullarenis* (formerly known as *Pasteurella tularensis*). The disease is transmitted through the bite of an infected deer tick or fly.[9] The disease also affects the skin, lymph nodes, eyes, and orophraynx.[10] Tularemic pneumonia is characterized by an acute fibrinous and necrotizing pneumonia with extensive necrosis of alveolar walls. The organisms may be demonstrated by immunofluorescent antibody staining.

Yersinia Pestis

Yersinia pestis (formerly *Pasteurella pestis*), a short, nonmotile gram-negative rod, is the causative organism of the bubonic plague. The plague is a zoonosis that is transmitted by the bite of a flea whose natural hosts are small animals, in particular rodents (especially rats). Plague was responsible for the death of millions of persons during the middle ages through to the 18th century, but it is very uncommon nowadays, and restricted to small rural areas in the southwest of the United States and certain parts of Africa, South America, and the Far East.[1] Pneumonia is one of the major manifestations of the disease. Lung involvement is characterized by a necrotizing and hemorrhagic pneumonia with extensive necrosis of alveolar walls. The terminal airways are filled with neutrophils but fibrin is conspicuously absent. Large numbers of organisms are seen in the alveolar lumens and can be demonstrated with silver stains such as Steiner, Whartin–Starry and Dieterle, or with the Brown and Hopps stain. The bacteria are bipolar and exhibit a "safety-pin" configuration, a feature best seen on touch imprints stained with the Gram stain. The organisms can be demonstrated by direct immunofluorescence on formalin-fixed deparaffinized sections.[11,12]

Melioidosis

Melioidosis is an infection caused by a gram-negative bacteria, *Burkholderia pseudomallei (Pseudomonas pseudomallei)*. The disease occurs exclusively in tropical regions and is endemic to Southeast Asia. The disease presents with skin abscesses, necrotizing pneumonia, and sepsis, but the main target organ is the lung.[13] The pneumonia may be acute, subacute, or chronic. The infection causes acute necrotizing bronchopneumonia with focal abscess formation.[14] The necrotizing pneumonia contains abundant neutrophils and macrophages. Some cases may display a mixture of acute inflammation and granulomatous inflammation manifested by a rim of palisaded histiocytes and giant cells at the edges of the necrotizing neutrophilic abscesses. The giant cells and macrophages usually contain dense clusters of bacilli called globi. Most of the organisms are intracellular and can sometimes be recognized in H&E tissue sections, but the diagnosis is best established based on bacterial cultures.

Malakoplakia

Malakoplakia is a distinctive inflammatory process that results from infection with various organisms, including *Rhodococcus equi, E. coli*, and *Acinetobacter*.[15,16] In the lungs, it is most commonly associated with *R. equi* infection. The infection has a predilection for immunocompromised patients, particularly AIDS patients.[17] *R. equi* is a gram-positive coccobacillus found in soil and in the feces of some animals, particularly horses. Infection is acquired through inhalation of contaminated aerosols. Lung infection generally results in areas of consolidation that may show focal cavitation. Histologically, the lesions are characterized by a dense histiocytic infiltrate with scattered plasma cells (Figs. 5.10 and 5.11). The hallmark of the lesion is the presence of scattered small, concentric calcifications known as Michaelis–Gutmann bodies measuring from 2 to 10 μm in diameter. These structures can be found within the cytoplasm of the histiocytes or within the interstitium (Fig. 5.12). On transbronchial

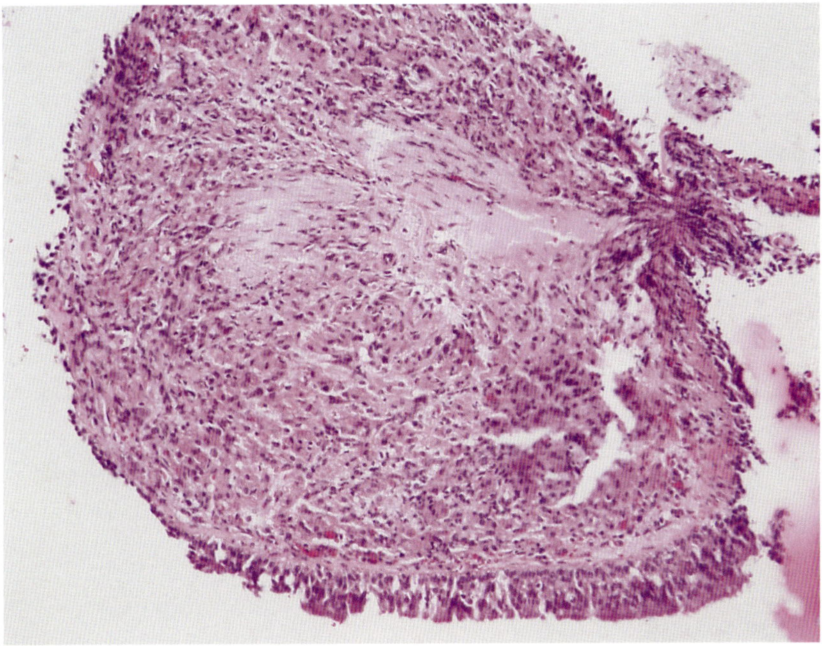

FIGURE 5.10 Transbronchial biopsy in patient with malakoplakia shows dense histiocytic infiltrate in the submucosa.

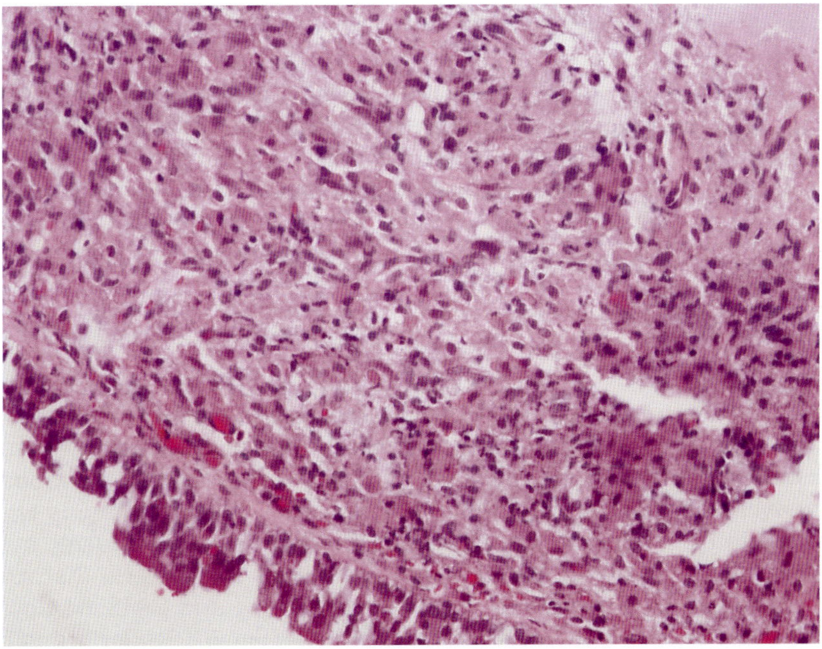

FIGURE 5.11 Higher magnification of the biopsy in patient with pulmonary involvement with malakoplakia shows abundant epithelioid histiocytes admixed with a few small lymphocytes and plasma cells.

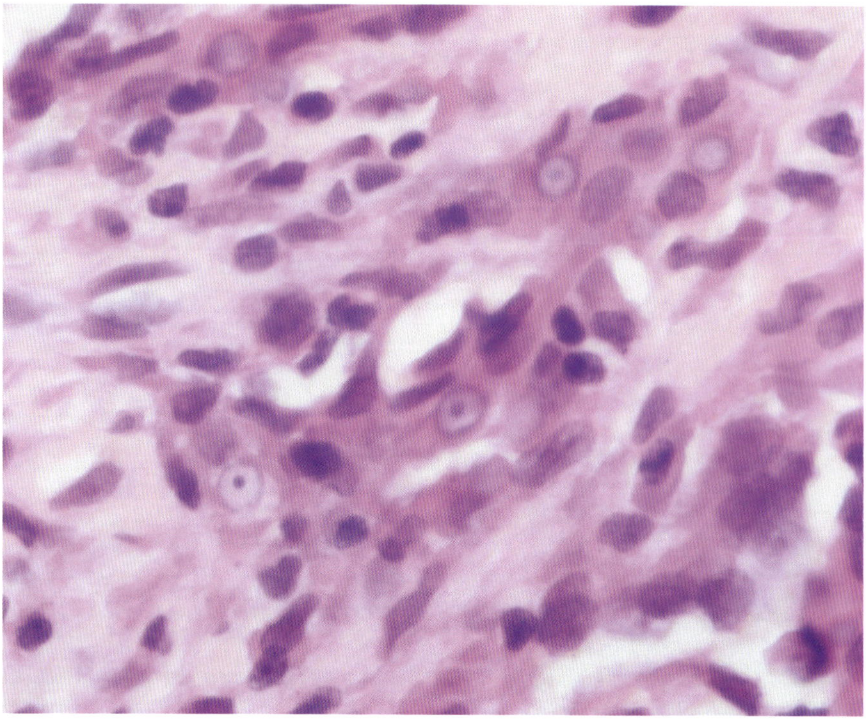

FIGURE 5.12 Small round concentric structures with central foci of calcification adopting a "targetoid" appearance characterize the Michaelis–Gutmann bodies in malakoplakia.

biopsies these structures may be few and difficult to find. Histochemical stains for calcium such as the von Kossa or Alizarin red stain will highlight them (Fig. 5.13). The bacteria can be identified in tissue sections with a tissue Gram stain such as Brown and Brenn, and they are also weakly acid fast and can be demonstrated with modified acid-fast stains such as the Fite–Faraco.

Whipple Disease

Whipple disease is a rare disorder caused by infection with the bacteria *Tropheryma whippelii.* The disease involves multiple organs, in particular the gastrointestinal tract, and usually presents with malabsorption, diarrhea, weight loss, and lymphadenopathy. Pulmonary involvement is extremely rare.[18–20] Histologically, the disease is characterized by sheets of macrophages with abundant clear, foamy cytoplasm (Fig. 5.14). The macrophages are filled with bacteria that stain positive with silver stains such as Whartin–Starry and GMS. The cytoplasm of the cells is strongly positive for PAS (Fig. 5.15). Peribronchial and peribronchiolar infiltrations are often seen as well as submucosal infiltration by the histiocytes. The histiocytic infiltrate in Whipple disease can be easily confused for infection with mybocaterium avium

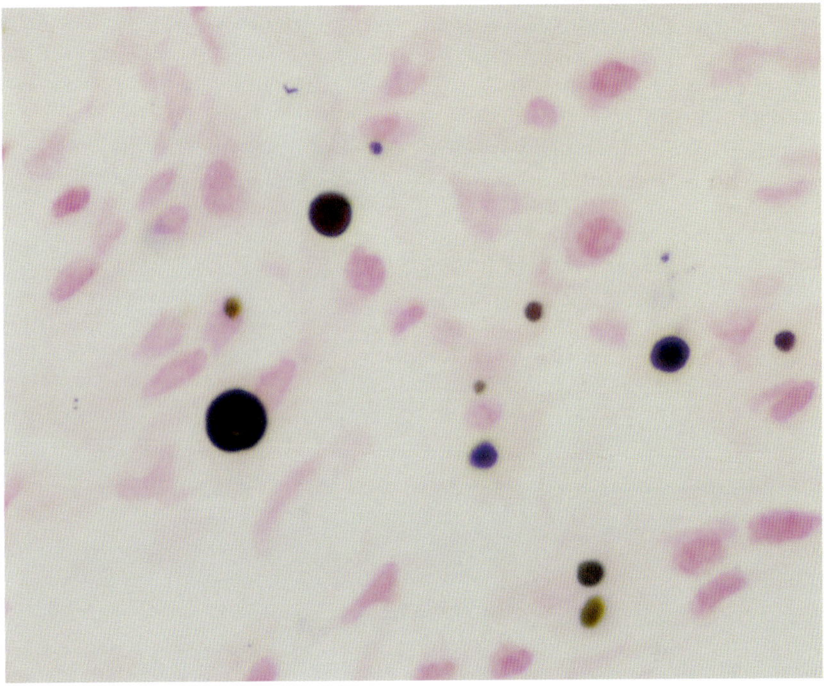

FIGURE 5.13 Von Kossa stain for calcium highlights the Michaelis–Gutmann bodies in pulmonary malakoplakia.

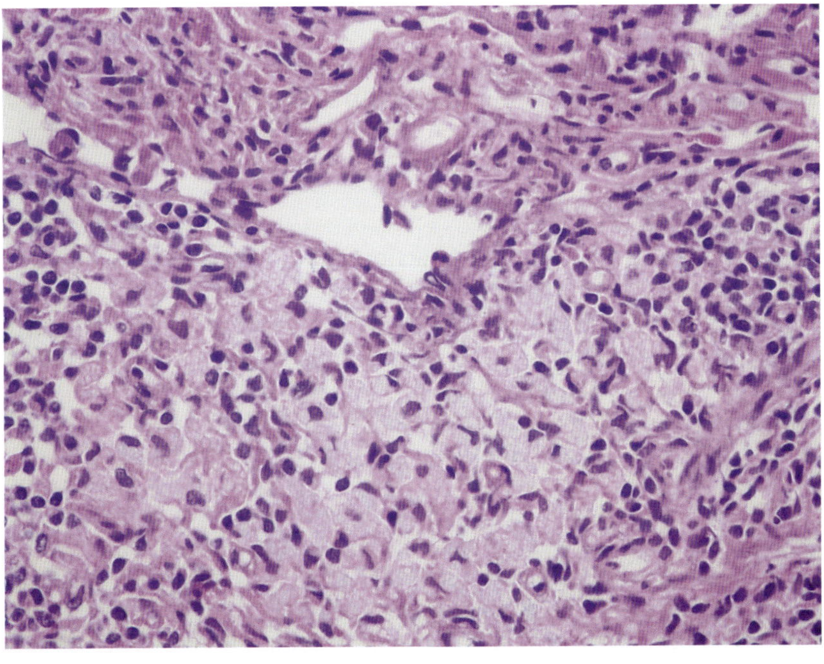

FIGURE 5.14 Sheets of vacuolated macrophages with a bubbly cytoplasm are seen in Whipple disease involving the lung.

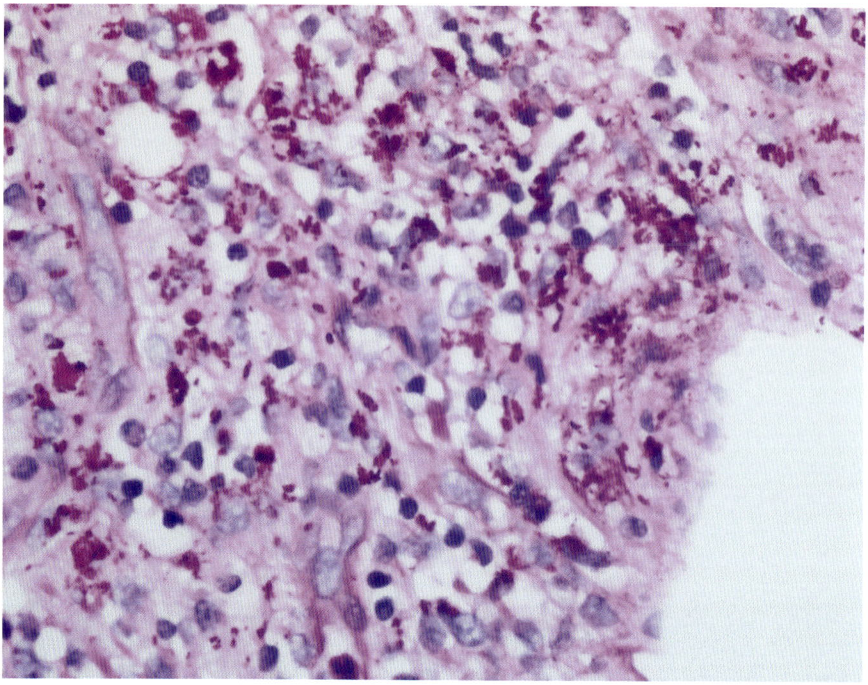

FIGURE 5.15 PAS stain showing abundant, intensely positive intracytoplasmic bacterial elements are seen in Whipple disease involving the lung.

intracellulare (MAI). Strong cytoplasmic positivity of the macrophages for PAS and negative staining of the organisms for the modified acid-fast stains such as Fite–Faraco will help distinguish between the two. Confirmation of the diagnosis requires demonstration of the organism by PCR.[21]

Bacillary Angiomatosis

Bacillary angiomatosis is a tissue reaction pattern comprising primarily an epithelioid vascular proliferation in response to an infection caused by a small coccobacillus, *Bartonella henselae* and *Bartonella quintana* (formerly *Rochalimea*). Cats are the most common hosts for the organisms, and transmission is through the cat flea. Immunocompromised patients are particularly prone to this infection. Bacillary angiomatosis most commonly affects the skin but can occur in almost all organs. Lung involvement has been reported in AIDS patients who presented with interstitial pneumonitis, lymphadenopathy, and polypoid endobronchial lesions.[22,23] Histologically, the lesions are characterized by a dense proliferation of small vessels lined by plump endothelial cells with abundant epithelioid cytoplasm (Fig. 5.16). Scattered inflammatory cells, particularly neutrophils and small lymphocytes, are often present forming discrete microabscesses (Fig. 5.17). The organisms can sometimes be visualized on H&E stains; they

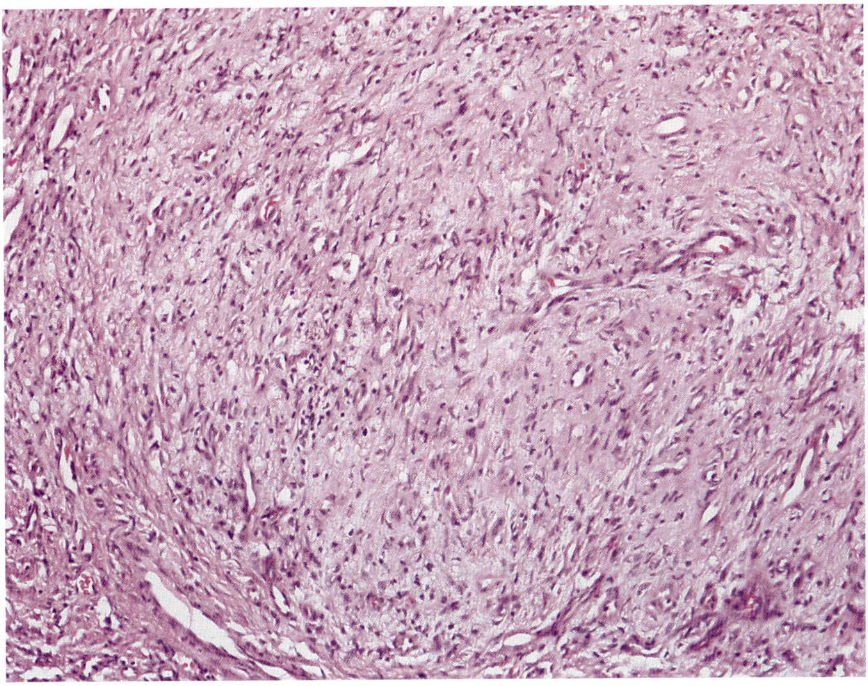

FIGURE 5.16 Proliferation of small vessels lined by plump epithelioid cells and admixed with inflammatory cells is seen in bacillary angiomatosis involving the lung.

show a tendency to cluster within the cytoplasm of the histiocyte imparting the lesions with a "dirty," purple appearance (eFigs. 5.5 and 5.6). The organisms are best visualized with a modified Whartin–Starry silver stain at a pH of 3.2. The organisms are negative for PAS and acid-fast stains. Both immunohistochemistry utilizing specific antibodies against *B. henselae* or detection by PCR can be used to confirm the diagnosis.

Botriomycosis

Botriomycosis is an infection caused by nonfilamentous bacteria that form "sulfur granules" similar to those seen in actinomycosis. The disease can affect almost any organ. The most common organism associated with botryomycosis is *S. aureus*, although other organisms can also result in the same lesions, including *P. aeruginosa, E. coli, Proteus, Streptococcus*, and others. Lung involvement is rare and can occur as bronchial infection complicating bronchiectasis, as focalized tumor-like lesions, or as diffuse bronchopneumonia.[8,24–26] The disease often presents in the setting of immunosuppression. The diagnosis is made when the distinctive "granules" measuring up to 2 mm in diameter are identified in tissue sections. These granules comprise nonfilamentous bacterial organisms, such as gram-positive cocci or gram-negative bacilli, and are typically located within areas of suppuration and necrosis (Fig. 5.18). The granules often

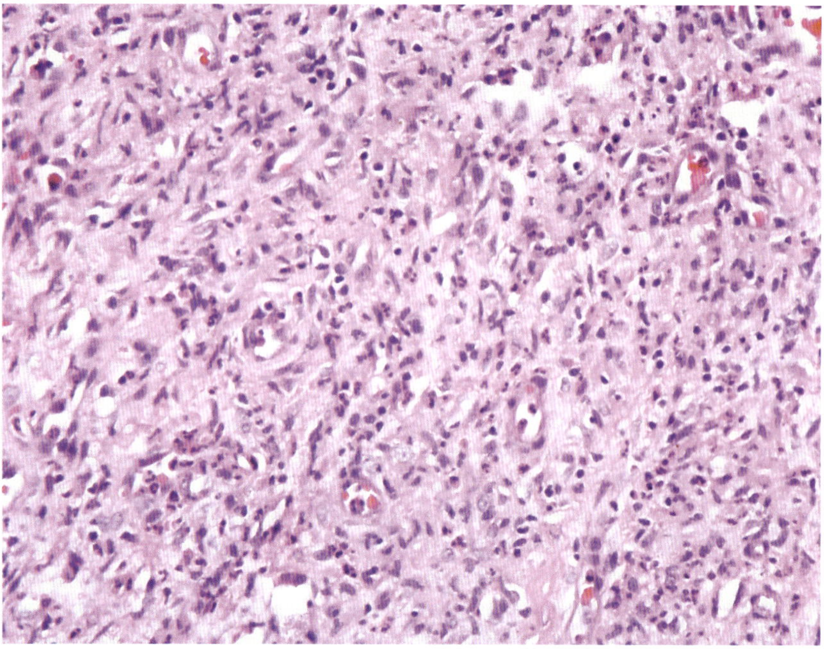

FIGURE 5.17 Higher magnification of bacillary angiomatosis showing a population of neutrophils and small lymphocytes surrounding the small vessels. The surrounding histiocytes have a "dirty" appearance and contain abundant organisms that are best appreciated with special stains.

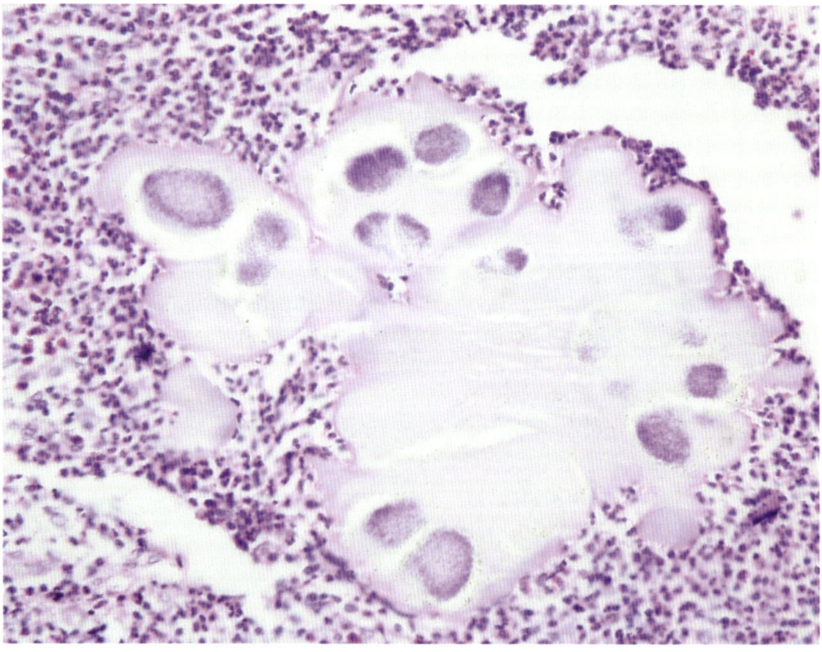

FIGURE 5.18 "Sulfur granule" comprising masses of nonfilamentous bacteria are seen in a case of botryomycosis involving the lung (tissue Gram stain; Brown and Brenn).

display the Splendore–Hoeppli phenomenon, with a layer of eosinophilic amorphous material deposited at the periphery of the bacterial colonies. The organisms are visualized on tissue Gram stains and characteristically grow forming grape-like cultures, hence the designation of "botryomycosis." The main differential diagnosis is with actinomycosis, but the organisms in botryomycosis do not show the filamentous branching seen in actinomycosis.

MYCOBACTERIAL PNEUMONIAS

Mycobacterial infection can be a frequent finding in the lungs of debilitated and immunosuppressed patients. The two main causative agents are *Mycobacterium tuberculosis* and the *Mycobacterium avium–intracellulare* complex. Although the incidence of infection with *M. tuberculosis* has decreased dramatically worldwide in developed countries owing to the use of antituberculous drugs, tuberculosis (TB) remains one of the most common infectious causes of death in underdeveloped countries. In the United States, the development of drug-resistant strains and the AIDS epidemic has seen resurgence in cases of TB. All mycobacteria share in common their acid-fast staining property caused by the high lipid content of the bacilli, a useful diagnostic feature.

Mycobacterium Tuberculosis

The lung is one of the main targets of TB and is characterized by chronic, recurrent infection that is transmitted through inhalation of aerosolized droplets containing the tubercule bacillus. TB is often associated with various underlying diseases such as diabetes, HIV infection, alcoholism, cancer, chronic renal failure, and drug abuse. It is clinically divided into primary and secondary (reactivation TB) infections. In primary TB, the initial response to the infection is a neutrophilic reaction followed by macrophages that engulf the organisms. The macrophages can spread to the regional lymph nodes, but they usually stay in the lungs and become localized to the upper half of the upper lobes ("Simon foci"). When the infection resolves, it undergoes fibrosis and calcification ("Ghon complex"). More than 90% of primary TB will heal spontaneously without progression. The patients will most often be asymptomatic, and the infection can be demonstrated only by a positive tuberculin skin test. Ten percent of patients will develop progressive disease characterized by hematogenous spread within the lungs to form a military pattern of involvement or foci of consolidation with tuberculous bronchopneumonia. Secondary TB occurs when a dormant focus of infection is reactivated causing reinfection. This will usually result in the characteristic cavitary lesions that can affect one or both upper lobes. This is the most common form of TB in adults.[27]

The pathologic findings in TB are mainly related to the destructive tissue reaction at the sites of infection. The most common reaction pattern is characterized by large, confluent necrotizing granulomas that show

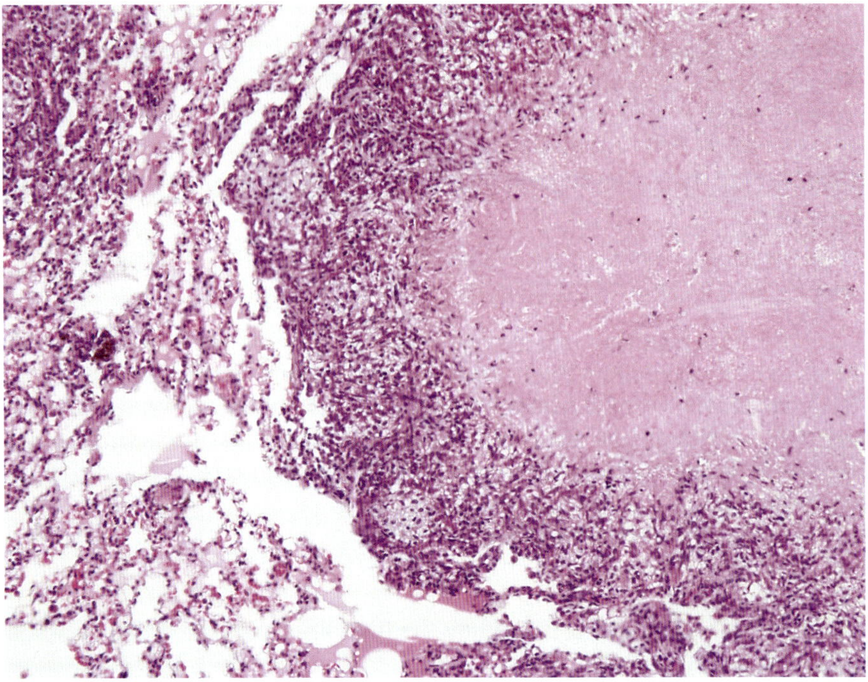

FIGURE 5.19 Necrotizing granuloma in lung infection with *Mycobacterium tuberculosis*. Notice peripheral palisading of histiocytes admixed with Langhans-type multinucleated giant cells surrounding necrotic center.

peripheral palisading of histiocytes, epithelioid histiocytes, and frequent Langhans-type multinucleated giant cells (Fig. 5.19) (eFigs. 5.7 and 5.8). A miliary pattern characterized by multiple small epithelioid granulomas can also be observed (Fig. 5.20). The lesions can sometimes be characterized by scattered microscopic granulomas and isolated Langhans giant cells distributed in peribronchial location (Fig. 5.21). The lesions contain bacilli mostly in the necrotic center, but they can also be identified within epithelioid histiocytes and multinucleated giant cells.[28] The bacilli are often few and difficult to identify and will require a diligent search, usually under oil-immersion. The organisms are best identified on acid-fast stains; Ziehl–Neelsen will stain the small, beaded and thin bacilli bright red (Fig. 5.22). Fluorescent staining, immunoperoxidase, and PCR methods can also be used to demonstrate the organism in tissues.[29,30] Long-standing lesions will tend to undergo fibrosis and calcification. Endobronchial spread occurs through lymphatic spread of organisms through the bronchial mucosa. The infection can also involve the pleura and regional lymph nodes. A rise in the incidence of TB has been observed in recent years, mainly related to the AIDS epidemic.[31]

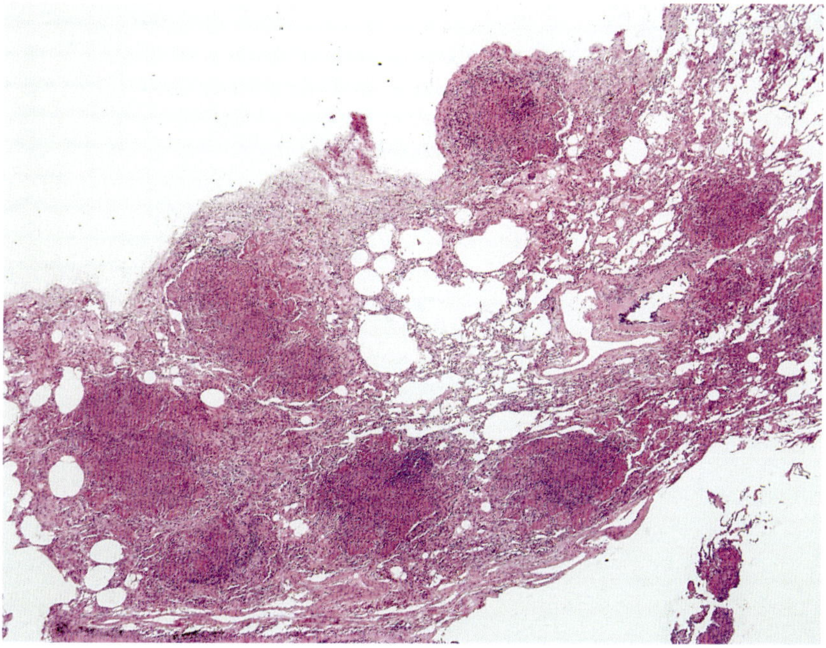

FIGURE 5.20 Miliary pattern in transbronchial lung biopsy in patients with tuberculosis.

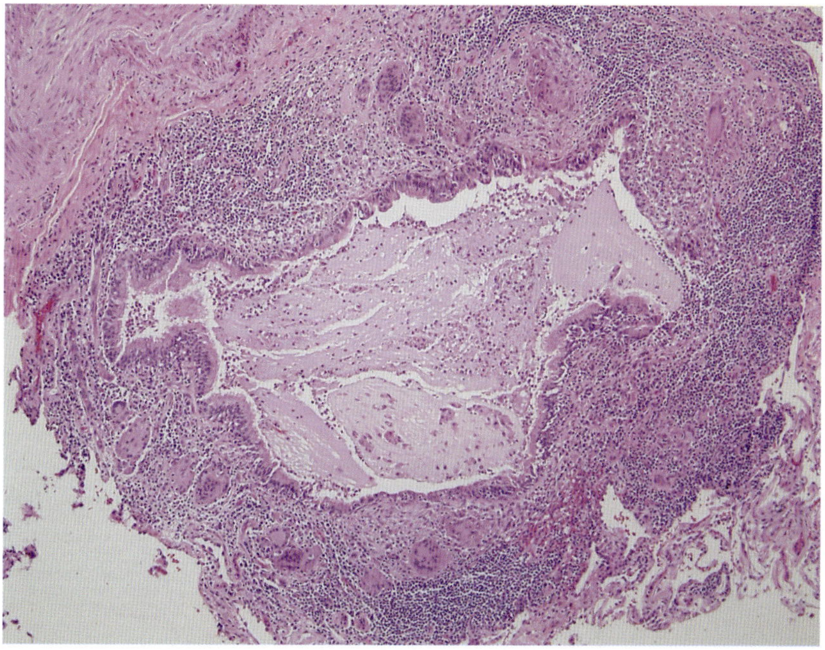

FIGURE 5.21 Granulomatous peribronchiolitis is seen in patient with tuberculosis. Notice small granulomas and scattered multinucleated giant cells surrounded by abundant lymphoid infiltrates.

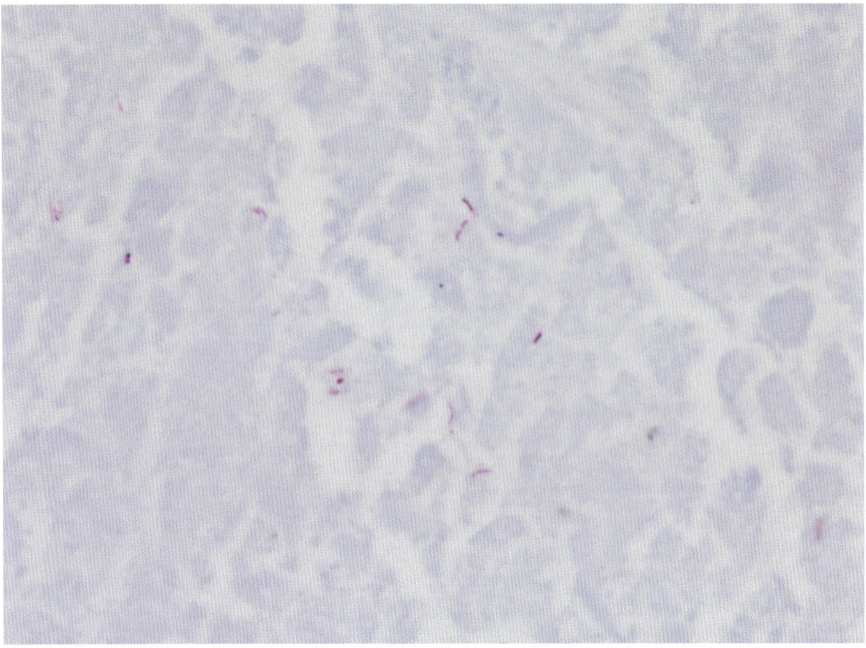

FIGURE 5.22 Few acid-fast bacilli are identified in areas of caseating necrosis within the granulomas of pulmonary tuberculosis (Ziehl–Neelsen stain).

Atypical Mycobacteria

Atypical, nontuberculous mycobacteria constitute a group of organisms that are found in soil, plants, fresh and salt water, and animals that cause infection directly from the environment rather than through human transmission. Atypical mycobacteria do not follow the same pattern of primary and secondary (reactivation) infections observed in TB. Primary infection of the lungs with atypical mycobacteria usually causes cavitary lung disease. In HIV-positive patients, the lung is considered to be the initial route of infection where the organisms lie dormant until the immunosuppression activates the organisms and dissemination takes place.[32] *M. avium* and *M. intracellulare* are closely related and are often grouped together and referred to as the *M. avium* complex (MAC) or MAI. The MAC is the most important atypical mycobacterial agent of human infection, with a high incidence in patients with AIDS.[33] *Mycobacterium kansasii* is another important cause of nontuberculous mycobacteriosis.[34] Although rarer, other types of atypical mycobacteria can be the source of infection in the lungs, including *M. abscessus, M. fortuitum*, and *M. chelonei.*

The histopathologic hallmark of atypical mycobacterial infection in the lung is the presence of nonnecrotizing epithelioid granulomas.[35–37] MAI also causes upper lobe cavitary lung lesions. The noncaseating

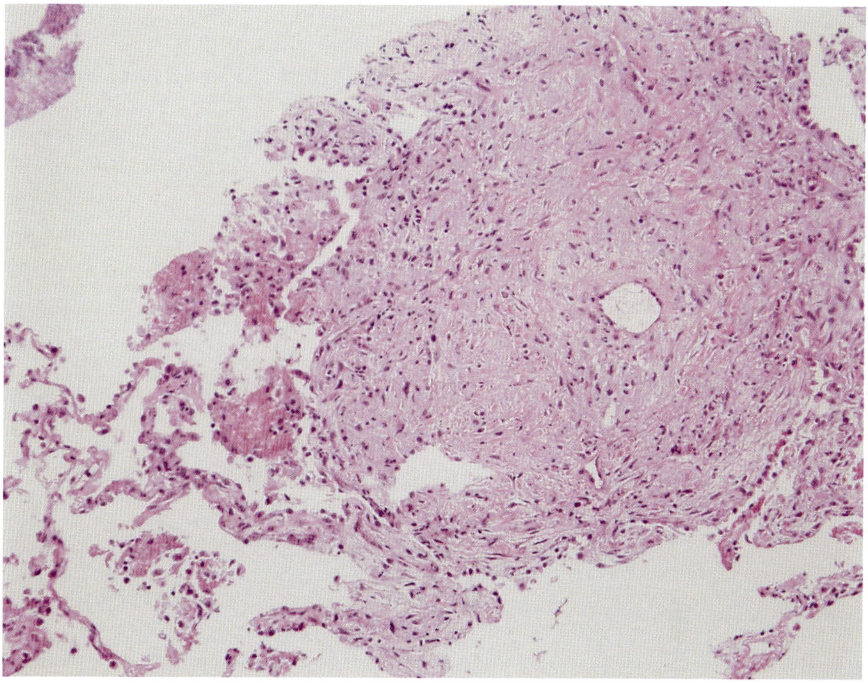

FIGURE 5.23 Transbronchial biopsy in immunosuppressed patient with MAI shows sheets of epithelioid histiocytes.

granulomas can resemble those seen in sarcoidosis. Transbronchial biopsies are quite helpful in diagnosing the condition (Fig. 5.23). The interstitium separating the alveolar septa show sheets of large epithelioid cells (Fig. 5.24); formation of well-defined granulomas may not always be present (eFig. 5.9). Higher magnification will show sheets of epithelioid histiocytes displaying a finely granular, "dirty" or cloudy cytoplasmic appearance (so-called pseudo-Gaucher cell) owing to the massive number of bacilli distending the cytoplasm (Fig. 5.25) (eFig. 5.10). The bacilli are easily visualized on Ziehl–Neelsen stains and are usually more slender and more abundant than in TB, particularly in AIDS patients.[32,38] The organisms can also be seen with PAS and GMS stains, and modified acid-fast stains such as Fite–Faraco, which will stain them intensely (Fig. 5.26). An unusual appearance that can be rarely encountered with MAC is the so-called mycobacterial spindle cell pseudotumor, a condition in which the histiocytes will adopt a spindled appearance with a fascicular growth pattern resembling a mesenchymal spindle cell proliferation.[39] Many of the spindled histiocytes, however, will display abundant "dirty" granular cytoplasm owing to the intracytoplasmic bacilli, which are easily highlighted by acid-fast stains.

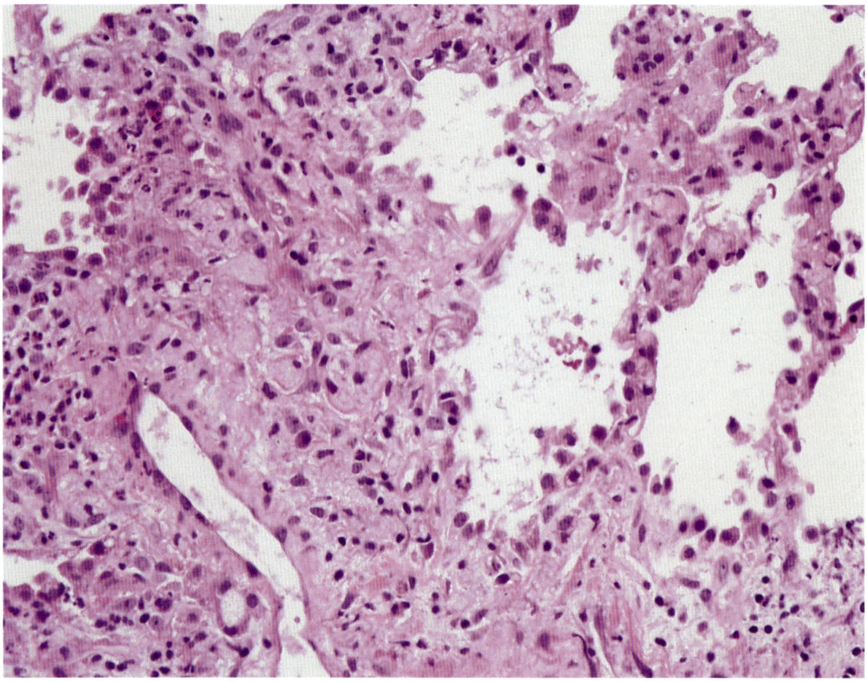

FIGURE 5.24 Lung involvement in MAI shows abundant epithelioid histiocytes admixed with other inflammatory elements in the interstitium.

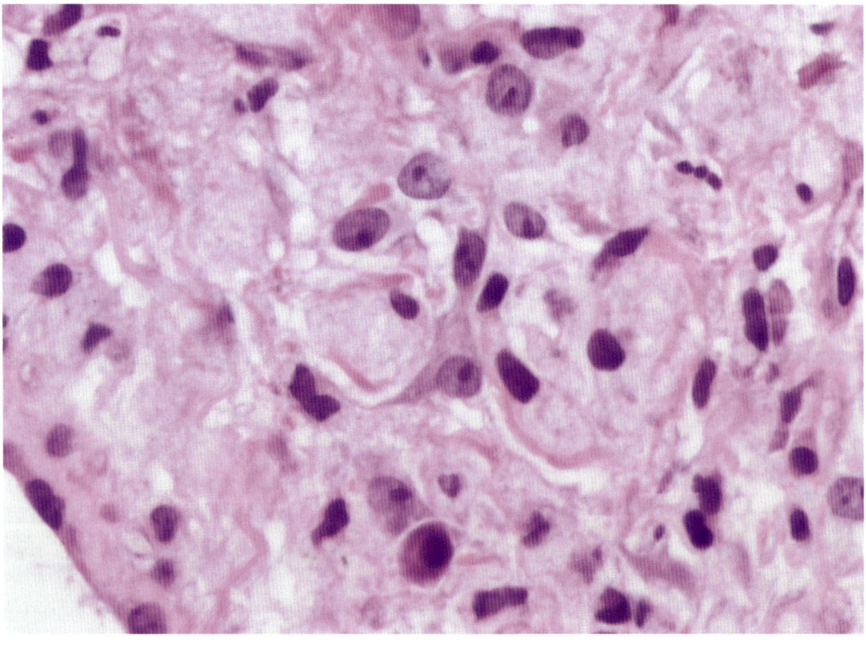

FIGURE 5.25 Higher magnification from preceding picture showing sheets of large, epithelioid histiocytes with "dirty" granular cytoplasm.

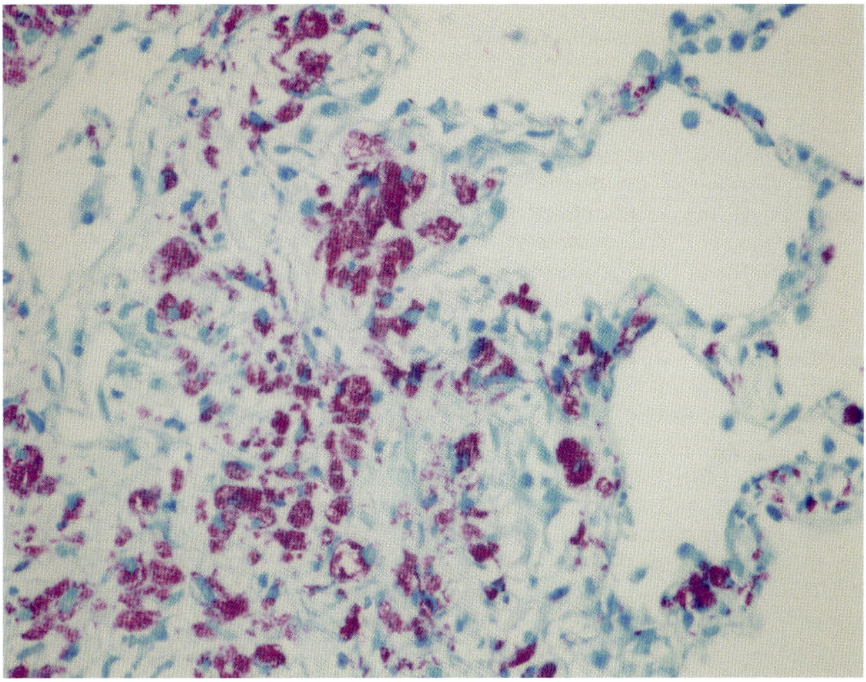

FIGURE 5.26 Modified acid-fast stain (Fite–Faraco) intensely stains the organisms in MAI. Notice the abundance of organisms and the larger size compared with those of *Mycobacterium tuberculosis*.

REFERENCES

1. Goetz MB, Finegold SM. Pyogenic bacterial pneumonia, lung abscess and empyema. In: Murray JF, Nadel JA, Mason RJ, et al, eds. *Textbook of Respiratory Medicine*. 3rd ed. Philadelphia, PA: WB Saunders Co; 2000:985–1041.
2. Chandler F. Approaches to the pathologic diagnosis of infectious diseases. In: Connor D, Chandler FW, Schwartz DA, et al, eds. *Pathology of Infectious Disease*. Stamford, CT: Appelton & Lange; 1997:3–7.
3. Weisenburger DD, Helms CM, Renner ED. Sporadic Legionnaires' disease. A pathologic study of 23 fatal cases. *Arch Pathol Lab Med*. 1981;105:130–137.
4. Fields BS, Benson RF, Besser RE. Legionella and Legionnaires' disease: 25 years of investigation. *Clin Microbiol Rev*. 2002;15:506–526.
5. Winn WC Jr, Myerowitz RL. The pathology of the Legionella pneumonias. A review of 74 cases and the literature. *Hum Pathol*. 1981;12:401–422.
6. Veza PR, Lack EE, Chandler FW. Legionellosis. In: Connor DH, Chandler FW, Manz HJ, et al, eds. *Pathology of Infectious Diseases*. Stamford, CT: Appelton & Lange; 1997:597–604.
7. Hayden RT, Uhl JR, Qian X, et al. Direct detection of *Legionella* species from bronchoalveolar lavage and open lung biopsy specimens: comparison of light cycler PCR, in-situ hybridization, direct fluorescence, antigen detection and culture. *J Clin Microbiol*. 2001;39:2618–2626.
8. De Montpreville VT, Nashashibi N, Dulmet EM. Actinomycosis and other bronchopulmonary infections with bacterial granules. *Ann Diagn Pathol*. 1999;3:67–74.

9. Evans ME, Gregory DW, Schaffner W, et al. Tularemia: a 30-year experience with 88 cases. *Medicine (Baltimore)*. 1985;64:251–269.
10. Miller RP, Bates JH. Pleuropulmonary tularemia. A review of 29 patients. *Am Rev Respir Dis*. 1969;99:31–41.
11. Johnson CC, Finegold SM. Pyogenic bacterial pneumonia, lung abscess and empyema. In: Murray JF, Nadel JA, eds. *Textbook of Respiratory Medicine*. 2nd ed. Philadelphia, PA: WB Saunders Co; 1994:1036–1093.
12. Smith JH, Reisner BS. Plague. In: Connor DH, Chandler FW, Manz HJ, et al, eds. *Pathology of Infectious Diseases*. Stamford, CT: Appelton & Lange; 1997:729–738.
13. Ip M, Osterberg LG, Chau PY, et al. Pulmonary melioidosis. *Chest*. 1995;108:1420–1424.
14. Greenwald KA, Nash G, Foley FD. Acute systemic melioidosis. Autopsy findings in four patients. *Am J Clin Pathol*. 1969;52:188–198.
15. Colby TV, Hunt S, Pelzmann K, et al. Malakoplakia of the lung: a report of two cases. *Respiration*. 1980;39:295–299.
16. Crouch E, White V, Wright J, et al. Malakoplakia mimicking carcinoma metastatic to the lung. *Am J Surg Pathol*. 1984;8:151–156.
17. Verville TD, Huycke MM, Greenfield RA, et al. Rhodococcus equi infections of humans. Twelve cases and a review of the literature. *Medicine (Baltimore)*. 1994;73:119–132.
18. Kelly CA, Egan M, Rawlinson J. Whipple's disease presenting with lung involvement. *Thorax*. 1996;51:343–344.
19. Pollock JJ. Pleuropulmonary Whipple's disease. *South Med J*. 1985;78:216–217.
20. Winberg CD, Rose ME, Rappaport H. Whipple's disease of the lung. *Am J Med*. 1978;65:873–880.
21. Misbah SA, Mapstone NP. Whipple's disease revisited. *J Clin Pathol*. 2000;53:750–755.
22. Foltzer MA, Guiney WB Jr, Wager CC, et al. Bronchopulmonary bacillary angiomatosis. *Chest*. 1993;104:973–975.
23. Slater LN, Min KW. Polypoid endobronchial lesions. A manifestation of bacillary angiomatosis. *Chest*. 1992;102:972–974.
24. Bersoff-Matcha SJ, Roper CC, Liapis H, et al. Primary pulmonary botryomycosis: case report and review. *Clin Infect Dis*. 1998;26:620–624.
25. Katapadi K, Pujol F, Vuletin JC, et al. Pulmonary botryomycosis in a patient with AIDS. *Chest*. 1996;109:276–278.
26. Speir WA Jr, Mitchener JW, Galloway RF. Primary pulmonary botryomycosis. *Chest*. 1971;60:92–93.
27. Hruban RH, Hutchin GM. Mycobacterial infections. In: *Pulmonary Pathology*. Dail DH, Hammar SP, eds. New York, NY: Springer-Verlag; 1994:331–350.
28. El Zammar OA, Katzenstein AL. Pathological diagnosis of granulomatous lung disease: a review. *Histopathology*. 2007;50:289–310.
29. Barbolini G, Bisetti A, Colizzi V, et al. Immunohistologic analysis of mycobacterial antigens by monoclonal antibodies in tuberculosis and mycobacetriosis. *Hum Pathol*. 1989;20:1078–1089.
30. Rish JA, Eisenach KD, Cave MD, et al. Polymerase chain reaction detection of Mycobacterium tuberculosis in formalin-fixed tissue. *Am J Respir Crit Care Med*. 1996;153:1419–1423.
31. Chaisson RE, Schecter GF, Theuer CP, et al. Tuberculosis in patients with the acquired immunodeficiency syndrome. Clinical features, response to therapy, and survival. *Am Rev Respir Dis*. 1987;136:570–584.
32. Hopewell PC, Bloom BR. Tuberculosis and other mycobacterial diseases. In: Murray JF, Nadel JA, Mason RJ, et al, eds. *Textbook of Respiratory Medicine*. 3rd ed. Philadelphia, PA: WB Saunders Co; 2000:1043–1105.

33. Wallace JM, Hannah JB. *Mycobacterium avium* complex infection in patients with the acquired immunodeficiency syndrome. A clinicopathologic study. *Chest.* 1988;93:926–932.
34. Christensen E, Dietz GW, Ahn C, et al. Initial roentgenographic manifestations of pulmonary *Mycobacterium tuberculosis, M. kansasii,* and *M. intracellulare* infections. *Chest.* 1981;80:132–147.
35. Contreras MA, Cheung OT, Sanders GE, et al. Pulmonary infection with non-tuberculous mycobacteria. *Am Rev Respir Dis.* 1988;137:149–156.
36. Farhi DC, Mason UG III, Horsburg CR Jr. Pathologic findings in disseminated *Mycobacterium avium-intracellulare* infection. A report of 11 cases. *Am J Clin Pathol.* 1986;85:67–71.
37. Marchevsky A, Damsker B, Gribetz A, et al. The spectrum of pathology of nontuberculous mycobacterial infections in open-lung biopsy specimens. *Am J Clin Pathol.* 1982;78:695–700.
38. Zakowski P, Fligiel S, Berlin GW, et al. Disseminated *Mycobacterium avium-intracellulare* infection in homosexual men dying of acquired immunodeficiency. *JAMA.* 1982;248:2980–2982.
39. Sekosan M, Cleto M, Senseng G, et al. Spindle cell pseudotumors in the lungs due to *Mycobacterium tuberculosis* in a transplant patient. *Am J Surg Pathol.* 1994;18:1065–1068.

6

FUNGAL LUNG INFECTIONS

Fungal infections are a common complication in immunocompromised patients. Transbronchial biopsies can be useful in the diagnosis of many fungal infections. Under certain circumstances, this may be the most rapid and effective method to diagnose fungal infection in an acutely ill patient in whom opportunistic infection is clinically suspected.[1] Histologic examination will often permit a rapid diagnosis and will allow the pathologist to assign the organism to a group or genus. Definitive speciation can be obtained later and confirmed by culture. Although some fungi are visible on hematoxylin and eosin (H&E), special stains such as periodic acid–Schiff (PAS), and silver stains such as Gomori methenamine silver (GMS) or Groccott stains are usually needed for proper identification.

Although more than 100 fungi have been identified in the lungs, only a small number are implicated as the source of human infection.[2] Fungi may be seen in the lungs as yeast (round spherules), hyphae (long tubular structures), and pseudohyphae (long tubular structures with regularly spaced constrictions). Fungal infections can cause several patterns of tissue damage in the lung, including necrotizing and nonnecrotizing granulomas, cavitary lesions, acute bronchopneumonia, and airway disease. The morphology of the organism can be a helpful clue for diagnosis; that is, septate mycelia with branching at 45° angles are typical of *Aspergillus* species, and large spherules with endospores are characteristic of *Coccidioides immitis*. It must be kept in mind, however, that atypical forms of many organisms may be encountered, and definitive speciation may require culture or other special techniques.[3–5] For ease of study, fungal diseases of the lung can be divided according to their morphologic appearances into fungi characterized by round yeast forms and fungi characterized by elongated hyphal or pseudohyphal forms, acknowledging the fact that an admixture of the two may be present in certain types of organisms.

FUNGI CHARACTERIZED BY ROUND YEAST FORMS

Histoplasmosis

Histoplasmosis is the most common fungal infection worldwide and is endemic to the Ohio and Mississippi river valleys in North America. It is also the most common opportunistic fungal infection in AIDS patients.[6] Histoplasmosis is caused by a dimorphic fungus *Histoplasma capsulatum* and can present as an asymptomatic, self-limited process that will pass clinically undetected, as an acute infection causing respiratory distress, a chronic process that may become progressive and disseminated, or may result in the formation of an asymptomatic, calcified pulmonary nodule. In its later stages, it may involve mediastinal lymph nodes and eventually progress to mediastinal fibrosis and sclerosing mediastinitis. The fungus lives in the soil and is contracted by inhalation of dust infected with bird droppings. Histologically, *H. capsulatum* infection results in necrotizing and nonnecrotizing granulomas that can present as large, solitary lesions, miliary nodules or cavitary lesions (Figs. 6.1 and 6.2) (eFigs. 6.1 to 6.3). In immunocompromised patients, intra-alveolar collections of foamy macrophages filled with organisms are seen. The process can progress to a life-threatening disseminated phase with fibrinopurulent exudates resembling a lobar pneumonia.[7] Chronic infection occurs most commonly in nonimmunosuppressed adults and resembles reinfection tuberculosis with cavitary lesions.

Morphologic diagnosis is based on identification of the yeast form of *H. capsulatum* in tissue sections. The organisms are characterized by small round to oval yeasts (2 to 4 μm), with narrow-based budding.

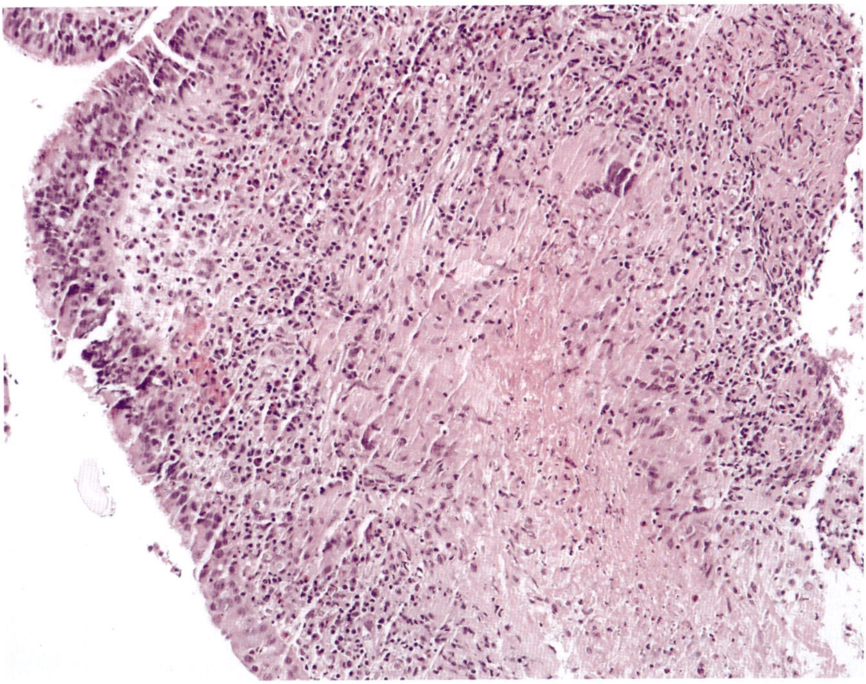

FIGURE 6.1 Bronchial biopsy showing *Histoplasma* granuloma with peripheral palisading of epithelioid histiocytes.

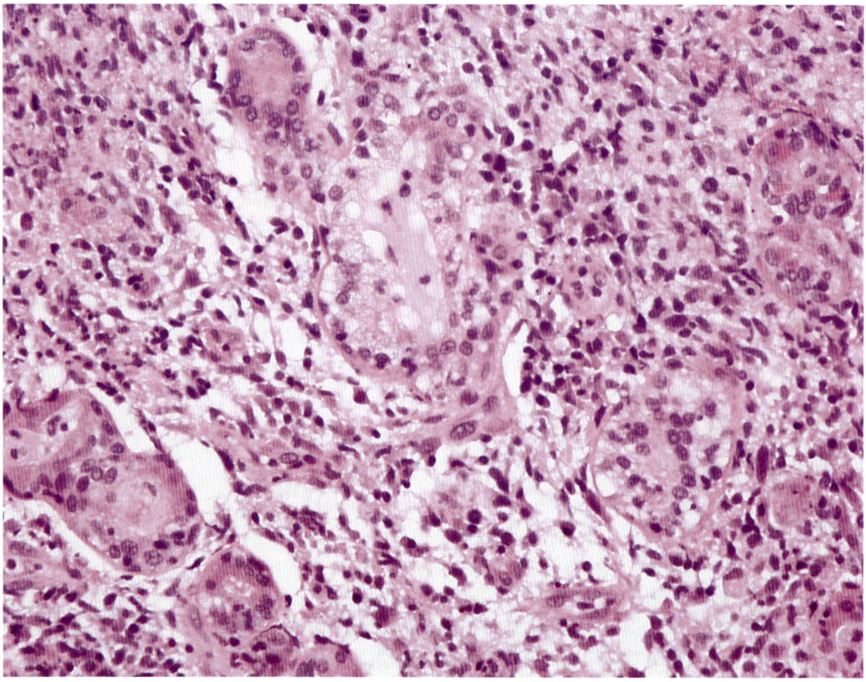

FIGURE 6.2 Higher magnification of *Histoplasma* granuloma showing round to oval, refractive structures within the cytoplasm of multinucleated giant cells.

When numerous, they can be seen on H&E stains as small refractive ovoid structures within macrophages; however, they are most often very difficult to visualize on routine staining and will require the use of silver stains (i.e., GMS) for identification (Fig. 6.3). Some of the organisms can show centrally placed, dot-like dark staining foci similar to those seen in *Pneumocystis carinii.* The diagnosis can also be established by direct immunofluorescence on histologic sections.[8] The number of organisms may vary widely depending on the stage of the lesion. Early lesions can contain abundant organisms, whereas in late stage, calcified or calcifying granulomas of the organisms may be very few or altogether absent. The small yeast of *H. capsulatum* need to be distinguished from *Pneumocystis,* capsule-deficient *Cryptococcus, Candida, Penicillium marneffei*, and *Blastomyces dermatidis* (Table 6.1).

Blastomycosis

Blastomycosis is a fungal infection caused by *B. dermatidis*, a dimorphic fungus found in the soil, most commonly in North America in the Mississippi, Missouri, and Ohio River valleys. The infection may be clinically asymptomatic or can be present as an acute pneumonia or chronic process.[9] The disease primarily affects the lungs but may spread to extrapulmonary sites, in particular to the skin and bone. In the lung,

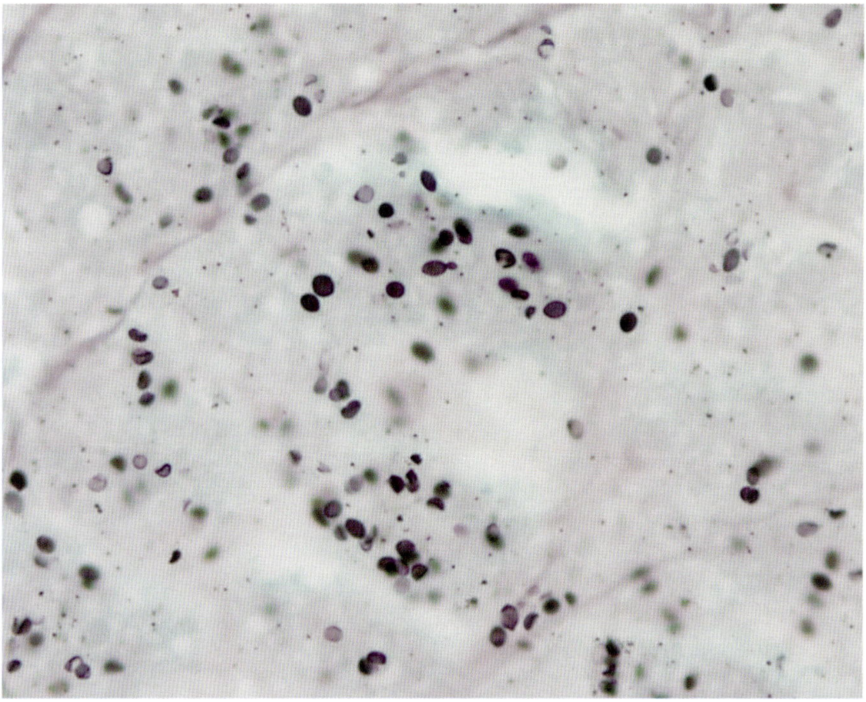

FIGURE 6.3 GMS highlights the organisms in pulmonary histoplasmosis.

the disease may cause focal or diffuse lung infiltrates primarily distributed in the upper lobes, diffuse alveolar damage, and solitary or multiple nodules. Focal involvement may manifest as a pulmonary mass that can be radiologically indistinguishable from lung cancer. Cavitation occurs in up to 20% of cases but calcification seldom ensues. The disease is not as common in immunocompromised patients but, when occurring in this setting, is more aggressive.[10] The clinical manifestations in patients with acute infection are similar to an acute bacterial pneumonia, and they can sometime lead to acute respiratory distress syndrome.[11] Chronic infection is more common and is characterized by necrotizing and nonnecrotizing granulomas.

The histologic appearance of *B. dermatidis* is that of round to oval yeast (8 to 15 μm), surrounded by thick, refractile walls with double contours (Fig. 6.4). The yeasts often show buds that are single and broad-based. Occasionally, the organisms may be much smaller (2 to 4 μm) resembling *H. capsulatum*. Larger forms (up to 30 μm) can be seen that can mimic the spherules in *Coccidioides*.[12] Organisms are highlighted by PAS and GMS stains (Fig. 6.5). Culture is the most definitive way to establish the diagnosis, but direct immunofluorescence on deparaffinized sections or immunohistochemistry can also be helpful.[8]

TABLE 6.1 Differential Diagnosis of Lung Infections Caused by Round Yeast-Like Fungi

Organism	Size	Shape	Lesions	Distinguishing Features
Histoplasma capsulatum	2–4 μm	Round to oval yeast Narrow-based budding Occasional dark staining foci Intracellular location within histiocytes	Histiocytic infiltrates filled with organisms (acute form) Necrotizing and nonnecrotizing granulomas (chronic form)	Uniform small yeast with narrow-based buds Positive for PAS and silver stains; negative for mucicarmine and Gram stains
Blastomyces dermatidis	2–4 and 8–15 μm	Round to oval yeast surrounded by thick, refractile walls Broad-based buds	Suppurative inflammation (acute) Necrotizing and nonnecrotizing granulomas (chronic)	Slightly larger yeast with broad-based buds and thick, refractile walls admixed with smaller yeast
Cryptococcus neoformans	2–20 μm	Round to oval yeast surrounded by thick halo Narrow-based buds Capsule-deficient forms	Necrotizing palisading granulomas or granulomatous pneumonia (in immunocompetent patients) Histiocytic and mucoid infiltrates devoid of inflammation (in immunocompromised patients)	Positivity for mucicarmine More variable size (2–20 μm) Absence of inflammatory reaction Capsule-deficient forms may be more difficult to diagnose
Candida albicans	2–6 μm	Round to oval yeast admixed with pseudohyphae (elongated branching structures without septae)	Suppurative, necrotizing inflammation No granulomas or foamy histiocytes	Presence of pseudohyphae without septae admixed with smaller yeast forms Positive for tissue Gram stain Extracellular location

Pneumocystis jiroveci	5–7 μm cysts	Round to oval cysts with grooves and folds, and dark-staining foci in the center of the cysts	Lymphocytic and fibrosing interstitial pneumonitis with foamy intra-alveolar exudates containing abundant organisms	Intra-alveolar location Foamy exudates Absence of budding walls Positive for GMS and with monoclonal antibodies by immunohistochemistry
Penicillium marneffei	2.5–5 μm	Round to oval yeast with transverse septum	Abundant macrophages filled with organisms	No budding forms Also shows short hyphae and elongated, oval and curved forms with rounded ends History of travel to Southeast Asia
Coccidioides immitis	30–100 μm	Large, round spherules with or without endospores	Necrotizing granulomas Fungus balls	Large round spherules with numerous endospores Spherules without endospores may be confused for large *Blastomyces* organisms
Paracoccidioides brazilensis	4–60 μm	Round yeast with multiple buds	Necrotizing granulomas	Distinguished from *Cryptococcus* by the multiple buds and lack of mucicarmine staining

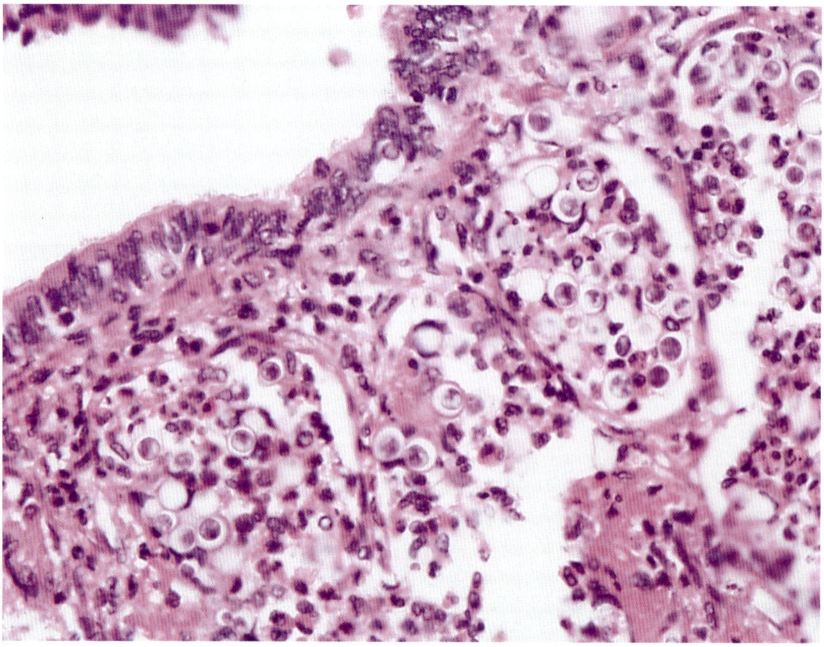

FIGURE 6.4 Endobronchial biopsy in *Blastomyces dermatidis* pneumonia shows round yeast surrounded by a thick refractile wall with double contours and occasional single, broad based buds.

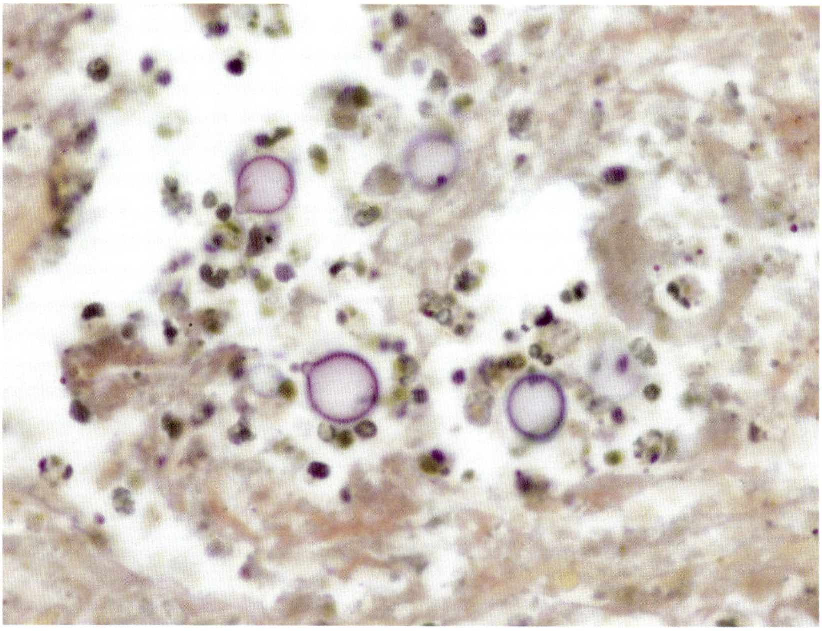

FIGURE 6.5 PAS stain in blastomycosis shows round to oval yeast surrounded by a thick refractile wall with small, broad-based single buds.

Cryptococcosis

Cryptococcosis is caused by the inhalation of spores of *Cryptococcus neoformans*, a yeast found worldwide in soil contaminated with pigeon droppings. There are two major clinical forms: pulmonary infection and leptomeningeal infection secondary to hematogenous spread from the lungs. Immunosuppressed patients are at higher risk for acquiring the infection. Primary lung infection is usually asymptomatic. Lung manifestations of the disease may be focal, including a nodule or mass lesion with ill-defined borders, multifocal peripheral pulmonary nodules or masses, or unilateral or bilateral parenchymal consolidation.[13] Immunocompromised patients most often exhibit disseminated disease with diffuse, bilateral interstitial infiltrates or miliary involvement that may progress to diffuse parenchymal consolidation and cavitation. In immunocompetent patients, the lesions most often manifest as necrotizing palisading granulomas or as granulomatous pneumonia (Fig. 6.6); in immunocompromised patients, the infiltrates are often histiocytic and mucoid and devoid of inflammation (Fig. 6.7).

On histology the organism are small, round to oval yeast (usually 4 to 6 μm) that may occasionally attain larger sizes (up to 20 μm) (eFig. 6.4). Single budding with a narrow base is a characteristic feature (Fig. 6.8). The organisms are best highlighted by silver stains (Fig. 6.9)

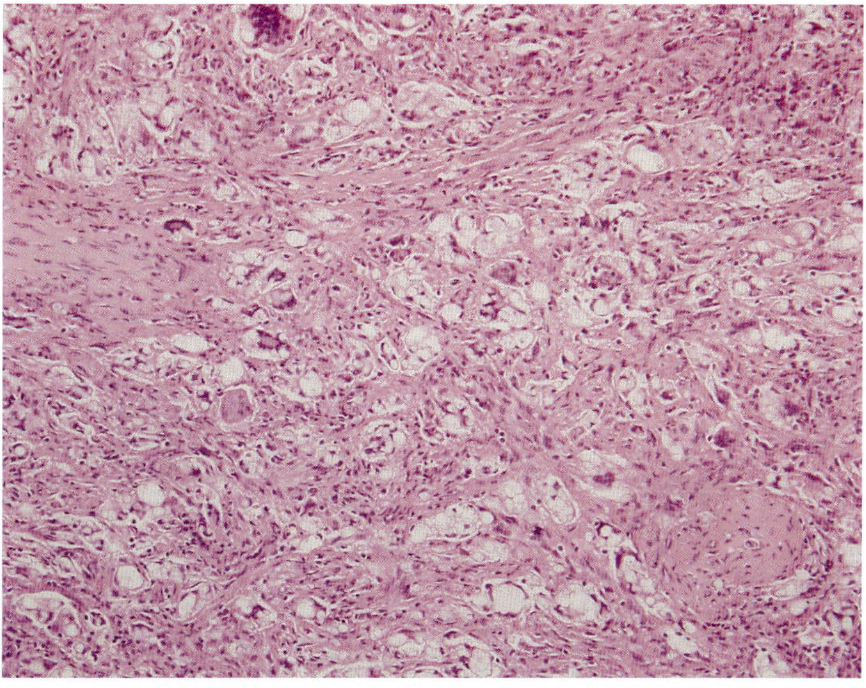

FIGURE 6.6 Granulomatous pneumonia in immunocompetent patient with cryptococcal infection.

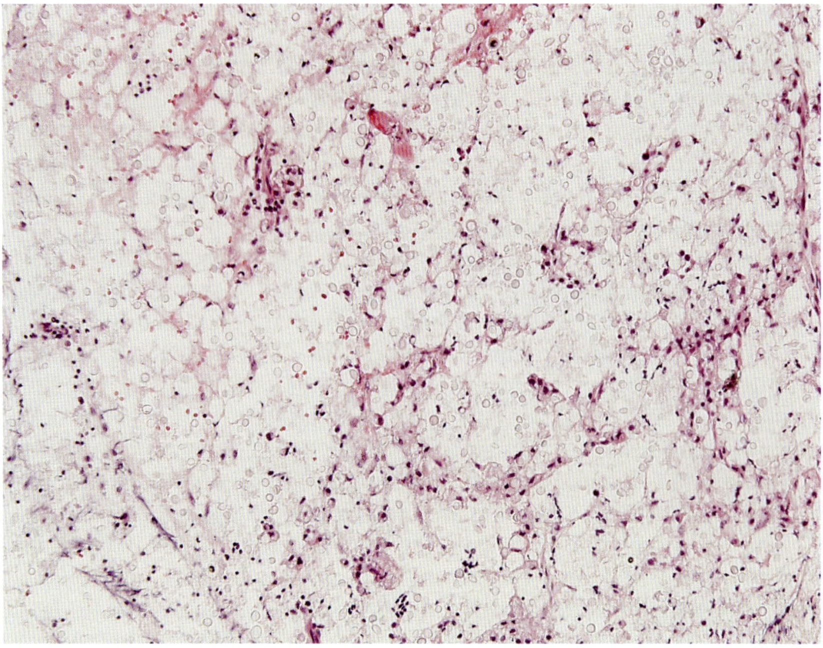

FIGURE 6.7 Immunocompromised patient with cryptococcal pneumonia. Notice the absence of inflammatory infiltrates and the abundance of organisms.

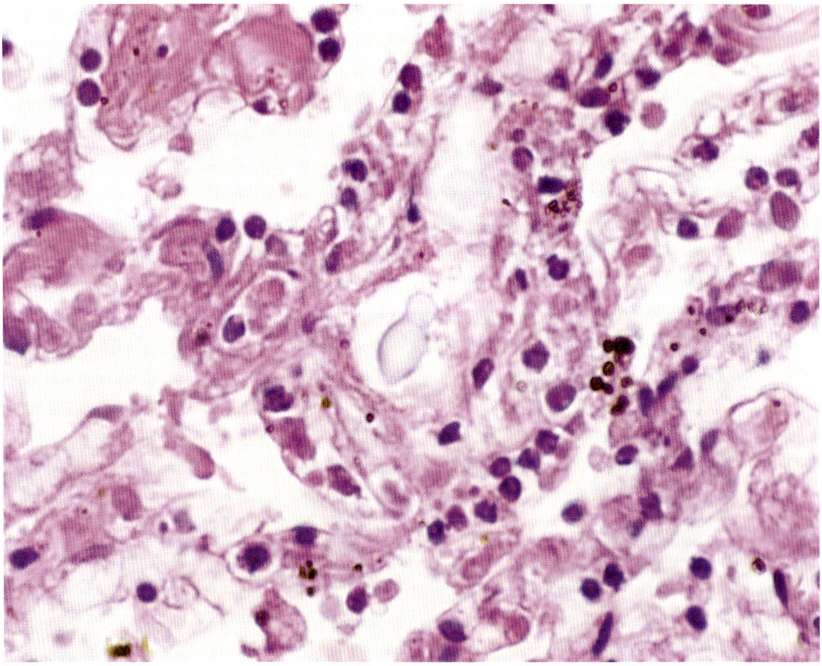

FIGURE 6.8 Lung biopsy in cryptococcal pneumonia showing oval yeast with narrow-based single budding.

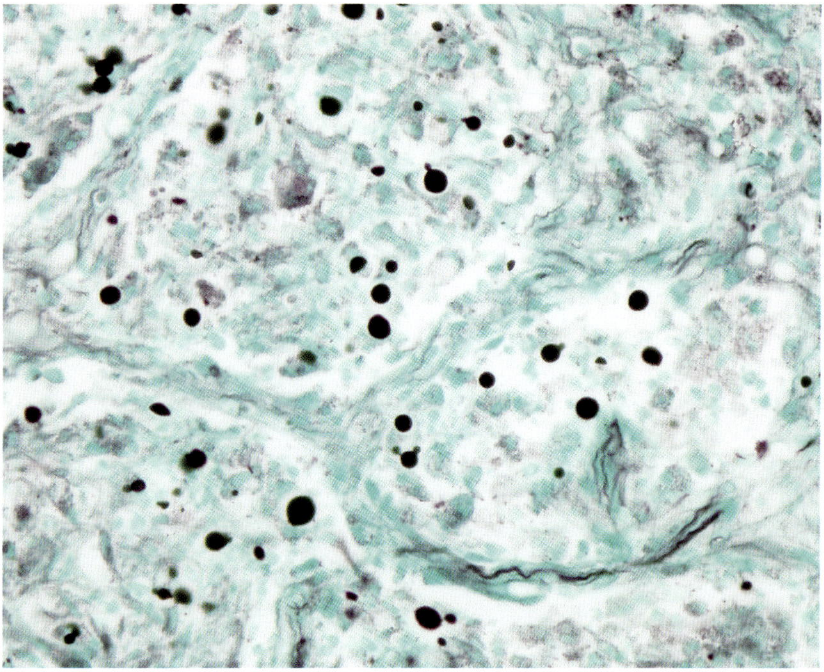

FIGURE 6.9 Methenamine silver stain in cryptococcal pneumonia shows numerous round to oval yeast with occasional single budding within alveolar spaces.

(eFig. 6.5). The cells appear to be surrounded by a thin halo, which actually corresponds to a mucinous capsule. This capsule is highlighted with mucin stains such as mucicarmine, a discriminating feature for diagnosis (Fig. 6.10) (eFig. 6.6). The organisms can also be highlighted with PAS and Fontana–Masson. A capsule-deficient form of *C. neoformans* has also been described and is typically found in immunocompromised patients. These forms may present a challenge for diagnosis as they will be negative or react only weakly with the mucicarmine stain. Culture or immunohistochemistry may be necessary to establish a definitive diagnosis.[4]

Candidiasis

Candidiasis is caused by yeast that is a normal commensal organism in the respiratory, gastrointestinal, and genitourinary tracts or normal individuals. In immunocompromised states, these organisms become pathogenic and invade into the tissues. The most common pathogenic organism in humans is *Candida albicans*. *Candida glabrata* (formerly *Torulopsis glabrata*) is also becoming increasingly recognized as a human pathogen. Pulmonary candidiasis usually manifests with unilateral or bilateral consolidation resulting in lobar, segmental, or patchy pneumonia.[14]

Candida species are small oval yeasts (2 to 6 μm) that show budding and are accompanied by pseudohyphae and occasionally true hyphae. The pseudohyphae are elongated structures that often tend to line up in chains

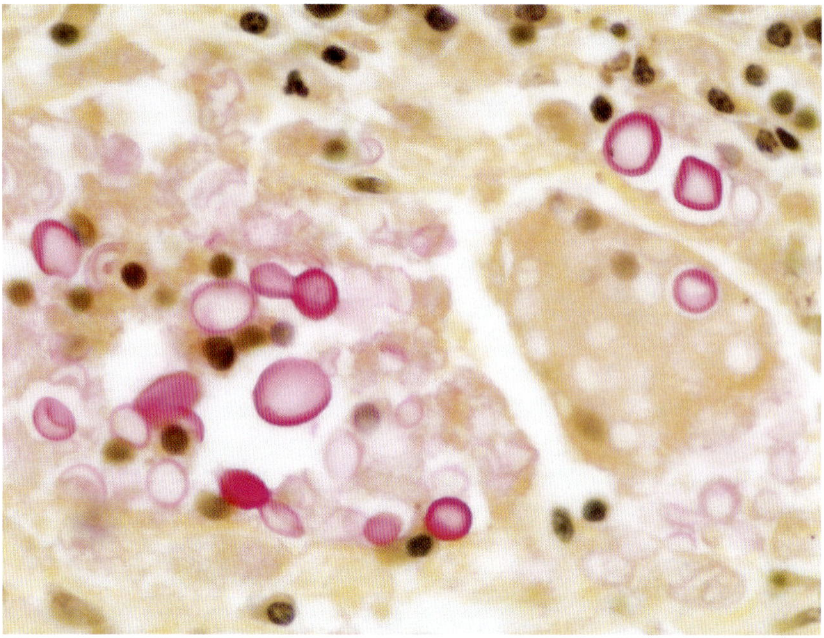

FIGURE 6.10 Mucicarmine stain in cryptococcal pneumonia shows round to oval yeast surrounded by a thick mucinous capsule and showing a few budding forms.

and show irregular branching at acute angles (Fig. 6.11). The pseudohyphae show constrictions at the points of attachment with other pseudohyphae but, unlike true hyphae, are not septated. The organisms are highlighted by PAS, GMS, and Gram stains. *C. glabrata* is characterized only by the yeast form and does not form hyphae or pseudohyphae. Histologically, *Candida* infection is characterized by necrotic and hemorrhagic nodules containing colonies of organisms admixed with fibrinopurulent exudate. Infarcts may occur secondary to vascular occlusion by organisms (eFigs. 6.7 and 6.8). Rarely, *Candida* may show very few pseudohyphae or present only the yeast form, closely resembling *Histoplasma*. Unlike the organisms in histoplasmosis, *Candida* organisms will stain positive with the tissue Gram stain. Furthermore, *H. capsulatum* characteristically shows an intracellular location within histiocytes, whereas *Candida* is always extracellular.

Pneumocystosis

Pneumocystosis is an important cause of opportunistic pneumonia in immunosuppressed patients.[15] Although formerly classified as a protozoan, *P. carinii* is currently classed as a fungus related to the *Saccharomyces*, and the species infecting humans has been renamed *Pneumocystis jirovesi*.[16,17] The organism is most likely acquired through airborne inhalation of respiratory secretions. Initial exposure causes subclinical infection followed by a latent state that develops into opportunistic infection when the patient

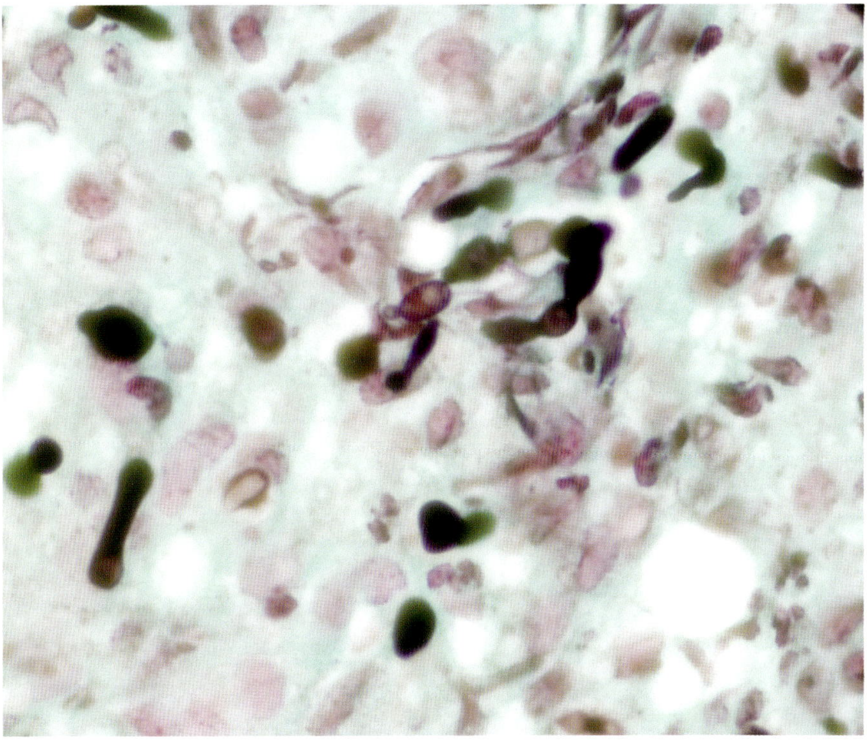

FIGURE 6.11 Silver stain in patient with *Candida* pneumonia shows small round to oval yeast admixed with pseudohyphae.

becomes immunosuppressed. Pneumocystosis can be reliably diagnosed by transbronchial lung biopsy, although equally effective approaches include cytologic examination of bronchoalveolar lavage fluid, bronchial washings, or sputum specimens. Clinically patients present with bilateral fine infiltrates in the perihilar region that progress to diffuse bilateral airspace consolidation involving mainly the lower lobes. AIDS patients may develop thin-walled bilateral cysts in the upper lobes in subpleural distribution.

Histologically, the typical lesion of *P. carinii* pneumonia comprises intra-alveolar foamy eosinophilic exudates containing the small organisms.[18] The frothy appearance of the eosinophilic exudate is caused by the accumulation of organisms (Figs. 6.12 and 6.13). The cysts of *Pneumocystis* are 5 to 7 μm in diameter and are round to oval. Collapsed and crescent-shaped forms are also seen. Small round, centrally placed dark-staining dots are often present within the cysts. Another distinctive feature is the presence of slender grooves or longitudinal folds in the cysts owing to collapse of the cyst wall. The best stain for demonstrating the cysts is the GMS stain (Fig. 6.14). Immunohistochemistry can also be performed in formalin-fixed paraffin-embedded tissue sections using a commercially available monoclonal antibody (Fig. 6.15).[19] The alveolar walls usually

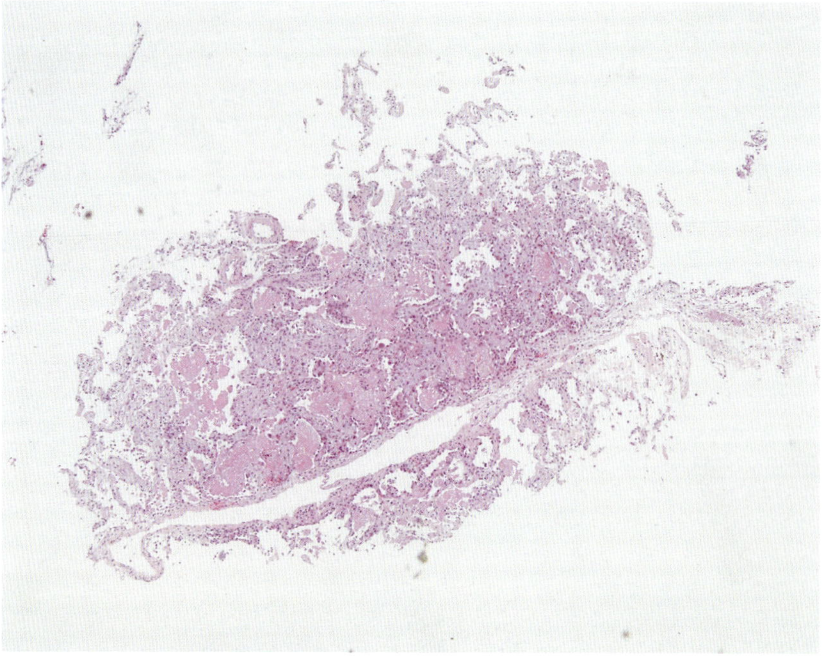

FIGURE 6.12 Transbronchial biopsy in AIDS patient with *Pneumocystis carinii* pneumonia. Notice eosinophilic exudates within alveolar lumens.

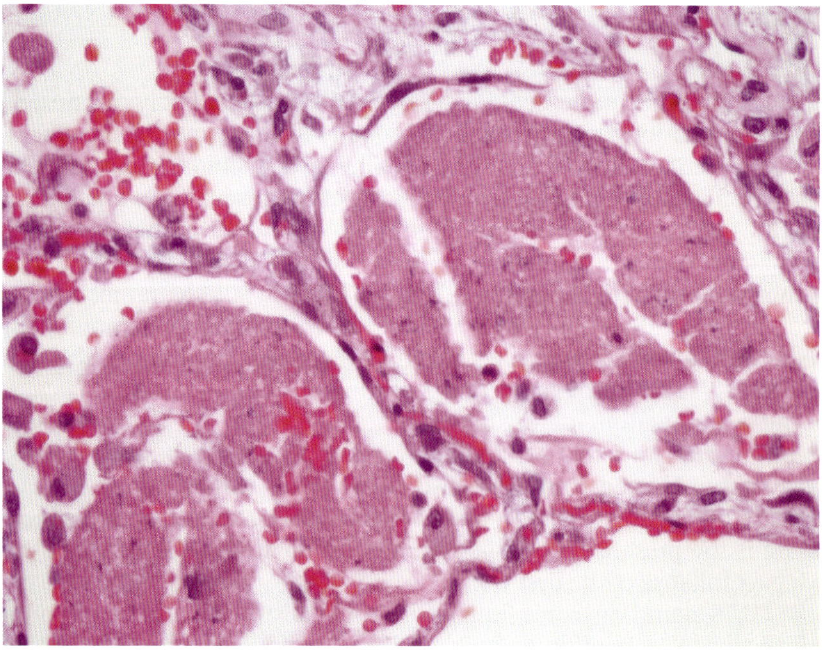

FIGURE 6.13 Higher magnification of lung biopsy with *Pneumocystis carinii* pneumonia showing granular eosinophilic exudates filling the alveolar lumens.

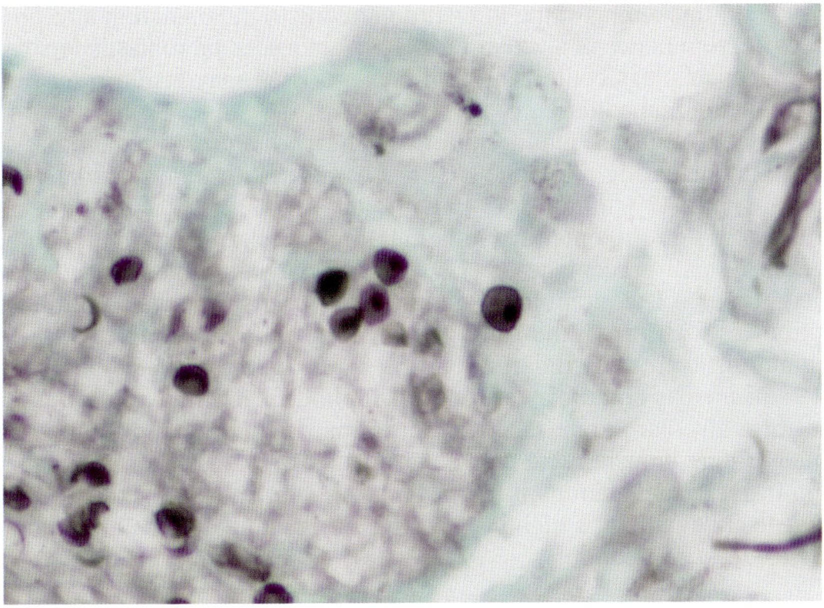

FIGURE 6.14 Silver stain (GMS) highlights the organisms of *Pneumocystis carinii* within the intra-alveolar exudates. The cysts are round to oval with centrally placed dark-staining dots but may also show collapsed or crescent-shaped forms.

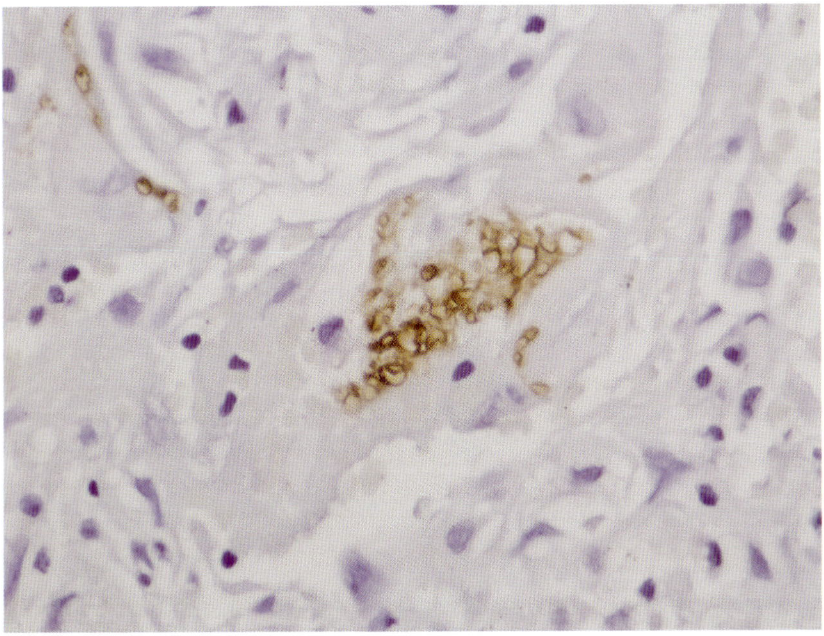

FIGURE 6.15 Immunoperoxidase stain with antibodies against *Pneumocystis carinii* shows positive-staining round organisms within the lumen of an alveolus.

show mild thickening of the interstitium owing to inflammation and fibrosis, with prominence of alveolar type II pneumocytes. Fibroblastic foci with intra-alveolar plugs comprising fibromyxoid tissue may result in an organized pneumonia pattern.

A few unusual manifestations of *Pneumocystis* pneumonia are worth underscoring. Absence of the characteristic foamy exudate may occur in up to 47% of non-HIV patients and in up to 19% of HIV-infected patients.[20,21] Granulomatous inflammation can be seen in lung biopsies in a small percentage of HIV-positive patients with *Pneumocystis* pneumonia.[22] The granulomas comprise clusters of small epithelioid histiocytes with or without multinucleated giant cells, admixed with the characteristic frothy exudates (Fig. 6.16). In malnourished infants, the interstitium may contain a very dense lymphocytic infiltrate that can mask the intra-alveolar exudates.[23] Calcifications are another unusual occurrence in lung biopsies where alveolar exudates are absent or inconspicuous. In fact, calcifications in lymph nodes, liver, spleen, or kidney in an HIV-positive patient is highly suggestive of disseminated extrapulmonary *Pneumocystis* infection.[24]

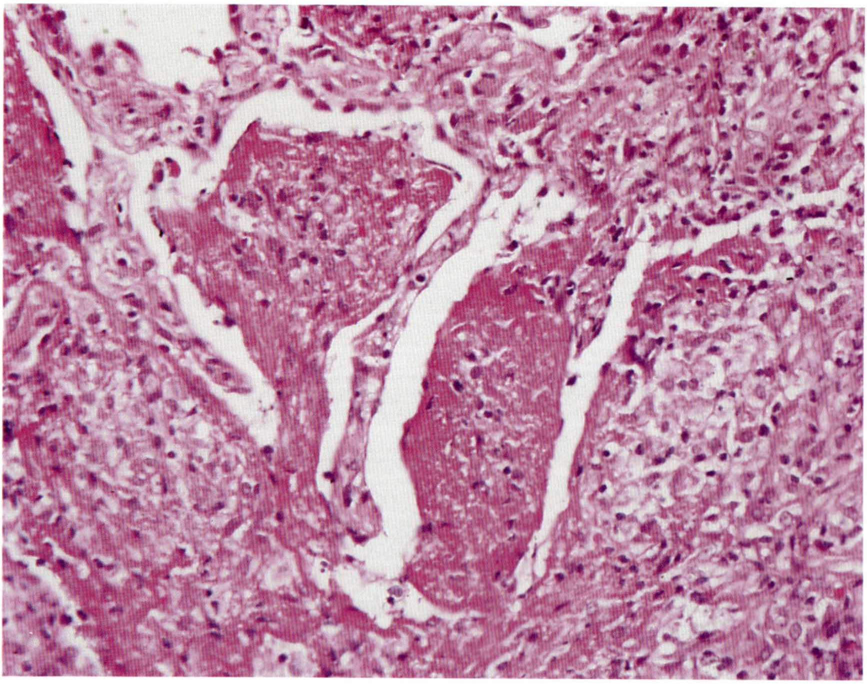

FIGURE 6.16 Granulomatous *Pneumocystis carinii* lung infection characterized by clusters of epithelioid histiocytes surrounding the frothy exudates. A high level of clinical suspicion and use of silver stains should lead to the correct diagnosis in such cases.

Penicilliosis

Penicilliosis is caused by a dimorphic fungus that is endemic to Southeast Asia, where it represents one of the commonest opportunistic infections in AIDS patients. It is seldom seen in the United States, except in immunocompromised patients who have traveled to endemic areas.[25] Lung infection is caused by inhalation of contaminated air. The organisms cause acute necrotizing pneumonia. The airspaces are stuffed with alveolar macrophages containing abundant organisms (Fig. 6.17). The organisms are round or oval yeast (2.5 to 5 μm) characterized by a single transverse septum. Short hyphal forms and elongated, curved sausage-shaped forms may also be seen in necrotic and cavitary lesions.

Coccidiodomycosis

Coccidiodomycosis is a fungal disease endemic to the southwestern United States (where it is also known as San Joaquin Valley fever) caused by a soil fungus, *C. immitis*. The fungus thrives in hot, dry climates and desert soil.[26] The disease shows a wide spectrum of morphologic manifestations in the lungs, including asymptomatic primary

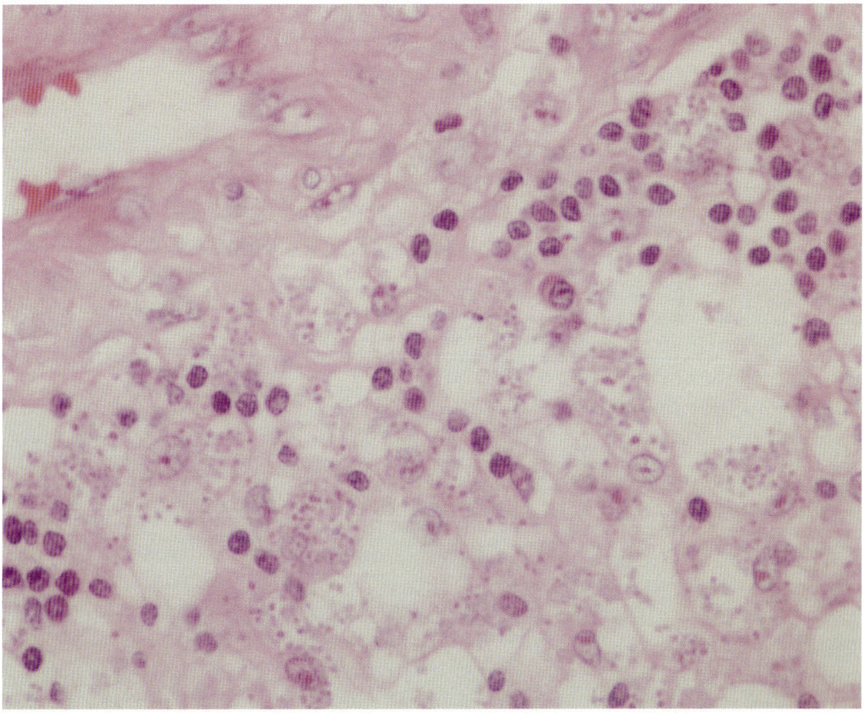

FIGURE 6.17 Numerous small round or oval yeast are present within alveolar macrophages in patient with pulmonary penicilliosis.

infection, solitary parenchymal nodules, acute bronchopneumonia, eosinophilic pneumonia, chronic progressive disease with miliary and cavitary lesions, and systemic dissemination.[27] Histologically, the hallmark of the infection is the production of necrotizing and nonnecrotizing granulomas (Fig. 6.18). Mycetomas (fungus balls) may occur within cavitary lesions.[28] In tissue sections, *Coccidioides* is seen as mature or immature spherules and endospores (eFig. 6.9). The spherules are large (30 to 100 μm), round to oval, and contain multiple endospores that measure from 2 to 5 μm (Fig. 6.19). The diagnosis of the disease requires the identification of the endosporulating organism. Immature spherules lack endospores. The mature spherules have a thick refractile wall. When mature spherules rupture, they spill their endospores into the surrounding tissues; the endospores stain with GMS and PAS stains (Fig. 6.20). Vegetative forms may also be seen in tissue sections and comprise 2 to 4 μm-thick septate hyphae that produce chains of barrel-shaped arthroconidia. The latter are usually present in cavitary lesions and in fungus balls and may cause problems for distinguishing from other hyphae-producing fungi (Table 6.2). When endospores cannot be identified in the spherules, definitive diagnosis may require culture, serologic testing, or immunofluorescence.[29]

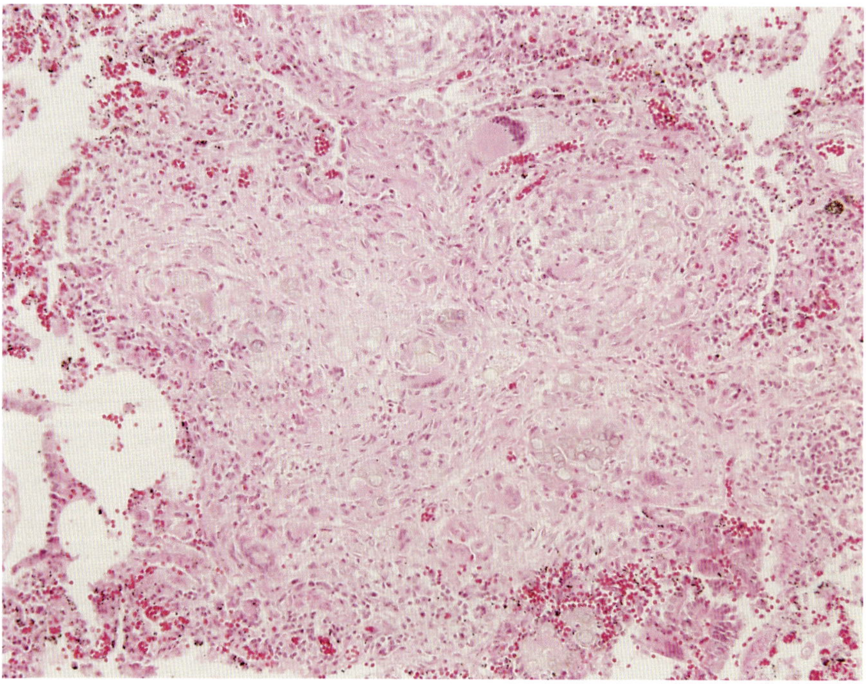

FIGURE 6.18 Granulomatous pneumonitis in coccidioidomycosis. Notice the epithelioid granulomas containing numerous fungal organisms within multinucleated giant cells.

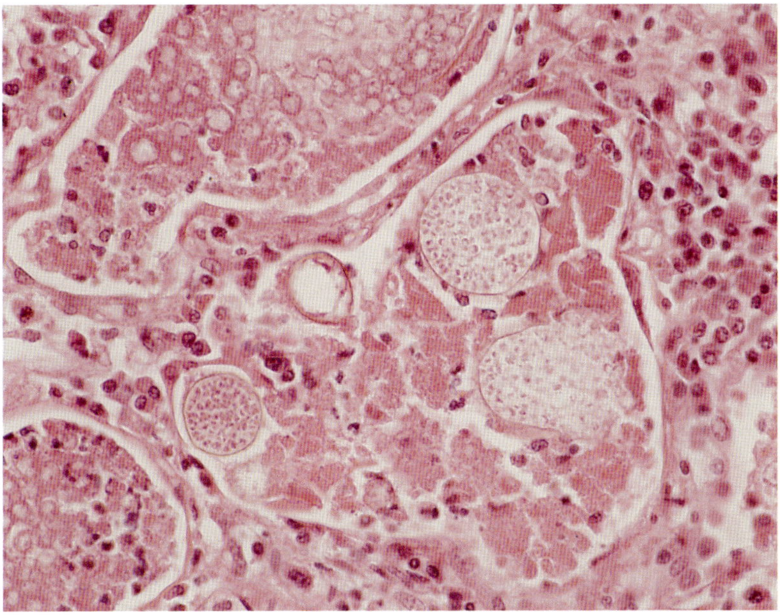

FIGURE 6.19 Higher magnification of lung infection with *Coccidiodes immitis* shows abundant spherules within multinucleated giant cells. Some of the spherules are large and contain multiple endospores.

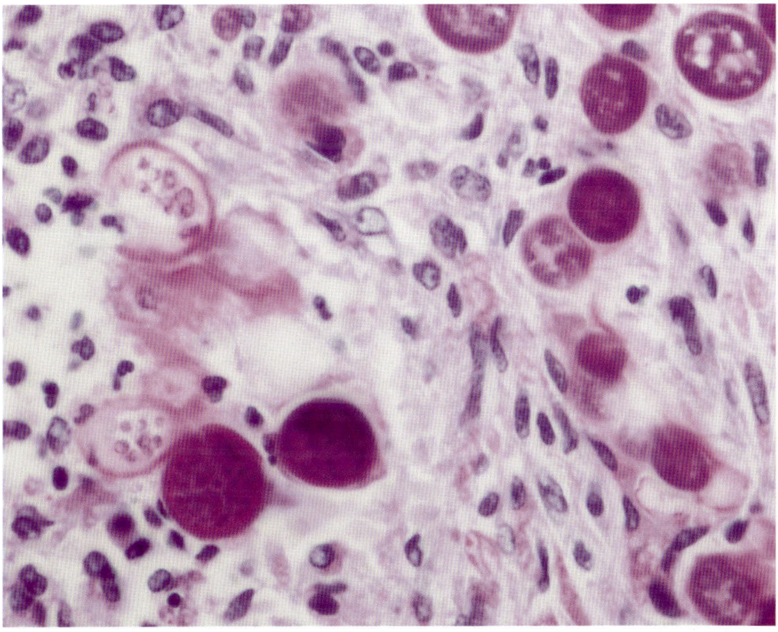

FIGURE 6.20 PAS stain highlights the spherules in coccidioidomycosis. Notice that some of the spherules contain abundant small endospores.

TABLE 6.2 Differential Diagnosis of Lung Infections Caused by Elongated Hyphal Organisms

Organism	Size	Shape	Lesions	Distinguishing Features
Candida albicans	2–6 μm width	Round to oval yeast admixed with pseudohyphae (elongated branching structures without septae)	Suppurative, necrotizing inflammation No granulomas or foamy histiocytes	Pseudohyphae without septae admixed with smaller yeast forms Gram positive Extracellular location
Aspergillus	3–6 μm width	Elongated septate hyphae with dichotomous branching Fruiting bodies and conidial heads	Necrotizing inflammation with angioinvasion	Septate hyphae with regular branching at acute angles May show swelling of hyphae resembling zygomycosis PAS and GMS positive
Zygomycetes	5–25 μm width	Broad, thin-walled hyphae with few septae and irregular branching at wide angles	Necrotizing inflammation with angioinvasion	Thick hyphae with irregular branching at wide angles GMS positive
Vegetative forms of Coccidioides	2–4 μm width	Septate hyphae and chains of barrel-shaped arthroconidia	Necrotizing inflammation in cavitary lesions	Need to find large spherules with endospores for definitive diagnosis

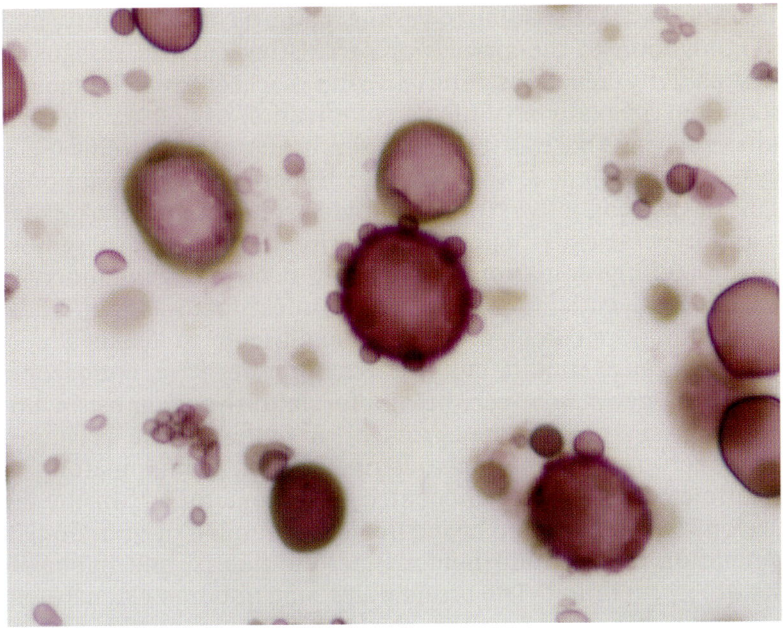

FIGURE 6.21 Pulmonary infection by *Paracoccidioides brazilensis* shows large yeast with multiple buds resembling a mariner's wheel (GMS stain).

Paracoccidioidomycosis

Paracoccidioidomycosis, also known as South American blastomycosis, is a fungal infection caused by *Paracoccidioides brazilensis*. The disease is endemic to tropical regions of South America and is caused by inhalation of the organisms.[30] The lungs are the primary site of infection but in more than 60% of patients the disease becomes systemic. Pulmonary infection may be acute or chronic and can mimic those of tuberculosis and sarcoidosis. The main histologic manifestation is that of necrotizing granulomas. The histologic hallmark of the disease is the presence of yeasts (blastoconidia) with multiple buds. The organisms are large round yeast of varying sizes (4 to 60 μm) surrounded by a thick wall. Multiple buds are seen in the periphery of the yeast imparting them with the distinctive "mariner's wheel" or "ship's wheel" appearance (Fig. 6.21). In tissues the organisms are best demonstrated with GMS stains.

FUNGI CHARACTERIZED BY ELONGATED HYPHAL FORMS

Aspergillosis

Aspergillosis is an infection caused by a mold, *Aspergillus*, of ubiquitous distribution. The most common types are *Aspergillus fumigatus*, *Aspergillus flavus*, and *Aspergillus niger*. The molds are inhaled into the respiratory tract, leading to various patterns of lung injury, including colonization of the airways or preexisting cavities (fungus ball), hypersensitivity reactions, and invasive aspergillosis. Fungus balls (aspergilloma) usually result from colonization of preexisting cavitary lesions, such as those of tuberculosis, bronchiectasis, chronic lung abscess, histoplasmosis, and cancer.[31] Hypersensitivity reactions can present in the lung in two forms: allergic bronchopulmonary aspergillosis and hypersensitivity pneumonitis. Acute invasive aspergillosis is a life-threatening condition that usually occurs in immunocompromised patients. Patients present with clinical features that resemble acute bacterial pneumonia. It can be difficult to make a correct diagnosis because sputum cultures are often negative; endoscopic or open lung biopsy may be very helpful for definitive diagnosis. Chronic necrotizing aspergillosis, the chronic form of the disease, is characterized by necrotizing granulomatous pneumonia, granulomatous bronchiectatic cavities, or bronchocentric granulomatosis.[32] In the latter, the lesions develop around bronchioles surrounded by granulomatous inflammation and contain mucus, necrotic debris, and hyphal fragments of *Aspergillus*.[33] The bronchioles may undergo extensive squamous metaplasia owing to the chronic irritation by the organisms (Fig. 6.22).

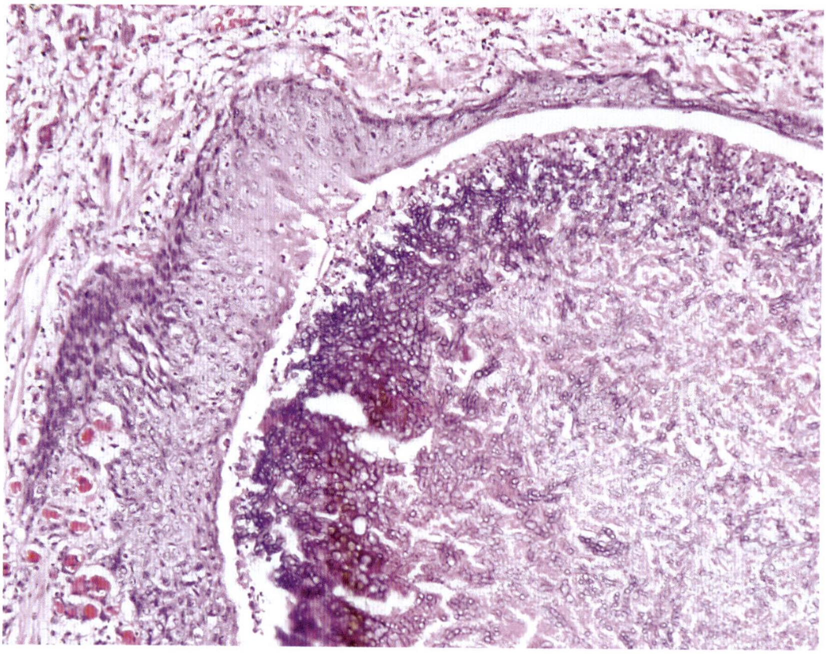

FIGURE 6.22 Extensive squamous metaplasia of a bronchiole is observed in this biopsy. The lumen of the bronchiole is filled with septate, branching hyphae of *Aspergillus*.

Aspergillus species is characterized in tissue sections by elongated, septate, and branching hyphae that are 3 to 6 μm in width. The hyphae tend to grow in an orderly, parallel fashion and show septa at regular intervals without constrictions at the points of septation. The branches of the hyphae are dichotomous, that is, the size of the branches is the same as the parent hyphae, and they are usually seen at acute angles (45°) (Fig. 6.23). The hyphae may show degenerative changes such as swelling of hyphal segments, making them difficult to distinguish them from that of other fungi such as mucormycosis. The organisms are easily visualized on H&E stains but are better highlighted with PAS or GMS stains (Fig. 6.24). *Aspergillus niger* is associated with deposits of calcium oxalate crystals. When the organisms are found in cavities exposed to air, they can develop fruiting bodies and conidial heads, which consist of a central vesicle surrounded by sterigmata and chains of conidia resembling a flower in bloom (Figs. 6.25 and 6.26). In chronic granulomatous lesions, the hyphae may be surrounded by the Splendori–Hoeppli phenomenon comprising radiating eosinophilic material at the periphery of the fungal mass. In acute invasive aspergillosis, there is extensive infarction of lung parenchyma with invasion of vessel walls and vascular occlusion by the organisms.

The diagnosis of pulmonary aspergillosis is usually straightforward in most cases; however, degenerative changes can make definitive diagnosis

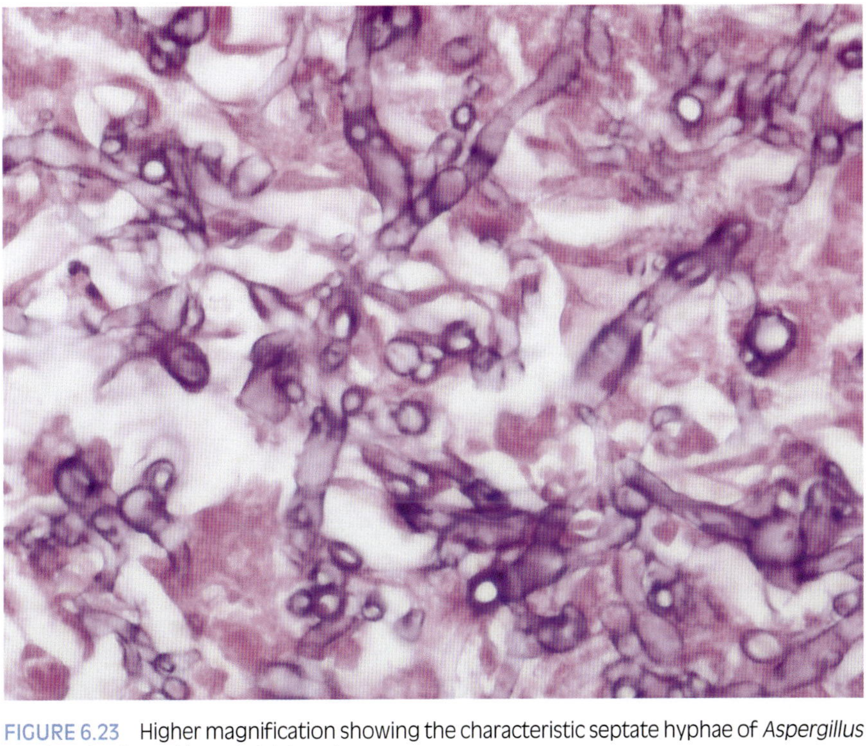

FIGURE 6.23 Higher magnification showing the characteristic septate hyphae of *Aspergillus* sp. showing branching at right angles.

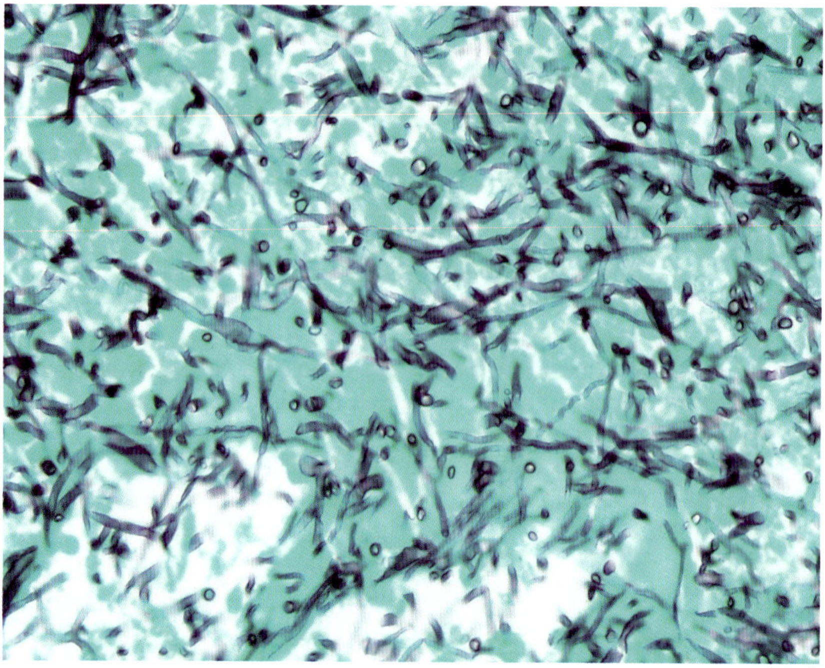

FIGURE 6.24 Silver stain (GMS) highlights the organisms in invasive aspergillosis. Notice branching septate hyphae.

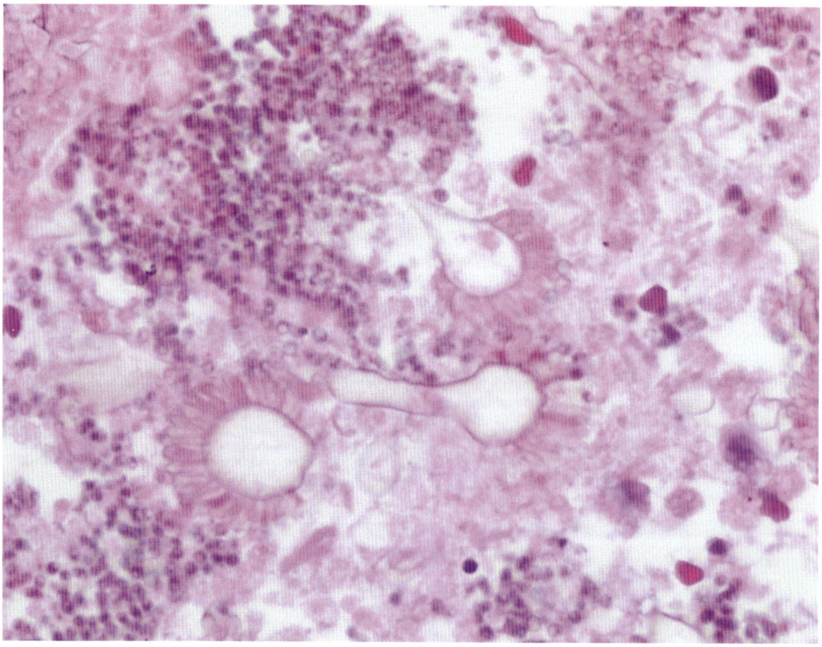

FIGURE 6.25 Fruiting bodies and conidial heads are seen in pulmonary aspergilloma. Notice central vesicles surrounded by multiple sterigmata resembling the petals of a flower.

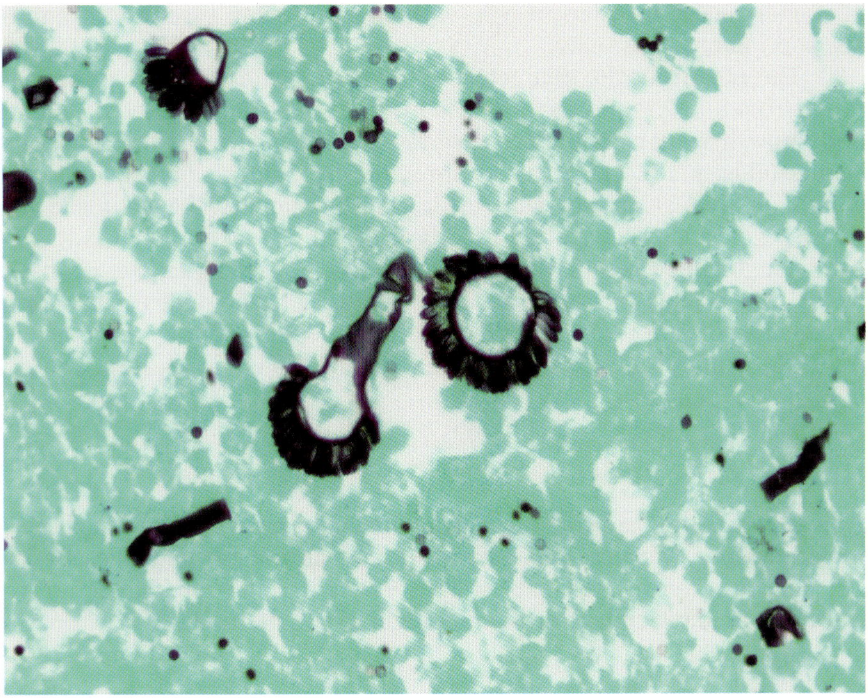

FIGURE 6.26 GMS stain in pulmonary aspergilloma highlights fruiting bodies and conidial heads.

difficult in some cases (Table 6.2). In particular, it can be difficult to separate *Aspergillus* from zygomycetes, *Fusarium,* and *Pseudoallescheria boydii*, requiring confirmation of the diagnosis by culture or immunologic methods.

Zygomycosis

Zygomycosis are fungi belonging to the class of *Zygomycetes* that share with *Aspergillus* the capacity for angioinvasion leading to hemorrhagic infarcts. There are two orders of *Zygomycetes*: the Mucorales and the Enteromophthorales; however, the majority of human disease is caused by the Mucorales, which includes the genera *Absidia, Rhizopus, Rhizomucor,* and *Mucor*, among others. Despite the fact that historically, the taxonomically incorrect term "mucormycosis" has been used for these infections, the majority of cases are caused by *Absidia* and *Rhizopus.*[34] Pulmonary infection occurs by inhalation of the spores or by percutaneous routes and is most often seen in the setting of immunosuppression, hematopoietic malignancies, and diabetes mellitus with acidosis.[35] There is a broad spectrum of pulmonary disease that includes solitary or multiple nodular lesions, segmental or lobar consolidation, cavitary lesions, infarcts and formation of fungus balls.[36] The lesions can undergo direct extension into the chest cavity and organs. Pulmonary zygomycosis is characterized by invasive growth, with angioinvasion, vascular thrombosis, and infarcts (Fig. 6.27).

The organisms are characterized by broad, thin-walled hyphae that range from 5 to 25 μm in width. The hyphae are usually twisted or folded and show irregular branching at wide angles and few or inconspicuous septae (eFig. 6.10). On cross sections, the hyphae can appear as large, round, or oval structures with clear centers that may be confused for other organisms. The hyphae usually stain very weakly with H&E and can be highlighted with GMS stain (Fig. 6.28). In cavitary lesions exposed to air, the hyphae may develop large, spherical, or ovoid, thick-walled chlamydospores at their ends. These are densely basophilic and positive for PAS. Culture or immunohistochemical methods are the best way to confirm the diagnosis.

OTHER RARE FUNGAL DISORDERS

A number of other less common fungal infections can be seen in the lungs, including sporotrichosis, phaeohypomycosis, fusariosis, psedoallescheriasis, adiaspiromycosis, and malassesiasis. These are quite rare and definitive diagnosis requires culture or immunologic testing methods.[37]

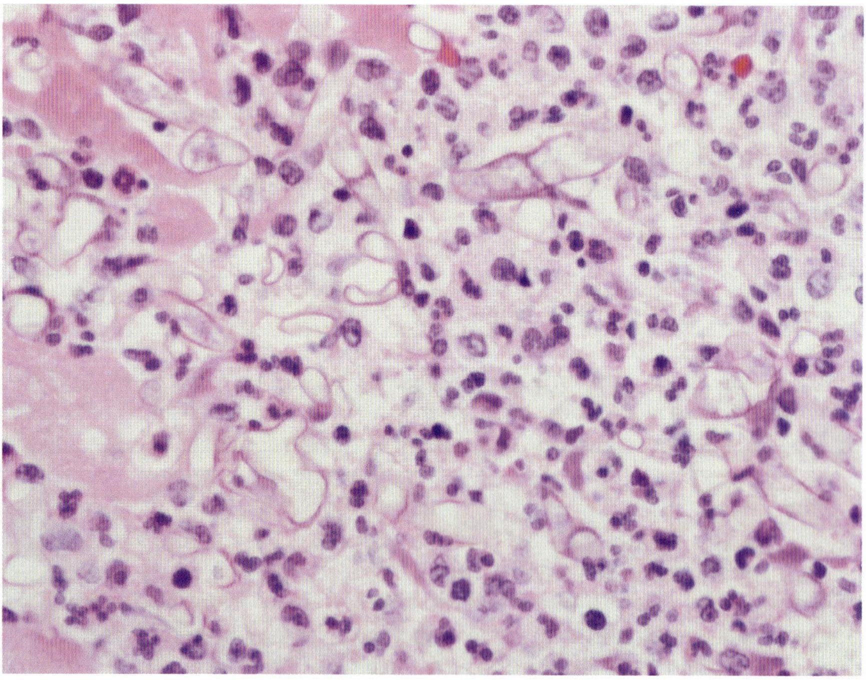

FIGURE 6.27 Necrotizing pneumonitis in zygomycosis owing to *Mucor* species shows broad, thin-walled hyphae that show irregular twisting and folding and show irregular branching.

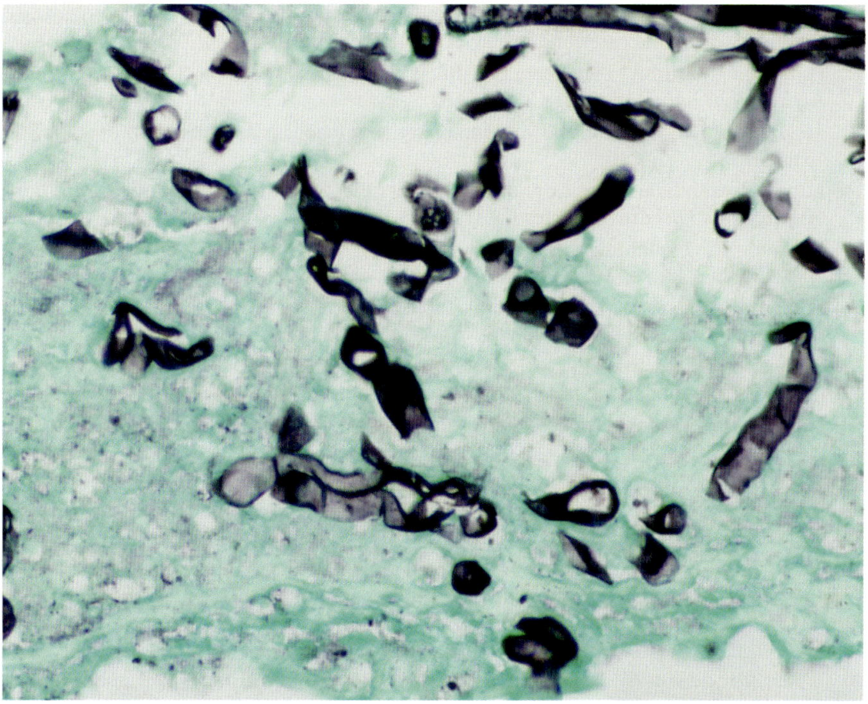

FIGURE 6.28 GMS stain highlights the organisms in pulmonary infection by Zygomycetes.

REFERENCES

1. El-Zammar OA, Katzenstein AL. Pathological diagnosis of granulomatous lung disease: a review. *Histopathology*. 2007;50:289–310.
2. Saubolle M. Fungal pneumonias. *Semin Respir Infect*. 2000;15:162–177.
3. Watts JC, Chandler FW. Morphologic identification of mycelia pathogens in tissue sections: a caveat. *Am J Clin Pathol*. 1998;109:1–2.
4. Cartun RW. Use of immunohistochemistry in the surgical pathology laboratory for the diagnosis of infectious disease. *Pathol Case Rev*. 1999;4:260–265.
5. Wolk D, Mitchell S, Patel R. Principles of molecular microbiology testing methods. *Infect Dis Clin North Am*. 2001;15:1157–1204.
6. Wheat J. Endemic mycoses in AIDS: a clinical review. *Clin Microbiol Rev*. 1995;8: 146–159.
7. Goodwin RA Jr, Shapiro JL, Thurman GH, et al. Disseminated histoplasmosis: clinical and pathologic correlations. *Medicine (Baltimore)*. 1980;59:1–33.
8. Chandler FW, Watts JC. *Pathologic Diagnosis of Fungal Infections*. Chicago, IL: American Society of Clinical Pathologists; 1987.
9. Lemos LB, Baliga M, Guo M. Blastomycosis: the great pretender can also be an opportunist. Initial clinical diagnosis and underlying disease in 123 patients. *Ann Diagn Pathol*. 2002;6:194–203.
10. Glassroth J. Fungal infections complicating HIV infection. In: Sarosi GA, Davies SF, eds. *Fungal Diseases of the Lung*. 3rd ed. Philadelphia, PA: Lippincott Williams & Wilkins; 2002:213–218.

11. Lemos LB, Baliga M, Guo M. Acute respiratory distress syndrome and blastomycosis: presentation of nine cases and review of the literature. *Ann Diagn Pathol.* 2001;5:1–9.
12. Hussain Z, Martin A, Youngberg GA. *Blastomyces dermatitidis* with large yeast forms. *Arch Pathol Lab Med.* 2001;125:663–664.
13. McDonnell JM, Hutchins GM. Pulmonary cryptococcosis. *Hum Pathol.* 1985;16: 121–128.
14. Luna MA. Candidiasis. In: Connor D, Chandler FW, Schwartz DA, et al, eds. *Pathology of Infectious Diseases.* Stamford, CT: Appleton and Lange; 1997:953–964.
15. Feldman C. Pneumonia associated with HIV infection. *Curr Opin Infect Dis.* 2005;18:165–170.
16. Edman JC, Kovacs JA, Masur H, et al. Ribosomal RNA sequence shows *Pneumocystis carinii* to be a member of the fungi. *Nature.* 1988;334:519–522.
17. Stringer JR, Beard CB, Miller RF, et al. A new name (*Pneumocystis jirovesi)* for pneumocystis from humans. *Emerg Infect Dis.* 2002;8:891–896.
18. Schliep TC, Yarrish RL. *Pneumocystis carinii* pneumonia. *Semin Respir Infect.* 1999;14:333–343.
19. Blumenfeld W, Kovacs JA. Use of a monoclonal antibody to detect *Pneumocystis carinii* in induced sputum and bronchoalveolar lavage fluid by immunoperoxidase staining. *Arch Pathol Lab Med.* 1988;112:1233–1236.
20. Travis WD, Pittaluga S, Lipschick GY, et al. Atypical pathologic manifestations of *Pneumocystis carinii* pneumonia in the acquired immune deficiency syndrome. Review of 123 lung biopsies from 76 patients with emphasis on cysts, vascular invasion, vasculitis and granulomas. *Am J Surg Pathol.* 1990;14:615–625.
21. Weber WR, Askin FB, Dehner LP. Lung biopsy in *Pneumocystis carinii* pneumonia: a histopathologic study of typical and atypical features. *Am J Clin Pathol.* 1977;67:11–19.
22. Cupples JB, Blackie SP, Road JD. Granulomatous *Pneumocystis carinii* pneumonia mimicking tuberculosis. *Arch Pathol Lab Med.* 1985;113:1281–1284.
23. Dutz W. *Pneumocystis carinii* pneumonia. *Pathol Annu.* 1970;5:309–341.
24. Feuerstain IM, Francis P, Raffeld M, et al. Widespread visceral calcifications in disseminated *Pneumocystis carinii* infection: CT characteristics. *J Comput Assist Tomogr.* 1990;14:149–151.
25. Deng ZL, Connor DH. Progressive disseminated penicilliosis caused by *Penicillium marneffei*: report of eight cases and differentiation of the causative organism from *Histoplasma capsulatum. Am J Clin Pathol.* 1985;84:323–327.
26. Davis SF, Sarosi GA. Fungal infections. In: Murray JF, Nadel JA, Mason RJ, et al, eds. *Textbook of Respiratory Medicine.* 3rd ed. Philadelphia, PA: WB Saunders Co; 2000:1107–1141.
27. Ampel NM. Coccidioidomycosis. In: Sarosi GA, Davis SF, eds. *Fungal Diseases of the Lung.* 3rd ed. Philadelphia, PA: Lippincott Williams & Wilkins; 2000:59–78.
28. Winn RE, Johnson R, Galgiani JN, et al. Cavitary coccidioidomycosis with fungus ball formation. Diagnosis by fiberoptic bronchoscopy with coexistence of hyphae and spherules. *Chest.* 1994;105:412–416.
29. Kaplan W, Kraft DE. Demonstration of pathogenic fungi in formalin-fixed tissues by immunofluorescence. *Am J Clin Pathol.* 1969;52:420–432.
30. Taborda AB, Arechavala AI. Paracoccydioidomycosis. In: Sarosi GA, Davies SF, eds. *Fungal Diseases of the Lung.* 3rd ed. Philadelphia, PA: Lippincott William and Wilkins; 2000:79–90.
31. Regnard JF, Icard P, Nicolosi M, et al. Aspergilloma: a series of 89 surgical cases. *Ann Thorac Surg.* 2000;69:898–903.
32. Yousem SA. The histological spectrum of chronic necrotizing forms of pulmonary aspergillosis. *Hum Pathol.* 1997;28:650–656.

33. Tron V, Churg A. Chronic necrotizing pulmonary aspergillosis mimicking bronchocentric granulomatosis. *Pathol Res Pract.* 1986;181:621–626.
34. Ribes JA, Vanover-Sams CL, Baker DJ. Zygomycetes in human disease. *Clin Microbiol Rev.* 2000;13:236–301.
35. Kontoyiannis DP, Wessel VC, Bodey GP, et al. Zygomycosis in the 1990s in a tertiary-care cancer center. *Clin Infect Dis.* 2000;30:851–856.
36. McAdams HP, Rosado-de-Christenson ML, Templeton PA, et al. Thoracic mycoses from opportunistic fungi: radiologic–pathologic correlation. *Radiographics.* 1995;15: 271–286.
37. Travis WD, Colby TV, Koss MN, et al. Non-neoplastic disorders of the lower respiratory tract. In: *Atlas of Nontumor Pathology.* Vol 2. Washington, DC: Armed Forces Institute of Pathology; 2002:592–638.

7

PARASITIC LUNG INFECTIONS

Pulmonary parasitic infections are rare and are hardly ever encountered in lung biopsy samples. Tourism and increased travel to endemic areas, however, can expose patients to a variety of parasites, thus posing a challenge for diagnostic surgical pathologist unfamiliar with these conditions. Several species of parasites migrate through the lungs as part of their life cycle, but few actually infect the lung. Most parasitic infections in the lung result from systemic dissemination in immunocompromised patients. Some of the more common parasitic lung pathogens are listed in Table 7.1. When parasites migrate to lung tissue, they usually elicit an intense inflammatory reaction with neutrophils, eosinophils, lymphocytes, and plasma cells that may produce various patterns of lung injury, including eosinophilic pneumonia, small or large nodular lesions, bronchitis, and bronchiolitis, and abscess cavities and cysts.

PROTOZOAL INFECTIONS

Amebiasis

Amebiasis is one of the most common parasitic infections in underdeveloped tropical countries caused by *Entamoeba histolytica*. The disease is primarily acquired through ingestion of contaminated water and food and can also be transmitted sexually among homosexual men. The disease causes gastrointestinal infection with mucosal ulceration that may spread to the liver causing amebic liver abscess. Pleuropulmonary complications of amebiasis occur in up to 20% of patients with hepatic infection. The organisms can reach the lung through direct invasion owing to rupture of a hepatic abscess into the lung or by hematogenous spread from the liver.[1] Rupture of an amebic liver abscess into the thoracic cavity may also cause a bronchopulmonary fistula. Pulmonary amebiasis is characterized by the formation of multiple abscesses that contain yellow–brown fluid.[2] The center of the abscess shows inflammatory cells admixed with necrotic debris and contains scattered trophozoites (Fig. 7.1) (eFig. 7.1). In histologic sections, the trophozoites measure approximately 15 to 25 μm in diameter and display a sharply defined cell membrane with clear to lightly eosinophilic cytoplasm that may contain red blood cells or other cellular debris and a small nucleus showing accentuation

TABLE 7.1 Common Lung Parasitic Infections

Protozoa	Amebiasis
	Toxoplasmosis
	Cryptosporidiosis
	Microsporidiosis
Nematodes	Dirofilariasis
	Filariasis
	Strongyloidiasis
Trematodes	Paragonimiasis
	Schistosomiasis
Cestodes	Echinococcosis

of the nuclear membrane. The cytoplasm also contains abundant glycogen that stains strongly with periodic acid–Schiff (PAS) stain (Fig. 7.2). The trophozoites may be difficult to visualize on routine examination and can be confused with histiocytes, but they have smaller nuclei and are slightly larger than histiocytes.

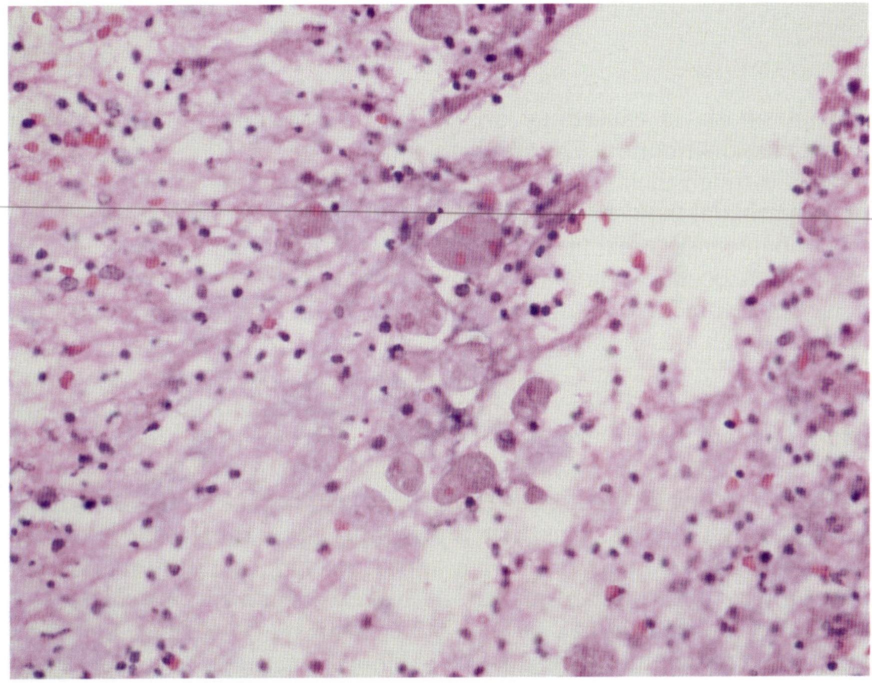

FIGURE 7.1 Pulmonary abscess caused by amebiasis. Notice scattered necrotic debris and large trophozoites with sharply defined cell membranes, abundant lightly eosinophilic cytoplasm, and occasional ingested red blood cells.

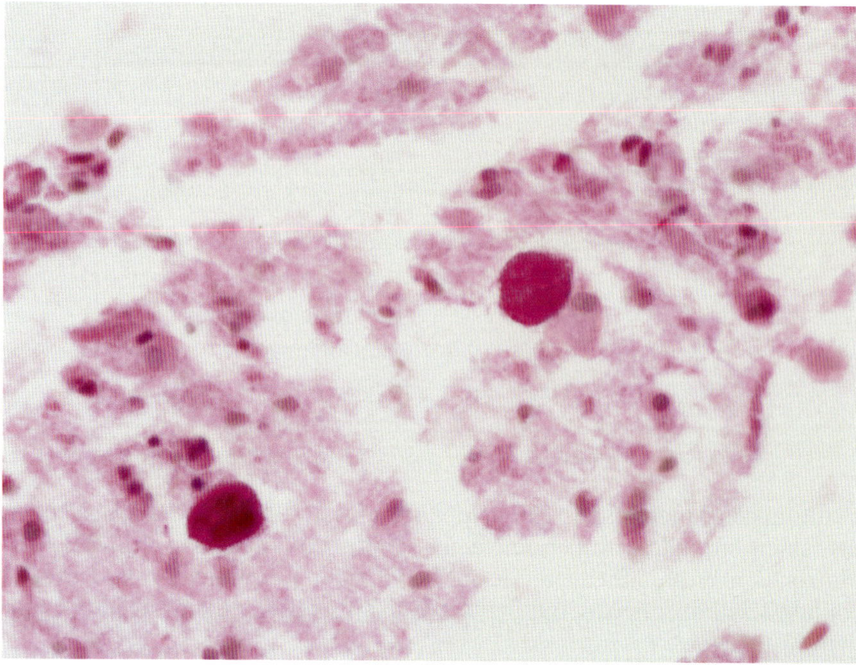

FIGURE 7.2 PAS stain highlights the organisms in amebic abscess of the lung.

Toxoplasmosis

Toxoplasmosis is caused by an obligate intracellular protozoan with worldwide distribution, *Toxoplasma gondii*. The infection is transmitted by cats through their feces but can also be acquired by eating raw meat or by perinatal exposure from an infected mother. Acute toxoplasmosis most often causes a painless, self-limited lymphadenopathy. Systemic dissemination occurs in immunocompromised patients or in patients with defective cell-mediated immunity.[3] The organisms are transported to the lungs through the bloodstream and lymphatics. In the lung, the organisms cause diffuse acute bronchopneumonia with occasional cavitation. Toxoplasmosis is a common opportunistic infection in AIDS patients.[4] In AIDS patients, the diffuse pulmonary opacities caused by toxoplasmosis must be distinguished from pneumocystosis. Histologically, the organisms (tachyzoites) invade the host cells and grow within the cytoplasm forming cysts and pseudocysts. The cysts are slightly larger than histiocytes and contain numerous bradyzoites that appear as dark, uniform dots within the cytoplasm. The organisms can be readily visualized on hematoxylin and eosin (H&E) and can be highlighted with the PAS stain. Serologic tests are very helpful for diagnosis (Sabin–Feldman dye test; differential agglutination test). Immunohistochemistry using a monoclonal antibody or polymerase chain reaction (PCR) can also help identify the organism in tissue sections.

Cryptosporidiosis

Cryptosporidiosis is caused by an intestinal protozoan, *Cryptosporidium parvum*, which rarely affects the lungs. The main clinical manifestation is acute diarrhea owing to colonization of the gastrointestinal tract epithelium. It is a common opportunistic infection in AIDS patients; approximately 10% to 15% of AIDS patients will develop pulmonary cryptosporidiosis.[5]

Pulmonary involvement is rare and most likely secondary to aspiration associated with fecal–oral spread in debilitated patients. Respiratory infection is characterized by tracheitis, bronchitis, and bronchiolitis. There is usually a very mild chronic inflammatory reaction, but the organisms are most commonly seen in the luminal aspect of the respiratory mucosa.[6] The organisms comprise small (4 to 6 μm), round to oval, basophilic structures that can be very easily missed on cursory examination. They appear to be lying in a single row on the surface of the respiratory mucosa and can be highlighted with the PAS, Giemsa, or Gomori methenamine silver (GMS) stain. The biggest challenge for diagnosis is overlooking the organisms in tissue sections.

Microsporidiosis

Microsporidiosis is an infection caused by a protozoan, *Encephalitozoon* and *Enterocytozoon bieneusi*. Microsporidium is a well-recognized opportunistic pathogen in AIDS patients that can affect kidney, gastrointestinal and biliary tracts, cornea, and brain. In the lungs, the disease is most often the result of dissemination from the gastrointestinal or biliary tract.[7] The diagnosis is most often established by cytologic examination of bronchioalveolar lavage fluid.[8] PCR techniques are useful for identifying the species. In tissue sections from lung biopsies, the organisms are found within bronchial and bronchiolar epithelial cells, where they grow within vacuoles in the apical aspect of the cells. A mild acute and chronic inflammatory reaction is seen in the mucosa. The intracytoplasmic spores are very small (1 to 1.5 μm) and appear as slightly basophilic small dots on H&E stains. They are gram-positive and weakly acid-fast. Some organisms can also stain with GMS, but the Brown and Brenn stain is the most reliable for visualization in routine histologic sections. The parasites are also birefringent. Because of their small size and subtle appearance, it is very easy to miss them on cursory examination.

NEMATODES

Dirofilariasis

Dirofilariasis is a disease caused by a parasite of dogs and other mammals, *Dirofilaria immitis* (or dog heartworm). The disease is transmitted by mosquitoes who inject the larvae into the skin from where they migrate to the heart. The parasites enter the pulmonary arterial circulation and become implanted in the periphery of the lungs where they form a small nodule containing a central zone of infarction surrounded by a rim of fibrosis (eFigs. 7.2 to 7.4). A dead worm can be usually identified within the lumen of a vessel. The worm will elicit an intense granulomatous reaction (Fig. 7.3). The organism measures approximately 120 to 300 μm in diameter, is densely eosinophilic, and is surrounded by a smooth cuticle with prominent external striations (Figs. 7.4 and 7.5). The lesions are usually stable and do not progress over time. Because of their peripheral location, dirofilariasis is not diagnosed on endoscopic biopsies, but may be seen in core biopsies or video-assisted thoracoscopic surgery biopsies done to rule out malignancy.[9]

Filariasis

Filariasis is an infection of the lung caused by *Wuchereria bancrofti*, *Brugia malayi*, and *Onchocerca volvulus*. The parasites are transmitted by infected mosquitoes. Lymphadenopathy and the formation of subcutaneous nodules are the primary manifestation of the disease.[10] However, microfilaria can migrate to the lung and other internal tissues. Pulmonary involvement may take the form of eosinophilic pneumonia, or a pulmonary nodule can develop owing to the nodular infarcts caused by the adult

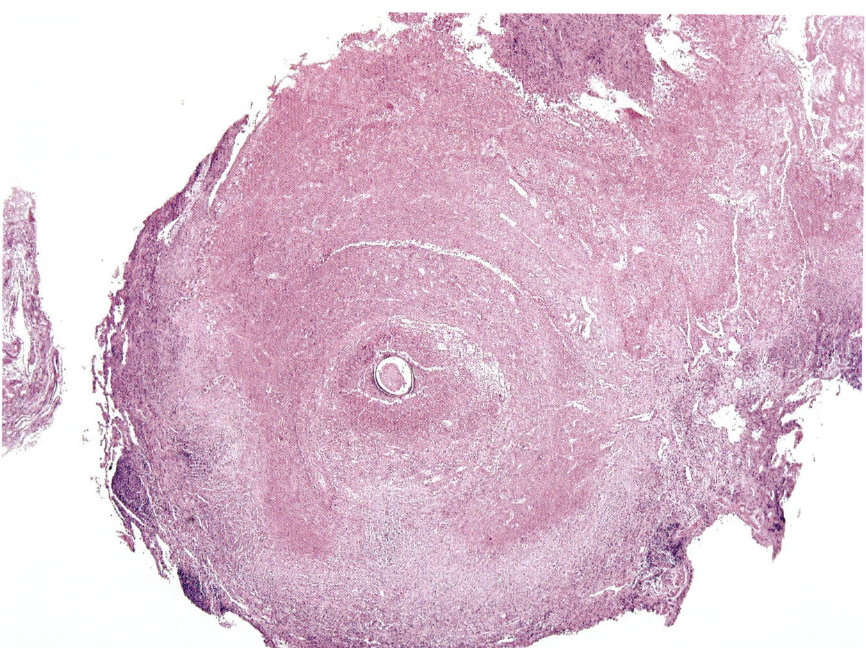

FIGURE 7.3 Pulmonary dirofilaria granuloma. Notice centrally necrotic granuloma surrounded by a rim of epithelioid histiocytes and a single dead worm in the center.

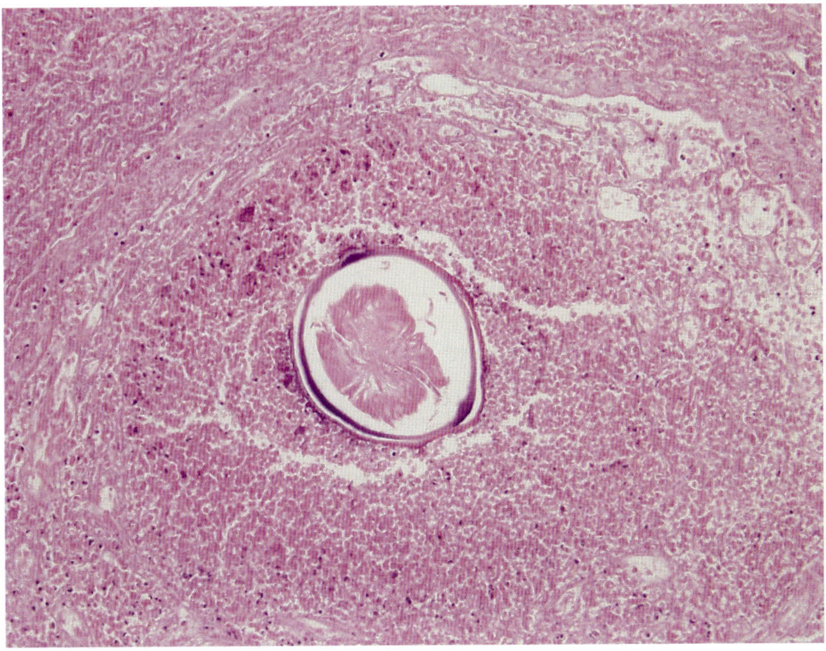

FIGURE 7.4 Higher magnification of dirofilaria granuloma showing cross section of dead worm in the center.

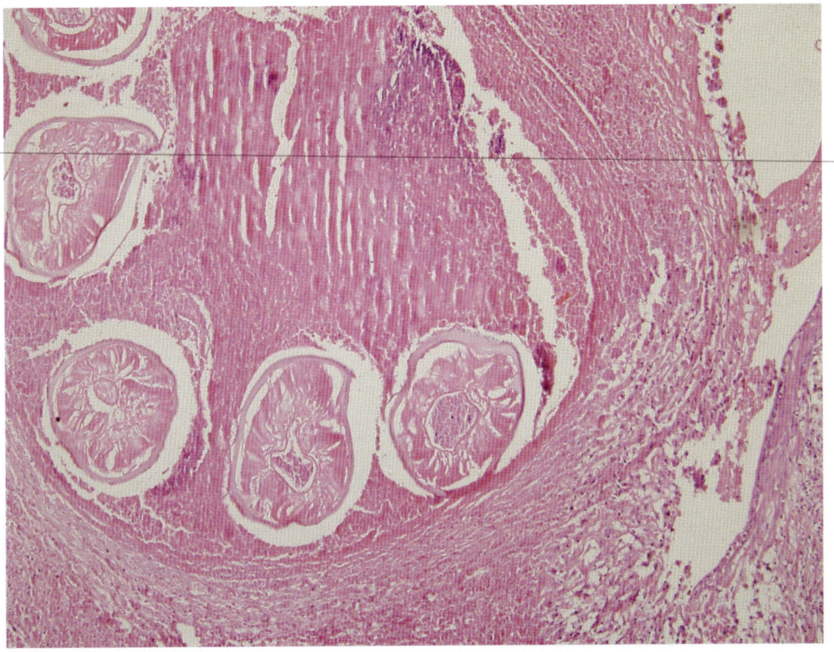

FIGURE 7.5 Another example of lung dirofilaria containing multiple organisms surrounded by a smooth cuticle and with extensive tissue necrosis of the surrounding parenchyma.

worm (eFigs. 7.5 and 7.6). The worms range from 100 to 250 μm in length and show tight coils with multiple cross sections that are surrounded by a thin, finely striated cuticle (Figs. 7.6 to 7.8). In the diffused form, the histologic appearance is that of an eosinophilic pneumonia; microfilariae showing a fine, pointed tail can sometimes be identified within lymphatics.

Strongyloidiasis

Strongyloidiasis is an infection caused by the threadworm, *Strongyloides stercoralis*. The organism penetrates the skin from the soil, and the larvae migrate through the bloodstream into the lungs and then to the gastrointestinal tract where they mature and produce rhabditiform (noninfective) and filariform (infective) larvae. Hyperinfection owing to endogenous reinfection can lead to massive larval infection of the lungs leading to consolidation and acute respiratory distress.[11] Histologically, diffuse alveolar damage and pulmonary hemorrhage are seen. The filariform larvae are 300 to 600 μm long and 10 to 20 μm wide, basophilic, S-shaped, and usually found within the alveolar spaces or bronchioles (Fig. 7.9). Pulmonary strongyloidiasis can be effectively diagnosed on open lung biopsy.[12]

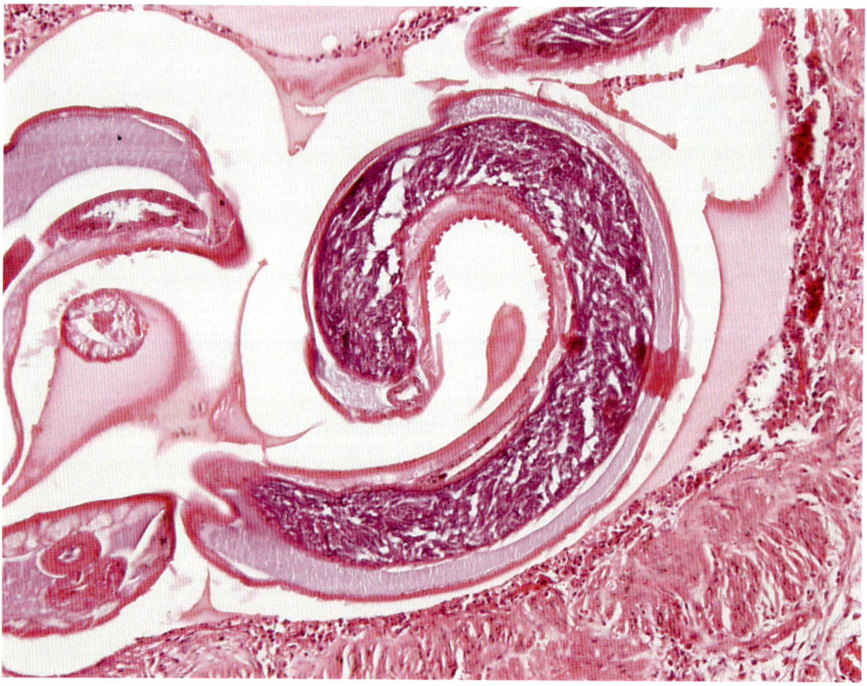

FIGURE 7.6 Pulmonary involvement by *Wuchereria bancrofti* shows coiled adult worm. Notice thin eosinophilic cuticle surrounding the organism.

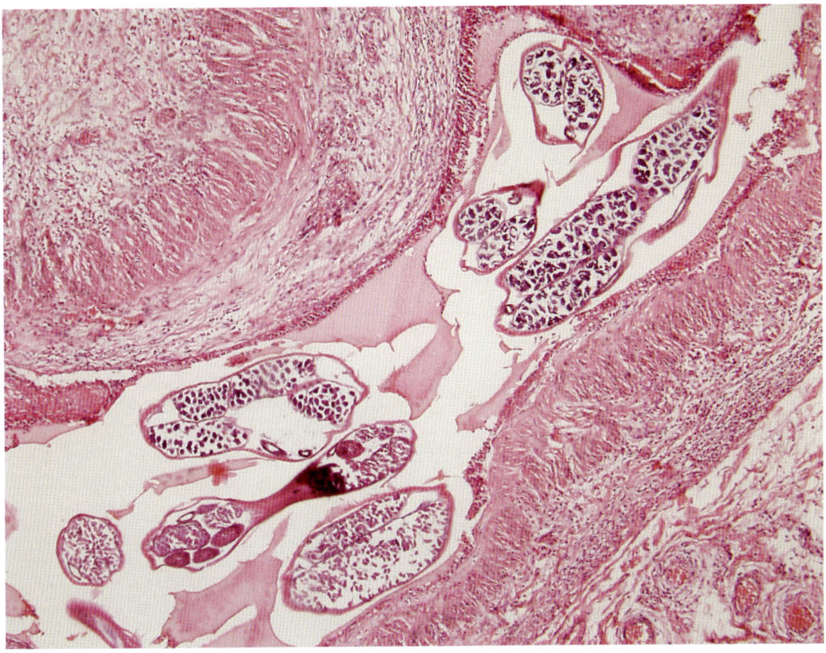

FIGURE 7.7 Another example of pulmonary filariasis showing multiple worms in cross section surrounded by thin eosinophilic cuticles.

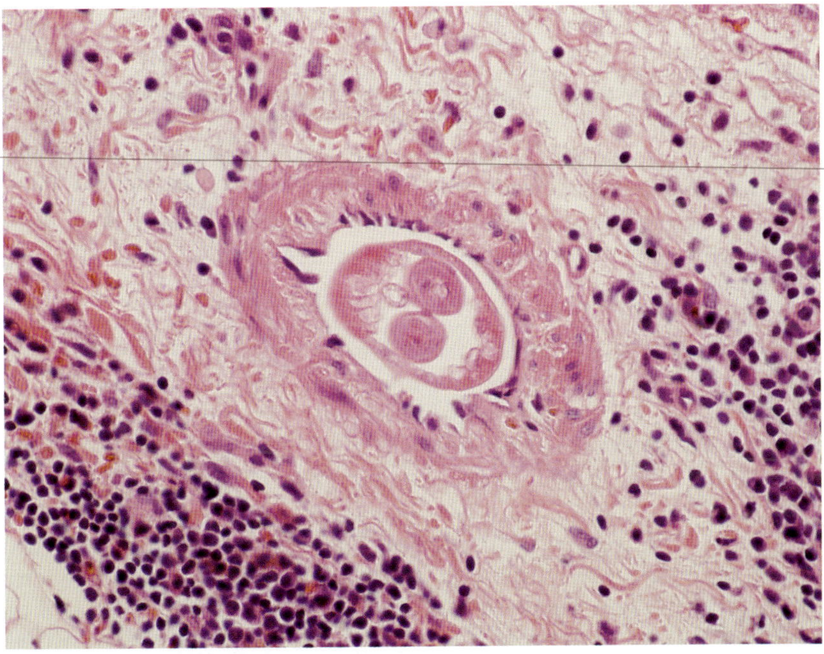

FIGURE 7.8 Cross section of a worm in filariasis owing to *Wuchereria bancrofti* lying within the lumen of small pulmonary vessel.

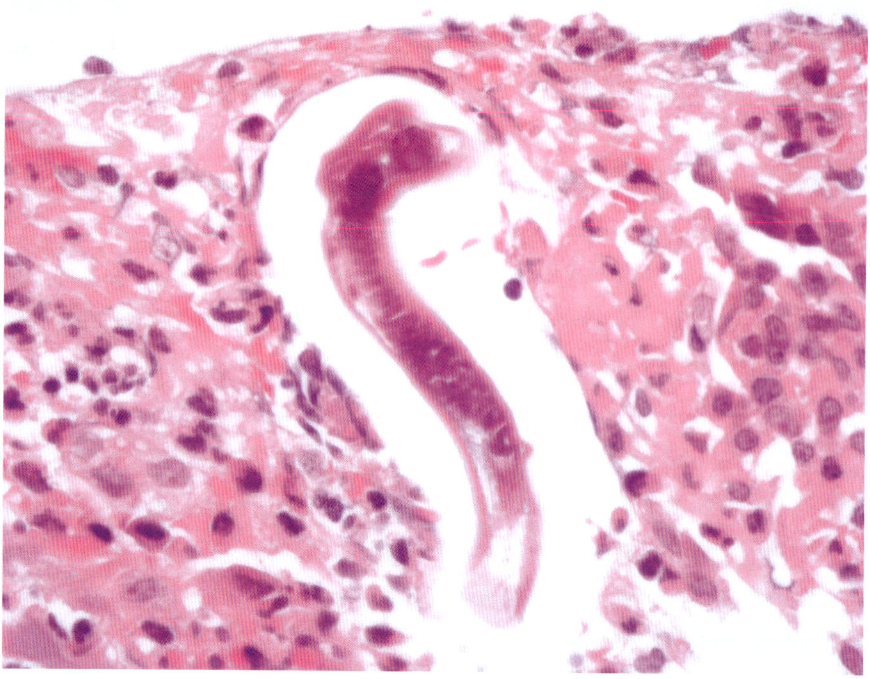

FIGURE 7.9 Larval infection of the lung by *Strongyloides stercoralis* showing S-shaped, basophilic filiform larva lying within alveolar space.

TREMATODES

Paragonimiasis

Paragonimiasis is an infection caused by the oriental lung fluke, *Paragonimus westermani*. Infection is acquired by eating raw or undercooked crabs or crayfish and is most common in Asia. The life cycle starts with a snail that infects a crustacean, where the cercaria develop into cysts (metacercaria), which are later ingested by the definitive host leading to human infection. The larvae pass from the intestines into the peritoneum, through the diaphragm into the chest cavity, and from there to the lungs. In the lungs, the worms are found adjacent to large bronchioles and are surrounded by fibrinopurulent exudate admixed with eosinophils and fibrosis forming a cyst.[13] The cysts are 1.5 cm in diameter and can rupture into the airways spilling eggs that will elicit a granulomatous and fibrosing reaction (Fig. 7.10). The eggs measure 75 to 100 μm, are yellow to brown and oval, have a flattened operculum at one end and a thick birefringent shell, a feature that permits distinction from nonbirefringent schistosoma eggs.

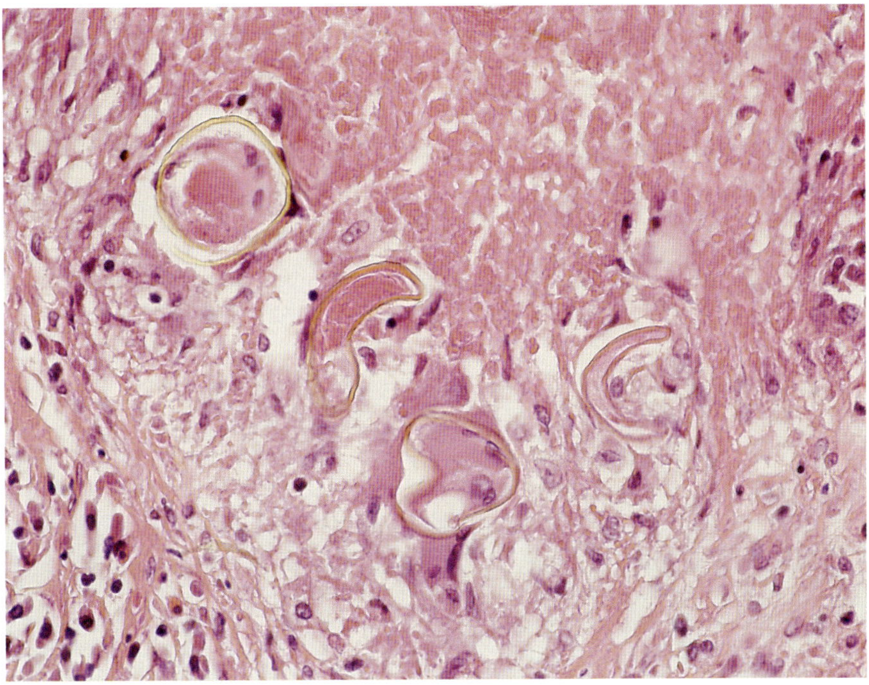

FIGURE 7.10 Cyst of *Paragonimus westermani* in the lung shows oval eggs with thick birefringent shell surrounded by granulomatous and fibrosing reaction.

Schistosomiasis

Schistosomiasis is an infection caused by tropical flukes, namely *Schistosoma mansoni, Schistosoma japonicum*, and *Schistosoma haematobium*. Human infection occurs through exposure to contaminated water infected with cercariae. The cercariae enter the circulation through the skin where they mature into adult worms. The female worm produces eggs that migrate into tissue causing disease. The eggs of *S. mansoni* and *S. japonicum* infect the gut, liver, and lung, whereas the eggs of *S. hematobium* reside mostly in the bladder, ureter, and pelvis. Larval pneumonitis can occur following heavy cercarial exposure and presents with peripheral eosinophilia and basilar patchy consolidation.[14] Chronic disease can present in the form of miliary nodular infiltrates. Histologically, in chronic infection the *Schistosoma* eggs are seen in association with a granulomatous reaction and fibrosis (Fig. 7.11).[15] The eggs are usually deposited in perivascular location and can be recognized by their morphology (Fig. 7.12) (eFig. 7.7). The eggs in *S. hematobium* are characterized by a terminal spine; those of *S. mansoni* have a large lateral spine; and those of *S. japonicum* have a small lateral spine. The eggs may range in size from 100 to 170 μm in diameter. They can be distinguished from those of *Paragonimus* by the smaller size, birefringence of the capsule, and absence of a spine in the latter.

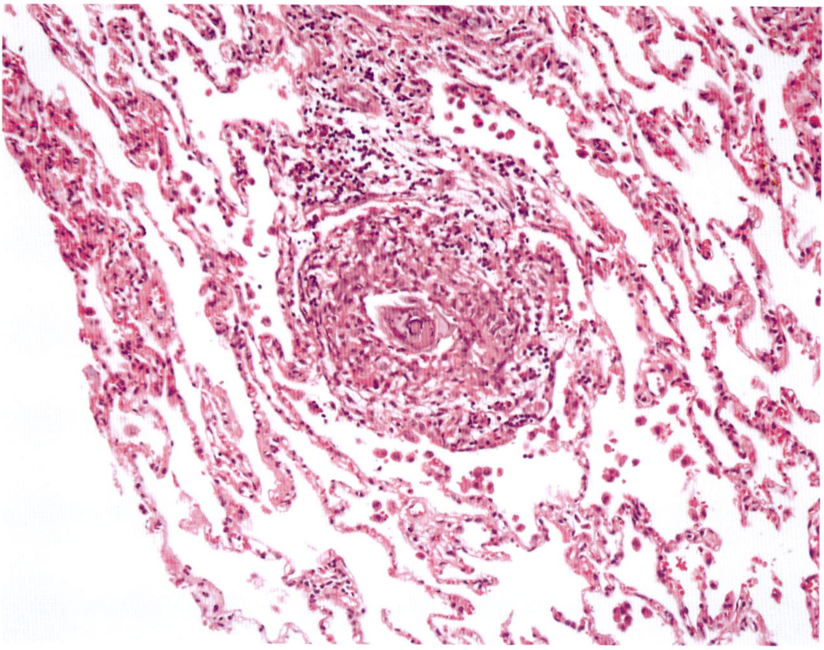

FIGURE 7.11 Pulmonary involvement in schistosomiasis shows pulmonary parenchyma containing a small egg surrounded by prominent granulomatous reaction.

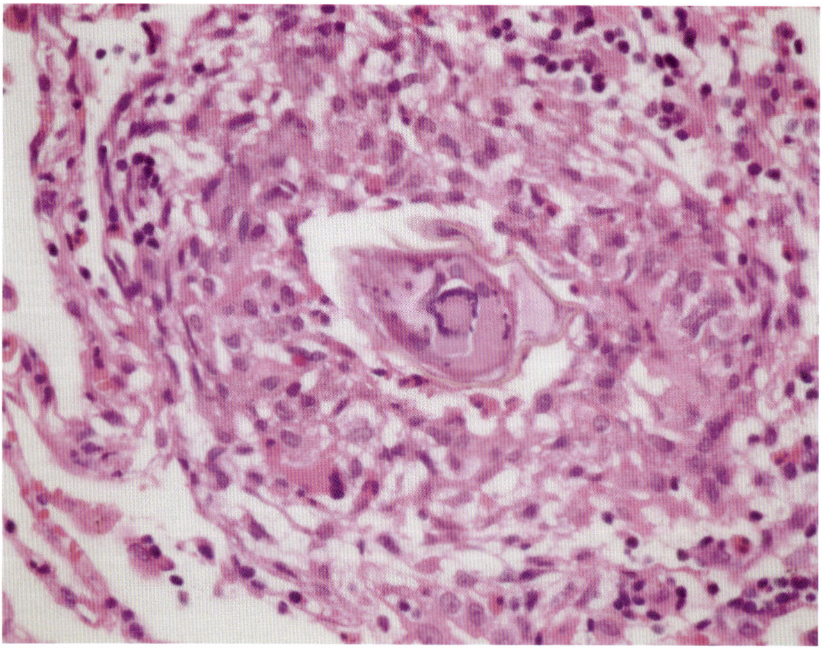

FIGURE 7.12 Higher magnification of schistosoma granuloma showing the organism with a birefringent capsule and a short lateral spine.

CESTODES

Echinococcosis

Echinococcosis, also known as hydatic disease or hydatidosis, is an infection of the lung caused by the larval tapeworms *Echinococcus granulosus*, *Echinococcus multilocularis*, and *Echinococcus vogeli.* The dog/sheep strain of *E. granulosus* is the most common. The most frequent site of infection following ingestion of the parasites is the liver, followed by the lung. In the lung, the echynoccocal cyst presents as a unilocular or multilocular cyst that can vary in size from a few millimeters to 20 cm.[16] The cyst wall in *E. granulosus* is thick with a hyaline appearance and is lined by a laminated germinal layer that is approximately 1 mm thick (Fig. 7.13) (eFig. 7.8). Attached to the germinal layer are multiple brood capsules that contain protoscolices (Figs. 7.14 and 7.15) (eFigs. 7.9 and 7.10). The protoscolices may lose their teeth-like hooklets that can be found floating in the vicinity of the cyst wall (Fig. 7.16). The hooklets are best identified by lowering the condenser in the microscope, which highlights their refringent appearance. The cyst wall may elicit a necrotizing granulomatous response in the surrounding lung parenchyma.

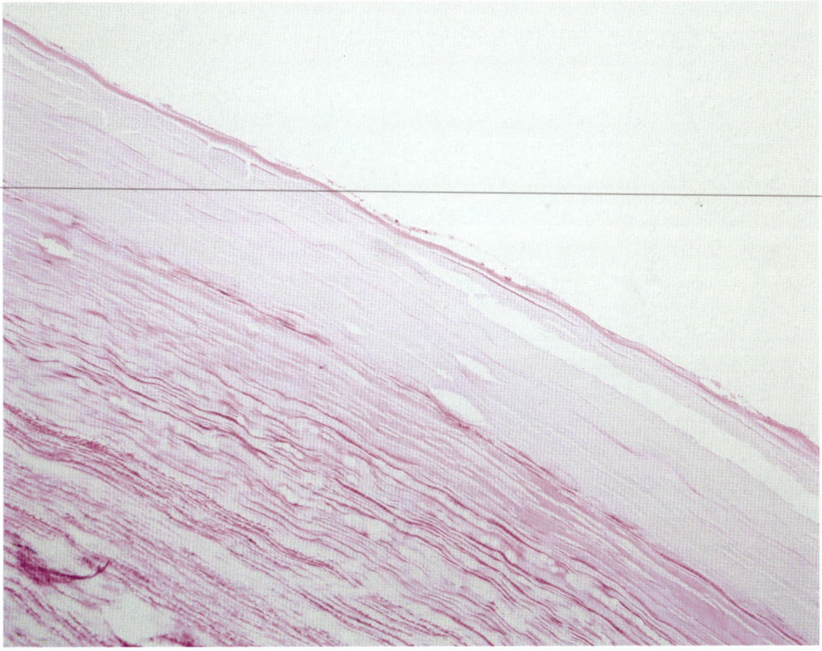

FIGURE 7.13 Hidatid disease of the lung owing to *Echinococcus granulosus* showing characteristic thick hyaline wall of the cyst. Occasionally, this may be the only structure identified in the biopsy.

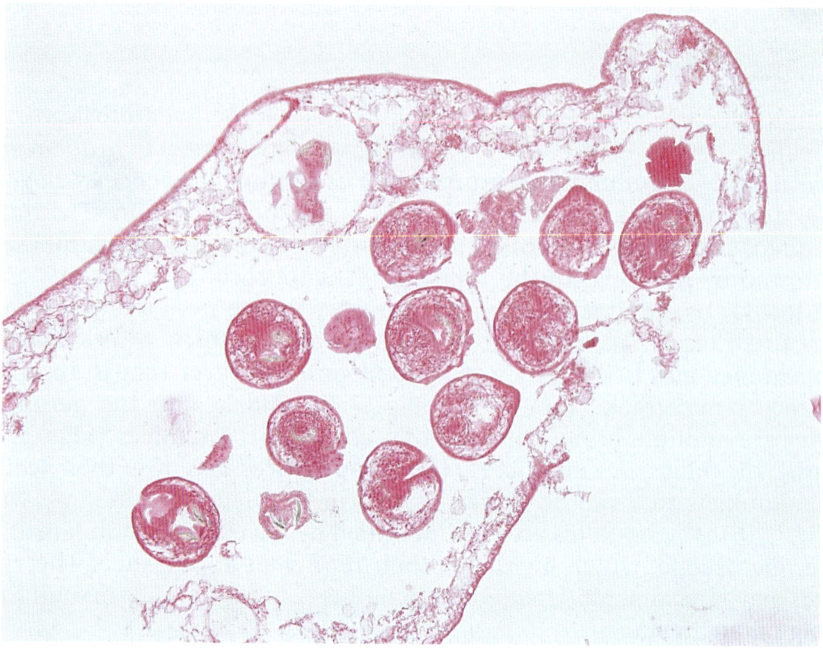

FIGURE 7.14 Fragment of the wall in hydatid cyst lined by hyaline germinal layer and multiple brood capsules.

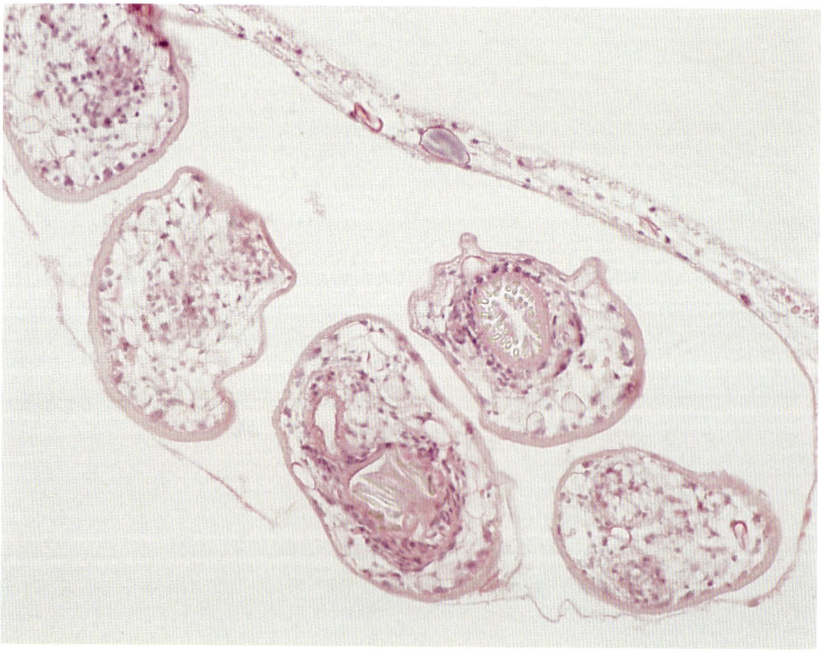

FIGURE 7.15 Higher magnification of brood cysts in hidatidosis showing protoscolices with multiple hooklets.

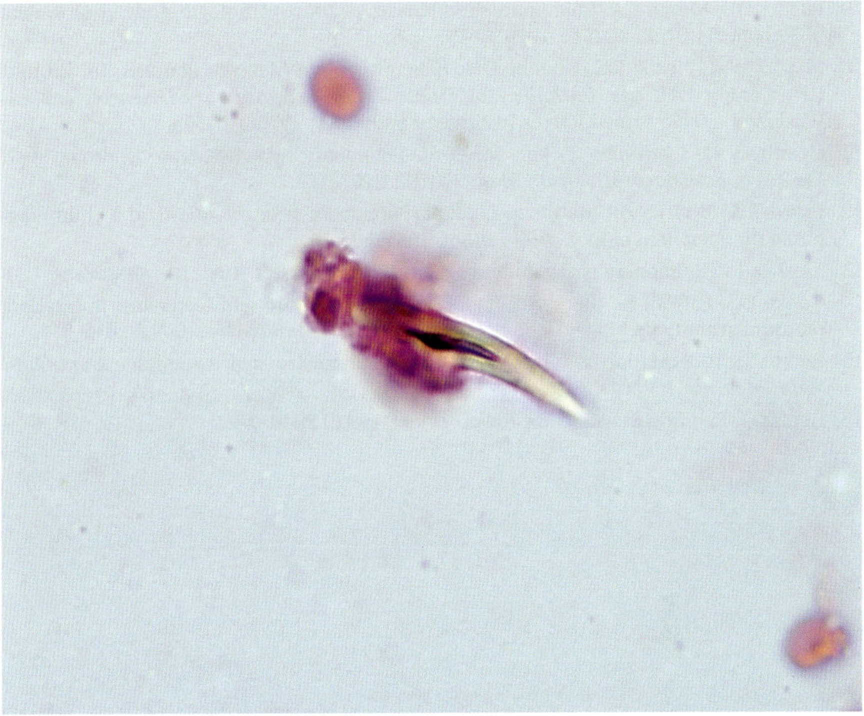

FIGURE 7.16 Tooth-like hooklet in pulmonary hydatidosis. In the absence of brood cysts, hooklets may be the only clue to the nature of the process.

REFERENCES

1. Gopinath R, Nutman TB. Parasitic diseases. In: Murray JF, Nadel JA, Mason RJ, et al., eds. *Textbook of Respiratory Medicine.* 3rd ed. Philadelphia, PA: WB Saunders Co; 2000:1143–1171.
2. Lyche KD, Jensen WA. Pleuropulmonary amebiasis. *Semin Respir Infect.* 1997;12: 106–112.
3. Pomeroy C, Filice GA. Pulmonary toxoplasmosis: a review. *Clin Infect Dis.* 1992;14: 863–870.
4. Nash G, Kerschmann RL, Herndier B, et al. The pathological manifestations of pulmonary toxoplasmosis in the acquired immunodeficiency syndrome. *Hum Pathol.* 1994;25:652–658.
5. Soave R, Johnson WD Jr. *Cryptosporidium* and *Isospora belli* infections. *J Infect Dis.* 1988;157:225–229.
6. Ma P, Villanueva TG, Kaufman D, et al. Respiratory cryptosporidiosis in the acquired immune deficiency syndrome. Use of modified cold Kinyoun and Hemacolor stains for rapid diagnoses. *JAMA.* 1984;252:1298–1301.
7. Weber R, Bryan RT, Schwartz DA, et al. Human microsporidial infections. *Clin Microbiol Rev.* 1994;7:426–461.
8. Remadi S, Dumais J, Wafa K, et al. Pulmonary microsporidiosis in a patient with the acquired immunodeficiency syndrome. A case report. *Acta Cytol.* 1995;39:1112–1116.

9. Flieder DB, Moran CA. Pulmonary dirofilariasis: a clinicopathologic study of 41 lesions in 39 patients. *Hum Pathol.* 1999;30:251–256.
10. Meyers WM, Neafie RC, Connor DH. Bancroftian and Malayan filariasis. In: Binford CH, Connor DH, eds. *Pathology of Tropical and Extraordinary Diseases.* 2nd ed. Washington, DC: Armed Forces Institute of Pathology; 1976:340–355.
11. Upadhyay D, Corbridge T, Jain M, et al. Pulmonary hyperinfection syndrome with *Strongyloides stercoralis. Am J Med.* 2001;111:167–179.
12. Byard RW, Bourne AJ, Matthews N, et al. Pulmonary strongyloidiasis in a child diagnosed on open lung biopsy. *Surg Pathol.* 1993;5:55–61.
13. Kagawa FT. Pulmonary paragonimiasis. *Semin Respir Infect.* 1997;12:149–158.
14. Cooke GS, Lalvani A, Gleeson FV, et al. Acute pulmonary schistosomiasis in travelers returning from Lake Malawi, sub-Saharan Africa. *Clin Infect Dis.* 1999;29:836–839.
15. Bethlem EP, Schettino GdeP, Carvalho CR. Pulmonary schistosomiasis. *Curr Opin Pulm Med.* 1997;3:361–365.
16. Bhatia G. Echinococcus. *Semin Respir Infect.* 1997;12:171–186.

8

VIRAL LUNG INFECTIONS

Viruses are a common cause of infection in the upper and lower respiratory tracts. Although most respiratory viral infections are self-limited, serious, life-threatening disease can also be caused by these agents in both previously healthy and immunocompromised individuals. Outbreaks of respiratory illness are caused every year by certain viruses, including influenza, parainfluenza, respiratory syncytial virus (RSV), and adenovirus.[1] These can be responsible for serious, life-threatening disease in the elderly and immunocompromised patients. Certain viruses, however, are more commonly associated with respiratory infections in immunocompromised patients, such as cytomegalovirus (CMV) and herpes simplex virus.

Viral infection of the pulmonary tract may manifest in a variety of ways, with several possible patterns of lung injury, including diffuse alveolar damage (DAD), acute bronchitis, organizing pneumonia, and diffuse interstitial pneumonia. The histopathologic diagnosis of specific viral infections, however, can be made only by recognizing their characteristic cytopathic effects, including nuclear and cytoplasmic alterations as seen on hematoxylin- and eosin-stained histologic slides on routine light microscopy.[2] Several specific antibodies have been developed for use by immunohistochemistry to identify several common pulmonary viral pathogens.

The most common pattern of lung injury owing to viruses is DAD. However, this is a very nonspecific injury pattern in the lung that can be caused by many other insults, including infections by bacteria, mycobacterial and fungal pneumonias, various forms of lung toxicity, drugs, and inhalation of toxic fumes. A careful search for viral cytopathic effect as well as correlation with the clinical history is indispensable for correct interpretation. The commonest cytopathic effect caused by viruses in the lung is the presence of cytoplasmic or intranuclear inclusions within the infected cells. A summary of the various types of inclusions in the lung is presented in Table 8.1. It is of note that some viral infections affecting the lung, such as hantavirus, influenza virus, and severe acute respiratory syndrome (SARS) coronavirus, do not produce any inclusions that are discernible on routine histologic examination.

TABLE 8.1 Cytopathic Effect in Pulmonary Viral Infections

Virus	Location	Cytopathic Effect
Cytomegalovirus	Nuclear and cytoplasmic	Large cells containing large, round, or oval eosinophilic to basophilic intranuclear or cytoplasmic inclusions
Herpes simplex virus (Varicella–zoster)	Intranuclear	Ground glass amphophylic intranuclear inclusion (early stage); single eosinophilic intranuclear inclusion surrounded by a halo (later stage)
Adenovirus	Intranuclear	Eosinophilic intranuclear inclusion (early stage); basophilic smudged nucleus (later stage)
Respiratory syncytial virus	Cytoplasmic	Syncytial giant cells with small eosinophilic inclusions
Measles	Intranuclear	Giant cells with intranuclear eosinophilic inclusions surrounded by a halo

CMV INFECTION

Cytomegalovirus (CMV) infection represents an acquired infection that is generally asymptomatic in healthy children and adults but can lead to severe and sometimes fatal illness in immune-deficient individuals. The organism is a double-stranded DNA herpesvirus that replicates in the host cell nucleus. CMV is one of the most common opportunistic viral infections in patients with the acquired immunodeficiency syndrome and in organ transplant patients.[3,4] Lung infection by CMV can be very minimal with only a few scattered alveolar lining cells showing the cytopathic viral changes, or it may progress to a hemorrhagic and necrotizing pneumonia. There are four main patterns of lung infection: minimal infection with isolated viral inclusions, a miliary pattern of lung involvement, a diffuse interstitial pneumonia pattern, and hemorrhagic pneumonia. The diffuse interstitial pattern may range from mild to severe DAD (Fig. 8.1). In the mild form, there is interstitial chronic inflammation with pneumocyte hyperplasia and intra-alveolar macrophages (Fig. 8.2). In the severe form, the main findings are those of DAD with abundant intra-alveolar fibrin

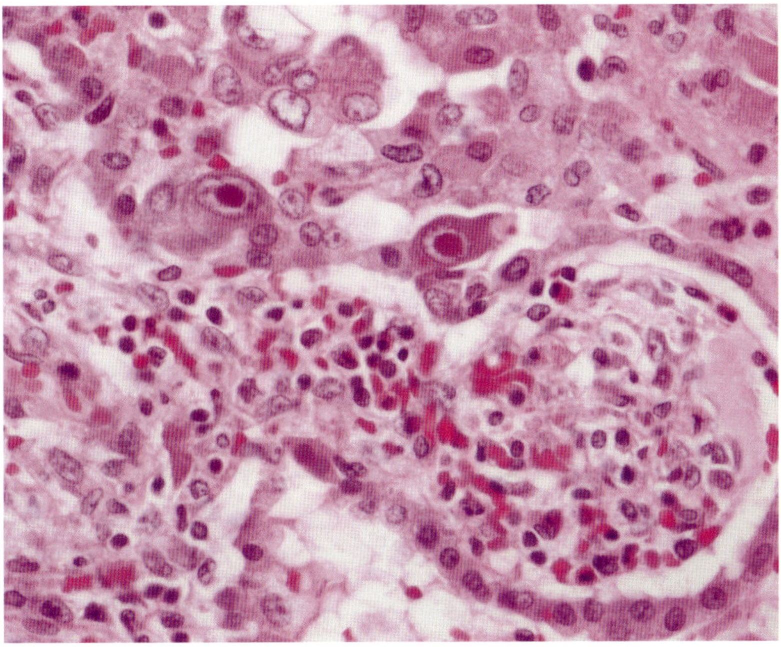

FIGURE 8.1 Diffuse interstitial pattern of lung involvement in CMV infection. There is DAD with organizing pneumonia and scattered pneumocytes containing eosinophilic viral inclusions.

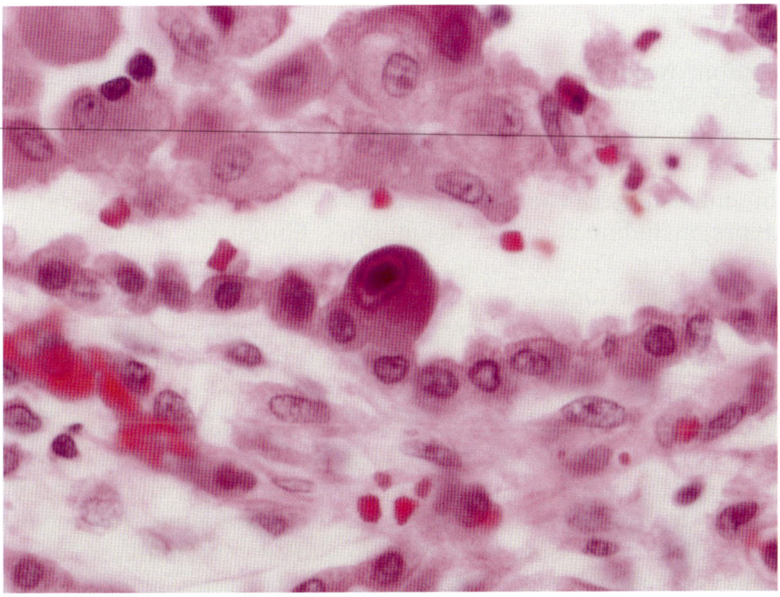

FIGURE 8.2 Mild form of CMV infection of the lung showing isolated infected cells in a minimally damaged lung.

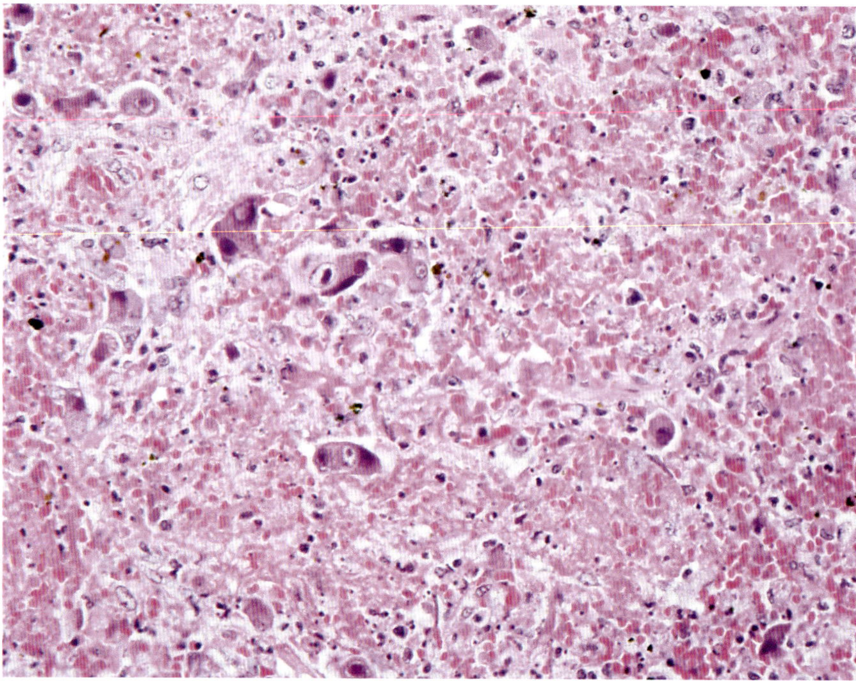

FIGURE 8.3 Severe form of CMV pneumonitis with extensive hemorrhagic and necrotizing pneumonia with scattered cells containing viral inclusions.

deposition, hyaline membranes, fibroblastic proliferation, and necrosis (Fig. 8.3). In some immunocompromised patients, the infection can be quite massive with sheets of infected cells against a background of necrotizing bronchopneumonia (Fig. 8.4). Diagnosis requires the identification of the characteristic viral inclusions. CMV can infect a wide variety of cell types, including alveolar pneumocytes, fibroblasts, macrophages, and endothelial cells. The cytopathic effects of CMV can be present in both the nucleus and the cytoplasm of infected cells (eFigs. 8.1 to 8.3). Infected cells usually show marked enlargement. The characteristic nuclear inclusions are large, single, and measure approximately 20 μm in diameter (Fig. 8.5). The cytoplasmic inclusions are usually much smaller and more difficult to identify; they can be stained with periodic acid-Schiff and Gomori methenamine silver (Fig. 8.6). The intranuclear inclusions are usually round to oval and may be basophilic or eosinophilic; they usually show a peripheral clear halo with accentuation of the nuclear membrane. The inclusions are easy to visualize using antibodies to CMV by immunohistochemistry (Fig. 8.7). In patients treated with antiviral agents the inclusions may be very scant and difficult to identify on routine microscopy; use of anti-CMV antibodies by immunohistochemistry is recommended in such cases for adequate identification.

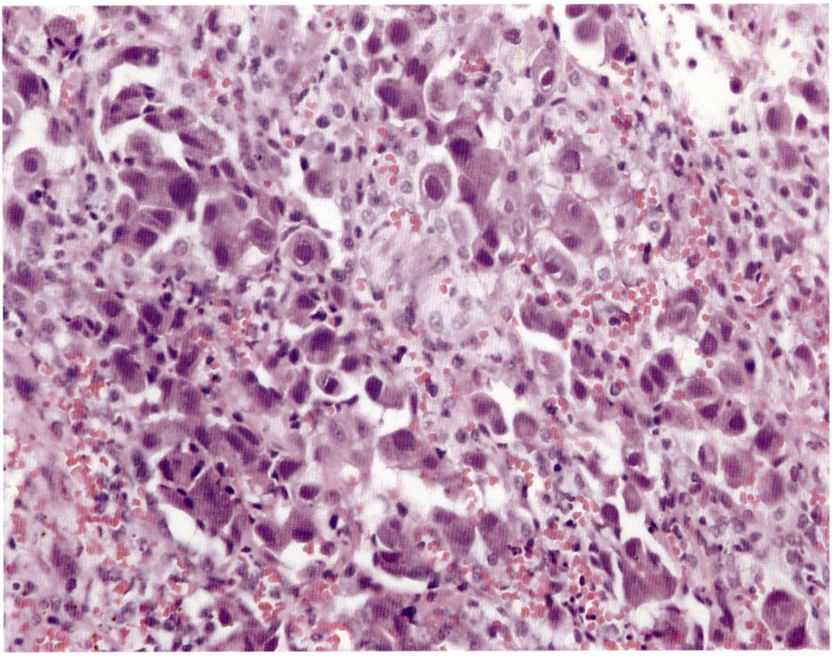

FIGURE 8.4 Massive infection by CMV in immunocompromised patient showing dense sheets of virally infected cells with large eosinophilic inclusions.

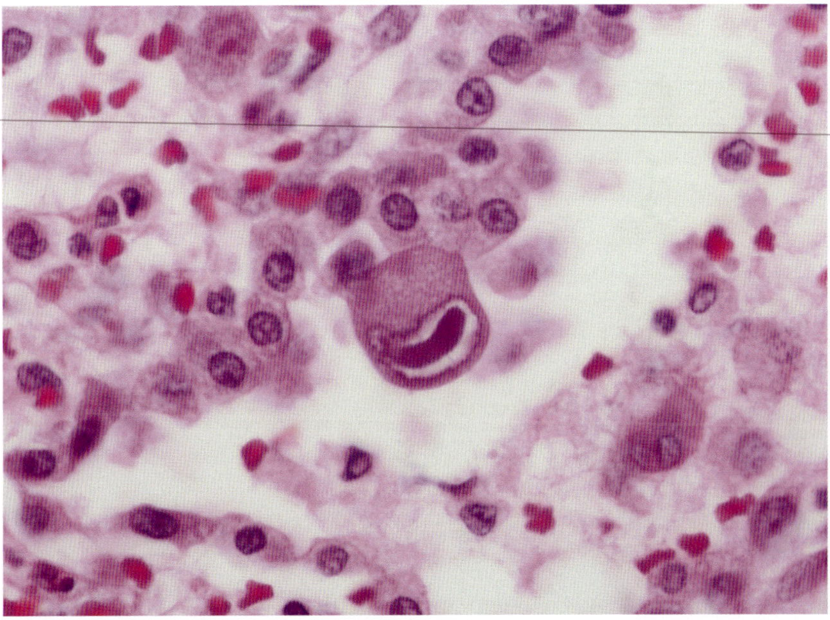

FIGURE 8.5 Characteristic intranuclear eosinophilic inclusion in CMV pneumonia. Notice the peripheral clear halo surrounding the inclusion.

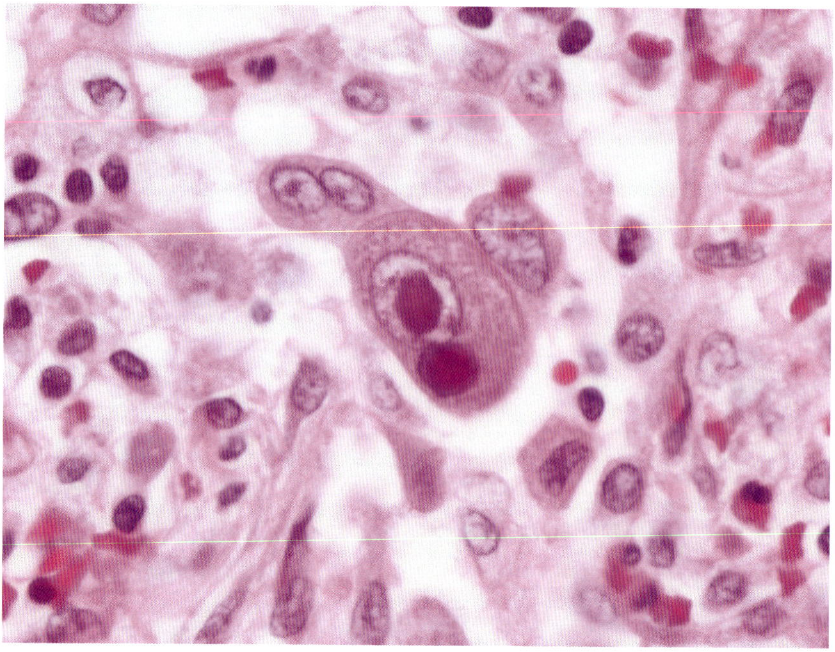

FIGURE 8.6 CMV-infected cell showing both nuclear and cytoplasmic inclusions.

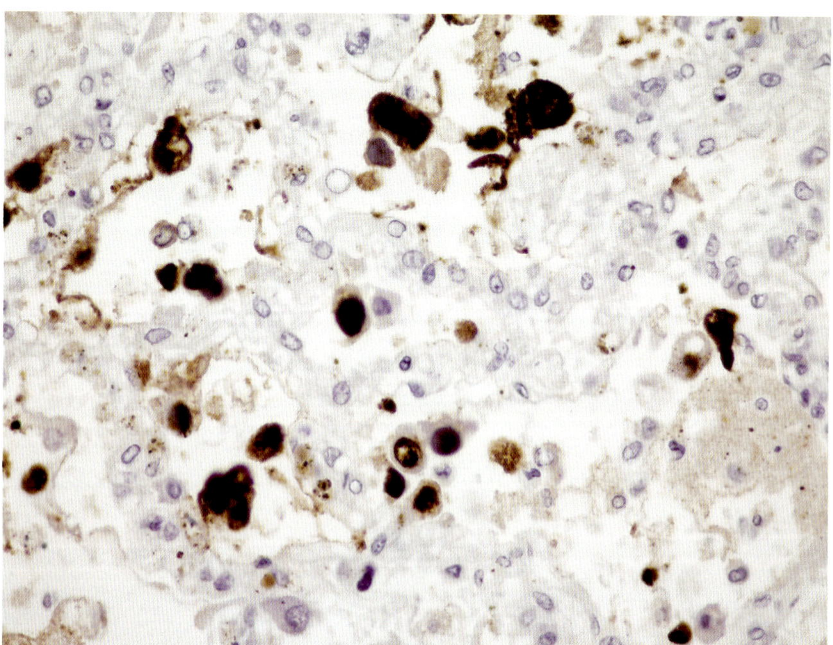

FIGURE 8.7 Immunohistochemical stain with anti-CMV antibodies highlights infected cells in CMV pneumonitis.

HERPES SIMPLEX PNEUMONIA

Herpes simplex pneumonia is caused by HSV-1, a double-stranded DNA virus that measures 100 nm in diameter. HSV pneumonia is seen in neonates as well as in adults who are immunosuppressed.[5] The organisms usually reach the lungs through contiguous spread from mucocutaneous lesions in the oral cavity and upper airways. There are three principal patterns of involvement in the lungs: necrotizing tracheobronchitis, necrotizing pneumonia, and interstitial pneumonitis.[6] Necrotizing tracheobronchitis owing to HSV is usually manifested by extensive ulceration and necrosis of the surface mucosa with production of abundant fibrinopurulent exudate (Fig. 8.8) (eFigs. 8.4 and 8.5). Necrotizing HSV pneumonia is usually distributed around the bronchi and is characterized by extensive suppurative necrosis of the surrounding lung parenchyma (Fig. 8.9). The diffuse interstitial pneumonitis pattern of HSV infection shows the histologic features of DAD, with interstitial edema, interstitial inflammation, and hyaline membrane formation.

The viral inclusions of HSV can be either large, eosinophilic, and surrounded by a halo or homogeneous and glassy (amphophylic) (Fig. 8.10). The infected epithelial cells may be multinucleated and contain multiple viral nuclear inclusions (eFig. 8.6). The intranuclear

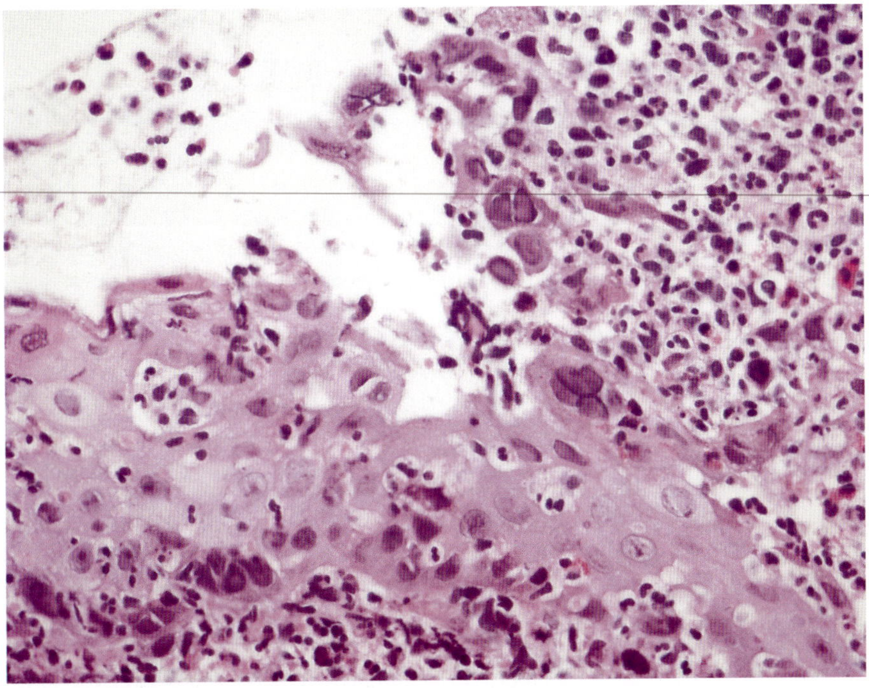

FIGURE 8.8 Necrotizing HSV tracheobronchitis. Notice the hyaline nuclear inclusions in the infected cells.

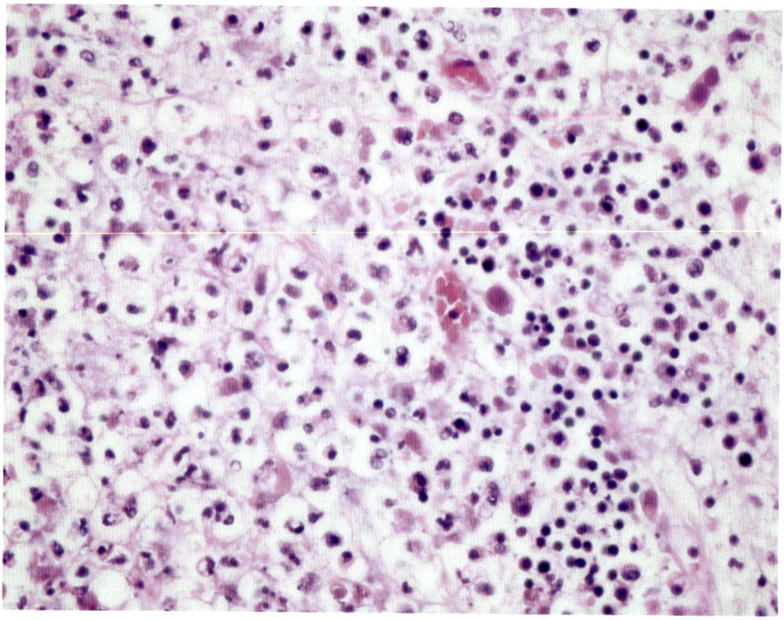

FIGURE 8.9 Necrotizing HSV pneumonia showing DAD with inflammation and scattered infected cells containing eosinophilic viral inclusions.

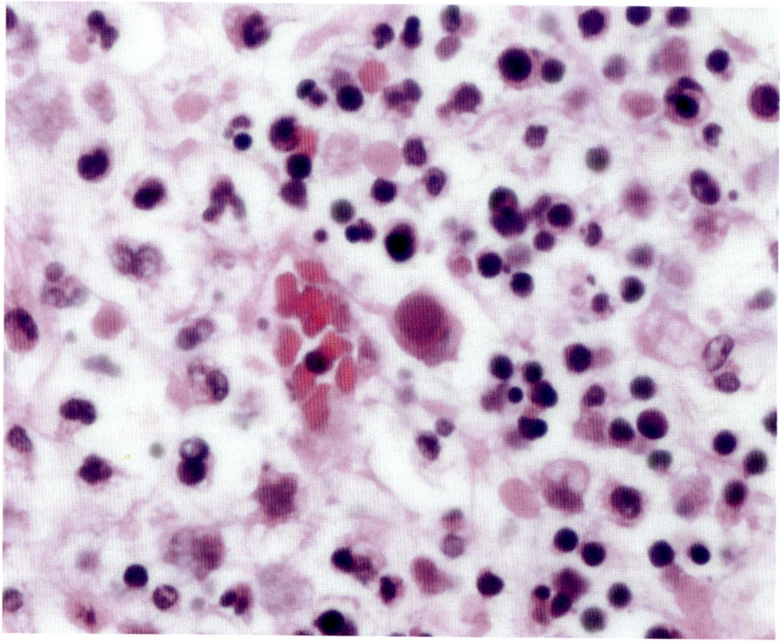

FIGURE 8.10 Higher magnification of HSV pneumonitis showing large eosinophilic inclusion surrounded by a halo.

inclusions are best appreciated in cells located at the periphery of the necrotic foci. The inclusions can closely resemble those of adenovirus. Immunohistochemical staining can be extremely useful for properly identifying the viral inclusions of HSV, particularly in cases with extensive necrosis.

Varicella–zoster pneumonia is a lung infection caused by a virus that is structurally very similar to HSV. Infection with the varicella–zoster virus (VZV) causes two clinical syndromes: varicella (chickenpox) and herpes zoster (shingles). In children and adults with impaired cell-mediated immunity, particularly bone marrow transplant recipients and acute leukemia patients, disseminated infection including pneumonia can occur. The pathologic findings are very similar to those of HSV lung infection. The viral inclusions are identical to those of HSV but may be harder to identify. A more specific diagnosis can be attained by the use of specific antibodies by immunohistochemistry against VZV or by the polymerase chain reaction (PCR) for viral nucleic acid. Isolation of the virus in cell culture, however, remains the gold standard for identification.

ADENOVIRUS

Adenovirus is a cause of respiratory infection owing to a double-stranded DNA virus found normally in the upper respiratory tract of humans. There are more than 50 known serotypes. In adults, the most common serotypes involved in causing pneumonia are 3, 4, and 7. The virus may cause latent infection that becomes reactivated during immunosuppression. The infection can spread quickly and be the cause of epidemics, particularly in military personnel, day care, school, and college students. Lung involvement with adenovirus can display acute necrotizing pneumonia with severe bronchitis and bronchiolitis, or an interstitial pattern characterized by DAD with hemorrhage and necrosis (Figs. 8.11 and 8.12).[7] Admixtures of the two are common. Involvement of secondary or medium-sized bronchi is characteristic and usually leads to striking necrosis with karyorrhexis and abundant cellular debris (Fig. 8.13). The intranuclear inclusions in adenoviral pneumonia closely resemble those of HSV and are characterized by small, dense eosinophilic round or oval inclusions surrounded by a clear halo (Figs. 8.14 and 8.15) (eFigs. 8.7 to 8.9). As the infection progresses, the inclusions become larger and more basophilic, and the halo disappears leading to a blurring of the margins between the inclusion and the nuclear membrane resulting in a smudged appearance (so-called smudge cell) (Fig. 8.16). The inclusions may be hard to find and are best identified at the leading edge of the necrotic zones. Infected cells can be easily identified by the use of specific antibodies by immunohistochemistry on routine formalin-fixed paraffin-embedded tissues, or by use of PCR (Fig. 8.17) (eFig. 8.10).

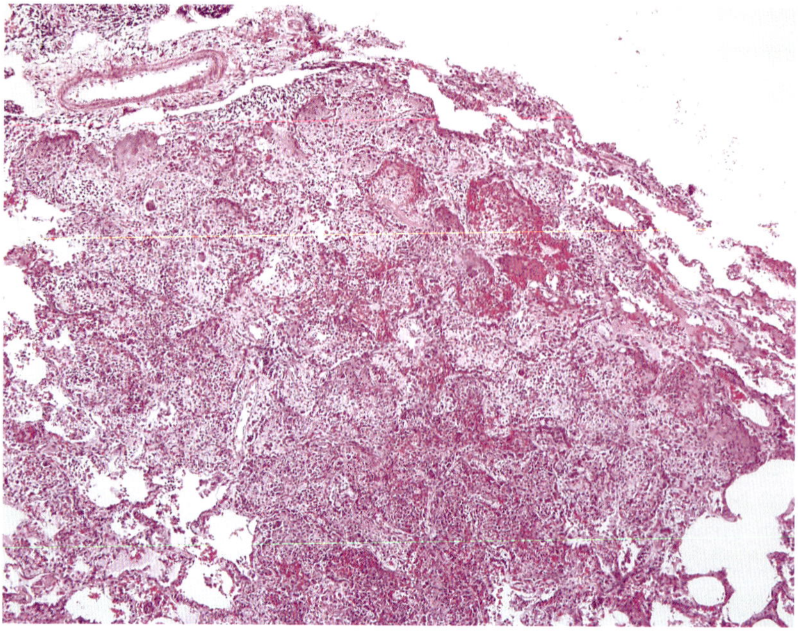

FIGURE 8.11 Acute necrotizing pneumonia in adenovirus infection characterized by extensive hemorrhage and diffuse alveolar damage.

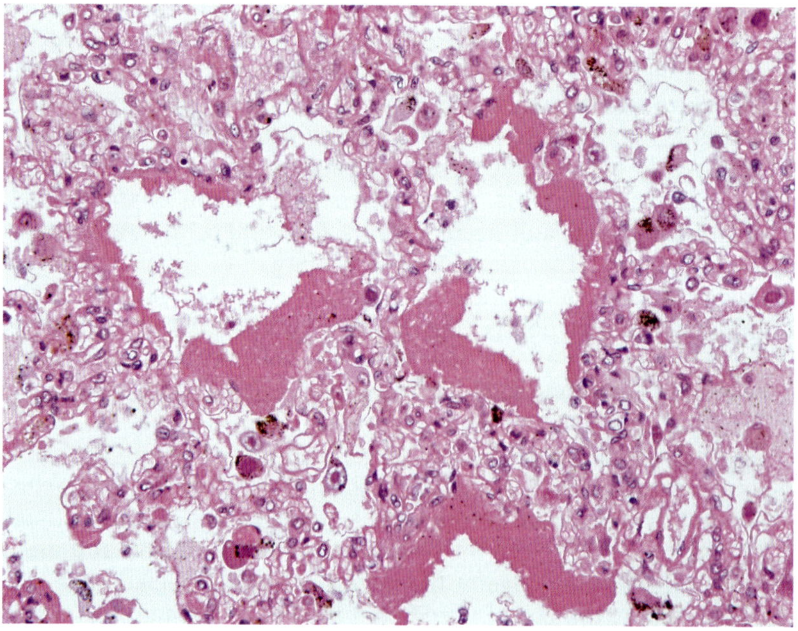

FIGURE 8.12 Interstitial pattern of involvement in adenoviral pneumonia showing fibrin deposition in alveolar lumens with hyaline membrane formation and scattered infected cells containing viral inclusions.

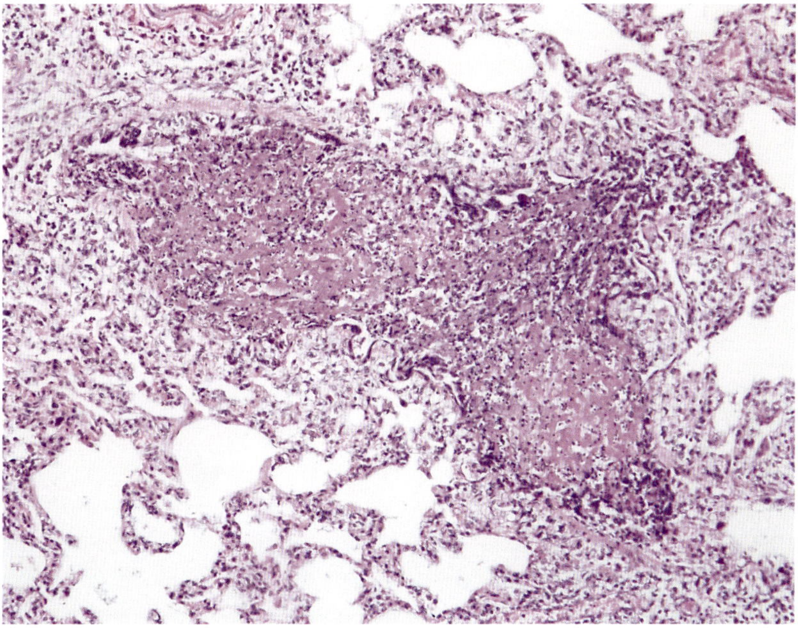

FIGURE 8.13 Adenoviral pneumonia showing acute necrotizing bronchiolitis.

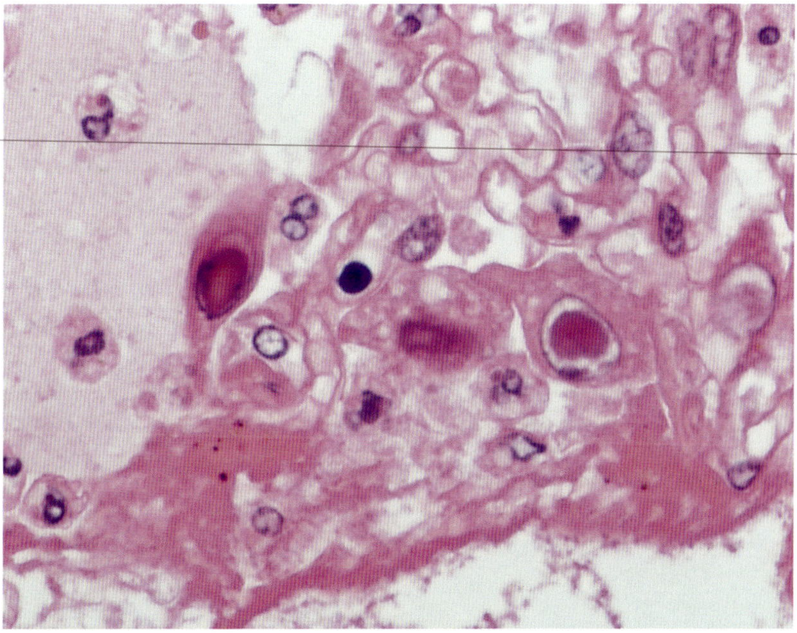

FIGURE 8.14 Small, dense, and eosinophilic round or oval inclusions surrounded by a halo are seen in the early lesions of adenovirus pneumonia.

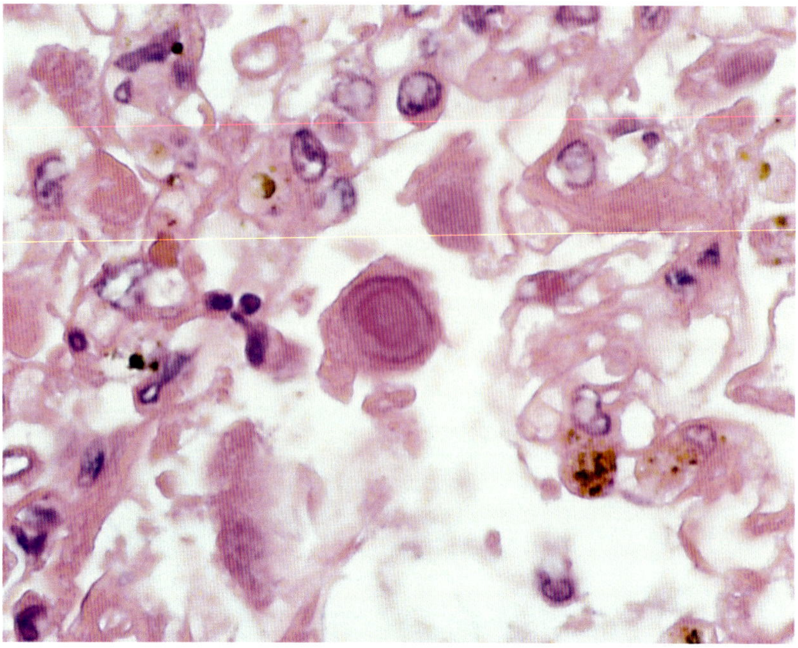

FIGURE 8.15 Characteristic adenovirus inclusion showing round eosinophilic structure surrounded by a distinct clear halo.

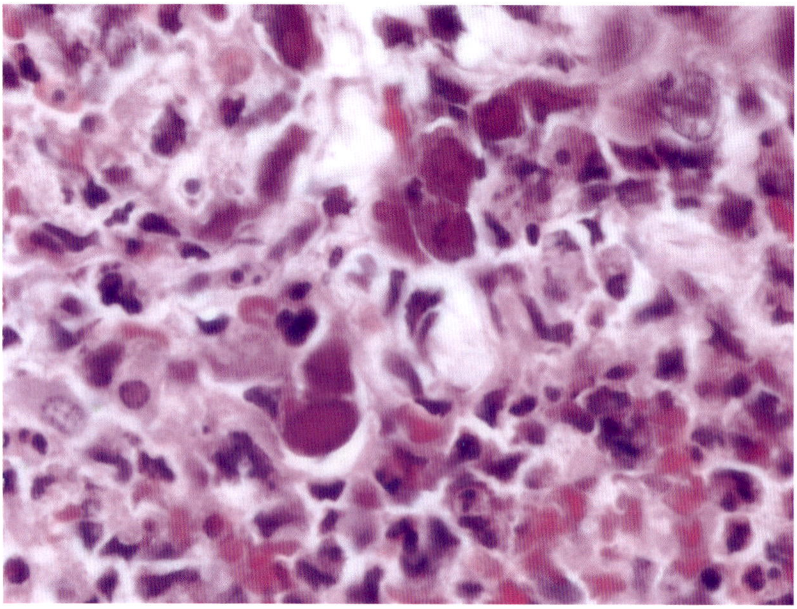

FIGURE 8.16 Late adenovirus inclusions are larger, more basophilic, and without a halo (smudge cells).

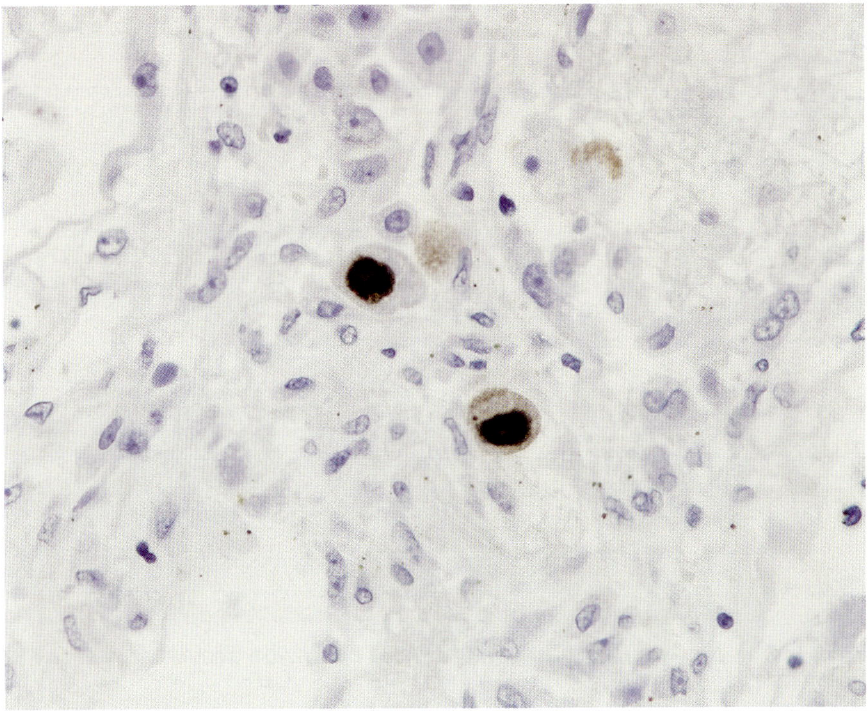

FIGURE 8.17 Immunohistochemical staining in adenoviral pneumonia highlights the viral cytopathic inclusions.

RESPIRATORY SYNCYTIAL VIRUS

RSV is a single-stranded RNA paramyxovirus that is a common cause of bronchiolitis and pneumonia in infants and children under 1 year of age. The two most common patterns of injury to the lung caused by RSV are necrotizing bronchiolitis and interstitial giant cell pneumonia.[8] The involved bronchial lumens and airways are usually filled with inflammatory infiltrates and necrotic debris (Fig. 8.18). The terminal bronchioles show severe peribronchiolar inflammation comprising mainly lymphocytes. Some cases may show features of giant cell interstitial pneumonia with prominent DAD. The syncytial giant cells comprise enlarged epithelial cells that line the alveolar walls and show multiple nuclei and may contain eosinophilic inclusions (Fig. 8.19). The inclusions in RSV are characteristically intracytoplasmic rather than nuclear and are usually small, eosinophilic, and paranuclear and surrounded by a clear halo. Specific diagnosis can be made by direct detection of viral antigens in clinical specimens by immunofluorescence, immunohistochemistry, or PCR. The differential diagnosis involves other viral pneumonias that produce multinucleated giant cells, including parainfluenza and measles.

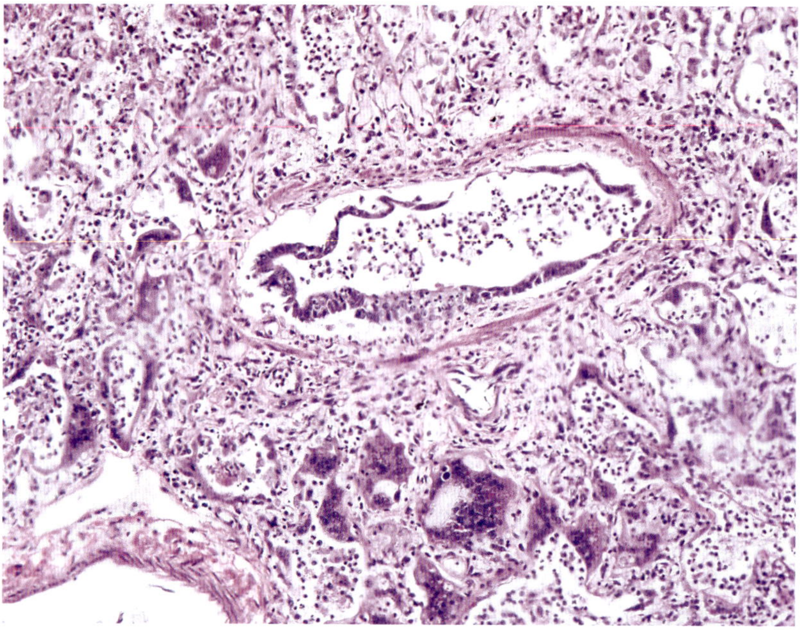

FIGURE 8.18 Necrotizing bronchiolitis surrounded by syncytial giant cells is seen in RSV pneumonia.

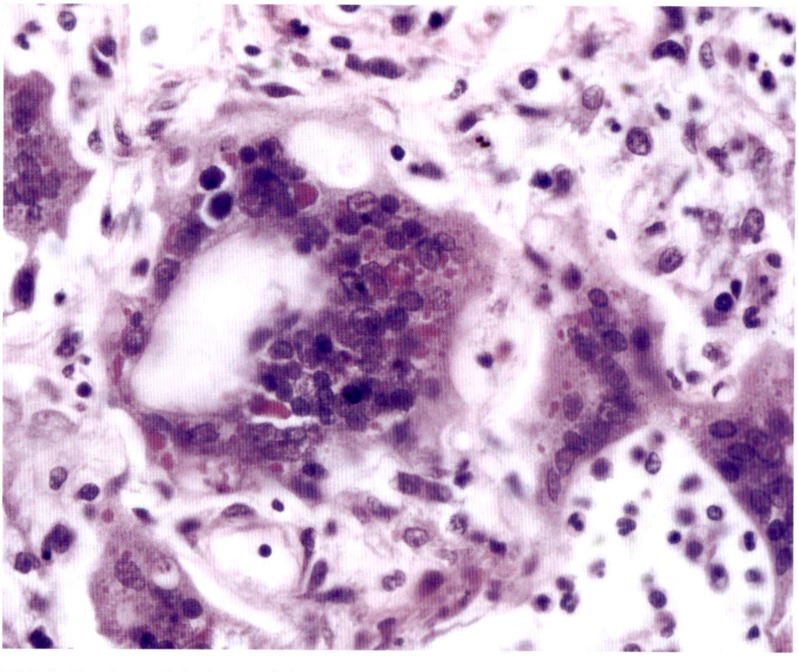

FIGURE 8.19 Syncytial giant cell in RSV pneumonia containing multiple small eosinophilic intracytoplasmic inclusions.

Human metapneumovirus (HMPV) is another recently described paramyxovirus that causes a very similar pattern of lung injury in children and adults as that of RSV.[9] Antibodies to HMPV are not yet widely available; most cases have been identified using reverse transcription PCR assays or by demonstration of a rise in HMPV-specific antibodies by serology.

MEASLES

Measles is caused by a single-stranded RNA paramyxovirus. The disease (rubeola) is an acute febrile viral illness characterized by fever, upper respiratory tract symptoms, and a maculopapular rash. The disease is highly contagious, spread through respiratory secretions and usually affects young children. Measles infection of the lungs can cause acute necrotizing bronchiolitis or a diffuse interstitial pneumonia with features of giant cell pneumonia.[10] The necrotizing bronchiolitis may be associated with regenerative changes of the epithelium including squamous metaplasia (Fig. 8.20). The interstitial giant cell pneumonitis will be characterized by DAD with prominent formation of syncytial giant cells (Fig. 8.21). The characteristic cytopathic change in measles pneumonia is the presence of large (100 μm) multinucleated epithelial cells in the bronchial mucosa and alveolar epithelium that have nuclear and cytoplasmic eosinophilic inclusions (Fig. 8.22). The nuclear inclusions are homogeneous and are

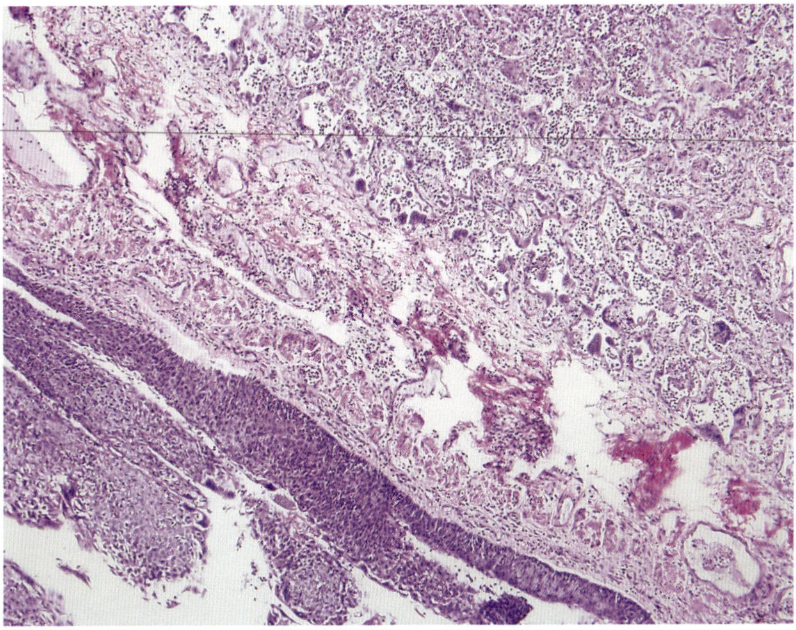

FIGURE 8.20 Measles pneumonia showing necrotizing bronchiolitis with prominent squamous metaplasia.

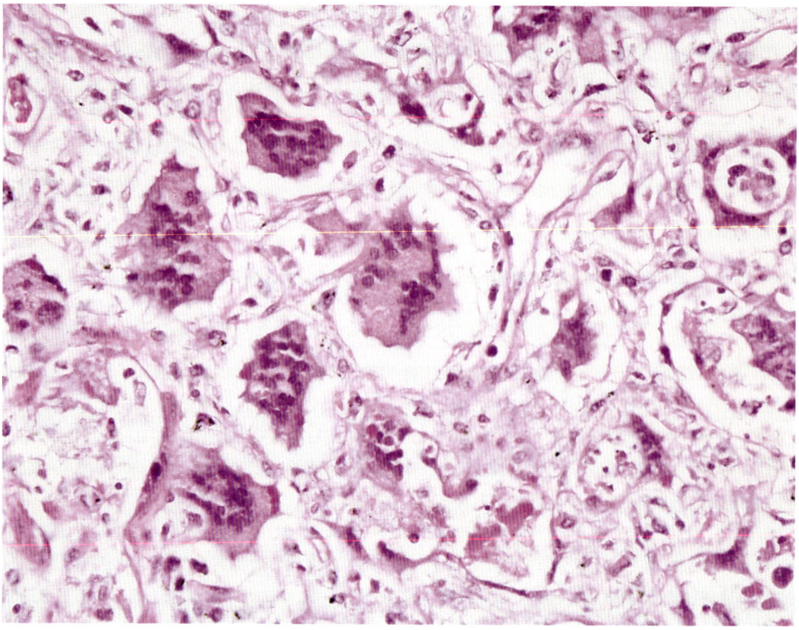

FIGURE 8.21 Measles giant cell interstitial pneumonia with multiple scattered multinucleated giant cells.

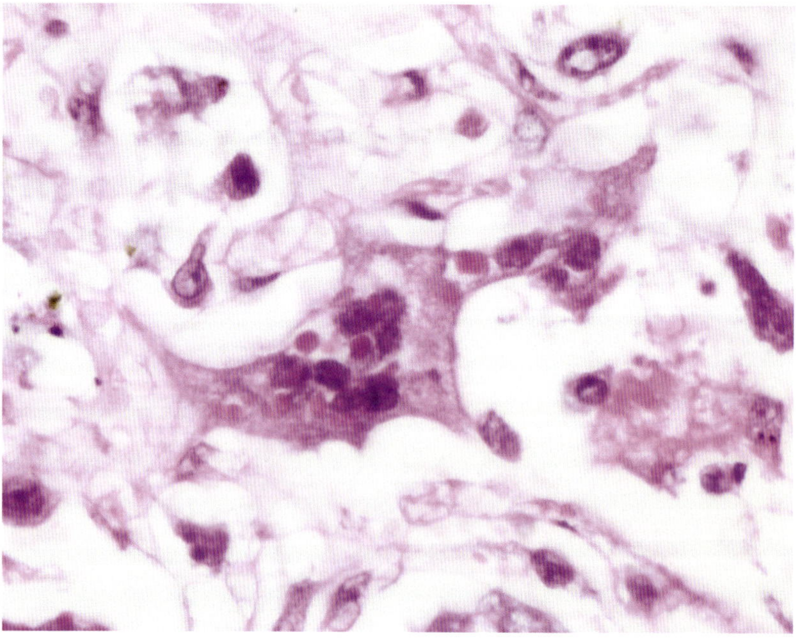

FIGURE 8.22 Higher magnification of multinucleated giant cell in interstitial pneumonia secondary to measles showing small, round eosinophilic inclusions similar to those seen in RSV pneumonia.

TABLE 8.2 Differential Diagnosis of Giant Cell Viral Pneumonias

Virus	Location	Features
Measles	Nuclear and cytoplasmic inclusions (numerous)	Large multinucleated epithelial cells with nuclear and cytoplasmic inclusions. Diagnosis can be confirmed by immunohistochemistry and in situ hybridization
Respiratory syncytial virus	Cytoplasmic inclusions (few)	Small, eosinophilic, paranuclear inclusions surrounded by a clear halo. Diagnosis can be confirmed by culture or immunofluorescent techniques
Herpes simplex virus–varicella–zoster virus	Nuclear inclusions (few). Giant cells are rare	Small, eosinophilic, or amphophylic, homogeneous and glassy. Diagnosis can be established by immunohistochemistry or PCR
Parainfluenza virus	Small cytoplasmic inclusions (numerous)	The cytoplasmic inclusions are very small and consist of aggregates of viral nucleocapsids. Diagnosis is established by cultures or immunofluorescent techniques

usually surrounded by a clear halo. The presence of the measles virus can be confirmed in tissues by immunohistochemistry or in situ hybridization.[11] The differential diagnosis of giant cell viral pneumonias involves RSV, VZV, and parainfluenza virus (PIV); the various features of these infections are compared in Table 8.2.

VIRUSES THAT DO NOT PRODUCE CYTOPATHIC EFFECTS

Several viruses that can affect the lungs will not produce any cytopathic effects. Identification of such viruses is more difficult to establish on biopsy material and will generally require epidemiologic, serologic, and other types of studies for confirmation including viral cultures, direct fluorescent antibody detection, PCR, or immunohistochemistry. These include the SARS virus, hantavirus, and influenza virus.

Severe Acute Respiratory Syndrome

SARS causes an influenza-like illness characterized by acute onset of fever, malaise, myalgia, dry cough, chills, and sore throat. The causative agent is a positive-strand RNA virus belonging in the genus *Coronavirus*. SARS was first recognized during a global outbreak originating in China in 2002, from where it spread to Asia, Europe, and the Americas.[12,13] The typical CT findings include peripheral subpleural ground-glass opacities or consolidation. The main histopathologic finding is DAD with scattered mononuclear cell infiltrates in the interstitium.[14] The affected parenchyma may also show intra-alveolar hemorrhage, suppurative inflammation, and organizing pneumonia. Multinucleated syncytial cells may be present in alveolar spaces, but no viral inclusions are identified. The histopathologic findings are entirely nonspecific, and diagnosis will require laboratory tests such as serology, viral cultures, PCR, or direct fluorescent antibody detection.

Influenza Virus

Influenza virus is a major cause of respiratory illness in adults and children. Uncomplicated influenza is characterized by the onset of constitutional symptoms, including chills, myalgia, fever, sore throat, headache, and malaise. The symptoms usually resolve after 3 to 7 days. When complications supervene, patients will develop secondary bacterial pneumonias and, less commonly, seizures, Reye's syndrome, encephalopathy, myositis, myocarditis, and pericarditis. Risk of death because of influenza is highest among children and the elderly. Radiologically the disease presents with patchy consolidation of lung parenchyma. The histologic features in the lung in patients with influenza include DAD, intra-alveolar hemorrhage, and necrotizing bronchitis.[15,16] No viral inclusions are present. The pathologic changes associated with the primary viral infection are often obscured by secondary bacterial pneumonia. Because the pathologic findings are so nonspecific, diagnosis will require laboratory tests such as direct fluorescent antibody, in situ hybridization, serology, or viral cultures.

A novel influenza A virus (H1N1) of swine origin was identified in 2009. After global spread, it was declared by the WHO the first influenza pandemic in 41 years. The disease causes respiratory illness that can progress to acute respiratory distress syndrome.[17] Fatal cases are characterized by tracheitis, bronchiolitis, and DAD. Influenza viral antigen can be detected in the epithelium of the tracheobronchial tree and alveolar epithelial cells by PCR.[18]

Hantavirus

Hantavirus is responsible for the hantavirus pulmonary syndrome (HPS), a disease characterized by malaise, fever, myalgia, headache, vomiting, weakness, and cough.[19] The initial phase is followed by acute pulmonary edema, respiratory distress, and shock. Large, bilateral pleural effusion is characteristic of HPS. The disease is caused by a negative-sense RNA virus of the genus *Hantavirus*. The pathologic findings include mild-to-moderate interstitial pneumonitis with prominent interstitial mononuclear cell infiltrates.[20] There may be focal hyaline membranes, but damage to the alveolar lining is not a prominent feature. No inclusions are seen. Specific diagnosis is done by serology, PCR, or immunohistochemistry with antibodies to hantaviral antigens. HPS should be suspected in cases of acute respiratory distress without a known precipitating cause among previously healthy individuals. Exposure to rodents in endemic areas also should raise the level of suspicion.

Viral Hemorrhagic Fever

Viral hemorrhagic fever (VHF) represents infection caused by a group of viruses transmitted to humans by rodents and arthropods. The syndrome of VHF is because of RNA viruses that may belong to four different families, including *Arenaviridae, Bunyaviridae, Flaviviridae,* and *Filoviridae.* Hemorrhagic fever can occur worldwide, and the diseases are usually named after the place where they were first described, such as Thailand hemorrhagic fever, and Crimean–Congo hemorrhagic fever. The oldest and best known is yellow fever; others include Ebola, Lassa, and dengue viruses.[21,22] The clinical manifestations of hemorrhagic fever are dominated by hemorrhage, which most commonly affects the mucosal surfaces. The most common findings in the lung include intra-alveolar hemorrhage, edema, interstitial pneumonia, and DAD. No viral inclusions are seen. The diagnosis is suspected in patients who have a history of travel to endemic areas. Definitive diagnosis can be made only by laboratory tests such as serology, cell culture, PCR, and immunohistochemistry.

REFERENCES

1. De Roux A, Marcos MA, Garcia E, et al. Viral community-acquired pneumonia in non-immunocompromised adults. *Chest.* 2004;125:1343–1351.
2. Fields BN, Knipe DM, Howley PM, eds. *Fields Virology.* 4th ed. Philadelphia, PA: Lippincott Williams and Williams; 2001.
3. Ison MG, Fishman JA. Cytomegalovirus pneumonia in transplant recipients. *Clin Chest Med.* 2005;26:691–705.
4. Ljungman P, Griffiths P, Paya C. Definitions of cytomegalic infection and disease in transplant recipients. *Clin Infect Dis.* 2002;34:1094–1097.
5. Singer DB. Pathology of neonatal herpes simplex virus infection. *Perspect Pediatr Pathol.* 1981;6:243–278.
6. Ramsey PG, Fife KH, Hackman RC, et al. Herpes simplex virus pneumonia: clinical, virologic, and pathologic features in 20 patients. *Ann Int Med.* 1982;97:813–820.
7. Becroft DM. Histopathology of fatal adenovirus infection of the respiratory tract in young children. *J Clin Pathol.* 1967;20:561–569.
8. Delage G, Brochu P, Robillard L, et al. Giant cell pneumonia due to respiratory syncytial virus. Occurrence in severe combined immunodeficiency syndrome. *Arch Pathol Mab Med.* 1984;108:623–625.
9. Van den Hoogen BG, de Jong JC, Groen J, et al. A newly discovered human pneumovirus isolated from young children with respiratory tract disease. *Nat Med.* 2001;7:719–724.
10. Radoycich GE, Zuppan CW, Weeks DA, et al. Patterns of measles pneumonia. *Pediatr Pathol.* 1992;12:773–786.
11. Sata T, Kurata T, Aoyama Y, et al. Analysis of viral antigens in giant cells of measles pneumonia by immunoperoxidase method. *Virchows Arch A Pathol Anat Histopathol.* 1986;410:133–138.

12. Ding Y, Wang H, Shen H, et al. The clinical pathology of severe acute respiratory syndrome (SARS): a report from China. *J Pathol.* 2003;200:282–289.
13. Chong PY, Chui P, Ling AE, et al. Analysis of deaths during the severe acute respiratory syndrome (SARS) epidemic in Singapore: challenges in determining a SARS diagnosis. *Arch Pathol Lab Med.* 2004;128:195–204.
14. Franks TJ, Chong PY, Chui P, et al. Lung pathology of severe acute respiratory syndrome (SARS): a study of 8 autopsy cases from Singapore. *Hum Pathol.* 2003;34:743–748.
15. Guarner J, Paddock CD, Shieh WJ, et al. Histopathologic and immunohistochemical features of fatal influenza virus infections in children during the 2003–2004 season. *Clin Infect Dis.* 2006;43:132–140.
16. Yeldandi AV, Colby TV. Pathologic features of lung biopsy specimens from influenza pneumonia cases. *Hum Pathol.* 1994;25:47–53.
17. Lai AR, Keet K, Yong CM, et al. Severe H1N1-associated acute respiratory distress syndrome: a case series. *Am J Med.* 2010;123:282–285.
18. Gill JR, Sheng ZM, Ely SF, et al. Pulmonary pathologic findings of fatal 2009 pandemic influenza A/H1N1 viral infections. *Arch Pathol Lab Med.* 2010;134:235–243.
19. Duchin JS, Koster FT, Peters CJ, et al. Hantavirus pulmonary syndrome: a clinical description of 17 patients with a newly recognized disease. The Hantavirus Study Group. *N Engl J Med.* 1994;330:949–955.
20. Nolte KB, Federsen RM, Foucar K, et al. Hantavirus pulmonary syndrome in the United States: a pathological description of a disease caused by a new agent. *Hum Pathol.* 1995;26:110–120.
21. Burke T. Dengue hemorrhagic fever: a pathological study. *Trans R Soc Trop Med Hyg.* 1968;62:682–692.
22. Walker DH, McCormick JB, Johnson KM, et al. Pathologic and virologic study of fatal Lassa fever in man. *Am J Pathol.* 1982;107:349–356.

9

INTERSTITIAL LUNG DISEASE

Involvement of the interstitial compartment of the lung, with or without compromise of the airspaces, can be seen in a wide variety of circumstances and represents a major cause of lung morbidity and mortality. Interstitial pneumonias can be categorized, in broad terms, into idiopathic interstitial pneumonias (IIPs) and into those for which a known precipitating cause or agent can be demonstrated (Table 9.1).

IDIOPATHIC INTERSTITIAL PNEUMONIAS

The IIPs are a group of relatively rare conditions of unknown etiology that are generally characterized by insidious onset and progressive interstitial fibrosis with inflammation. Secondary involvement of the airspaces can also occur, but the principal pathology is centered in the interstitium of the alveolar walls. Our understanding of idiopathic interstitial lung diseases has progressed slowly, from the initial description by Liebow,[1] to the classification proposed by Katzenstein,[2] to the more recent international workshop on the classification of these conditions.[3] IIP is generally a diffuse and bilateral process, and the various specific categories that comprise this spectrum of disorders represent various reaction patterns of lung parenchyma to the underlying injury. In general, such reaction patterns are nonspecific and often blend into each other or may show significant overlap. The diagnosis is established strictly on the basis of clinicopathologic and radiologic correlation and not on the basis of the histopathologic findings alone. Because the lesions are not localized but diffuse and also because there can be considerable variation in the stage of evolution of the lesions ("temporal heterogeneity"), proper evaluation of these disorders cannot be reliably accomplished by performing a single transbronchial biopsy.[4] The proper way to evaluate patients suspected of idiopathic interstitial lung disease is through multiple open lung wedge biopsies or video-assisted thoracoscopic lung biopsies. It is important to obtain at least three samples involving all lobes, taking care to avoid areas of scarring particularly in the apices or the lingula. The use of bronchoscopic or transbronchial biopsy for the diagnosis of idiopathic interstitial lung disease should be discouraged, as it will usually lead to equivocal or unreliable results. The damage in these conditions usually affects the periphery of the lungs, and these areas cannot be adequately sampled

TABLE 9.1 Types of Interstitial Lung Disease

Idiopathic Interstitial Pneumonias	Specific Interstitial Pneumonias
Idiopathic pulmonary fibrosis/UIP	Collagen-vascular disease-related interstitial pneumonia
Nonspecific interstitial pneumonia	Drug-mediated diffuse lung disease
Desquamative interstitial pneumonia	Hypersensitivity pneumonitis (extrinsic allergic alveolitis)
Lymphoid interstitial pneumonia	Respiratory bronchiolitis-Interstitial lung disease
Cryptogenic organizing pneumonia (Bronchiolitis obliterans organizing pneumonia)	Langerhans cell histiocytosis
Acute interstitial pneumonia	Giant cell interstitial pneumonia (hard metal disease)

through transbronchial biopsies. The changes described in this chapter will thus refer to those that can be observed in open or thoracoscopic wedge biopsies rather than in bronchoscopic or transbronchial biopsies.

Idiopathic Interstitial Fibrosis/ Usual Interstitial Pneumonia

Usual interstitial pneumonia (UIP) refers to a reaction pattern of inflammation and lung fibrosis that can be observed in a variety of conditions. The histopathologic changes observed are nonspecific and must be correlated with the clinical and radiologic changes before a diagnosis of UIP can be established. UIP changes can be observed in a variety of specific conditions, such as collagen-vascular disease (CVD), asbestosis, and drug reactions. The term *idiopathic interstitial fibrosis—UIP pattern* should be applied only when no underlying causes for the changes are observed clinically.[5] Patients are usually middle-aged adults who present with slowly progressive dyspnea and nonproductive cough. High-resolution computed tomography (HRCT) shows distinctive findings in more than 50% of cases. There is a predominantly reticular pattern of ground glass opacities with honeycombing showing basal and peripheral predominance.[6] The findings are patchy and heterogeneous in distribution. Traction bronchiectasis is another distinctive finding. If the characteristic HRCT findings are present, a diagnosis of idiopathic interstitial fibrosis can be made without a need for open lung biopsy. A lung biopsy should be undertaken only in patients suspected of UIP who do not have the characteristic HRCT findings. Chest X-ray in patients with UIP typically shows a bilateral reticular pattern predominantly involving the lung bases. A normal chest X-ray can be seen in some cases.

The histopathologic hallmark of UIP is the presence of areas of lung parenchyma showing the fibrosing and inflammatory changes adjacent

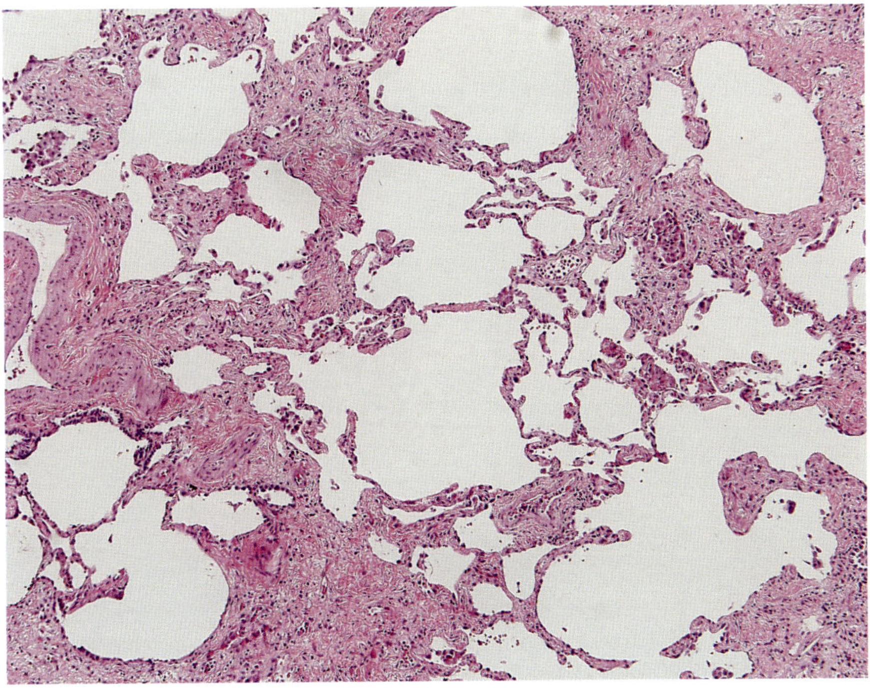

FIGURE 9.1 Scanning magnification of lung biopsy in UIP. Notice areas containing thickened and fibrotic alveolar septa alternating with areas of normal lung parenchyma.

to areas displaying early involvement or perfectly normal parenchyma (Fig. 9.1) (eFigs. 9.1 and 9.2). This has been referred to as "temporal heterogeneity," and refers essentially to the variegated appearance of the lung caused by areas showing lung parenchyma involved with the pathologic process in varying stages of evolution alternating with areas of uninvolved, normal lung parenchyma.[7] The fibrosis is usually subpleural and paraseptal. In the early stages of fibrosis, foci containing spindled fibroblasts or myofibroblasts admixed with loose connective tissue are usually present (so-called fibroblastic foci) (Fig. 9.2). Mild interstitial chronic inflammation and scattered lymphoid aggregates can also be found. Accumulation of alveolar macrophages can be seen focally resulting in a "DIP-like" appearance (Fig. 9.3). Marked thickening secondary to fibrosis with widening of the alveolar septa is seen in well-established lesions (Fig. 9.4) (eFig. 9.3). Bronchiolization ("lambertosis") and squamous metaplasia of alveolar spaces can be observed in the areas of scarring and fibrosis (Fig. 9.5) (eFigs. 9.4 and 9.5). Smooth muscle proliferation may accompany the scarring, a process referred to in the British literature as "muscular cirrhosis" (Fig. 9.6). The fibrosis may progress resulting in scarring and the formation of cystic spaces containing mucus or inflammatory cells, a process that has been termed *honeycombing* (Fig. 9.7) (eFig. 9.6). Episodes of acute exacerbation can be seen in patients with UIP, leading

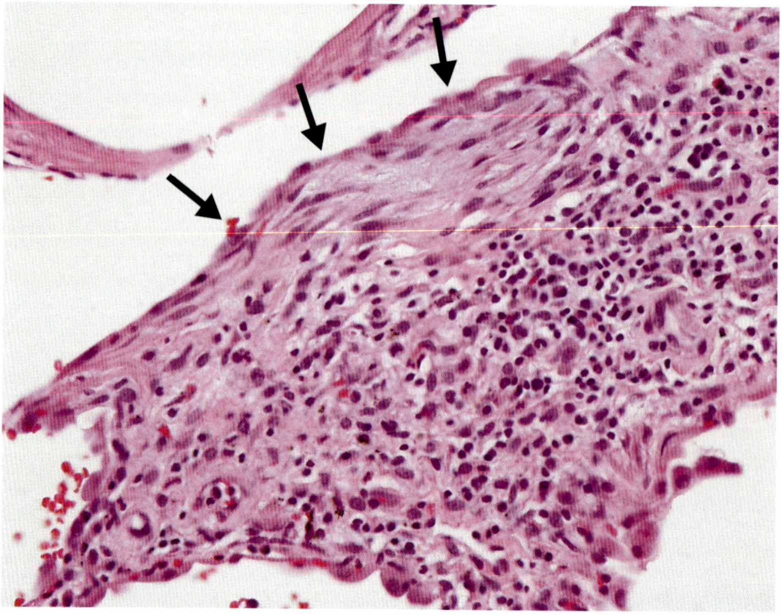

FIGURE 9.2 UIP showing thickening of the alveolar wall due to fibrosis and chronic inflammation with early fibroblastic focus comprising young fibroblasts admixed with a myxoid matrix (arrows).

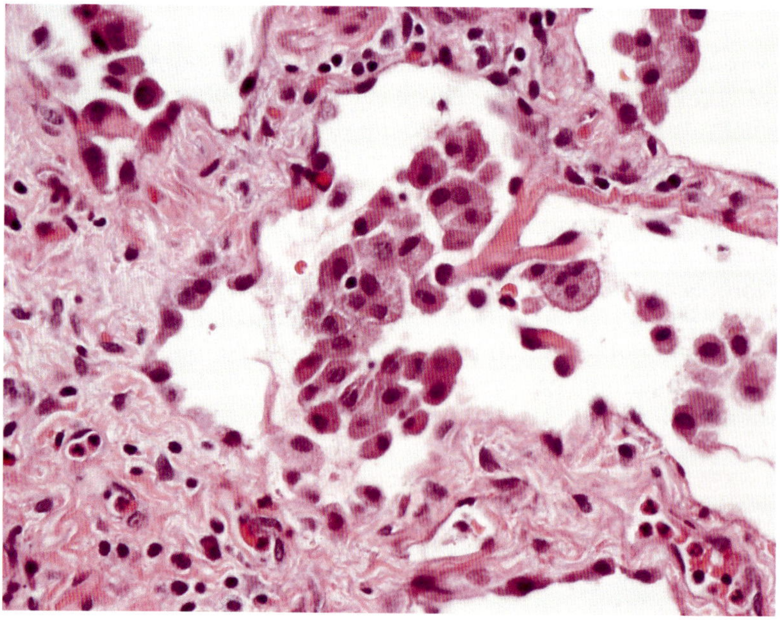

FIGURE 9.3 DIP-like changes can be seen in UIP, with accumulation of macrophages in alveolar lumina.

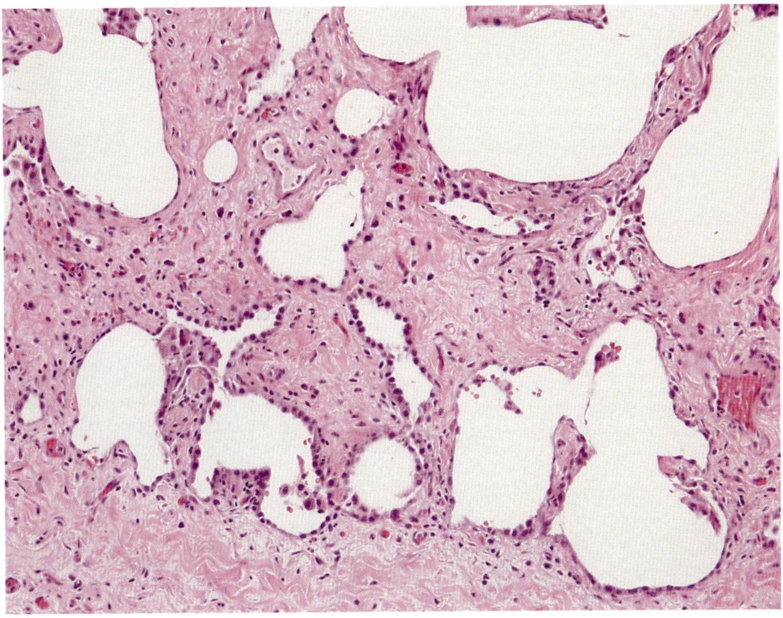

FIGURE 9.4 Marked thickening of alveolar septa due to fibroblastic proliferation and collagen deposition is seen in UIP. Notice focal hyperplasia of type II pneumocytes lining the alveolar spaces.

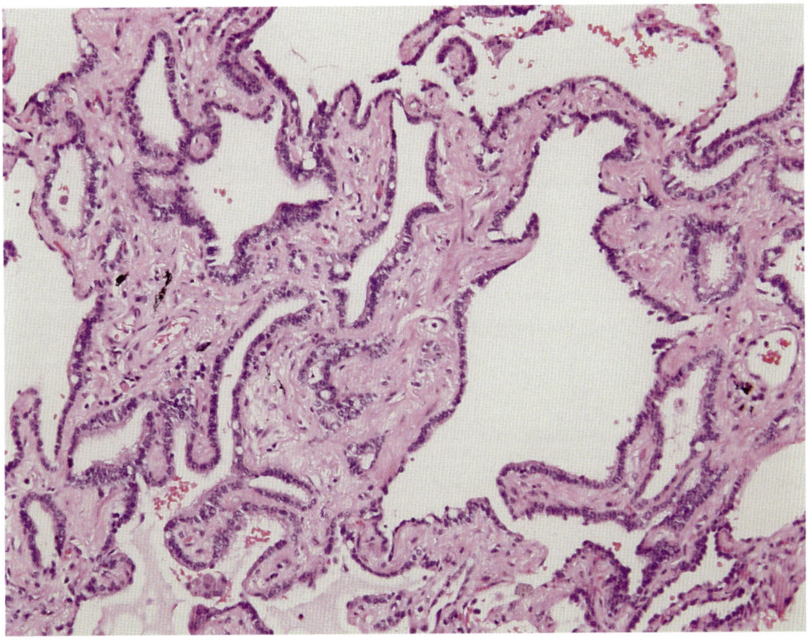

FIGURE 9.5 Extensive bronchiolization is seen in this example of UIP characterized by replacement of the alveolar lining by columnar ciliated epithelium.

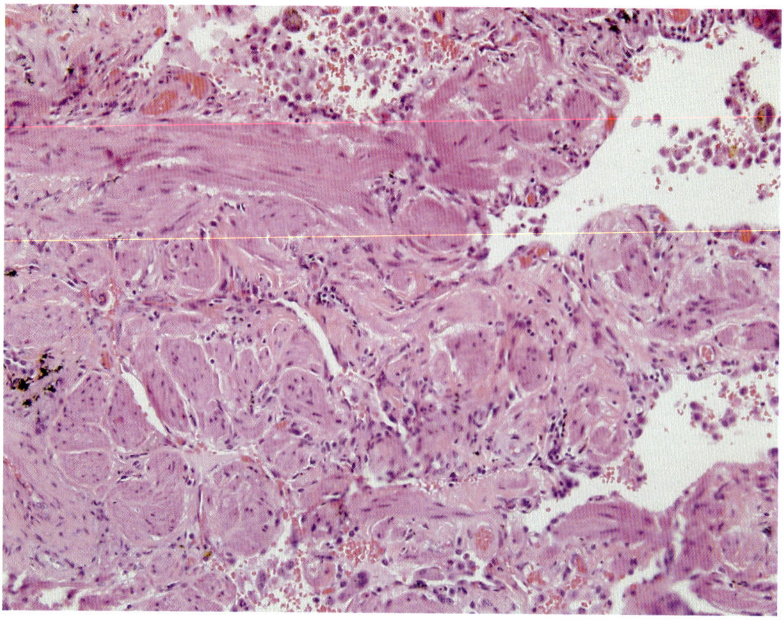

FIGURE 9.6 Prominent smooth muscle proliferation is seen in the walls of the alveolar septa in advanced stages of UIP.

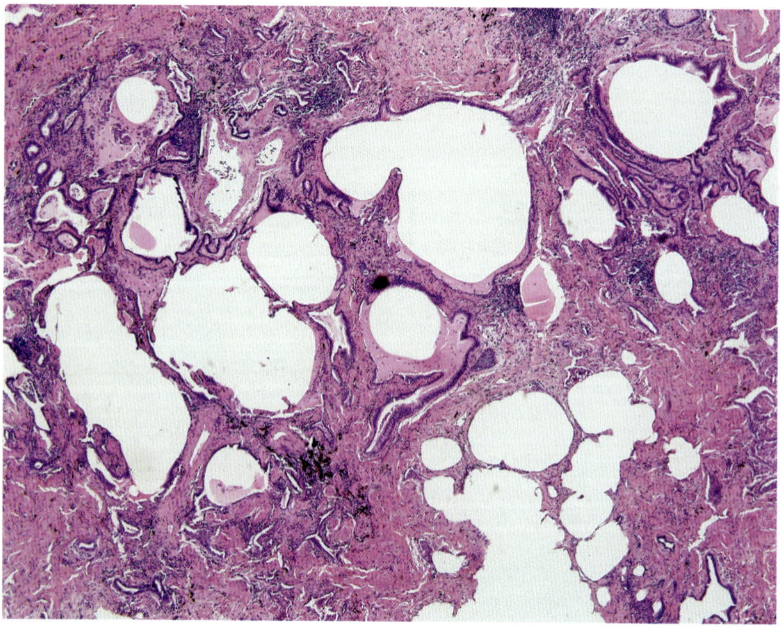

FIGURE 9.7 Extensive "honeycombing" of lung is seen in advanced stages of UIP characterized by cystic dilatation of alveolar spaces that sometimes become filled with mucin.

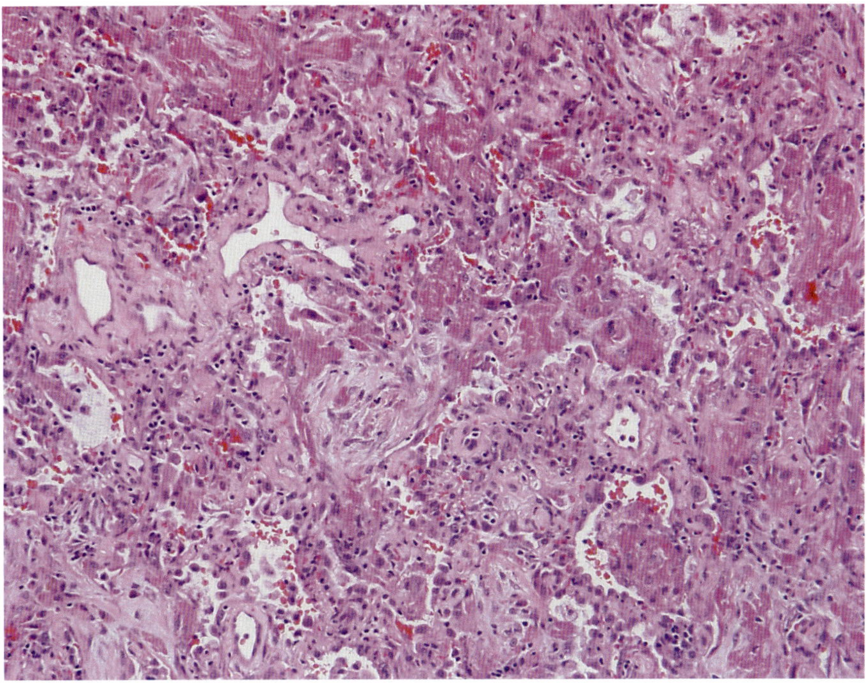

FIGURE 9.8 Acute exacerbation in UIP shows changes of diffuse alveolar damage superimposed in a background of alveolar wall fibrosis.

to the presence of diffuse alveolar damage superimposed on the chronic changes of UIP (Fig. 9.8). Idiopathic pulmonary fibrosis is a progressive disorder that leads to death as a result of respiratory failure in the majority of instances, with a median survival of less than 4 years from the time of initial diagnosis. The disease does not respond to treatment with immunosuppressants or corticosteroids.

Nonspecific Interstitial Pneumonia

The term *nonspecific interstitial pneumonia* (NSIP) was proposed in 1994 by Katzenstein and Fiorelli[8] for patients presenting with slowly progressive cough and dyspnea, bilateral interstitial infiltrates, and a histopathologic picture on open lung biopsy that differed significantly from UIP. In contrast with UIP, which is characterized by "temporal heterogeneity," NSIP is characterized by a temporally uniform pattern of changes. The inflammatory process in NSIP is diffuse and uniform and involves mainly the alveolar septa (Fig. 9.9). The interstitial inflammatory infiltrate mainly comprises plasma cells and small lymphocytes and can be accompanied by mild interstitial fibrosis (Fig. 9.10). Fibroblastic foci and honeycombing are not seen.[9] Advanced fibrosis is extremely rare in this condition and portends a worse prognosis. The prognosis for NSIP is much better than that for UIP, and most patients will respond

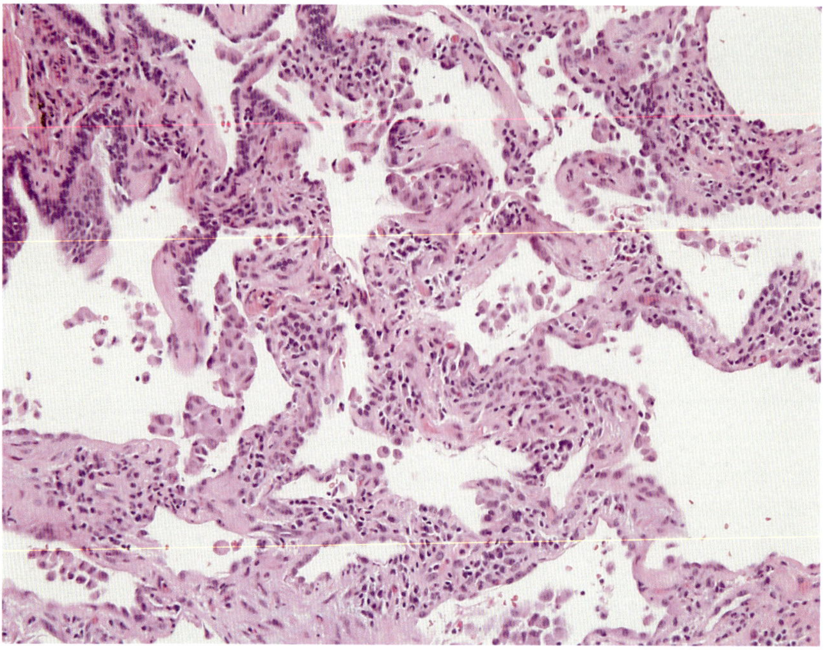

FIGURE 9.9 NSIP pattern showing uniform thickening and fibrosis of alveolar septa without intervening normal areas.

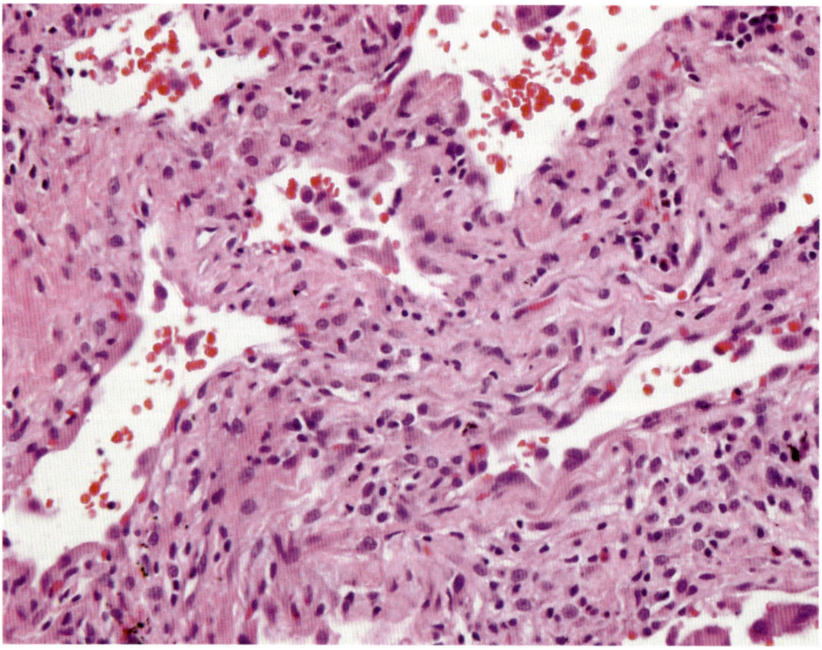

FIGURE 9.10 Higher magnification of NSIP showing dense inflammatory infiltrate and fibrosis producing widening of alveolar walls.

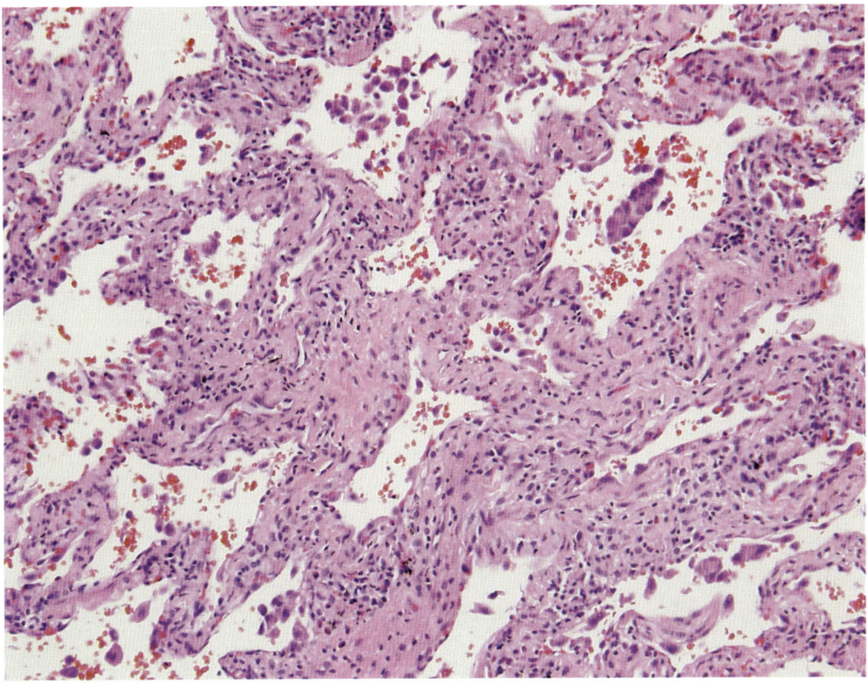

FIGURE 9.11 "Cellular" NSIP showing predominance of inflammatory cells in alveolar walls.

favorably to corticosteroid therapy. About 50% to 70% of patients will recover completely after treatment.[9] The prognosis for "cellular" NSIP (i.e., NSIP devoid of fibrosis) is much better than that seen in fibrosing NSIP (Figs. 9.11 and 9.12). The most important histologic feature of NSIP is the temporal uniformity of the changes (i.e., all lesions are in the same stage of evolution). The histologic picture is thus one of a uniform process throughout with identical findings in all areas of the biopsy (eFigs. 9.7 and 9.8). Small areas showing bronchiolitis obliterans organizing pneumonia-(BOOP-) like changes can be found in nearly half the cases. Focal, patchy accumulation of intra-alveolar macrophages can also be observed.

Desquamative Interstitial Pneumonia

Initially reported by Liebow[1] as a disease characterized by "desquamated" epithelial cells filling the alveolar lumens, desquamative interstitial pneumonia (DIP) represents a very rare lung process characterized by accumulation of macrophages within the airspaces. DIP occurs in patients at least 10 years younger than those with UIP. The process has an insidious onset and is associated with cigarette smoking.[10] Patients develop slowly progressive cough and dyspnea over several weeks or months, with mild restriction in lung function and moderate reduction in diffusing capacity. Digital clubbing can be seen in approximately half of the patients. Chest

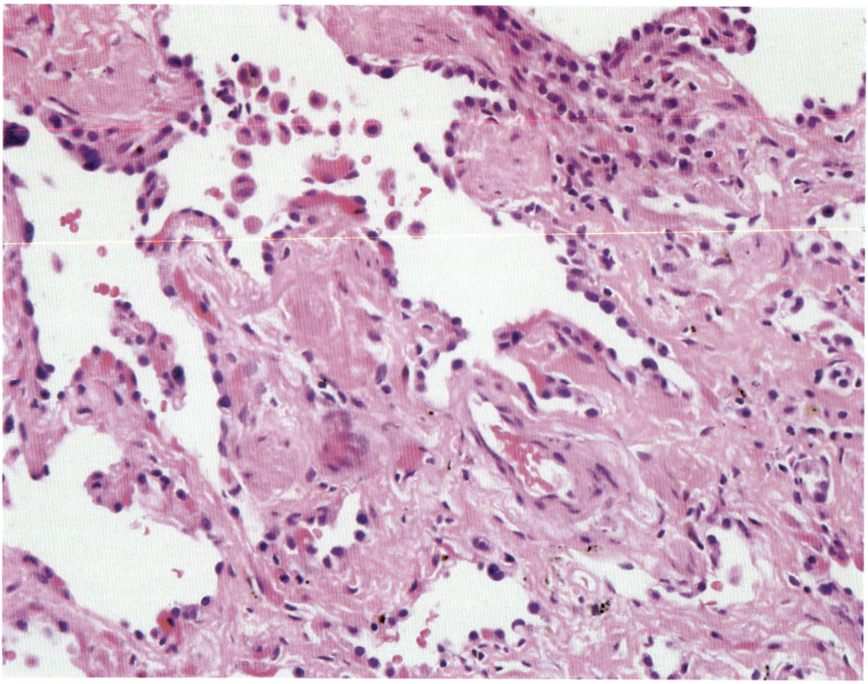

FIGURE 9.12 Fibrotic NSIP showing widening of alveolar septa secondary to fibrosis with scant inflammatory elements.

films and CT scans may be normal in some patients but more often show patchy areas of ground glass opacification in the lung bases and the periphery.[11] The most striking histologic finding is distention of the alveolar spaces by sheets of macrophages containing abundant eosinophilic cytoplasm (Figs. 9.13 and 9.14) (eFig. 9.9). The alveolar walls show mild thickening owing to fibrosis and chronic inflammation (Figs. 9.15 and 9.16). The histiocytic nature of the intra-alveolar infiltrate can be demonstrated by immunohistochemistry with antibodies to CD68 or CD163 (Fig. 9.17). The process shows an even and diffuse distribution throughout the lung fields with temporal uniformity (i.e., all lesions are in the same stage of evolution).[12] The prognosis for DIP is much better than that of UIP. A favorable response to steroids and complete recovery is observed in most patients. DIP-like reaction can be observed focally in other conditions, including UIP, Langerhans cell histiocytosis (LCH), and respiratory alveolitis-related interstitial pneumonia (RB-ILD). Proper distinction from these conditions is important because of the differences in prognosis and treatment.

Lymphoid Interstitial Pneumonia

Lymphoid interstitial pneumonia (LIP) is generally included among the IIPs for historical reasons, but it is generally accepted today that this

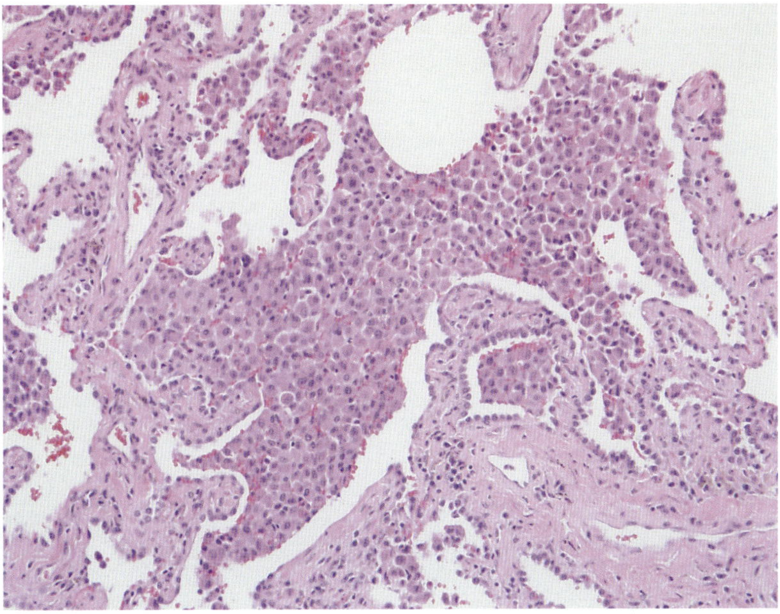

FIGURE 9.13 Scanning magnification of lung biopsy in DIP showing distention of alveolar spaces by macrophages.

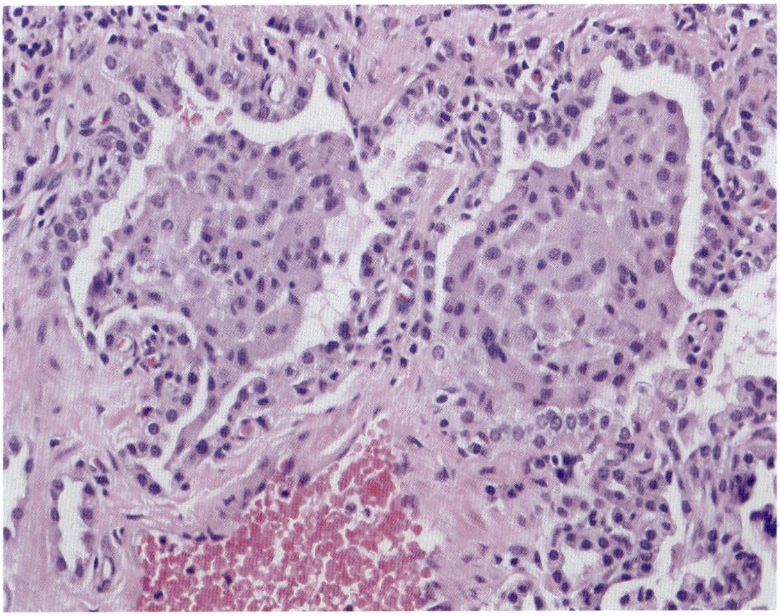

FIGURE 9.14 Higher power of DIP showing almost complete filling of alveolar lumina by monotonous population of macrophages. Mild thickening and fibrosis/inflammation of alveolar walls.

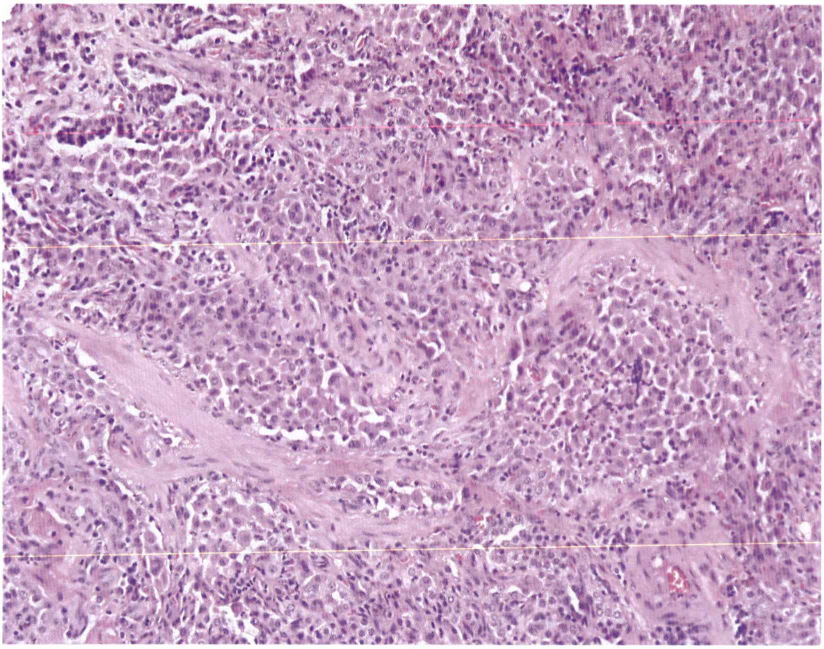

FIGURE 9.15 Another example of DIP showing mild thickening of alveolar septa by fibrosis.

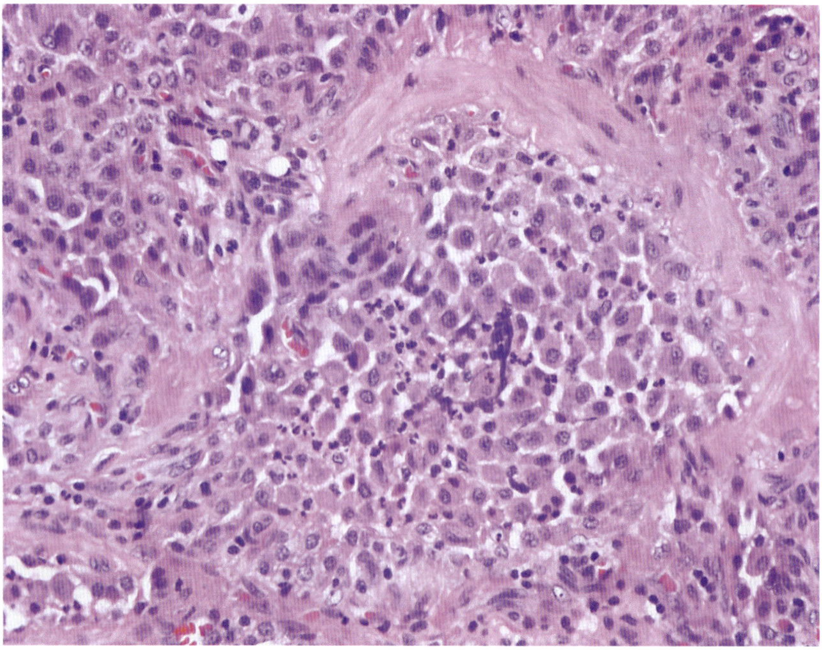

FIGURE 9.16 Higher magnification from the same field showing complete filling of the alveolar lumen by monotonous sheets of macrophages.

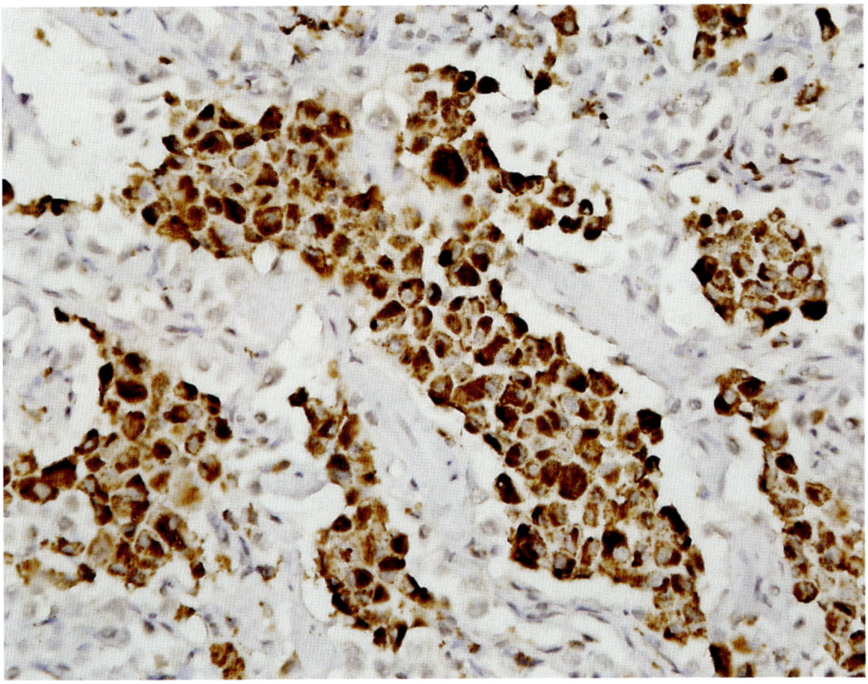

FIGURE 9.17 Immunohistochemical staining shows CD68+ (KP-1 macrophage marker) alveolar macrophages in DIP.

represents a precursor lesion to a lymphoproliferative disorder that may progress to a low-grade extranodal marginal zone lymphoma (so-called BALT-lymphoma).[13] As such, it will be discussed under the heading "lymphoproliferative disorders." Some cases categorized as examples of LIP may also overlap morphologically with cases of "cellular" NSIP.

Cryptogenic Organizing Pneumonia

The term *bronchiolitis obliterans organizing pneumonia* (BOOP) was first proposed for patients who presented with organizing pneumonia of unexplained etiology.[14] This pattern of airspace organization is an extremely common and nonspecific manifestation of lung injury that can be seen in a variety of conditions, from infections to neoplasia. Because of the nonspecific nature of the changes, the term *BOOP* has been increasingly abandoned in recent years and replaced by the term *cryptogenic organizing pneumonia* (COP) when the changes are extensive and no etiology can be recognized.[3] COP is associated with a favorable clinical evolution and responds well to corticosteroid administration. The term *COP* or *BOOP* should not be used in the setting of extensive interstitial fibrosis, as the finding in such instances is secondary to the underlying fibrosing process and will be associated with a poor prognosis. COP usually occurs after an upper respiratory tract infection with slowly progressive symptoms of cough and shortness of breath. Patients are usually middle aged and nonsmokers. Patchy airspace consolidation with ground glass attenuation is the most common radiologic finding. COP is histologically characterized by filling of the airspaces by plugs comprising loose fibroblasts admixed with a myxoid ground substance (Fig. 9.18). The surrounding alveolar walls may contain a mild interstitial inflammatory infiltrate made up of small lymphocytes, plasma cells, and histiocytes (Fig. 9.19). Fibrin may also be seen focally in association with the fibroblastic plugs, and more advanced lesions may display more prominent fibrosis (Fig. 9.20). Interstitial fibrosis and honeycombing should not be present in the idiopathic form of organizing pneumonia.

Acute Interstitial Pneumonia

Acute interstitial pneumonia (AIP) is a rapidly progressive form of interstitial pneumonia that affects young adults and is usually preceded by flu-like symptoms. The pathologic findings are similar to those seen in organizing diffuse alveolar damage and have been detailed in Chapter 2. The condition has also been termed *idiopathic adult respiratory distress syndrome*. The term *AIP* should not be used in cases where an inciting

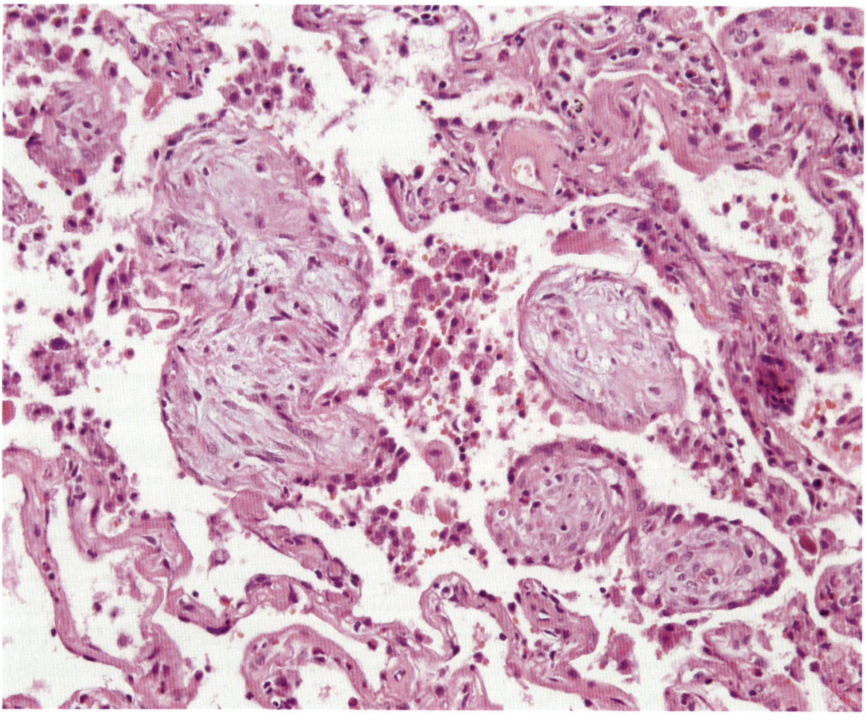

FIGURE 9.18 COP shows multiple fibroblastic plugs filling the alveolar lumens. Notice the absence of fibrosis in surrounding alveolar walls.

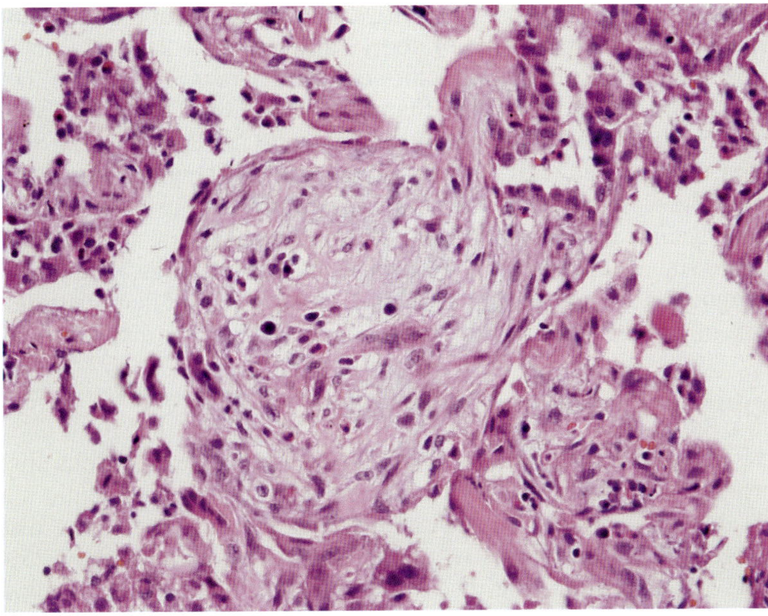

FIGURE 9.19 Early stage of organization in COP shows abundant myxoid matrix with granulation tissue plugging the alveolar space.

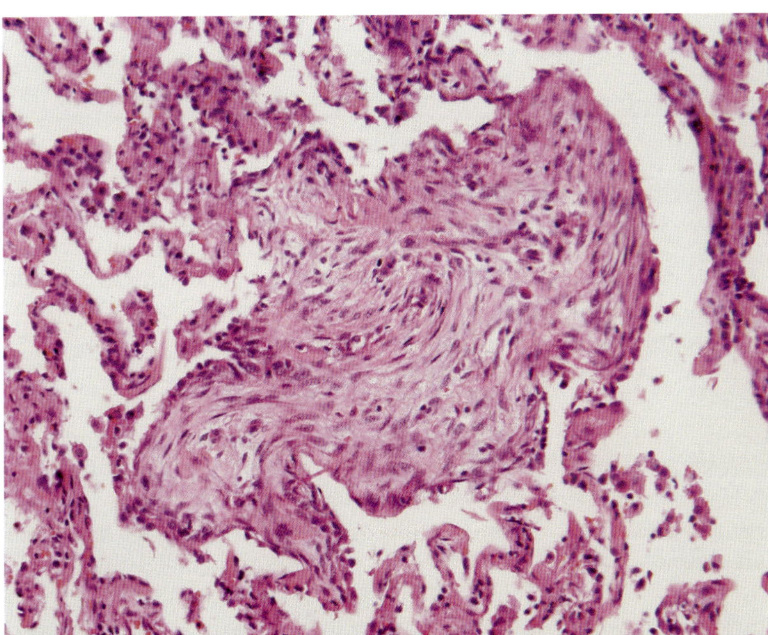

FIGURE 9.20 More advanced stage of COP shows plugging of alveolar lumens by predominantly fibroblastic proliferation with minimal inflammation.

event such as shock, sepsis, or drugs has been documented. Patients present with acute symptoms of short duration (1 or 2 days), including dyspnea, fever, and bilateral opacities on chest X-rays. The clinical course is rapidly progressive with more than 70% mortality. The histologic findings are characterized by thickening of alveolar septa due to fibroblastic proliferation admixed with chronic inflammation.[15] There is usually hyperplasia of alveolar pneumocytes with squamous metaplasia. There may be residual hyaline membranes lining alveolar spaces. The process closely resembles the organizing stage of diffuse alveolar damage. The diagnosis of AIP requires strict clinical–pathologic correlation and demonstration of absence of an underlying cause for the acute respiratory distress.

SPECIFIC INTERSTITIAL PNEUMONIAS

Diffuse interstitial lung disease may often be the result of various specific underlying conditions that are amenable to specific therapeutic strategies (Table 9.1). One of the commonest causes of diffuse lung disease is collagen-vascular disease, which accounts for approximately 25% of all cases of interstitial lung diseases and 2% of deaths from respiratory causes (Table 9.2).[16] The histopathologic findings in the acute and chronic phases of the various CVD have been detailed in Chapters 2 and 3, including rheumatoid arthritis, progressive systemic sclerosis, systemic lupus

TABLE 9.2 Diffuse Lung Manifestations of Systemic collagen-vascular disease

Disease	Pulmonary Manifestation
Rheumatoid arthritis	Follicular bronchiolitis, diffuse alveolar damage, organizing pneumonia, diffuse fibrosing interstitial pneumonia (UIP pattern), granulomatous interstitial pneumonia, vasculitis
Systemic lupus erythematosus	Follicular bronchiolitis, diffuse alveolar damage, organizing pneumonia, diffuse fibrosing interstitial pneumonia (UIP pattern), granulomatous interstitial pneumonia, vasculitis
Progressive systemic sclerosis	Diffuse alveolar damage, organizing pneumonia, diffuse fibrosing interstitial pneumonia (UIP pattern), vasculitis
Dermatomyositis/ polymyositis	Bronchiolitis, diffuse alveolar damage, organizing pneumonia, diffuse fibrosing interstitial pneumonia (UIP pattern),vasculitis
Sjogren syndrome	Follicular bronchiolitis, diffuse alveolar damage, organizing pneumonia, diffuse fibrosing interstitial pneumonia (UIP pattern), vasculitis

erythematosus, polymyositis/dermatomyositis, and Sjogren syndrome. The findings in these conditions can often be confused for UIP or other types of IIPs. Correlation with the clinical history and laboratory tests is indispensable for arriving at the correct diagnosis.

A similar situation applies to diffuse lung disease associated with drugs.[17,18] The various pathologic manifestations of drug-induced lung changes are detailed in Chapters 2 and 3, and include acute lung injury associated with drug administration, drug-mediated chronic diffuse lung disease, and vascular disease produced by medications. The most common offending agents include methotrexate, amiodarone, carmustine, busulfan and bleomycin.

Four other types of diffuse lung disease that can have a treatable and identifiable underlying cause will be dealt with here in more detail: hypersensitivity pneumonitis (extrinsic allergic alveolitis), RB-ILD, LCH, and giant cell interstitial pneumonia due to heavy metal exposure.

Hypersensitivity Pneumonitis

Hypersensitivity pneumonitis is a distinctive type of diffuse interstitial lung process caused by airway inhalation exposure to environmental antigens. Typical examples include "farmer's lung," caused by inhalation of actinomyces in hay, and "pigeon breeder's lung," caused by inhalation of avian antigens.[19,20] Hypersensitivity pneumonitis can manifest either as an acute reaction or as a chronic process. The acute form presents within hours after exposure to the inhaled antigen and will manifest with cough, dyspnea, fever, and chills, resembling a viral infection. The symptoms are exacerbated with recurrent exposure to the antigen. A chronic form may result from lower levels of exposure to antigens. The chronic form of the disease may be progressive and lead to death because of diffuse lung fibrosis. CT scans show diffuse ground glass infiltrates in the acute form that are mostly confined to the upper half of the lungs. In the chronic form, small nodules, irregular linear opacities, and ground glass changes may be seen, mostly in the middle lung zones with relative sparing of the apices and bases. In very late stages, honeycombing resembling that of UIP will be seen.

The pathologic features of hypersensitivity pneumonitis have been reviewed in Chapter 3, and include changes of chronic interstitial inflammation associated with the production of small, nonnecrotizing interstitial granulomas. The chronic interstitial inflammation resembles NSIP and other forms of cellular inflammatory interstitial pneumonias. The lung biopsy typically shows widening of the alveolar walls by a dense interstitial inflammatory infiltrate comprising small lymphocytes and plasma cells. Foci of organizing pneumonia with airspace fibroblastic plugs can be seen in more than half of cases. Focal bronchiolization of airspaces (lambertosis) can also result from chronic injury to airway spaces, as well as bronchiolitis with aggregates of plasma cells and small lymphocytes surrounding terminal airways. The chronic inflammatory changes will give rise to interstitial fibrosis, with dense collagen deposition and honeycombing resembling UIP resulting in

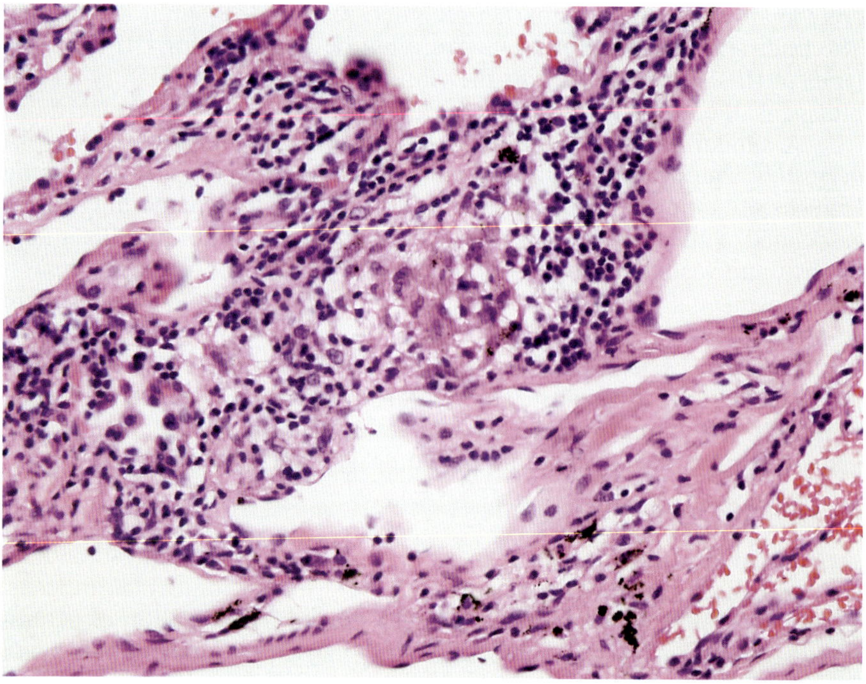

FIGURE 9.21 Thickening of alveolar septa by dense lymphoid infiltrate and incipient fibrosis in allergic extrinsic alveolitis. Notice the small, ill-defined epithelioid granuloma admixed with the lymphocytes within the alveolar wall.

end stages. An indispensable component of the process is the presence of small, ill-formed epithelioid granulomas in the interstitium (Fig. 9.21). The granulomas may be extremely subtle and easy to overlook on cursory examination.[21] Sometimes only scattered multinucleated giant cells will be seen in the interstitium, which should prompt a search for the microgranulomas. Refractile oxalate crystals may be found within giant cells; these should not be interpreted as evidence of aspiration pneumonia. Prominent, well-formed epithelioid granulomas should point in the direction of an alternate diagnosis. The differential diagnosis for hypersensitivity pneumonitis includes cellular interstitial pneumonias caused by drug reactions or atypical mycobacteria. Clinical correlation and special stains will be of help in separating these conditions. Treatment of the condition involves removal of exposure to the offending antigen. Patients may not respond well to corticoids if the offending antigen is not removed. Chronic cases may progress to lung fibrosis with potential fatal outcome.

Respiratory Bronchiolitis-Associated Interstitial Lung Disease

RB-ILD is a disorder strictly related to cigarette smoking that leads to a mild form of interstitial lung disease.[22] This process is currently believed to be closely related to DIP and LCH. Respiratory bronchiolitis (RB) is a microscopic incidental finding in the small airways of cigarette smokers characterized by mild peribronchiolar inflammation with deposition of pigment-laden macrophages within the lumen of the bronchioles. In some patients, an exuberant form of this process will develop leading to clinical and radiographic manifestations of disease. RB, RB-ILD, and DIP have been regarded by some as a continuous spectrum of disease, with RB representing the asymptomatic end of the spectrum and DIP corresponding to the other end.[23] Patients with RB-ILD are usually 10 years younger than those with DIP (30 to 40 years old) and present with symptoms of shortness of breath and cough. Chest X-rays and CT scans will show ground glass opacities. Histologic changes of RB-ILD can be seen in smokers in the vicinity of other processes and may represent an incidental finding. A diagnosis of RB-ILD should be established only in the appropriate clinical and radiographic contexts. The main histologic findings comprise mild chronic inflammation around bronchioles with variable numbers of hemosiderin-laden macrophages in the lumen, and metaplastic bronchiolar epithelium extending into the alveolar ducts (Fig. 9.22). Scant peribronchiolar fibrosis may also be present (Fig. 9.23). RB-ILD has an excellent prognosis, and the symptoms usually subside with cessation of smoking.[24]

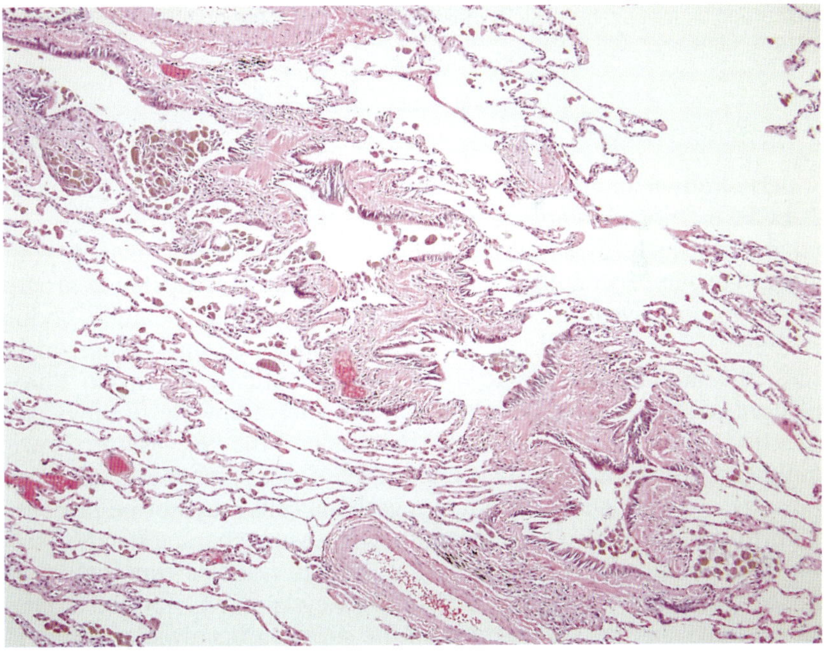

FIGURE 9.22 Lung changes in RB-ILD characterized by mild chronic peribronchiolar inflammation with metaplastic bronchiolar epithelium extending into alveolar ducts and collections of hemosiderin-laden macrophages.

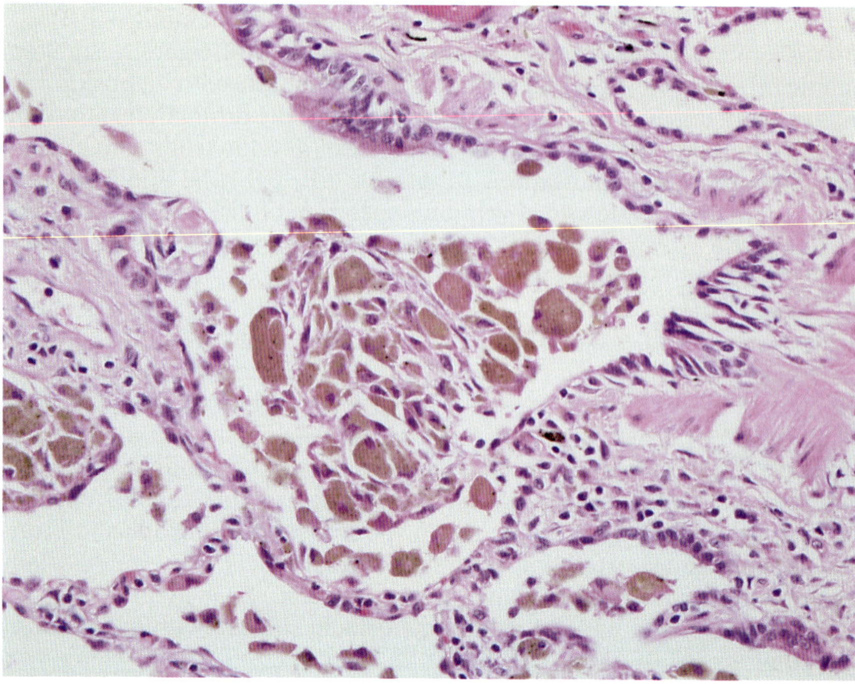

FIGURE 9.23 Higher magnification in lung biopsy from patient with RB-ILD showing RB characterized by mild peribronchiolar inflammation with variable numbers of hemosiderin-laden macrophages in the lumen.

Langerhans Cell Histiocytosis

Formerly known as pulmonary eosinophilic granuloma or "histiocytosis-X," LCH is another smoking-related condition.[25,26] The disease occurs almost exclusively in smokers. Affected individuals are usually young adults, between 20 and 40 years of age, and present with slowly progressive cough and dyspnea. Imaging studies show small, bilateral nodules distributed in the upper lobes in the early stages of the disease; in late stages, the nodules are replaced by cysts, eventually ending in fibrosis and honeycombing. The histology mirrors the radiologic findings, with the early lesions showing a cellular process and the late lesions showing mainly fibrosis. In the late stages, the disease can be very difficult to recognize because the characteristic Langerhans cells may not be present in the fibrotic areas. The cellular form of the disease is characterized on scanning magnification by small, irregular, stellate nodules centered on the small airways (Fig. 9.24) (eFig. 9.10). Small cysts may be formed adjacent to the nodules because of traction on the surrounding alveolar walls. The nodules comprise eosinophils in variable numbers admixed with a population of Langerhans cells and small lymphocytes (Fig. 9.25). Langerhans cells are characterized by pale, irregular nuclei displaying striking nuclear

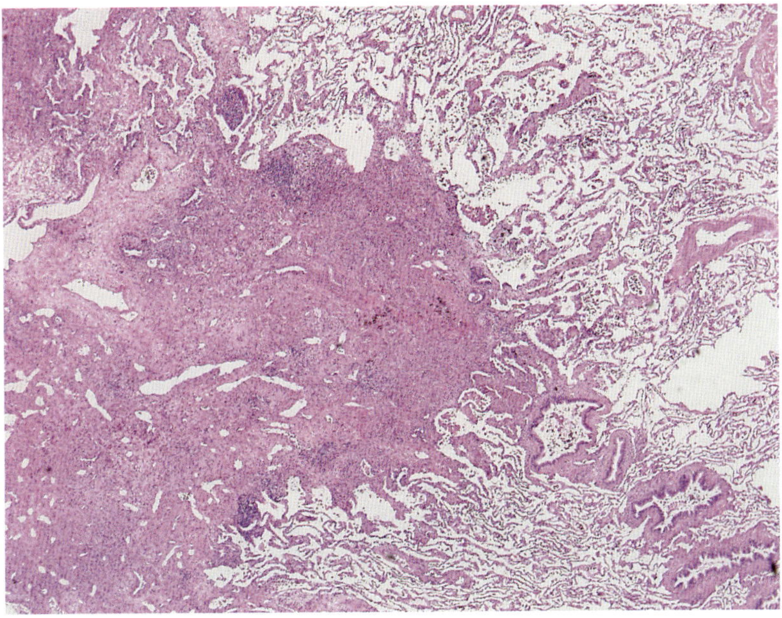

FIGURE 9.24 Scanning magnification in lung biopsy of patient with LCH showing stellate scar adjacent to the small airways.

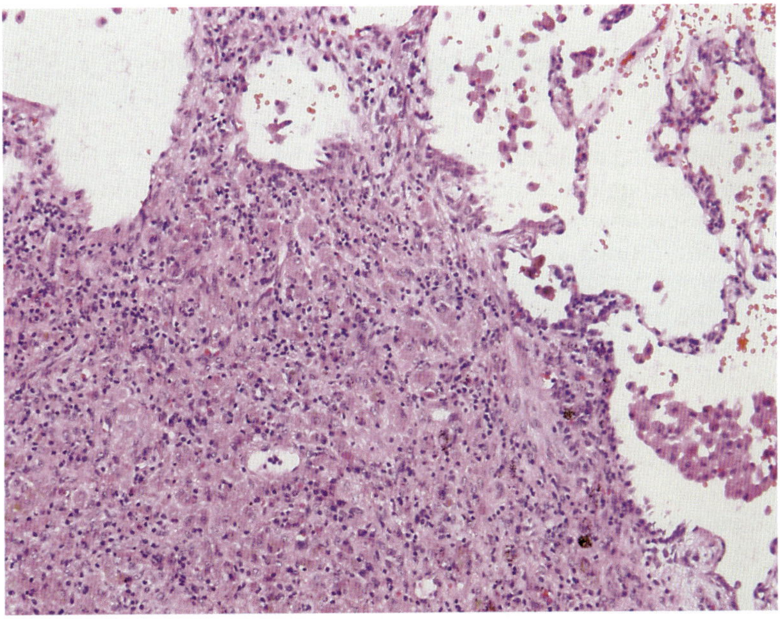

FIGURE 9.25 Higher magnification from fully developed lesion in LCH of the lung shows dense population of inflammatory and mononuclear cells admixed with histiocytes.

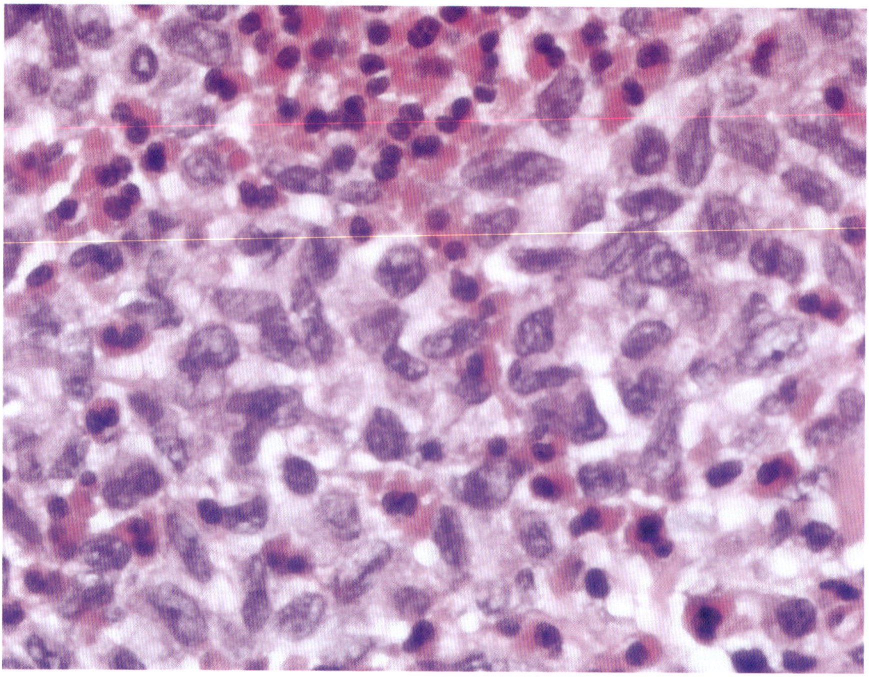

FIGURE 9.26 High power of LCH showing eosinophils admixed with Langerhans cells. The latter are characterized by their striking nuclear convolutions, longitudinal nuclear grooves, and small inconspicuous nucleoli.

convolutions and infoldings imparting them a "cerebriform" appearance (Fig. 9.26). The cytoplasm of the Langerhans cells is mildly eosinophilic with indistinct cell borders. The surrounding small airways may display features of RB. The Langerhans cells can be highlighted by the use of immunohistochemical stains. Antibodies to CD1a and S-100 protein will stain these cells very strongly, facilitating the diagnosis (Fig. 9.27). The late, fibrotic lesions are characterized by residual stellate, parenchymal scars that may be completely depleted of Langerhans cells. Smoking cessation is the most effective treatment and usually results in disappearance of the symptoms. Some have utilized immunosuppressive agents with or without the addition of a cytotoxic agent. Most patients recover spontaneously; however, some cases may progress to fibrosis with development of honeycomb lung.

Giant Cell Interstitial Pneumonitis due to Hard Metal Pneumoconiosis

Originally described as "giant cell interstitial pneumonia" by Liebow,[27] this disorder has now been found to be related to inhalation of dust containing hard metal particles, such as tungsten carbide, titanium,

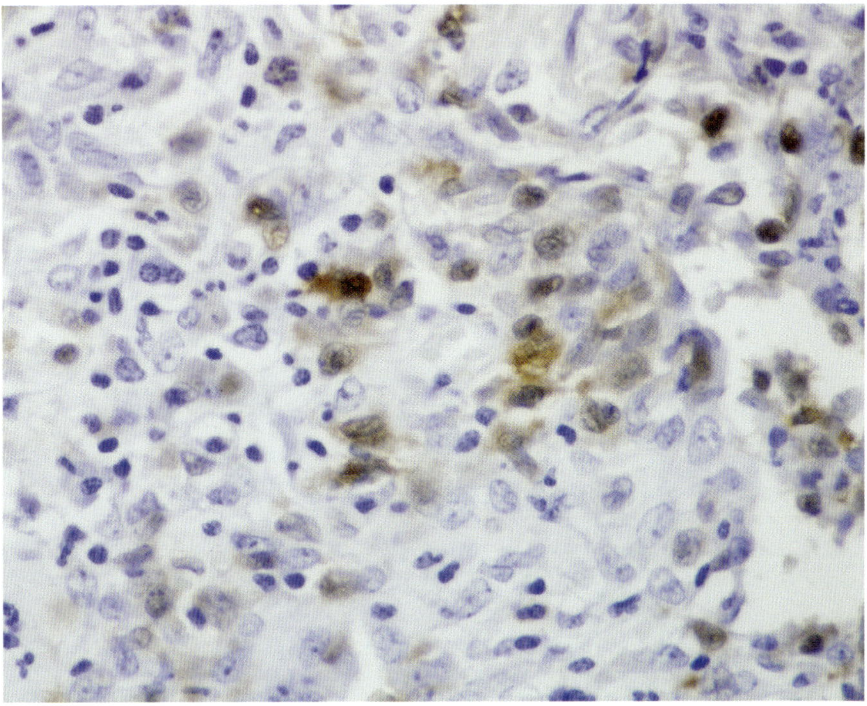

FIGURE 9.27 Immunohistochemical stain for S-100 protein highlights a cluster of Langerhans cells in LCH of the lung.

and cobalt. Exposure can occur during the manufacturing process of products containing hard metals or in certain industries such as the diamond-polishing industry. Patients usually present with progressive dyspnea. Cessation of the exposure is usually effective in controlling the symptoms and leads to full recovery in most patients. In a few cases, the disease may follow a progressive course to death. It is believed that the pathogenetic mechanism of disease is because of hypersensitivity; less than 1% of those exposed to hard metals develop the disease. Histologic findings include thickening of alveolar septa secondary to fibrosis, chronic inflammation, and hyperplasia of type II alveolar pneumocytes. The most distinctive feature, however, is the presence of abundant multinucleated giant cells within the alveolar lumens and lining the alveolar septa (Fig. 9.28). The giant cells are found admixed with numerous macrophages, resulting in a histologic appearance that is reminiscent of DIP. In advanced stages, there is severe interstitial fibrosis with bronchiolar metaplasia and honeycombing resembling UIP. The metal particles can be observed only by using analytical electron microscopy.[28] Transbronchial biopsy and bronchioloalveolar lavage may be useful in the diagnosis of this condition.[29]

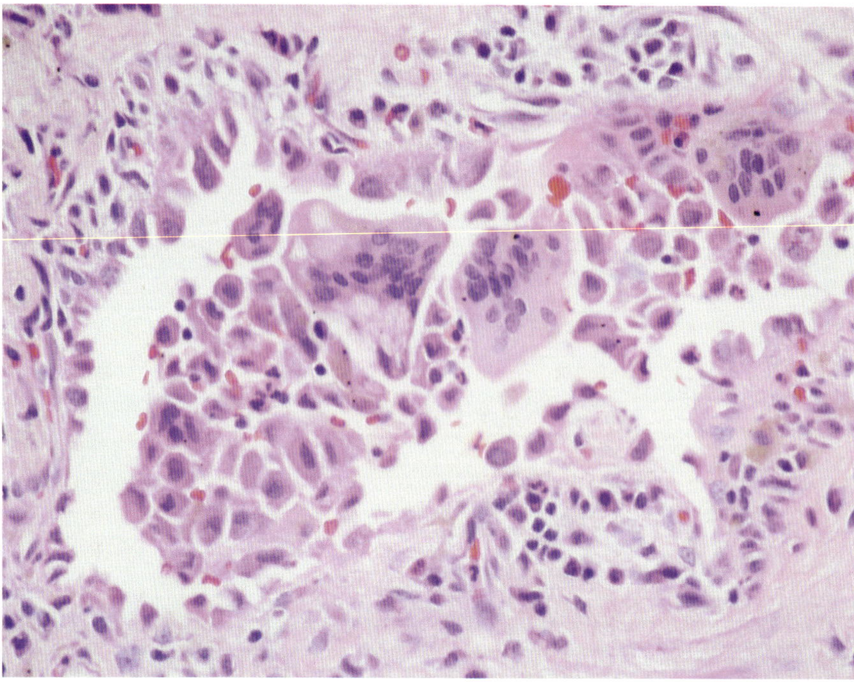

FIGURE 9.28 Lung biopsy in patient with giant cell interstitial pneumonia due to exposure to dust with hard metal particles (hard metal pneumoconiosis) showing abundant macrophages within alveolar lumen admixed with large, multinucleated giant cells.

REFERENCES

1. Liebow A, Carrington C. The interstitial pneumonias. In: Simon M, Potchen E, LeMay M, eds. *Frontiers of Pulmonary Radiology: Pathophysiologic, Roentgenographic and Radioisotopic Considerations*. Orlando, FL: Grune & Stratton; 1969:109–141.
2. Katzenstein AL. Idiopathic interstitial pneumonia: classification and diagnosis. *Monogr Pathol.* 1993;36:1–31.
3. Travis W, King TJ, Bateman E, et al. American Thoracic Society/European Respiratory Society international multidisciplinary consensus classification of the idiopathic interstitial pneumonias. *Am Rev Respir Crit Care Med*. 2002;165:227–304.
4. Wall CP, Gaensler EA, Carrington CB. Comparison of transbronchial and open biopsies in diffuse infiltrative lung disease. *Am Rev Respir Dis*. 1981;123:280–285.
5. Crystal R, Fulmer J, Roberts W, et al. Idiopathic pulmonary fibrosis. Clinical, histologic, radiographic, physiologic, scintigraphic, cytologic and biochemical aspects. *Ann Intern Med*. 1976;85:769–788.
6. Muller N, Staples C, Miller R, et al. Disease activity in idiopathic pulmonary fibrosis. CT and pathologic correlation. *Radiology*. 1987;165:731–743.
7. Katzenstein A-L A. Idiopathic interstitial pneumonia/idiopathic pulmonary fibrosis. *Katzenstein and Askin's Surgical Pathology of Non-Neoplastic Lung Disease*. 3rd ed. Philadelphia, PA: WB Saunders; 1990:48–80.

8. Katzenstein AL, Fiorelli RF. Nonspecific interstitial pneumonia/fibrosis: histologic features and clinical significance. *Am J Surg Pathol.* 1994;18:136–147.
9. Danil ZD, Gilchrist FC, Nicholson AG, et al. A histologic pattern of nonspecific interstitial pneumonia is associated with a better prognosis than usual interstitial pneumonia in patients with cryptogenic fibrosing alveolitis. *Am J Respire Crit Care Med.* 1999;160:899–905.
10. Carrington CB, Gaensler EA, Coutu RE, et al. Natural history and treated course of usual and desquamative interstitial pneumonia. *N Engl J Med.* 1978;298:801–803.
11. Hartman TE, Primack SL, Swensen SJ, et al. Desquamative interstitial pneumonia: thin-section CT findings in 22 patients. *Radiology.* 1993;187:787–790.
12. Carrington CB, Gaensler EA, Coutu RE, et al. Usual and desquamative interstitial pneumonia. *Chest.* 1976;69(S):261–263.
13. Herbert A, Walters MT, Crawley MI, et al. Lymphocytic interstitial pneumonia identified as lymphoma of mucosa associated lymphoid tissue. *J Pathol.* 1985;146:129–138.
14. Epler GR, Colby TV, McLoud TC, et al. Bronchiolitis obliterans organizing pneumonia. *N Engl J Med.* 1985;312:152–158.
15. Olsen J, Colby TV, Elliot C. Hamman-Rich syndrome revisited. *Mayo Clin Proced.* 1998;65:1538–1101.
16. Black I, Katz S. *Respiratory Disease: Task Force Report on Problems, Research Approaches, Needs.* Bethesda, MD: National Heart and Lung Institute; 1977.
17. Cooper JA Jr. Drug-induced lung disease. *Adv Intern Med.* 1997;42:231–268.
18. Camus PH, Foucher P, Bounniaud PH, et al. Drug-induced infiltrative lung disease. *Eur Respir J.* 2001;32(S):93–100s.
19. Braun SR, Pico GA, Tsiatis S, et al. Framer's lung disease: long-term clinical and physiologic outcome. *Am Rev Respir Dis.* 1979;119:185–191.
20. Suda T, Sato A, Ida M, et al. Hypersensitivity pneumonitis associated with home ultrasonic humidifiers. *Chest.* 1995;107:711–719.
21. Coleman A, Colby TV. Histologic diagnosis of extrinsic allergic alveolitis. *Am J Surg Pathol.* 1988;12:514–518.
22. Niewoehner D, Kleinerman J, Rice D. Pathologic changes in the peripheral airways in young cigarette smokers. *N Eng J Med.* 1974;291:755–758.
23. Heyneman LE, Ward S, Lynch DA, et al. Respiratory bronchiolitis, respiratory bronchiolitis-associated interstitial lung disease, and desquamative interstitial pneumonia: different entities or part of the spectrum of the same disease process? *Am J Roentgenol.* 1999;173:1617–1622.
24. Myers J, Veal C, Shin M, et al. Respiratory bronchiolitis causing interstitial lung disease. A clinicopathologic study of six cases. *Am Rev Respir Dis.* 1987;135:880–884.
25. Vasallo R, Ryu JH, Colby TV, et al. Pulmonary Langerhans'-cell histiocytosis. *N Eng J Med.* 2000;342:1969–1978.
26. Travis WD, Borok Z, Roum JH, et al. Pulmonary Langerhans cell granulomatosis (histiocytosis X). A clinicopathologic study of 48 cases. *Am J Surg Pathol.* 1993;17:971–986.
27. Liebow AA. Definition and classification of interstitial pneumonias in human pathology. *Prog Resp Res.* 1975;8:1–33.
28. Stettler LE, Groth DH, Platek SF. Automated characterization of particles extracted from human lungs: three cases of tungsten carbide exposure. *Scanning Electron Microsc.* 1983;I:439–448.
29. Tabatowski K, Roggli VL, Fulkerson WJ, et al. Giant cell interstitial pneumonia in a hard-metal worker: cytologic, histologic and analytical electron microscopic investigation. *Acta Cytolog.* 1988;32;240–246.

10

LUNG TRANSPLANT PATHOLOGY

Lung transplantation has been utilized over the past years for the management of advanced stage lung disease, including emphysema, cystic fibrosis, chronic obstructive pulmonary disease, primary pulmonary hypertension, and idiopathic pulmonary fibrosis. Unlike some other transplant organs, complications of lung transplants occur with high frequency and about half of the patients suffer chronic rejection. The figures for 5-year survival in lung transplant patients were below 50% in 2001.[1] Several complications can ensue after lung transplant, including vascular complications, airway anastomosis complications, and ischemia–reperfusion injury. Vascular complications include acute post-surgical obstruction of the arterial or venous anastomosis by thrombus, which constitutes a medical emergency, or chronic obstruction due to organizing thrombosis with progressive stenosis. The site of anastomosis may develop a superimposed infection with necrosis or dehiscence of the anastomosis. Ischemia–reperfusion injury can occur in up to 20% of patients, resulting in endothelial injury and pulmonary edema with or without alveolar damage. Recovery occurs in a few days in most patients with supportive therapy alone. Complications of lung transplant can occur immediately in the early postoperative period, within the first month of transplant or later (Table 10.1). The commonest complication of lung transplant, however, is allograft rejection.

Transbronchial lung biopsy is the method of choice for evaluating pulmonary complications in transplant patients.[2] Bronchioloalveolar lavage fluid should also be obtained at the time of the procedure and stained with silver stains and Gram stain for the identification of fungi, *Pneumocystis*, and bacteria. Obtaining adequate tissue samples by the endoscopist is critical for proper evaluation of the process. Multiple tissue samples are preferable and should contain sufficient alveoli and at least one bronchiole in each fragment for proper evaluation. Biopsies of the site of anastomosis are also recommended if infection is suspected to evaluate whether fungal or bacterial infection is present.

TABLE 10.1 Complications of Lung Transplantation

Period	Complication
Immediate (0–5 days)	Primary graft failure
	Vascular complications (bleeding, obstruction)
	Ischemia–reperfusion injury
	Hyperacute rejection
Early (7–30 days)	Infection
	Dehiscence of anastomosis
	Acute rejection
Late (>30 days)	Acute rejection
	Lung infection
	Airway stenosis
	Chronic rejection
	Posttransplant lymphoproliferative disease

REPERFUSION INJURY

Reperfusion injury occurs early in the transplant process as a result of capillary injury leading to noncardiogenic pulmonary edema. The injury is produced by the ischemia induced during the procedure, but becomes manifested only when the circulation to the lung is reestablished. This complication has been observed clinically in up to 80% of patients undergoing lung or lung–heart transplant.[3] This condition manifests clinically within the first 4 days posttransplant with worsening oxygenation and decreased lung compliance. Imaging studies show diffuse alveolar and perihilar interstitial infiltrates. Transbronchial biopsy may be required to exclude acute rejection. The main histologic finding is that of diffuse alveolar damage (DAD), with congestion, interstitial edema, hyperplasia of alveolar type II pneumocytes, and hyaline membrane formation (Fig. 10.1).[4] A few neutrophils can be observed in the interstitium. In the healing phase of reperfusion injury, the hyaline membranes are replaced by intra-alveolar plugs of loose fibrous tissue with myxoid matrix (Masson bodies) with fibrous thickening of the alveolar septa (Fig. 10.2). The features of reperfusion injury can also occur in conjunction with acute rejection and can mask the rejection process. The presence of small lymphocytes in the interstitium, particularly when showing a dense perivascular location and in association with eosinophils should raise the suspicion of acute rejection superimposed on reperfusion injury (Fig. 10.3). Severe acute rejection typically contains a component of DAD; however, acute rejection generally manifests after the first week posttransplant. Attention to the time of the biopsy is therefore critical to

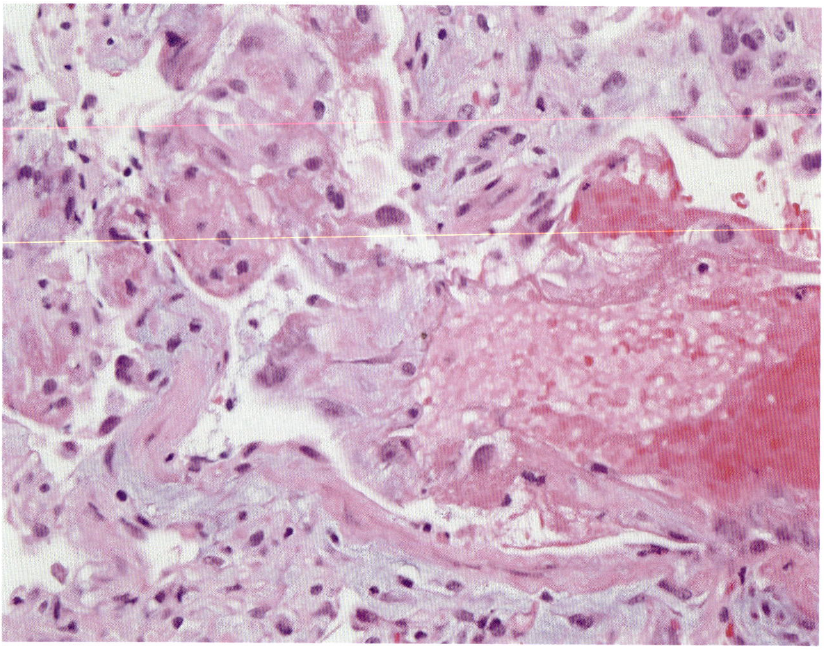

FIGURE 10.1 Reperfusion injury in heart–lung transplant showing diffuse alveolar damage with hyaline membranes and scattered neutrophils.

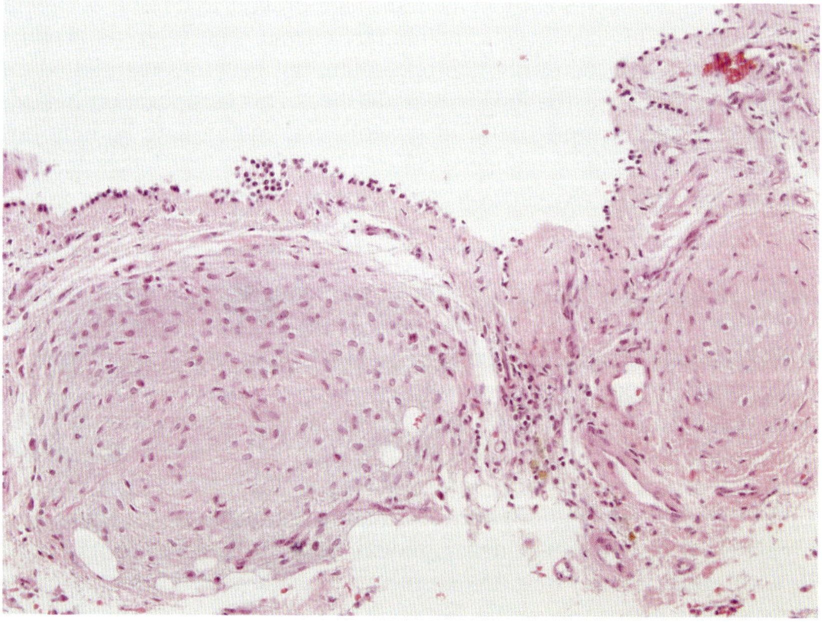

FIGURE 10.2 Healing phase of reperfusion injury showing intra-alveolar plugs of fibromyxoid tissue with fibrous thickening of alveolar septa.

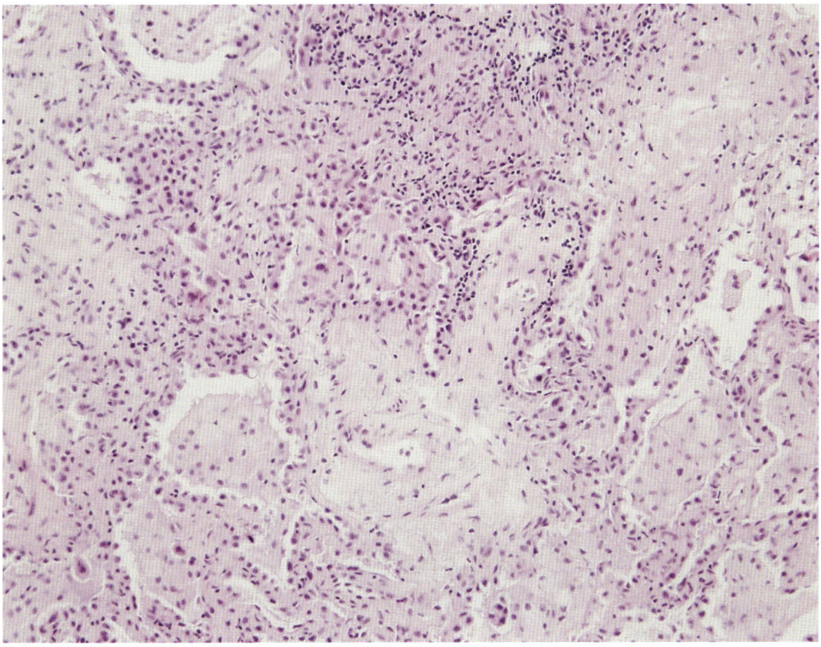

FIGURE 10.3 Acute rejection superimposed on reperfusion injury showing dense interstitial lymphoid infiltrate in alveolar septa.

assess the presence of DAD in the biopsy sample. Biopsies taken early in the course of the first week posttransplant and that show DAD with lymphoid infiltrates restricted to perivascular areas with minimal interstitial component most likely correspond to combined reperfusion injury with mild rejection. When the lymphoid infiltrates are perivascular and also extend prominently into the interstitium, the process most likely corresponds to severe acute rejection. If the biopsy is done after 2 weeks posttransplant, reperfusion injury would be highly unlikely and the process will most likely correspond to acute rejection. Fortunately, acute rejection is becoming less frequent in the immediate posttransplant period. Infection is another cause of DAD and should also be considered in such cases. Use of appropriate stains to rule out organisms and microbiologic cultures is also indicated.

HYPERACUTE REJECTION

Hyperacute rejection represents a hyperacute response to the lung transplant and occurs within minutes to a few hours after transplantation. It is a rare, but potentially fatal complication of lung transplant caused by a humoral-mediated response by antibodies generated against the donor that develop in the recipient before transplantation. Recipients with high titers of these antiendothelial antibodies are at the highest risk for developing hyperacute rejection.[5] Clinical features include respiratory failure and pulmonary edema with complete opacification of the transplanted lung on imaging studies. The diagnosis is based on the clinical findings and a positive donor-specific IgG crossmatch.[5] Histologic features of hyperacute rejection may be variable and include DAD, neutrophilic infiltration, vasculitis, and fibrin thrombi (Fig. 10.4).[5,6] Immunofluorescent studies will show deposition of IgG and complement in the alveolar septa.[5]

ACUTE REJECTION

Acute rejection refers to a cell-mediated response that causes rejection of the allograft and is common in the first 3 to 6 months after lung transplantation. A revised working formulation for the classification of pulmonary allograft rejection was proposed in 1996, which is currently regarded as the accepted standard for the grading of pulmonary rejection.[7] The immune cell activation in acute rejection causes the release of chemokines with progressive infiltration of the graft by host mononuclear cells. Patients can experience multiple episodes of acute rejection. The symptoms include cough, fever, and shortness of breath, but some patients can be asymptomatic. The most important challenge lies in distinguishing acute rejection from infection. Endobronchial biopsy is the method of choice for establishing this distinction.[8] Imaging studies show nonspecific

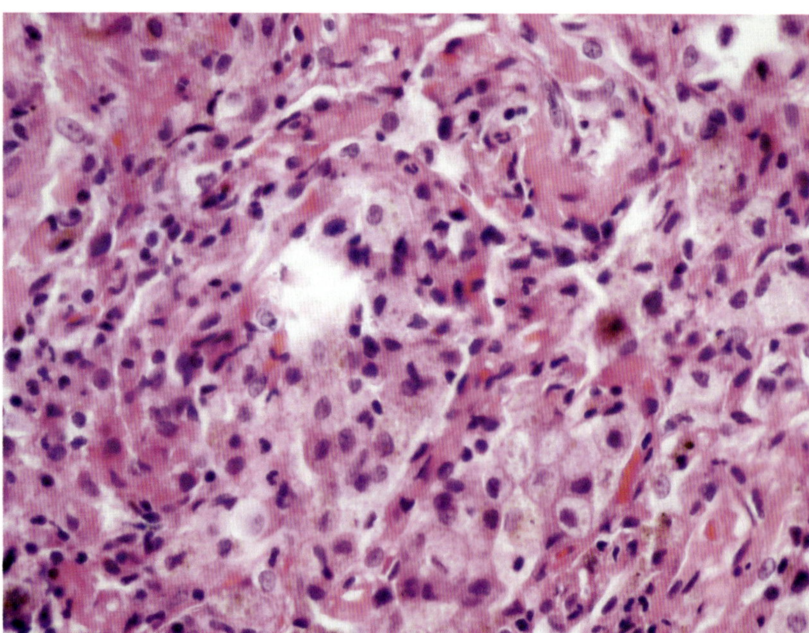

FIGURE 10.4 Acute injury with diffuse alveolar damage and capillaritis in humoral response to hyperacute rejection. The diagnosis is established by demonstrating IgG and complement deposition in the alveolar septa by immunofluorescence.

changes that simulate those of interstitial pulmonary edema. There can be pleural effusion, and up to 50% of patients may show normal radiographic findings. Minimal rejection does not require treatment, but mild-to-severe rejection is treated by increasing the immunosuppression.

Histologically, acute rejection is generally graded on the basis of the intensity and composition of the lymphoid infiltrates[7] (Table 10.2).

The earliest manifestation of acute rejection is perivascular lymphoid infiltrates. The infiltrate comprises small lymphocytes and occasional immunoblasts and may show admixed plasma cells and eosinophils. In minimal acute rejection (A1), the perivascular mononuclear cell infiltrate is usually less than three cells thick (Figs. 10.5 to 10.7). This is normally not readily identified on scanning magnification, and careful examination of vessels is indicated (eFigs. 10.1 and 10.2). A single involved vessel is sufficient to establish the diagnosis. Mild acute rejection (A2) is characterized by increased density of the perivascular mononuclear cell infiltrate that can be up to seven or eight cells thick (Fig. 10.8) (eFig. 10.3). Moderate acute rejection (A3) shows extension of the mononuclear cell infiltrate into the alveolar septa and airspaces (Figs. 10.9 and 10.10) (eFig. 10.4), in addition to the features of A2. In severe acute rejection (A4), the mononuclear cell infiltrate is dense and is associated with pneumocyte damage

TABLE 10.2 Grading of Acute Rejection

Grade	Histologic Features	Cell Composition
A0—(None)	Normal lung parenchyma	—
A1—Minimal	Perivascular mononuclear cell infiltrates, 2–3 cells thick (not apparent on scanning magnification)	Small lymphocytes, plasma cells, occasional larger, transformed lymphocytes
A2—Mild	Perivascular mononuclear cell infiltrates, more than three cells thick (already visible at scanning magnification)	Same as A1, with macrophages and eosinophils
A3—Moderate	Perivascular mononuclear cell infiltrates more than three cells thick with extension into alveolar septa and air spaces	Same as A2, with occasional neutrophils
A4—Severe	Diffuse mononuclear cell infiltrates similar to A3, with prominent pneumocyte damage (DAD)	Same as A3

Reproduced by permission from Yousem SA, Berry GJ, Cagle PT, et al. Revision of the 1990 working formulation for the classification of pulmonary allograft rejection: Lung Rejection Study Group. The International Society for Heart Transplantation. *J Heart Lung Transplant.* 1996;15:1–15.

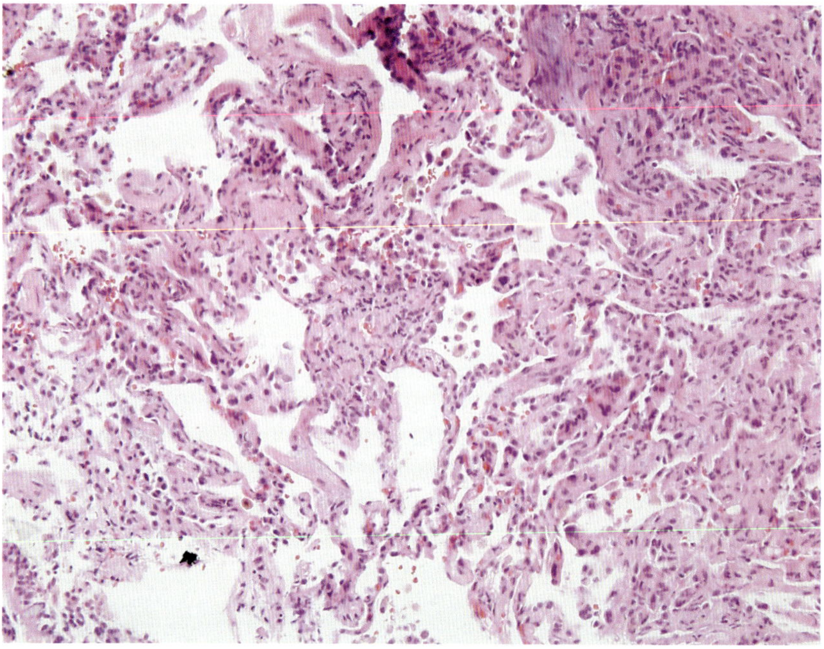

FIGURE 10.5 Scanning magnification in patient with minimal acute rejection (A1) does not reveal any significant abnormalities.

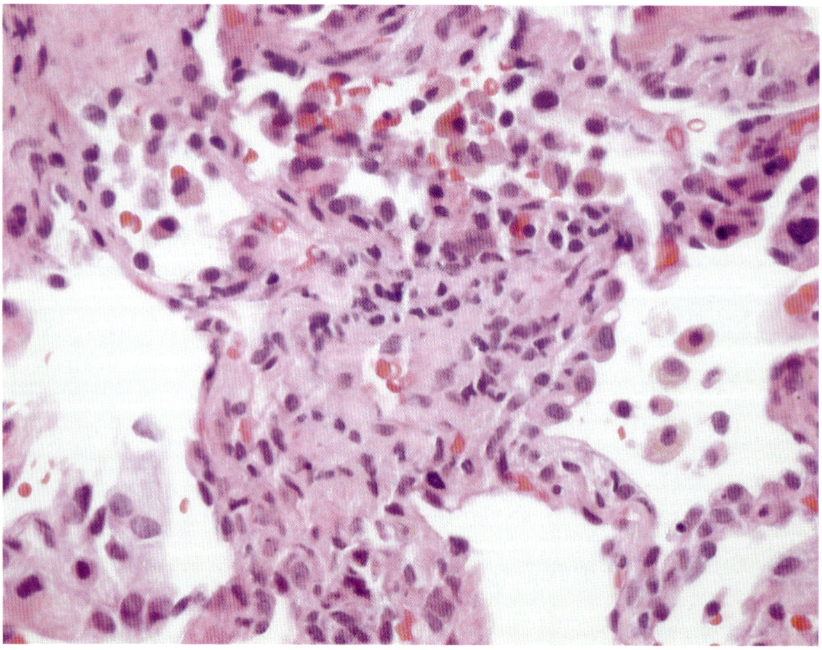

FIGURE 10.6 Higher magnification from preceding field shows a small vessel (center) displaying mild perivascular lymphoid cell infiltrate less than three cells thick.

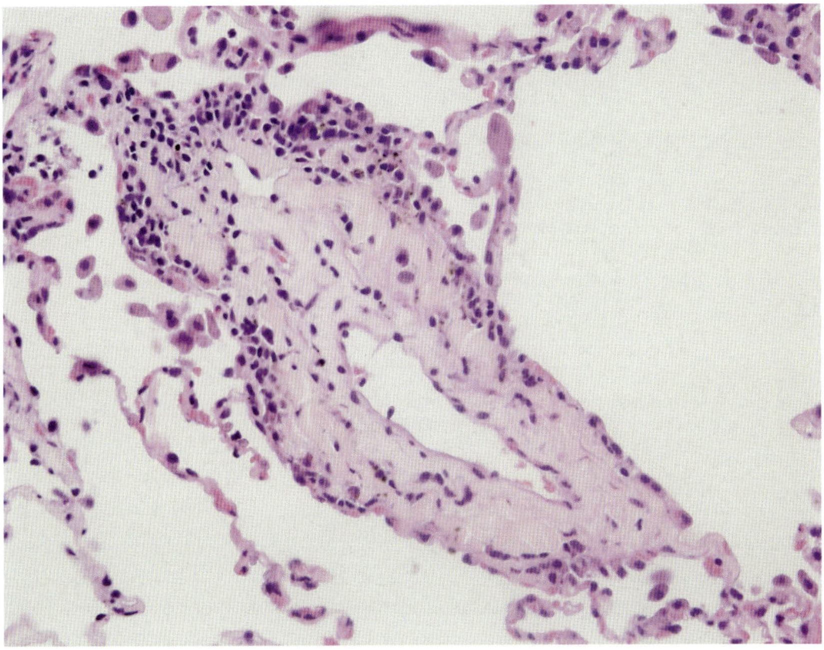

FIGURE 10.7 Another example of minimal acute rejection (A1) showing small blood vessel surrounded by small lymphocytes that are less than three cells in thickness.

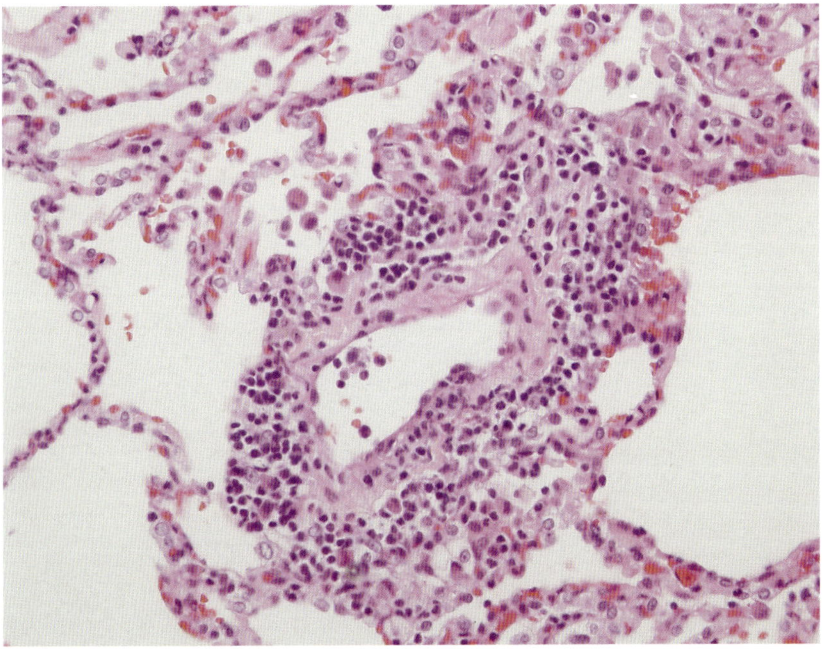

FIGURE 10.8 Mild acute rejection (A2) showing small vessel surrounded by lymphoid cell infiltrate that is more than three cells thick.

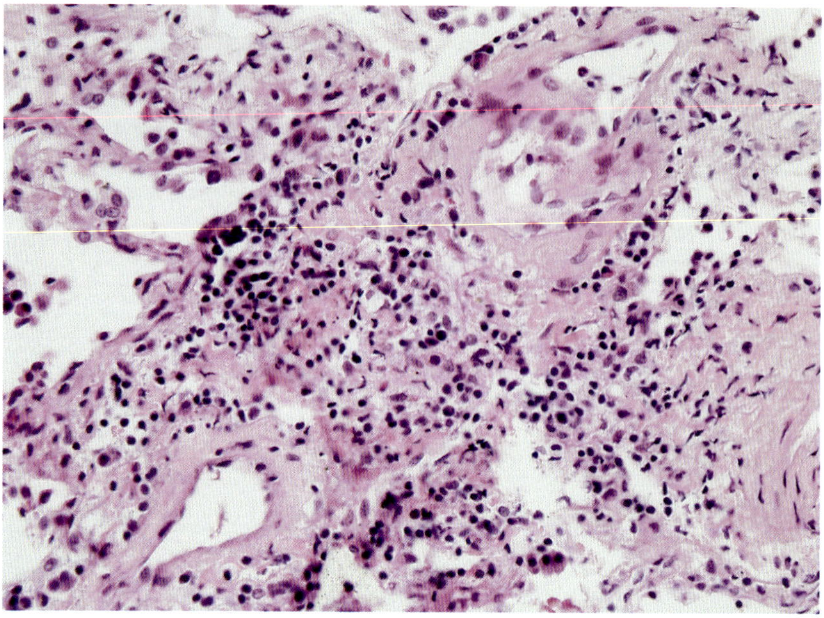

FIGURE 10.9 Moderate acute rejection shows vessel wall surrounded by mononuclear cell infiltrate thicker than three cells and with extension into the surrounding alveolar septa and airspaces.

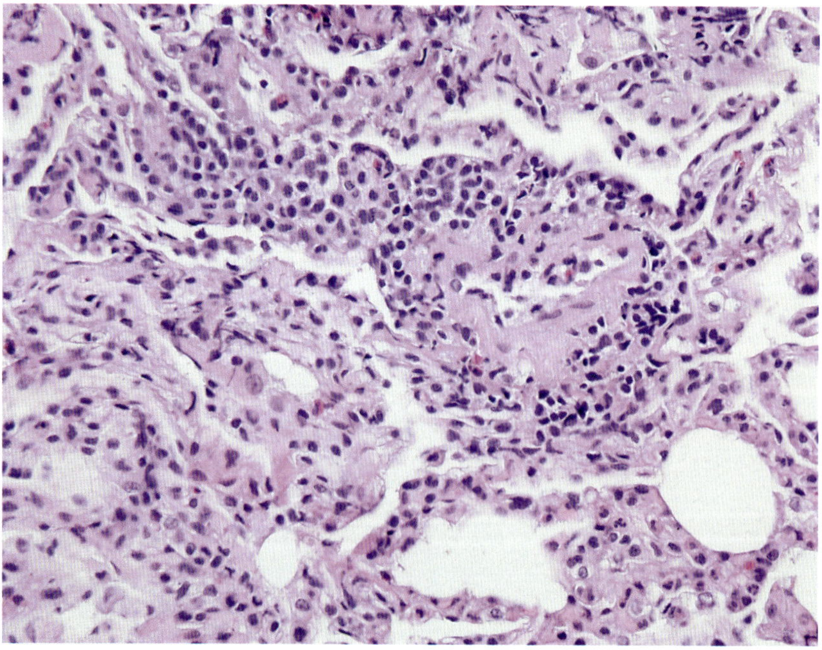

FIGURE 10.10 Another example of moderate acute rejection showing thick cuff of lymphocytes surrounding the vessel wall and extending into adjacent alveolar septa.

that essentially shows the features of DAD, with severe interstitial edema, fibrin deposition, and hyaline membranes (Fig. 10.11). The cell composition of the infiltrate also varies in the different stages. In the early stages, the infiltrate primarily comprises small lymphocytes, plasma cells, and occasional larger, transformed lymphocytes (lymphoblasts) (Figs. 10.12 and 10.13) (eFigs. 10.5 and 10.6). As the process advances, the infiltrate will also display macrophages, eosinophils, and neutrophils. Grade A2 or higher acute rejection can also be accompanied by lymphocytic bronchitis or bronchiolitis, with variable subepithelial lymphocytic infiltrates in the submucosa of the bronchial or bronchiolar walls, which may occasionally extend into the epithelium (Fig. 10.14). In high-grade rejection, the inflammatory infiltrate can permeate through the vessel walls to cause endothelialitis. A rare and unusual variant of acute rejection is characterized by dense eosinophilic infiltration, which can obscure the mononuclear cells in the perivascular infiltrates.

Acute rejection is diagnosed only after infection is excluded.[9] Perivascular lymphoid infiltrates are not specific for rejection and can also be seen in infection with *Pneumocystis* and cytomegalovirus (CMV). Special stains for organisms need to be routinely performed in cases of lung transplant patients to distinguish infection from acute rejection.

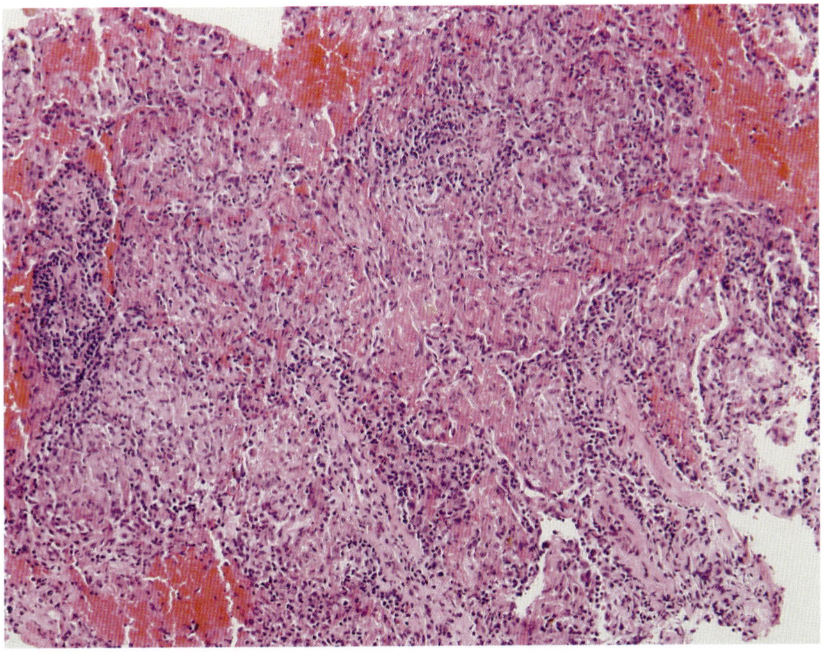

FIGURE 10.11 Severe acute rejection (A4) shows dense perivascular lymphoid infiltrates (left) associated with diffuse alveolar damage in surrounding parenchyma.

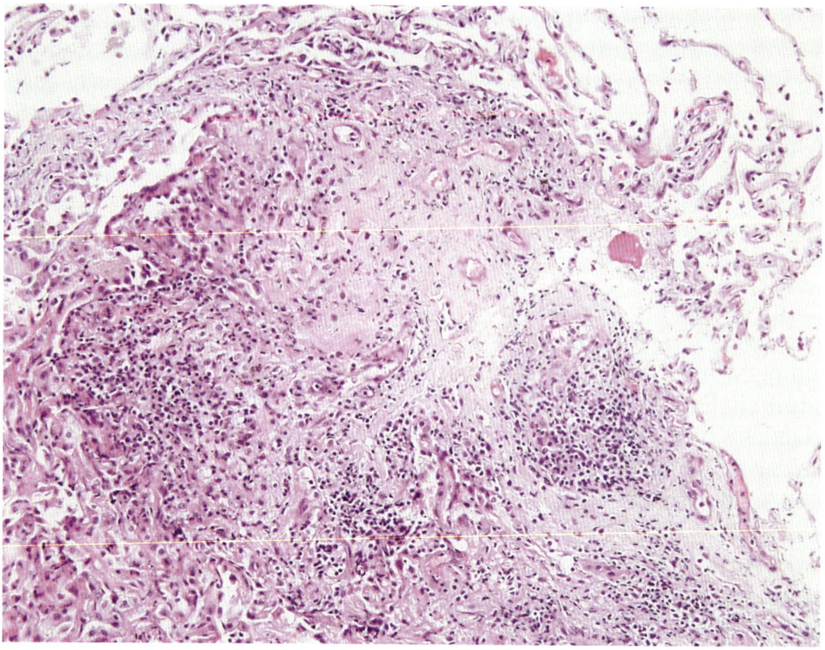

FIGURE 10.12 Another example of severe acute rejection (A4) showing dense perivascular mononuclear cell infiltrates with interstitial edema and fibrin deposition.

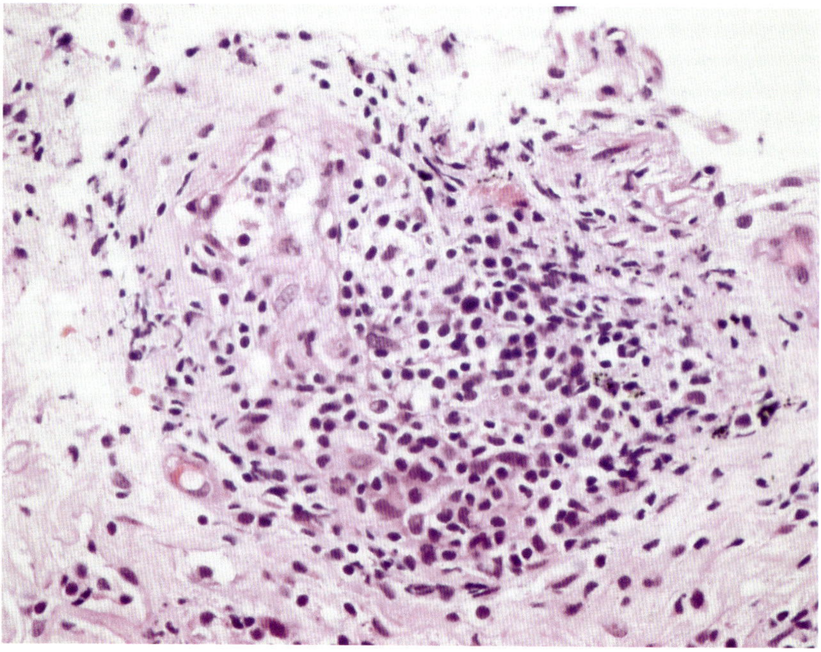

FIGURE 10.13 Higher magnification from preceding field shows small vessel with dense perivascular cuff of lymphocytes admixed with plasma cells and histiocytes.

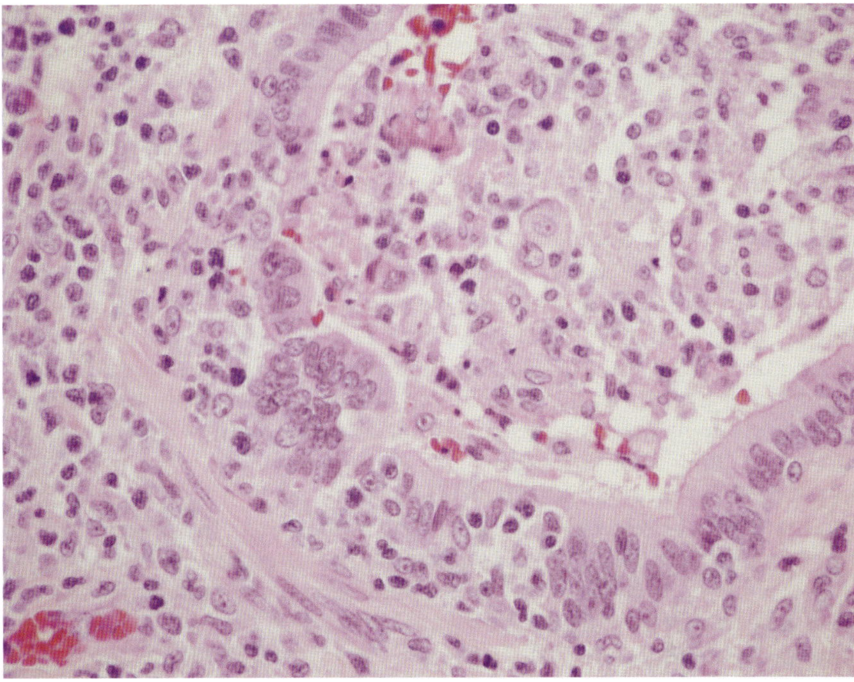

FIGURE 10.14 Severe acute rejection (A4) showing lymphocytic bronchiolitis causing destruction of the bronchiolar wall with infiltration of the mucosa.

CHRONIC REJECTION (BRONCHIOLITIS OBLITERANS)

Chronic rejection (bronchiolitis obliterans, or BO) generally develops between 9 and 12 months posttransplant. The frequency and severity of episodes of acute rejection have been regarded as the most important risk factors for the subsequent development of chronic rejection.[10] Chronic rejection occurs in 30% to 50% of lung transplant patients and has been associated with a 25% mortality rate.[11] The term *BO* has been adopted in the transplantation literature to refer to the histologic changes in chronic rejection. Similar lesions in nontransplant patients have been termed *obliterative bronchiolitis*.[12,13] BO of chronic rejection needs to be distinguished from bronchiolitis obliterans organizing pneumonia (BOOP), which is an unrelated process. Clinically, chronic rejection is characterized by an insidious onset with cough and general symptoms of malaise, followed by progressive shortness of breath.[14] Chest imaging studies will show changes once the process is well advanced, characterized by distal airway obstruction with proximal bronchiectasis and overinflation. The diagnosis is established by demonstrating the characteristic changes on transbronchial biopsy. Sampling can often be a significant issue in the evaluation of chronic rejection; in one study, the sensitivity of transbronchial biopsy for this process was only 28%.[15] Adequate sampling, including the presence of bronchioles, is therefore necessary for proper evaluation.

The histologic features of BO in chronic rejection include progressive deposition of fibrous tissue around the bronchioles with narrowing of the bronchiolar lumen as a result of fibrosis (Fig. 10.15) (eFig. 10.7). The term *active BO* has been proposed to refer to the presence of inflammatory cells admixed with the fibrosing process (Fig. 10.16), and *inactive BO* for those cases devoid of inflammation.[7] The submucosal fibrosis can be symmetrical and lead to concentric narrowing of the lumen, or asymmetric, causing bulging of the lumen with only partial obstruction. Elastic stains can be of aid in identifying late stages of peribronchiolar fibrosis by highlighting residual elastic fibers of bronchioles in areas showing extensive scarring.[16] Secondary changes can sometimes supervene, including mucostasis and endogenous lipid pneumonia. BO may be patchy in distribution and in severity. For this reason, the finding of a normal bronchiole does not entirely exclude the diagnosis. The main histologic differential diagnosis for BO is cryptogenic organizing pneumonia (i.e., BOOP), which is characterized by concentric fibrous and fibrinous plugs within the airways comprising fibroblasts embedded in loose myxoid matrix. A trichrome stain can be helpful in distinguishing

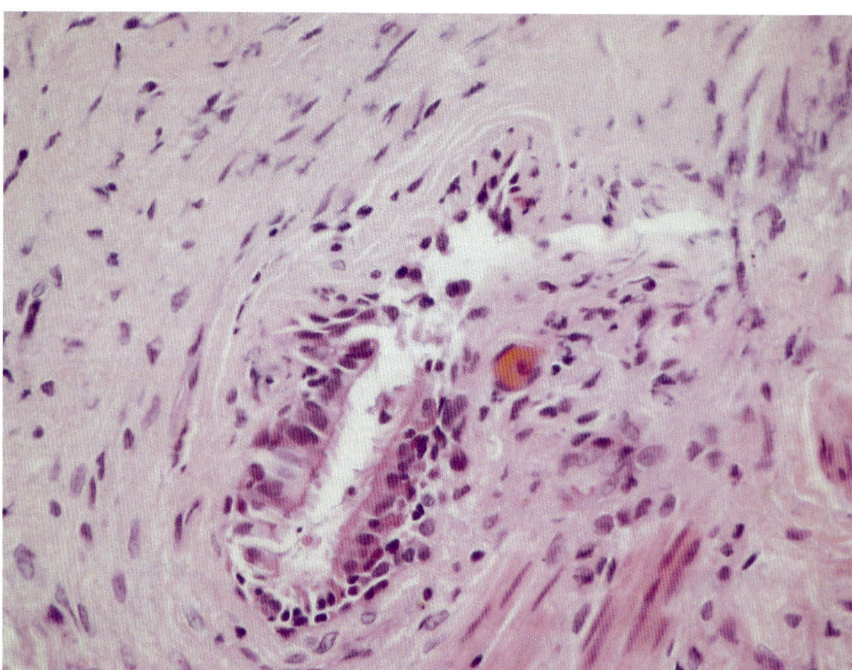

FIGURE 10.15 BO in chronic rejection is characterized by progressive deposition of fibrous tissue around the bronchiole with narrowing of the lumen.

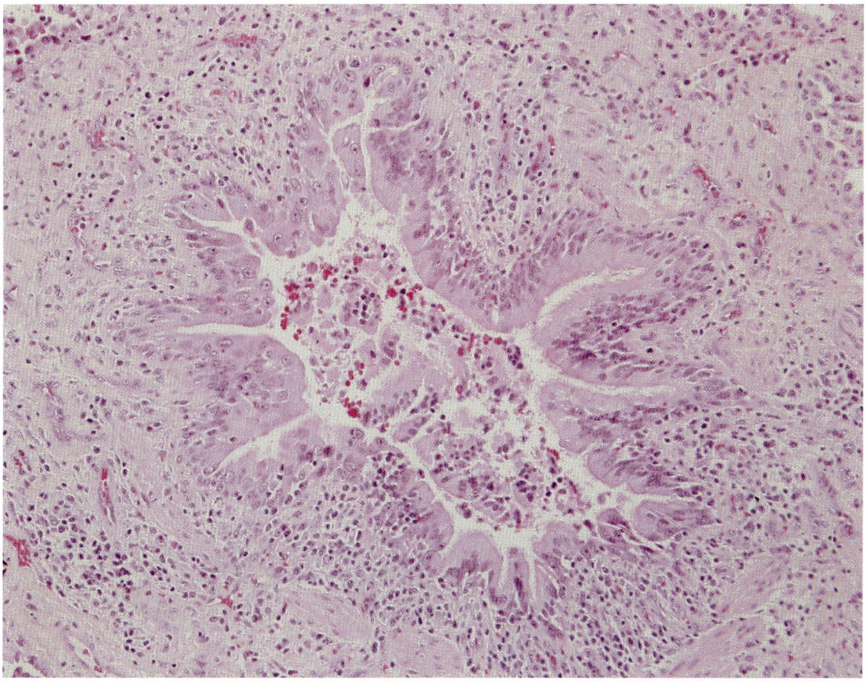

FIGURE 10.16 "Active" BO in chronic rejection is characterized by a dense inflammatory infiltrate around the wall of the bronchiole.

organizing pneumonia from BO, which is characterized by dense scar tissue surrounding the small airways rather than within the airspaces. Cryptogenic organizing pneumonia can occur in the setting of lung transplantation in patients with superimposed infection, following aspiration, or as a feature of acute rejection, but it is not generally associated with chronic rejection.[17,18]

Chronic vascular rejection with accelerated graft vascular sclerosis is another, but less frequent, manifestation of chronic rejection that can be seen accompanying chronic airway obstruction. The histologic features include fibrointimal and medial thickening of arteries and veins that may be accompanied by active lymphocytic inflammation (Fig. 10.17) (eFig. 10.8).[19] The significance of this finding is uncertain, but it is believed that it does not contribute significantly to allograft dysfunction.

The airway obstruction in chronic rejection is usually progressive and unresponsive to treatment; however, the course can be highly variable.[20] Increasing the immunosuppression has been shown to improve the BO in some patients. Currently, most efforts are in increasing the tolerance between donor and recipient and in applying preventive measures to avoid infections and airway ischemic injuries.

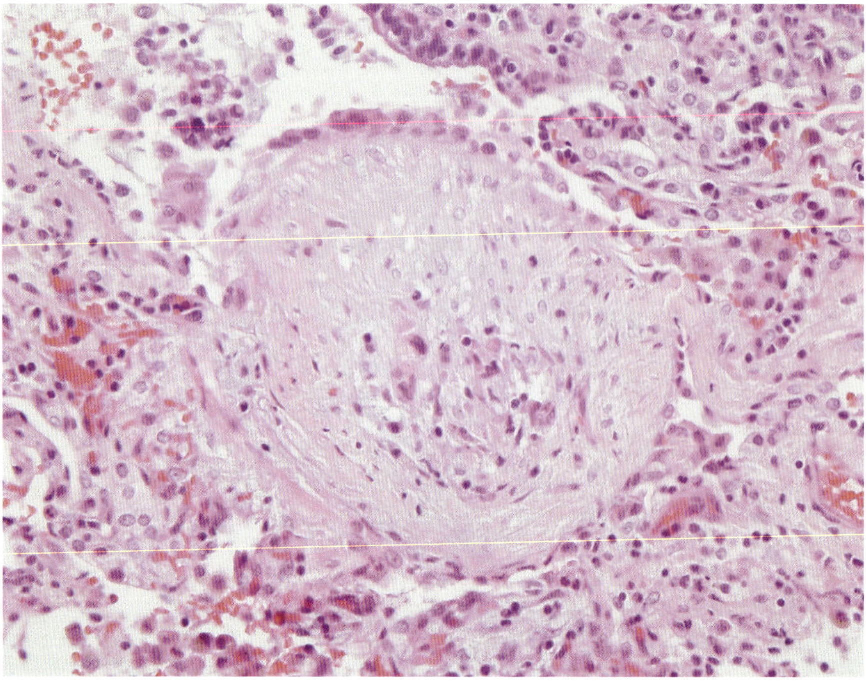

FIGURE 10.17 Sclerosing arteriopathy in chronic lung rejection shows thickening of the intima and the media of a small artery with chronic inflammation.

TRANSPLANT-RELATED INFECTION

Transplant-related infection represents a common complication of lung and heart–lung transplantations due to the immunosuppressed state of the individual.[21] Patients present with cough, fever, purulent sputum, dyspnea, and hypoxemia with peripheral leukocytosis. Bacterial infections have a tendency to be more common in the first month posttransplant, whereas viral and fungal infections tend to occur from 3 to 6 months following transplant. Distinguishing acute rejection from infection is of critical importance for patient management and can sometimes be problematic in transbronchial biopsies. Routine use of special stains for organisms is therefore recommended in all transplant patients.

Bacterial infections in lung transplant patients are characterized by neutrophilic infiltrates within alveolar spaces and involving the bronchial mucosa, often with mucosal ulceration. Tissue Gram stains can be of aid in identifying bacteria. The most common types of bacteria involved in transplant-related infection are gram-negative, particularly *Pseudomonas* species. Microbiologic cultures should be routinely done in such patients to identify microbiologic agents. The histologic findings are distinguished from acute rejection by the presence of neutrophils, instead of the perivascular mononuclear cells observed in acute rejection.

Viral infection by CMV is the commonest type observed in lung and heart–lung transplant patients, followed by herpes simplex virus (HSV).[22–24] Most cases of CMV infection are characterized by a diffuse lymphoid interstitial pneumonia containing a mixed lymphocytic and polymorphonuclear infiltrate or they may show acute necrotizing pneumonia with DAD (Fig. 10.18) (eFig. 10.9). The mononuclear cells will diffusely infiltrate the alveolar septa without perivascular accentuation. Careful search for the characteristic cytopathic effect with prominent nuclear and cytoplasmic eosinophilic inclusions is required for diagnosis. Use of immunohistochemical stains with anti-CMV antibodies can be helpful, particularly in treated cases in which the inclusions can become smudged and may be difficult to identify on routine microscopy. Areas of zonal necrosis may be observed with both CMV and HSV. The differential diagnosis with acute rejection is based on the identification of the characteristic cytopathic effects or the use of special stains.[9] Immunohistochemistry, in situ hybridization, and polymerase chain reaction techniques can be used effectively for identifying many viruses and can be used for definitive diagnosis. A subtle histologic difference between viral infection and acute rejection is the fact that the mononuclear cell infiltrate in viral infection is predominantly interstitial, whereas in acute rejection it is primarily perivascular.

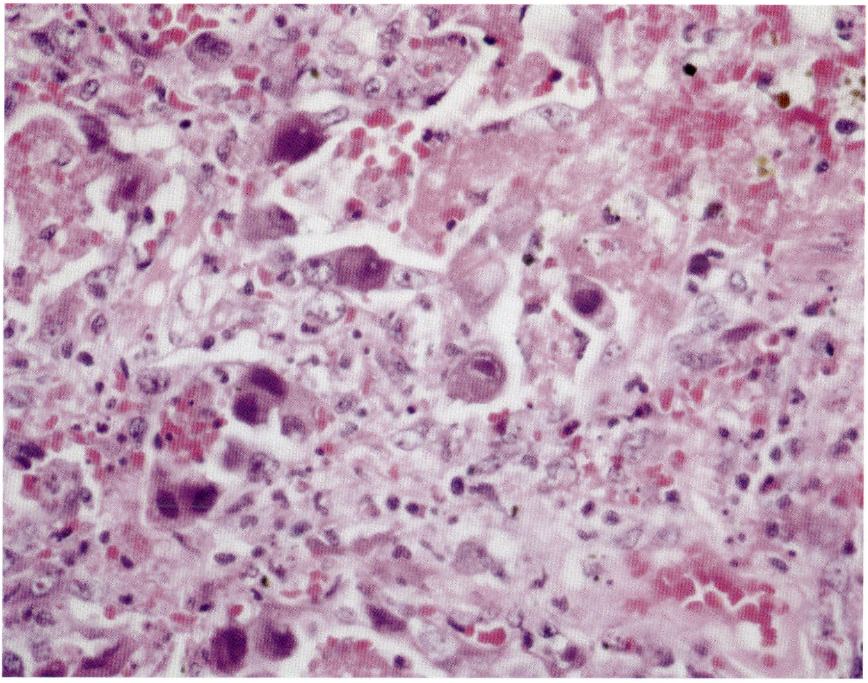

FIGURE 10.18 CMV infection in lung transplant patient shows numerous infected cells with cytomegalic inclusions against a background of necrotizing pneumonia with diffuse alveolar damage.

Fungal infection in lung and heart–lung transplant patients is less frequent than viral and bacterial infection, but is associated with a higher mortality when present. The most common organisms encountered in this setting are *Aspergillus* and *Candida*.[25,26] Other types of fungi have also been described, although less frequently.[26] The organisms can be cultured from bronchoalveolar lavage samples, blood, or other body fluids. Transbronchial biopsy may be the fastest way to obtain a diagnosis. The organisms are easily identified by morphology on routine microscopy, although special stains such as periodic acid–Schiff and Gomori methenamine silver may be of help in highlighting them in small biopsy samples.

Pneumocystis pneumonia is another complication of lung and heart–lung transplants. Without prophylaxis, *Pneumocystis* pneumonia occurs in nearly all transplant patients.[27] Routine prophylaxis, however, has made this a relatively rare complication.

POSTTRANSPLANT LYMPHOPROLIFERATIVE DISORDERS

Posttransplant lymphoproliferative disorders (PTLD) can occur in about 5% of all lung and heart–lung transplant patients, particularly among pulmonary allograft recipients. Most PTLD are associated with Epstein–Barr virus (EBV) infection and represent EBV-induced lymphoproliferations.[28] Approximately 20% of patients with PTLD can be EBV-negative. The disease can present clinically between 3 and 7 months posttransplant. Patients usually develop shortness of breath, or the disease can be discovered incidentally on chest X-rays. Radiographic findings include single or multiple pulmonary nodules with or without mediastinal adenopathy. Histologically, the lesions of PTLD can show a variable spectrum, ranging from lymphoid hyperplasia to full-blown lymphoma.[29,30] The most widely accepted classification for these disorders is that proposed by the WHO, which divides them into early lesions, polymorphic PTLD, monomorphic PTLD, and Hodgkin lymphoma-like PTLD.[31] Proper evaluation of PTLD in transplant patients requires adequate tissue for routine morphology, immunohistochemistry, flow cytometry, and molecular genetic studies.[32]

Early lesions of PTLD involve mainly lymph nodes and lymphoid tissue outside of the lung, and rarely involve pulmonary parenchyma. They include plasmacytic hyperplasia and infectious mononucleosis-like changes. The infiltrates comprise polyclonal B-cell admixed with plasma cells and reactive T cells.

Polymorphic PTLD are tissue destructive lesions comprising an admixture of mature lymphocytes, immunoblasts, plasma cells, and large transformed lymphocytes that show evidence of monoclonality by molecular testing (Fig. 10.19). The lesions are EBV-positive.

Monomorphic PTLD are lesions comprising a monomorphic population of atypical lymphoid cells indistinguishable from conventional types of lymphoma (Figs. 10.20 to 10.22). They are classified using the same classification for malignant lymphoma into diffuse large B-cell

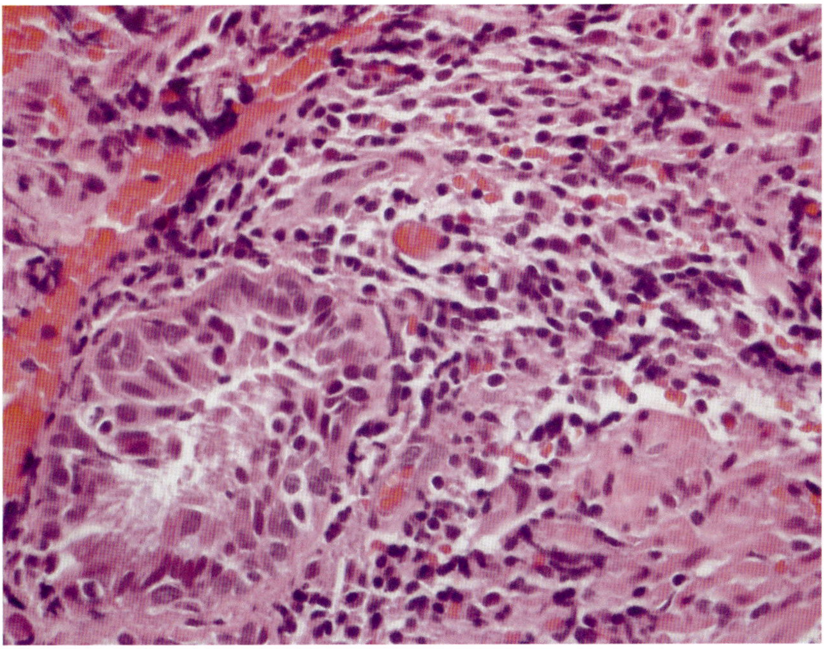

FIGURE 10.19 Polymorphic PTLD shows a polyclonal admixture of small lymphocytes, immunoblasts and plasma cells that are EBV-negative.

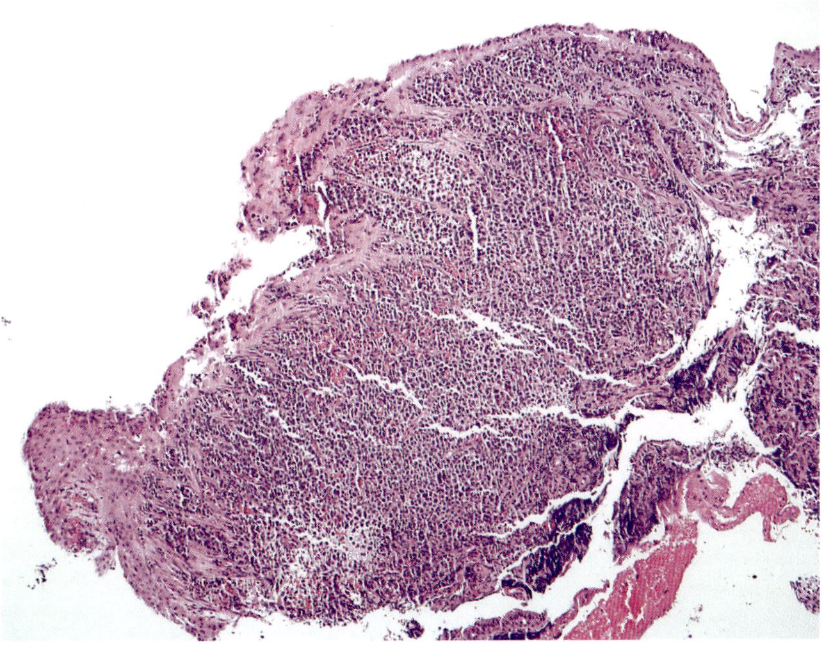

FIGURE 10.20 Transbronchial biopsy in patient with monomorphic PTLD shows a uniform, dense lymphoid cell population replacing the lung parenchyma.

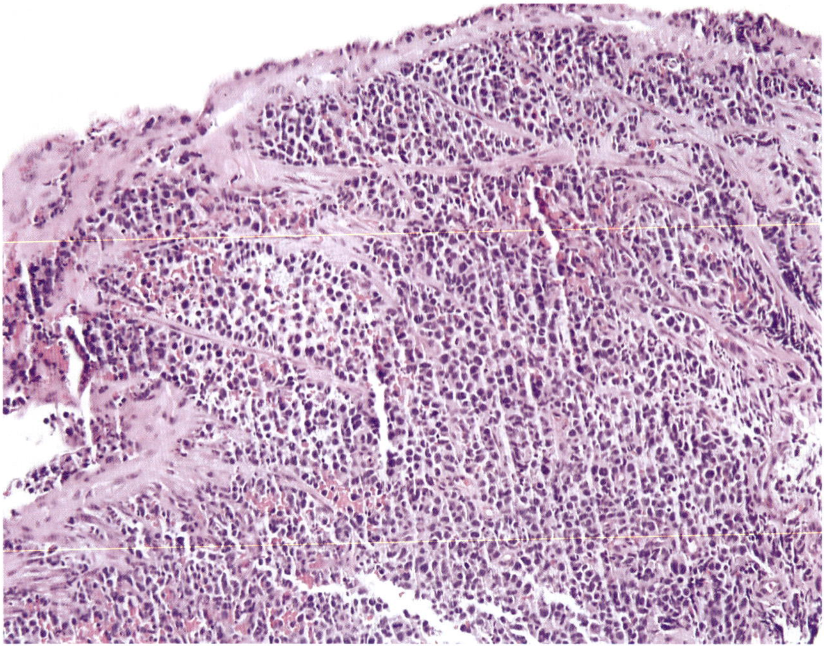

FIGURE 10.21 Higher magnification from preceding field shows large, atypical lymphocytes showing features of diffuse large cell lymphoma.

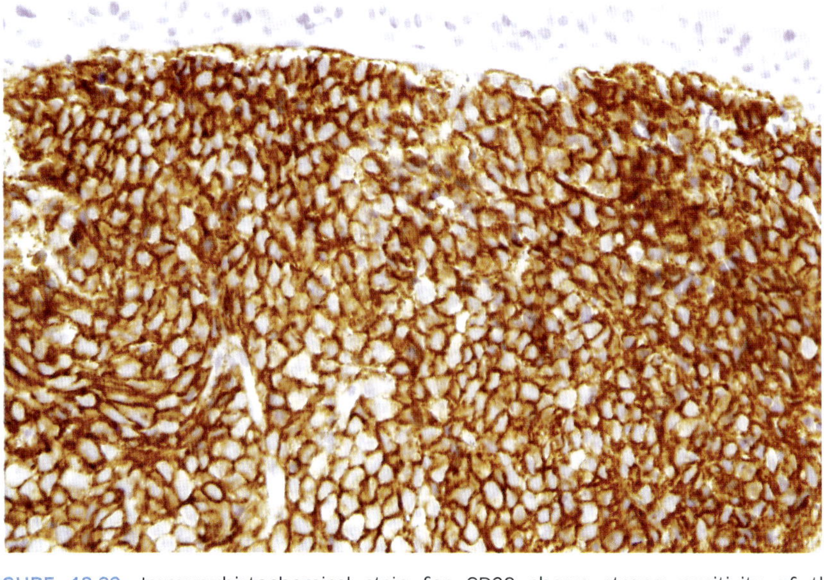

FIGURE 10.22 Immunohistochemical stain for CD20 shows strong positivity of the neoplastic lymphoid cells for this marker.

lymphoma, Burkitt and Burkitt-like lymphoma, plasma cell myeloma, peripheral T-cell lymphoma, and other types of lymphoma (eFig. 10.10). Most cases are monoclonal and demonstrate EBV-positivity (Fig. 10.23).

Hodgkin disease-type PTLD can show features of classical Hodgkin lymphoma or Hodgkin lymphoma-like PTLD with an atypical immunophenotype and B-cell antigen expression (Figs. 10.24 to 10.27). Virtually all cases are EBV-positive.

EBV can be identified in the atypical lymphocytes in the majority of polymorphic and monomorphic PTLD cases. EBV can be detected using immunohistochemistry for latent membrane protein (LMP-1) or by in situ hybridization for EBV-encoded nuclear RNA-1 (EBER). The latter test, however, is considered more reliable. EBV determination should be made in all lung transplant patients showing a suspicious dense polymorphic or monomorphic lymphoid infiltrate. In rare cases, early lesions may be confused with acute lung rejection; demonstration of EBV infection will help establish the diagnosis.[33] Early lesions of PTLD often regress spontaneously or with reduction of immunosuppressive therapy. Monomorphic lesions can progress and will require cytotoxic chemotherapy. The overall mortality of PTLD in solid organ allograft recipients has been approximately 60%.

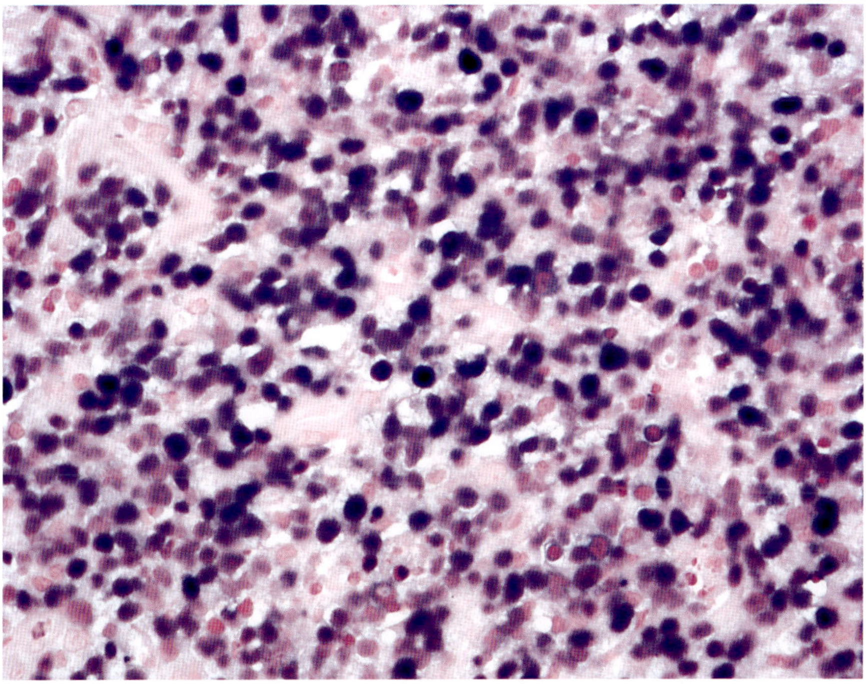

FIGURE 10.23 In situ hybridization for EBV-encoded RNA (EBER-1) shows positive signal in the majority of the tumor cells.

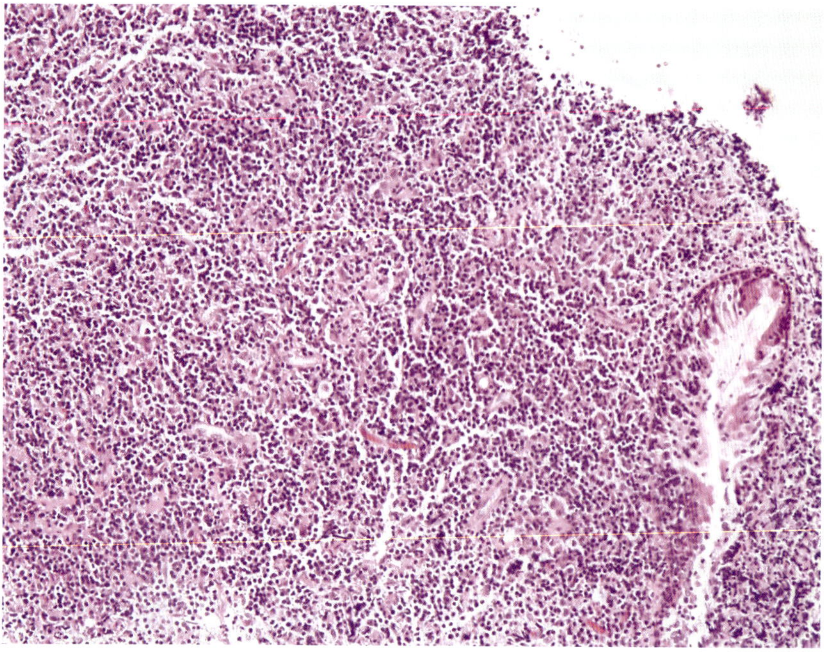

FIGURE 10.24 Transbronchial biopsy in patient with Hodgkin-type PTLD showing mixed population of cells effacing underlying lung parenchyma.

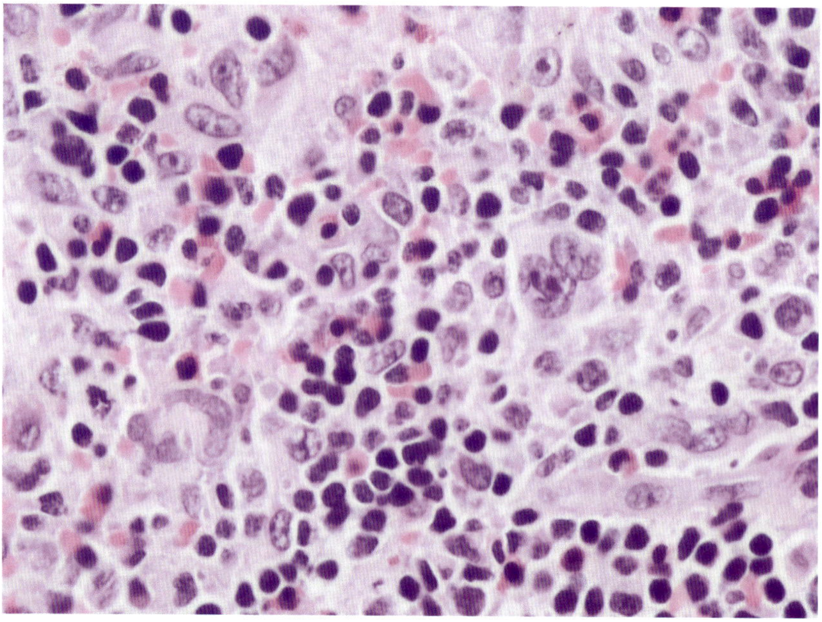

FIGURE 10.25 Higher magnification showing mixed infiltrate comprising small lymphocytes, plasma cells, and scattered larger mono- and multinucleated cells with features of Reed–Sternberg cells.

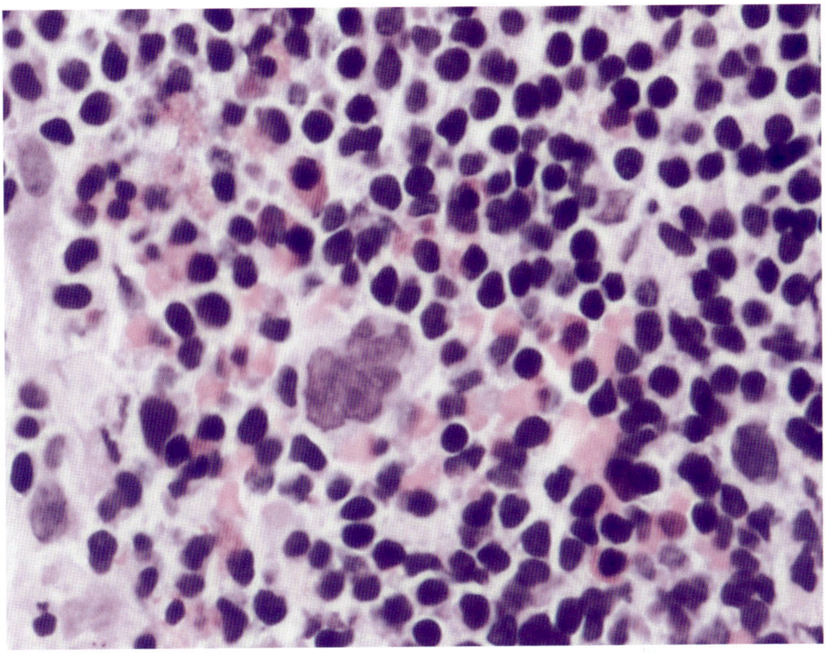

FIGURE 10.26 A multinucleated Reed–Sternberg cell is seen in the center of the field showing prominent eosinophilic nucleoli.

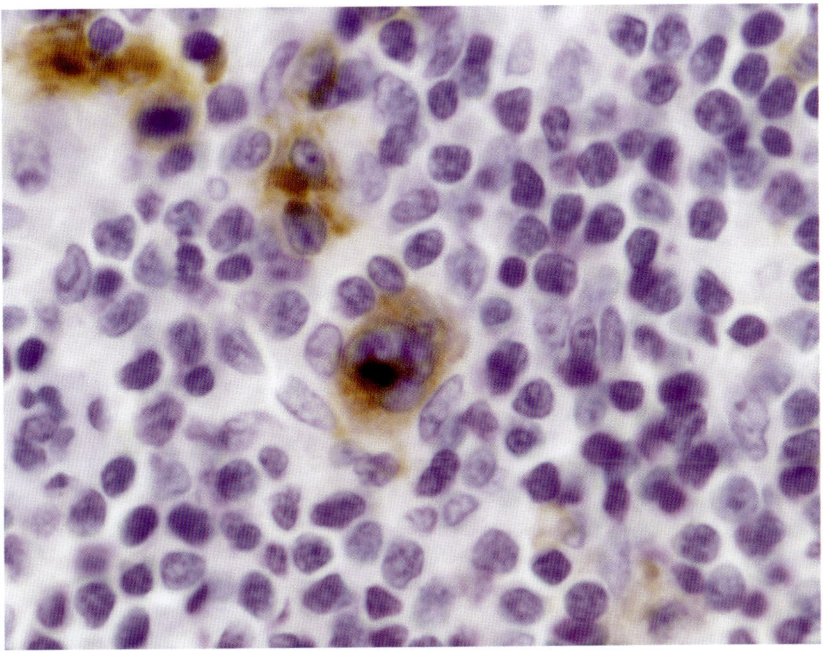

FIGURE 10.27 Immunohistochemical stain for CD30 shows characteristic membranous and dot-like paranuclear staining in Reed–Sternberg cell.

OTHER COMPLICATIONS

Other complications include graft versus host disease and recurrence of the primary disease in the allograft.

Pulmonary graft versus host disease is essentially analogous to lung transplant rejection because the same basic underlying mechanism operates in both, that is, host immune competent cells reacting against antigens in the transplanted lung allograft. The histologic findings are identical to those of acute and chronic lung transplant rejection.

Recurrence of the primary disease occurs in a small percentage of lung transplant patients. The most common disease that recurs in this setting is sarcoidosis.[34] Other conditions that have been reported to recur in lung transplant recipients include lymphangioleiomyomatosis, diffuse panbronchiolitis, desquamative interstitial pneumonia, giant cell pneumonitis, and bronchioloalveolar cell carcinoma. The diagnosis is made on transbronchial biopsy.

REFERENCES

1. Hisenpud JD, Bennett LE, Keck BM, et al. The Registry of the International Society for Heart and Lung Transplantation: eighteenth official report—2001. *J Heart Lung Transplant*. 2001;20:805–815.
2. Hopkins PM, Aboyoun CL, Chhajed PN, et al. Prospective analysis of 1,235 transbronchial lung biopsies in lung transplant recipients. *J Heart Lung Transplant*. 2002;21:1062–1067.
3. Bierman MI, Satein KL, Stuart RS, et al. Critical care management of lung transplant recipients. *J Intensive Care Med*. 1991;6:135–142.
4. Tazelaar HD, Yousem SA. The pathology of combined heart–lung transplantation: an autopsy study. *Hum Pathol*. 1988;19:1403–1416.
5. Choi JK, Kearns J, Palevski HI, et al. Hyepracute rejection of a pulmonary allograft. Immediate clinical and pathologic findings. *Am J Respir Crit Care Med*. 1999;160:1015–1018.
6. Frost AE, Jammal CT, Cagle PT. Hyperacute rejection following lung transplantation. *Chest*. 1996;110:559–562.
7. Yousem SA, Berry GJ, Cagle PT, et al. Revision of the 1990 working formulation for the classification of pulmonary allograft rejection: Lung Rejection Study Group. The International Society for Heart Transplantation. *J Heart Lung Transplant*. 1996;15:1–15.
8. Hasegawa T, Iacono AT, Yousem SA. The anatomic distribution of acute cellular rejection in the allograft lung. *Ann Thorac Surg*. 2000;69:1529–1531.
9. Nakleh RE, Bolman RM III, Henke CA, et al. Lung transplant pathology. A comparative study of pulmonary acute rejection and cytomegaloviral infection. *Am J Surg Pathol*. 1991;15:1197–1201.
10. Martinu T, Howell DN, Palmer SM. Acute cellular rejection and humoral sensitization in lung transplant recipients. *Semin Respir Crit Care Med*. 2010;31:179–188.
11. Bando K, Paradis IL, Similo S, et al. Obliterative bronchiolitis after lung and heart–lung transplantation. An analysis of risk factors and management. *J Thorac Cardiovasc Surg*. 1995;110:4–14.
12. Colby TV. Bronchiolitis. Pathologic considerations. *Am J Clin Pathol*. 1998;109:101–109.
13. Myers JL, Colby TV. Pathologic manifestations of bronchiolitis, constrictive bronchiolitis, cryptogenic organizing pneumonia, and diffuse panbronchiolitis. *Clin Chest Med*. 1993;14:611–622.

14. Paradis I, Yousem S, Griffith B. Airway obstruction and bronchiolitis obliterans after lung transplantation. *Clin Chest Med.* 1993;14:751–763.
15. Pomerance A, Madden B, Burke MM, et al. Transbronchial biopsy in heart and lung transplantation: clinicopathologic correlations. *J Heart Lung Transplant.* 1995;14:761–763.
16. Schlesinger C, Meyer CA, Veeraraghavan S, et al. Constrictive (obliterative) bronchiolitis: diagnosis, etiology, and a critical review of the literature. *Ann Diagn Pathol.* 1998;4:288–293.
17. Yousem SA, Duncan SR, Griffith BP. Interstitial and airspace granulation tissue reactions in lung transplant recipients. *Am J Surg Pathol.* 1992;16:877–884.
18. Abernathy ED, Hruban RH, Baumgartner WA, et al. The two forms of bronchiolitis obliterans in heart–lung transplant recipients. *Hum Pathol.* 1991;27:714–719.
19. Yousem SA, Paradis IL, Dauber JH, et al. Pulmonary arteriosclerosis in long-term human heart–lung transplant recipients. *Transplantation.* 1989;47:564–569.
20. Weigt SS, Wallace WD, Derhovanessian A, et al. Chronic allograft rejection: epidemiology, diagnosis, pathogenesis, and treatment. *Semin Respir Crit Care Med.* 2010;31:189–207.
21. Marchevsky A, Hartman G, Walts A, et al. Lung transplantation: the pathologic diagnosis of pulmonary complications. *Mod Pathol.* 1991;4:133–138.
22. Kramer MR, Marshall SE, Starnes VA, et al. Infectious complications in heart–lung transplantation. Analysis of 200 episodes. *Arch Intern Med.* 1993;153:2010–2016.
23. Gould FK, Freeman R, Taylor CE, et al. Prophylaxis and management of cytomegalovirus pneumonitis after lung transplantation: a review of experience in one center. *J Heart Lung Transplant.* 1993;12:695–699.
24. Shah PD, McDyer JF. Viral infections in lung transplant recipients. *Semin Respir Crit Care Med.* 2010;31:243–254.
25. Cahill CB, Hibbs JR, Savik K, et al. Aspergillus airway colonization and invasive disease after lung transplantation. *Chest.* 1997;112:1160–1164.
26. Kanj SS, Welty-Wolf K, Madden J, et al. Fungal infections in lung and heart–lung transplant recipients. Report of 9 cases and review of the literature. *Medicine (Baltimore).* 1996;75:142–156.
27. Gryzan S, Paradis IL, Zeevi A, et al. Unexpectedly high incidence of *Pneumocystis carinii* infection after lung–heart transplantation. Implications for lung defense and allograft survival. *Am Rev Respir Dis.* 1988;137:1268–1274.
28. Randhawa PS, Yousem S, Paradis IL, et al. The clinical spectrum, pathology, and clonal analysis of Epstein–Barr virus-associated lymphoproliferative disorders in heart–lung transplant recipients. *Am J Clin Pathol.* 1989;92:177–185.
29. Nalesnik MA, Jaffe R, Starzl TE, et al. The pathology of posttransplant lymphoproliferative disorders occurring in the setting of cyclosporine A-prednisone immunosuppression. *Am J Pathol.* 1988;133:173–192.
30. Knowles DM, Cesarman E, Chadburn A, et al. Correlative morphologic and molecular genetic analysis demonstrates three distinct categories of posttransplant lymphoproliferative disorders. *Blood.* 1995;85:552–565.
31. Harris NL, Swerdlow SH, Frizzera G, et al. Post-transplant lymphoproliferative disorders, In: Jaffee ES, Harris NL, Stein H, Vardiman JW, eds. *Pathology and Genetics of Tumors of Hematopoietic and Lymphoid Tissues.* Lyon, France: IARC Press; 2001.
32. Chadburn A, Chen JM, Hsu DT, et al. The morphologic and molecular genetic categories of posttransplantation lymphoproliferative disorders are clinically relevant. *Cancer.* 1998;82:1978–1987.
33. Rosendale B, Yousem SA. Discrimination of Epstein–Barr virus-related posttransplant lymphoproliferations from acute rejection in lung allograft recipients. *Arch Pathol Lab Med.* 119:418–423, 1995.
34. Collins J, Hartman MJ, Warner TF, et al. Frequency and CT findings of recurrent disease after lung transplantation. *Radiology.* 2001;219:503–509.

11

LYMPHOID LESIONS OF THE LUNG

Lymphoid lesions involving the lung are relatively rare and span the entire spectrum from benign to malignant processes. Significant changes in our understanding of these disorders have occurred during the past few years owing to advances in the application of immunologic and molecular tools for diagnosis in this family of tumors. The modern evaluation of lymphoproliferative disorders relies heavily on immunophenotypic analysis of the cell type for correct and specific classification. These findings often need to be integrated with the results of molecular genetic analyses to arrive at a definitive diagnosis.[1] Immunohistochemistry, flow cytometry, and molecular genetic techniques now form a part of the routine armamentarium in the evaluation of lymphoproliferative disorders and play a critical role in their diagnosis. The lung may be involved in various lymphoproliferative processes (Table 11.1). Benign lymphoid proliferations include follicular bronchiolitis (FB), nodular lymphoid hyperplasia (NLH), and diffuse lymphoid hyperplasia (DLH). Malignant conditions include extranodal marginal zone lymphoma, diffuse large B-cell lymphoma (DLBCL), anaplastic large cell lymphoma (ALCL), lymphomatoid granulomatosis (LYG), pulmonary Hodgkin lymphoma (HL), plasmacytoma, and posttransplant lymphoproliferative disorder (PTLD). The latter was discussed in the chapter 10 dealing with transplant pathology and will not be further discussed here.

BENIGN/HYPERPLASTIC LYMPHOID PROCESSES

Our understanding of benign hyperplastic lymphoid proliferations of the lung has evolved significantly over the past 15 years. Historically, the process we now designate as DLH was regarded by Liebow[2] as a distinctive type of idiopathic interstitial pneumonia. Although some experts still propose that we continue to include DLH among the group of idiopathic interstitial pneumonias for historical reasons, it is now widely recognized that there may be great deal of overlap between the DLH and the "cellular" form of nonspecific interstitial pneumonia (NSIP) as well as with other lymphoid interstitial infiltrates observed in several specific autoimmune conditions, such as acute lupus pneumonitis. The term DLH or diffuse bronchial associated lymphoid tissue (BALT) hyperplasia is therefore currently favored. The term "pseudolymphoma" was also used in previous years to refer to

TABLE 11.1 Pulmonary Lymphoid Lesions

Benign/Borderline	Malignant
Follicular bronchiolitis	Marginal zone lymphoma
Nodular lymphoid hyperplasia	Diffuse large B-cell lymphoma
Diffuse lymphoid hyperplasia	Anaplastic large cell lymphoma
	Lymphomatoid granulomatosis
	Hodgkin lymphoma
	Plasmacytoma
	Posttransplant lymphoproliferative disorder

some of these conditions, particularly for the process we now designate as NLH. With the advent of modern immunohistochemical and molecular diagnostic testing, a thorough understanding has been obtained of these processes. It is now believed that some of these conditions may serve as precursor lesions to malignant lymphoproliferations in the lung, although most cases will regress spontaneously or follow an indolent clinical course.

Follicular Bronchiolitis

FB refers to a process in which lymphoid aggregates are deposited around or in the vicinity of the small airways. FB is more common in males than in females and usually involves the lungs bilaterally producing an interstitial pattern of involvement of lung parenchyma.[3] This process is often seen in association with immunodeficiency states, collagen vascular diseases, or in patients with chronic obstructive pulmonary disease[4,5] but may also be present as a secondary finding in patients with chronic lung disorders. Symptoms may include progressive dyspnea and cough, and chest X-rays will show bilateral reticular or reticulonodular infiltrates. The histologic hallmark of FB is the accumulation of dense aggregates of mature small lymphocytes in the vicinity or at the periphery of bronchioles that may compress or distort the bronchiolar lumens (Fig. 11.1). The lymphoid aggregates are usually small and well delimited and do not extend into the surrounding alveolar septa, and they may or may not show well-developed germinal centers. The CD20+ small lymphocytes are polytypic and do not show evidence of light chain restriction. CD21 may highlight residual follicular dendritic cells within the nodules. FB is most often diagnosed in open lung biopsy or video-assisted thoracoscopic surgery (VATS) specimens, although occasionally may be encountered in transbronchial lung biopsies.

Nodular Lymphoid Hyperplasia

NLH, also known as nodular BALT hyperplasia, is a reactive process characterized by follicular lymphoid hyperplasia with interfollicular

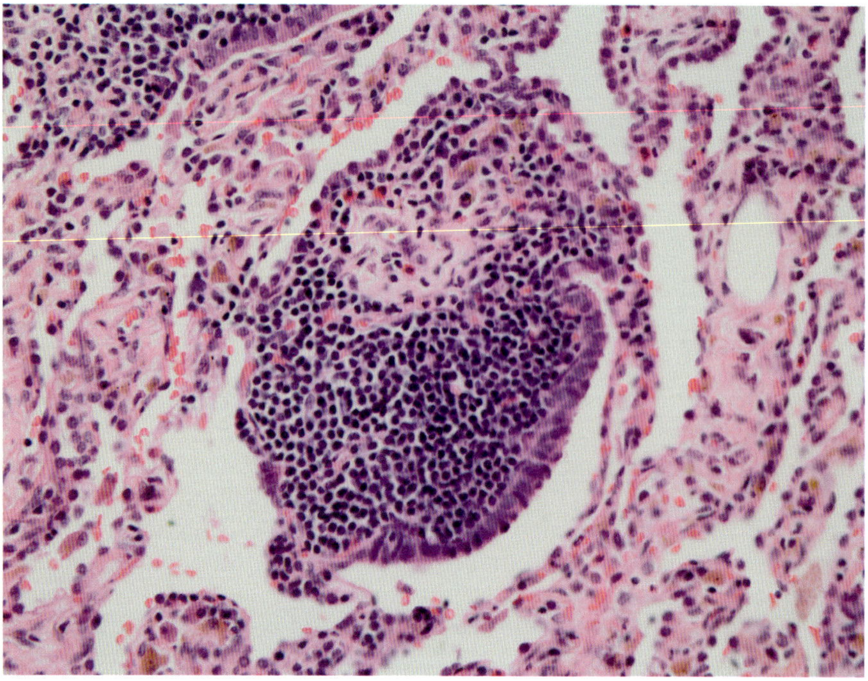

FIGURE 11.1 Small lymphoid follicle is seen adjacent to the lining of a bronchiole in FB. Notice that the lymphoid follicle is located in the alveolar wall and is compressing the lumen of the bronchiole.

plasmacytosis and prominent reactive germinal centers. In the past, lesions with these features were termed "pseudolymphoma," an outdated term that is no longer in use.[6] NLH is most common in adults between 40 and 70 years of age (average, 55 years) and may be associated with collagen-vascular disorders or autoimmune diseases.[6,7] Chest X-rays and CT scans will show a solitary nodule or, in some instances, multiple confluent nodules that can measure up to 5 cm in greatest diameter. Histologically, the process is characterized by a well-demarcated area of the lung showing replacement of the parenchyma by a proliferation of multiple enlarged lymphoid follicles with reactive germinal centers. The germinal centers in the nodules display prominent polarity and are surrounded by a well-developed mantle zone. There is striking interfollicular lymphoplasmocytosis, but atypical cells or transformed lymphocytes are not a feature of the process. The lesions are sharply demarcated from the surrounding lung parenchyma and do not extend along alveolar septa or into the alveolar walls.[8] Immunohistochemical analysis will stain the lymphocytes in the germinal centers positive for CD20 and negative for bcl-2. The interfollicular lymphocytes primarily comprise small T-cells that are CD3- and CD5-positive. The lymphocytes will also show a polyclonal pattern of expression for κ and λ light chains. The diagnosis of NLH is best made in open lung biopsy specimens (wedge resections or nodulectomy specimens). The nodular pattern of the lesion may not be appreciated in core biopsy specimens or transbronchial biopsies, and the best diagnostic offering under such circumstances is to indicate that the lymphoid infiltrate does not demonstrate evidence of monoclonality by immunophenotypic studies.

Diffuse Lymphoid Hyperplasia

DLH, also known as diffuse BALT hyperplasia, and formerly designated as lymphoid interstitial pneumonia is a reactive process characterized by a polyclonal proliferation of lymphocytes and plasma cells occupying the pulmonary interstitium and distending the alveolar walls.[3,8] DLH is a common manifestation in the lung of patients with a number of collagen vascular diseases (i.e., Sjogren syndrome, rheumatoid arthritis, systemic lupus erythematosus), autoimmune disorders, and immunodeficiency conditions (such as AIDS and common variable immunodeficiency syndrome). It is a common manifestation in children with AIDS.[9,10] It can also be associated with certain infections, such as *Pneumocystosis* and *Legionella* infection. Clinical symptoms include dyspnea and cough, and it is often accompanied by polyclonal gammopathy or hypergammaglobulinemia. Chest X-rays show patchy, bilateral reticulonodular infiltrates with predilection for the lower lobes. The process is histologically characterized by a dense, predominantly interstitial proliferation of small lymphocytes that distend the alveolar walls (Fig. 11.2) (eFig. 11.1). Small follicles with residual germinal centers showing a distribution reminiscent of FB may be seen admixed with the diffuse lymphoid infiltrates. The interstitial infiltrate may also contain scattered plasma cells and histiocytes, but no atypical or transformed lymphocytes are present. Focal infiltration of bronchial epithelium by small lymphocytes may lead to the formation of lymphoepithelial lesions. Immunohistochemical stains will highlight a predominant population of CD3+/CD5+ small T-lymphocytes in the interstitium admixed with a polyclonal lymphoplasmacytic small B-cell population.[11] Cases occurring in the context of AIDS will show immunoreactivity for the p21 protein of the HIV. Immunoglobulin (IG) heavy chain gene rearrangement studies will yield a polyclonal pattern of expression. In some instances, DLH may act as a precursor lesion that can progress to mucosa-associated lymphoid tissue (MALT) lymphoma. DLH may be very difficult to diagnose in small biopsy specimens (transbronchial or core biopsies) and will require immunohistochemical, flow cytometric, or other support to rule out monoclonality. Lung involvement by chronic lymphocytic leukemia (CLL) may also be indistinguishable from DLH. The lymphoid cells in CLL coexpress CD5, CD20, CD23, and CD43 and are negative for T-cell markers. The process may be impossible to separate morphologically from DLH in the absence of a clinical history.

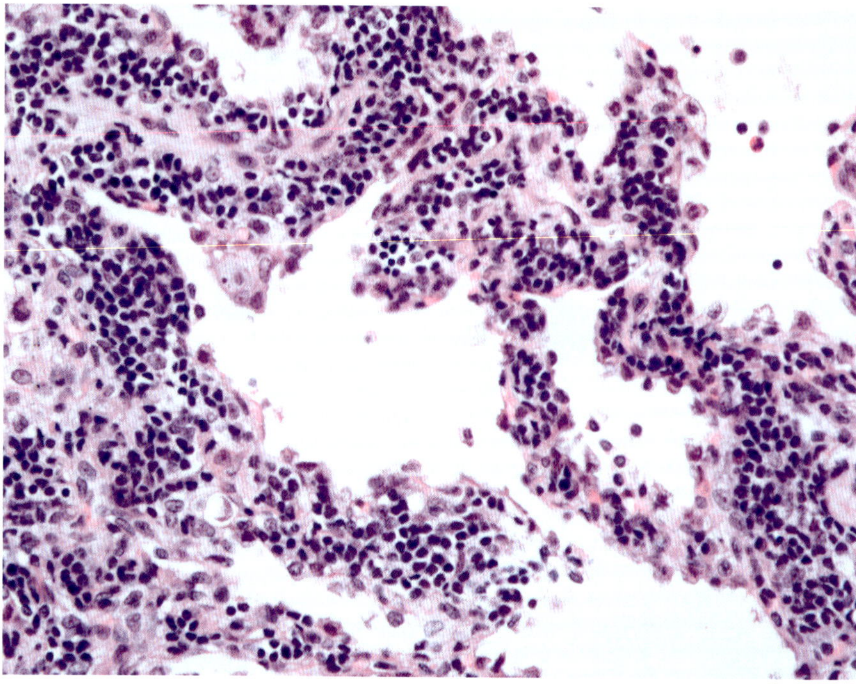

FIGURE 11.2 Diffuse interstitial lymphoid infiltrate is seen distending the alveolar walls in DLH. The lymphoid infiltrate is distinguished from a low-grade MALT lymphoma by the polyclonality of the lymphoid cells. Some authors still designate this process as "lymphoid interstitial pneumonia."

MALIGNANT LYMPHOID PROCESSES

The lung is a common site for primary extranodal lymphomas and may be often involved secondarily in advanced systemic nodal-based disease. Primary lung lymphoma is diagnosed when the disease is confined or restricted to the lungs.[12,13] Malignant pulmonary lymphoid processes include marginal zone B-cell lymphoma of bronchial Mucosa-Associated Lymphoid Tissue, Diffuse Large B-cell Lymphoma, Hodgkin lymphoma, Anaplastic Large Cell Lymphoma, Lymphomatoid Granulomatosis, plasmacytoma, PostTransplant Lymphoproliferative Disorder, and secondary involvement of the lung by leukemia and lymphoma. Adults are more commonly affected by primary lymphoma of the lung. Diagnosis is usually made by a combination of imaging studies and histologic examination of biopsy material or resection specimens. Application of immunohistochemical stains and molecular studies now form an integral and critical part of the evaluation of these tumors.[14] Flow cytometry immunophenotyping, when adequately preserved tissue with good cell viability is obtained, is another important tool for making a definitive and specific diagnosis. Endoscopic biopsies may yield variable results depending on the preservation of the tissue and amount of crush artifact but are often sufficient to formulate a differential diagnosis that will prompt an additional, more definitive diagnostic procedure. VATS or open biopsies are the most ideal vehicle for obtaining adequate and representative tissue and for maximizing the opportunity for rendering a specific diagnosis. Procurement of fresh frozen tissue for gene-rearrangement studies and other molecular studies is always recommended when there is a suspicion of a malignant lymphoproliferative process.

Marginal Zone B-Cell Lymphoma of MALT

Marginal zone lymphoma of the lung or MALT lymphoma is an extranodal lymphoma of B-lymphocytes presumably derived from the marginal zones of lymphoid follicles. The tumors comprise a heterogeneous population made up primarily of small lymphocytes, which may range from mature small lymphocytes, to small lymphocytes with abundant rim of cytoplasm resembling monocytoid B-cells, to small lymphocytes with plasmacytoid features or plasmacytic differentiation. The tumors are characterized on scanning magnification by numerous reactive lymphoid follicles; in the past many such lesions were regarded as examples of "pseudolymphoma" because of the prominence of lymphoid follicles with reactive germinal centers.[15] MALT lymphomas account for approximately 80% to 90% of all primary pulmonary lymphomas. The majority of patients are in their fifth or sixth decade of life, with a slight male predilection.[16] The disease can also be seen in younger patients who are immunosuppressed. The most common presentation is as a solitary parenchymatous nodule discovered incidentally on chest X-ray. The lesions can also be multiple and bilateral and present as well-defined masses or alveolar opacities associated with air bronchograms on high-resolution CT scans. The diagnosis can often be made on transbronchial biopsy, although an open biopsy is the ideal vehicle for making a definitive diagnosis. Core needle biopsies can also yield a diagnosis of malignant lymphoma when supported by adequate ancillary studies and demonstration of monoclonality but may be often difficult to subtype into a specific lymphoma category (Fig. 11.3). The prognosis for these tumors is excellent and bilateral or diffuse lesions can be followed without treatment with a 5-year survival that often exceeds 90%.[17,18] Localized lesions respond well to surgical excision. A small percentage of MALT lymphomas can progress to DLBCL.[16]

Histologically, pulmonary MALT lymphoma is characterized by a diffuse infiltrate of small B-lymphocytes that surrounds reactive lymphoid follicles (eFigs. 11.2 and 11.3).[19] The infiltrate is centered in the marginal zone of the follicles and usually extends into and expands the interfollicular areas (Fig. 11.4) (eFigs. 11.4 and 11.5). The follicles may be often obscured by overgrowth of the neoplastic small lymphocytes, a phenomenon described as "colonization" of the follicles. A prominent feature in these tumors is infiltration by the small lymphocytes of bronchial, bronchiolar, or alveolar epithelium resulting in the formation of "lymphoepithelial lesions" (Fig. 11.5). The latter are quite distinctive but not pathognomonic and may be also seen occasionally in reactive processes. When the infiltrate becomes dense

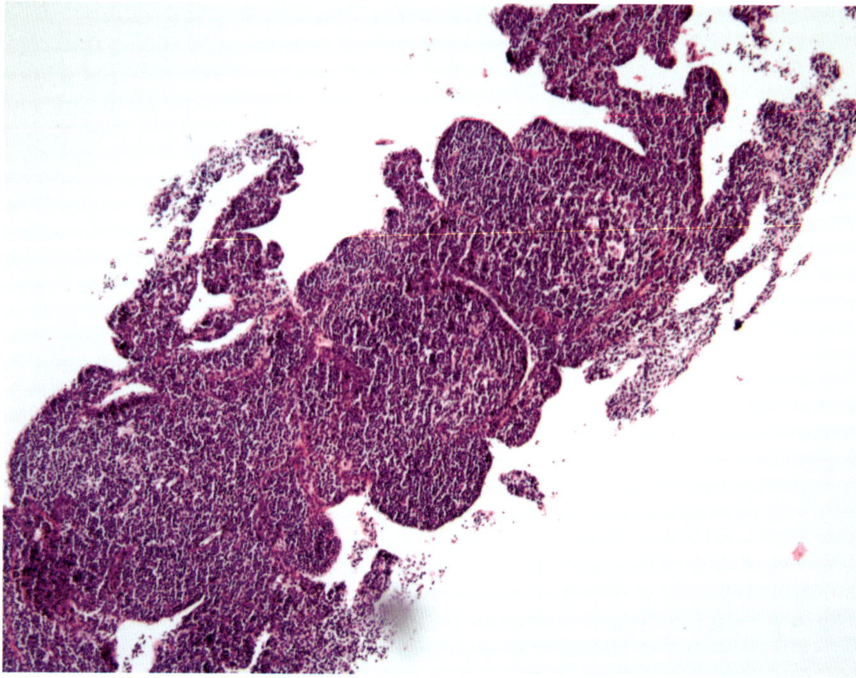

FIGURE 11.3 Percutaneous core biopsy of MALT lymphoma of the lung shows marked widening of alveolar septa by monotonous population of small lymphoid cells with a few residual germinal centers.

and confluent it can consolidate and replace the lung parenchyma and may undergo prominent stromal sclerosis. Peripheral lesions may show pleural infiltration. Poorly formed epithelioid granulomas can also be occasionally found. The lesions rarely give rise to tumor necrosis or are associated with destruction of the airways. The neoplastic cell population in the interfollicular areas may comprise sheets of monotonous mature small lymphocytes with minimal nuclear irregularities, cells with prominent plasmacytoid features, and mature plasma cells as well as "monocytoid" cells characterized by small, round-to-indented nuclei surrounded by an ample rim of amphophylic to lightly eosinophilic cytoplasm forming a perinuclear "halo." Cells containing prominent plasmacytic differentiation can be mistaken for plasmacytoma; ample sampling and identification of monocytoid cells or sheets of small lymphocytes forming lymphoepithelial lesions should permit correct identification of the process. Scattered larger cells resembling centroblasts or immunoblasts may also be present admixed with the small lymphocytes, but they are usually in the minority. Presence of sheets of large, atypical immunoblastic cells heralds the transformation to DLBCL. The neoplastic B-cell population is monoclonal and light chain restriction can usually be demonstrated either on fresh tissue or paraffin sections, although light chain restriction is most reliably established by flow cytometry. Amplification of the IG heavy chain can detect monoclonality in up to 60% of cases using

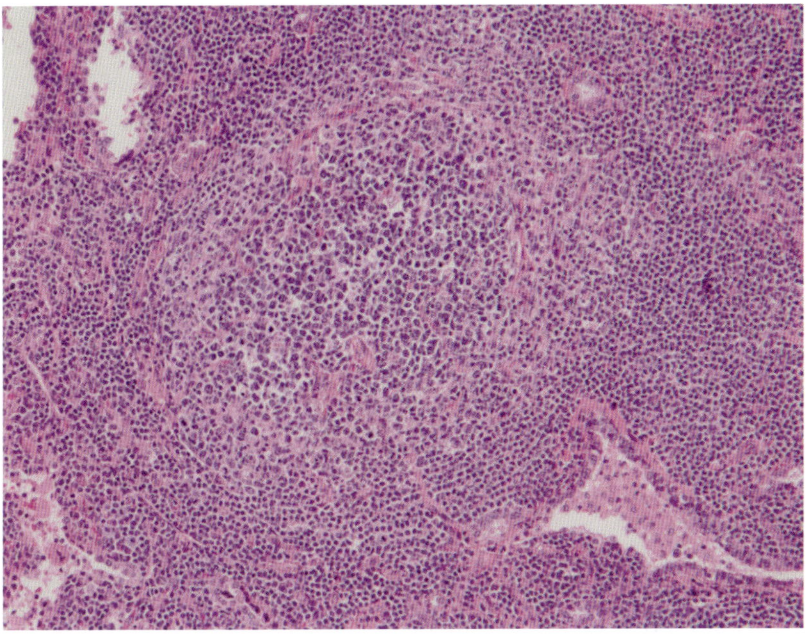

FIGURE 11.4 High magnification from open biopsy of MALT lymphoma shows lymphoid follicle with reactive germinal center surrounded by a dense, monotonous population of small lymphoid cells expanding the marginal zone of the follicle.

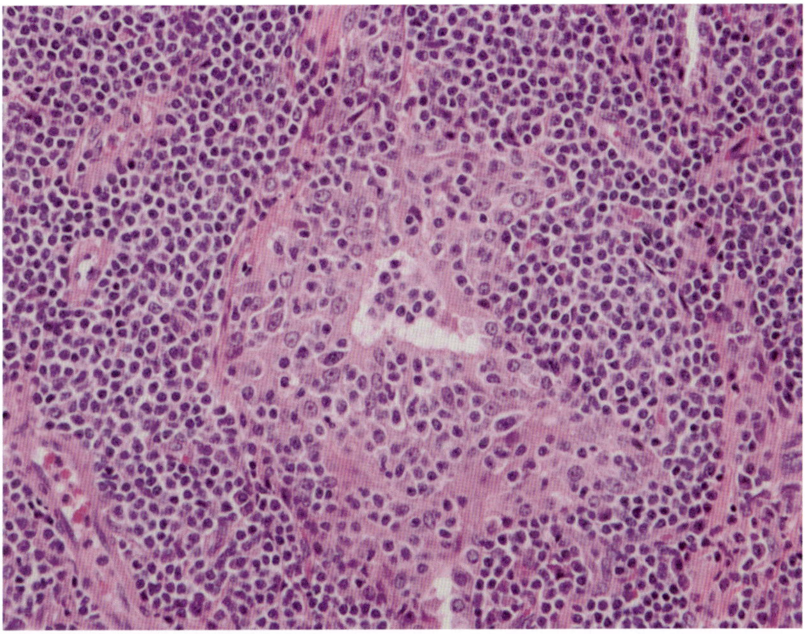

FIGURE 11.5 High magnification of MALT lymphoma shows characteristic lymphoepithelial lesion displaying extensive infiltration and expansion of the wall of a bronchiole by atypical small lymphocytes.

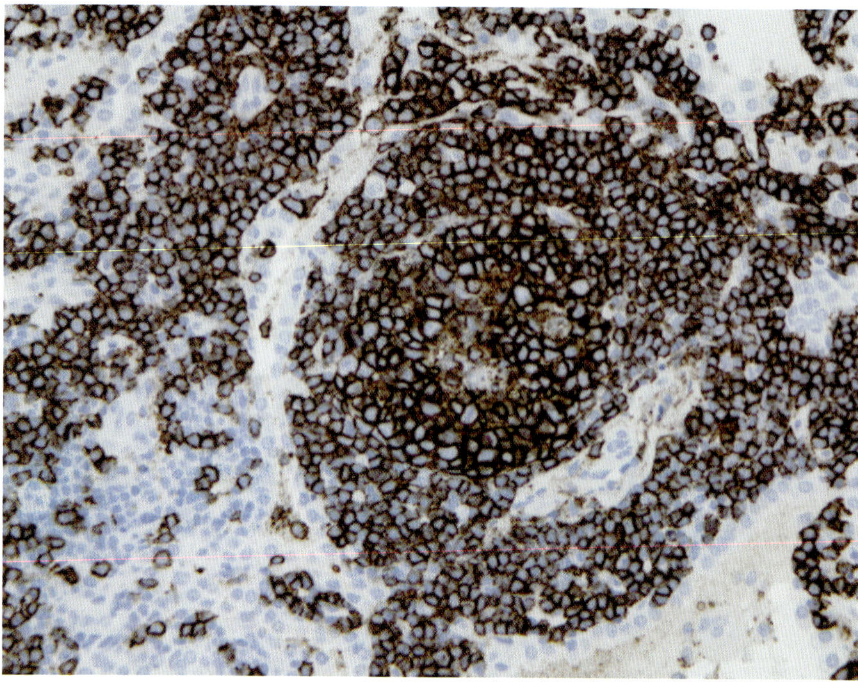

FIGURE 11.6 MALT lymphoma shows strong positivity of the small lymphoid cells for CD20 antibodies.

PCR in paraffin sections.[14] The tumor cells are strongly positive for CD20 and CD79a, and they also express bcl-2 (unlike reactive "monocytoid" B cells) (Fig. 11.6) (eFig. 11.5). The cells are negative for CD5, CD10, CD23, bcl-1, and bcl-6. Use of cytokeratin stains is useful for highlighting lymphoepithelial lesions (Fig. 11.7). Stains for CD21, CD23, and CD35 may be helpful for highlighting residual germinal centers overrun by the tumor cells by demonstrating an expanded network of follicular dendritic cells. A genetic abnormality comprising t(11;18)(q21;q21) is demonstrated in approximately 50% of marginal zone lymphomas.[20] The t(11;18) involves the API2 and MALT1 genes and will lead to the production of a fusion protein that can be detected by nuclear expression of bcl-10 in paraffin sections by immunohistochemistry. Trisomy 3 or t(1;14) have also been reported. The diagnosis of MALT lymphoma of the lung can be established with confidence on transbronchial biopsies when sheets of the characteristic small lymphoid cells expanding the interfollicular areas is seen that show the appropriate phenotype (CD20/CD79a/bcl-2+) and demonstrate light chain restriction by immunohistochemistry.

Diffuse Large B-Cell Lymphoma

These tumors account for approximately 10% of all primary lymphomas of the lung and comprise a diffuse proliferation of large B-cells that are

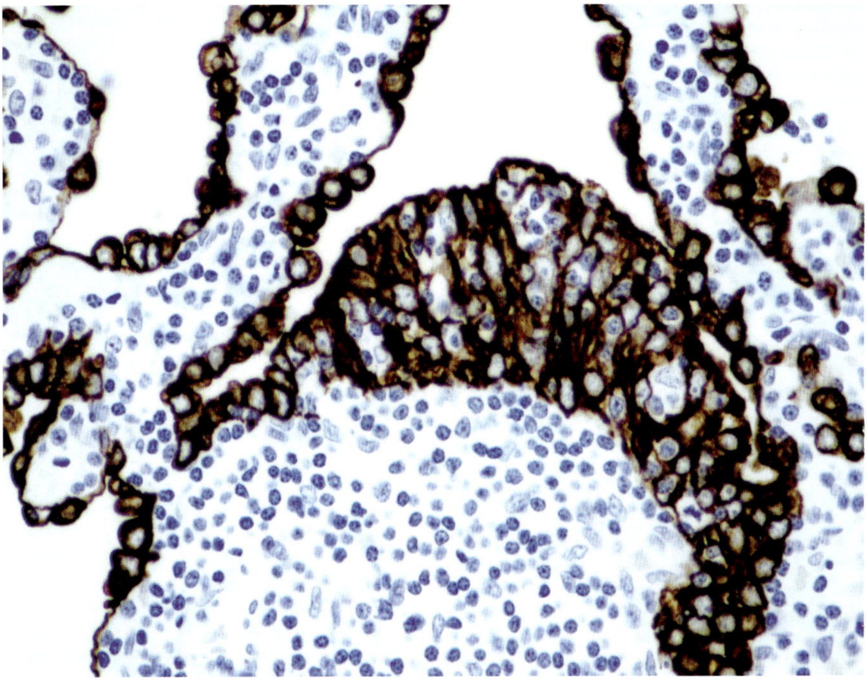

FIGURE 11.7 Cytokeratin (AE1/AE3) stain in MALT lymphoma highlights epithelial elements in a lymphoepithelial lesion. Notice the keratin-negative small lymphocytes percolating in-between the epithelial cells.

more than twice the size of a normal lymphocyte. Some authors have postulated that DLBCL of the lung may represent progression from a preexisting MALT lymphoma. The tumors show a tendency to arise in peripheral location. Patients are generally adults in their fifth or sixth decade of life, and the tumors occur more often in immunocompromised patients (HIV+, organ transplant patients) than in healthy individuals. Symptoms include cough, dyspnea, and hemoptysis, although the patients are more often asymptomatic. The prognosis for DLBCL of the lung is much worse than for MALT lymphoma with a median survival of 3 to 5 years in most instances, despite treatment with combination chemotherapy.[16] The tumors are usually single but may present as multiple discrete nodules that are sharply delimited from the surrounding lung parenchyma. Hilar lymph nodes may also be involved in some cases. Histologically, DLBCL of the lung comprises sheets of large, atypical lymphocytes displaying enlarged nuclei with coarse chromatin and prominent nucleoli and surrounded by a rim of amphophilic cytoplasm (Figs. 11.8 and 11.9) (eFigs. 11.6 to 11.8). Mitoses can be easily identified, and there are usually focal areas of necrosis with replacement and destruction of the underlying lung parenchyma. The tumors may invade the pleura or the bronchial walls and are usually sharply demarcated from the surrounding parenchyma

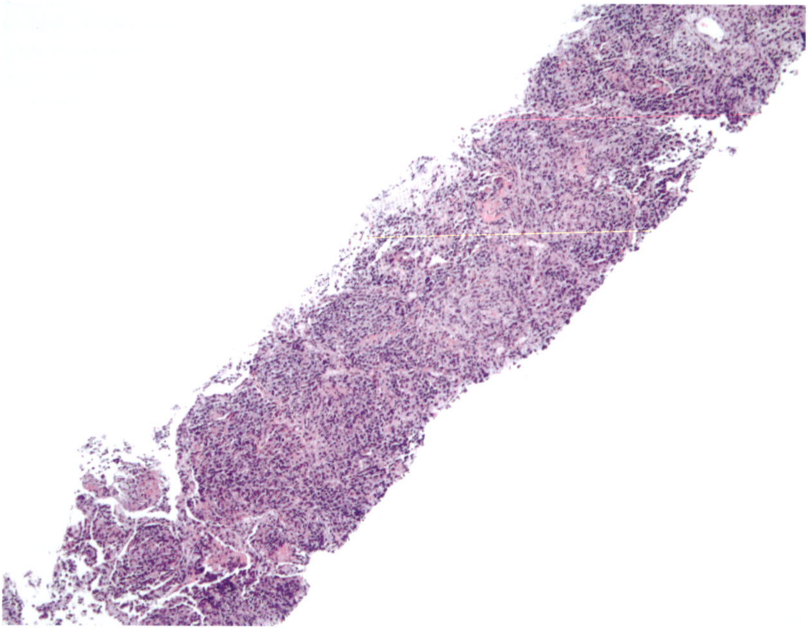

FIGURE 11.8 Core needle biopsy of peripheral mass in the lung shows DLBCL. Notice complete effacement of the underlying lung architecture.

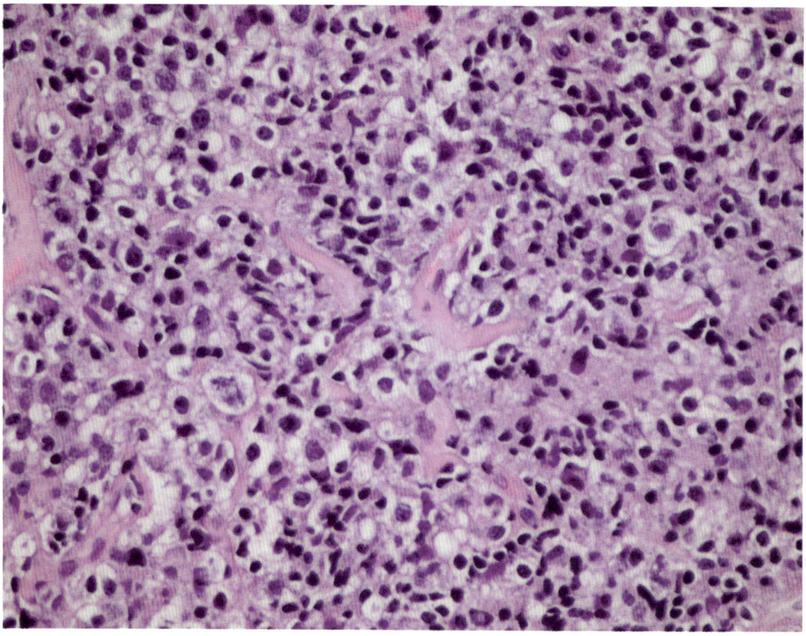

FIGURE 11.9 Higher magnification from core needle biopsy of diffuse large cell lymphoma of the lung showing atypical lymphoid cells with large nuclei and prominent nucleoli. The tumor cells showed strong CD20 positivity.

without displaying the lymphangitic pattern of spread observed in MALT lymphoma. Foci of low-grade MALT lymphoma can be usually identified in adequately sampled cases. In some cases, particularly on needle core biopsies, the tumor cells may suffer artifactual distortion and adopt a spindled appearance (Fig. 11.10). Immunohistochemical stains are of help in such instances by demonstrating the lymphoid nature of the cells. An immunoblastic variant of DLBCL can be observed that is characterized by large cells with vesicular nuclei, prominent eosinophilic nucleoli, and abundant rim of eosinophilic, plasmacytoid cytoplasm (Figs. 11.11 and 11.12). Cases with such features are generally associated with a more aggressive course. Immunohistochemical studies of DLBCL will demonstrate strong positivity of the tumor cells for CD20 and CD79a (Fig. 11.13). Background CD3+ small lymphocytes are usually absent or inconspicuous. Light chain restriction for κ or λ can be usually demonstrated by immunohistochemistry or by flow cytometry.[14] PCR assay for the IG heavy chain gene will demonstrate a clonal gene rearrangement in most cases. DLBCL is often diagnosed first on core needle biopsy specimens because of its predominantly peripheral location, but can also be diagnosed on endoscopic transbronchial biopsies when the tumor involves the bronchial wall. Sometimes the distinction

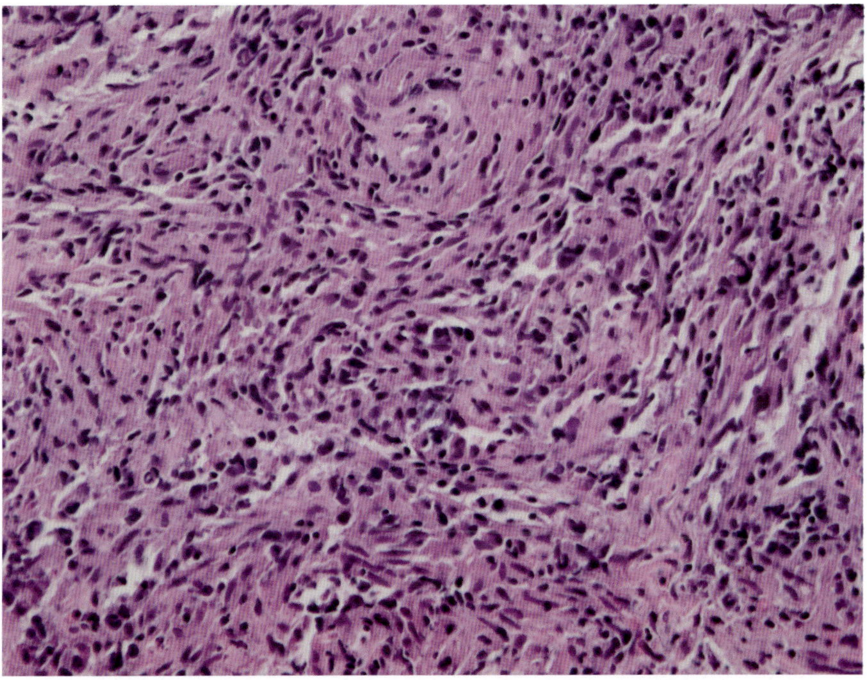

FIGURE 11.10 Core needle biopsy of the lung in patient with DLBCL shows artifactual distortion of the cells that adopt a vaguely spindled appearance. It is important not to mistake such cases for a spindle cell sarcoma; immunohistochemical staining for CD20 will strongly label the spindle cells in such instances.

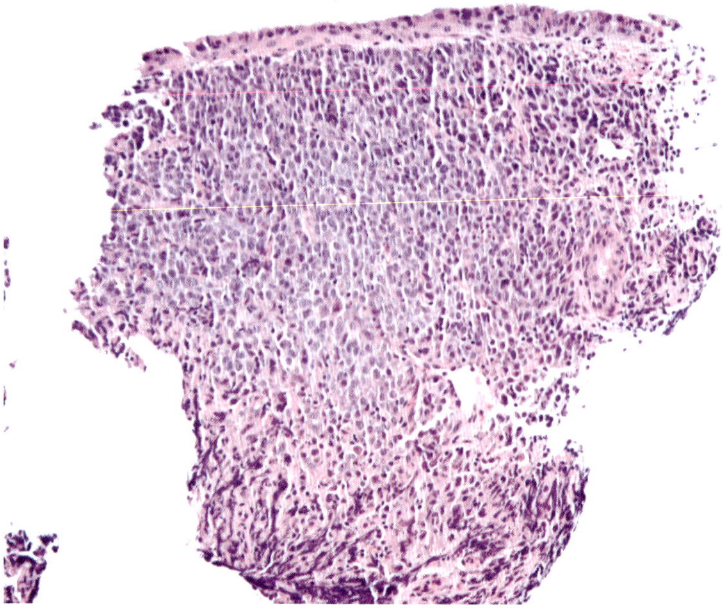

FIGURE 11.11 Endobronchial biopsy shows thin layer of bronchial respiratory mucosa (top) with replacement of the submucosa by a dense population of atypical round blue cells with large nuclei and scant stroma.

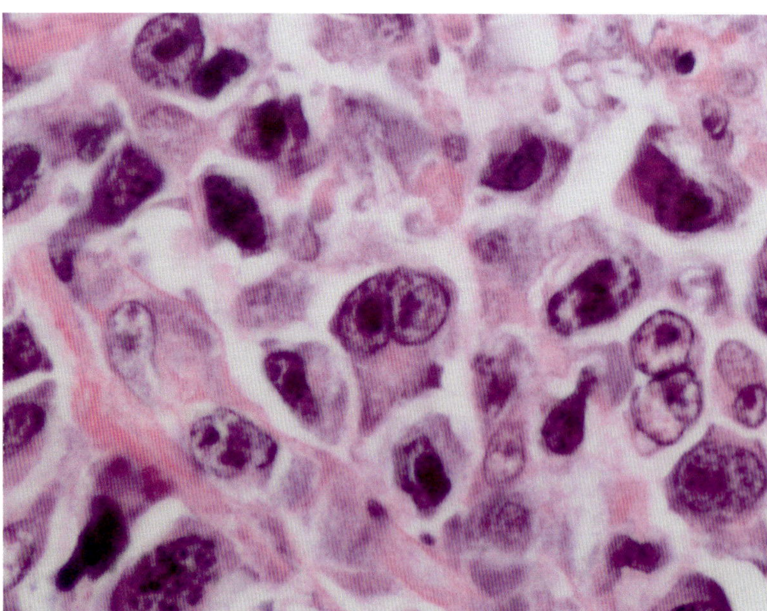

FIGURE 11.12 Higher magnification from endoscopic biopsy in patient with DLBCL, immunoblastic type, shows large tumor cells with hyperchromatic nuclei and abundant rim of plasmacytoid cytoplasm.

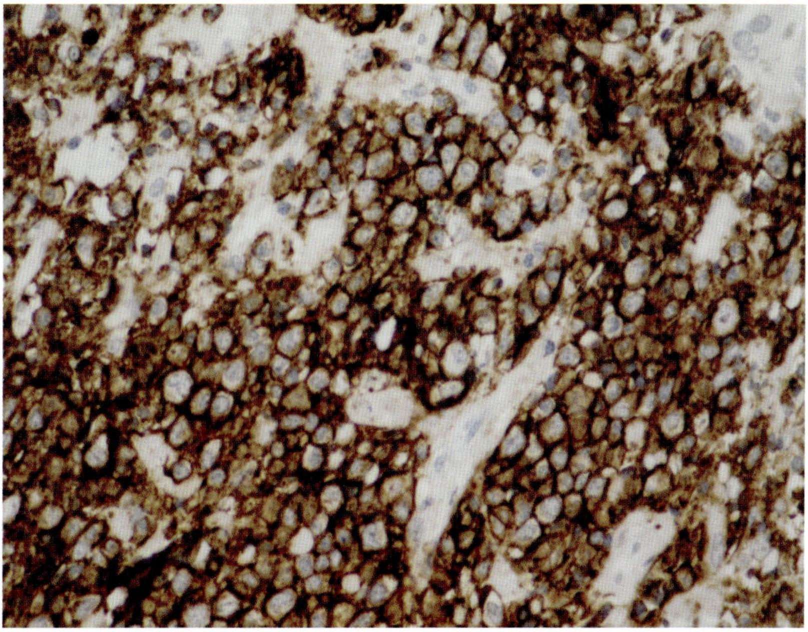

FIGURE 11.13 Immunohistochemical staining for CD20 shows strong cytoplasmic staining of the tumor cells in DLBCL (endoscopic biopsy).

between DLBCL and MALT lymphoma with focal transformation to DLBCL cannot be established with confidence on small endoscopic biopsies. Open or laparoscopic surgery with incisional biopsy, wedge resection, or lobectomy may be required for a more definitive diagnosis. DLBCL should be distinguished from anaplastic carcinoma or large cell neuroendocrine carcinoma; the distinction can sometimes be problematic on small endoscopic biopsies, particularly when there is prominent crush artifact (Figs. 11.14 and 11.15). Immunohistochemical stains, in particular negative results for cytokeratins and positive staining for leukocyte common antigen (LCA) and CD20 may be of help in this context. Distinction from high-grade LYG may also be quite difficult, particularly when the characteristic angiocentric pattern of involvement of LYG is not present in a small endoscopic biopsy. Demonstration of a significant population of CD3+ lymphocytes in the background and of Epstein–Barr virus (EBV) in the atypical B-cells will be of help to properly identify LYG.

Anaplastic Large Cell Lymphoma

ALCL has become increasingly recognized in the lung in the past few years.[21,22] The tumors may present as peripheral solitary nodules, although cases presenting as an endobronchial lesion have also been described.[23,24] The tumors can be single or multiple and generally present as well-circumscribed nodules. The clinical presentation is similar to that of DLBCL. Histologically, the tumors are characterized by sheets of large, anaplastic

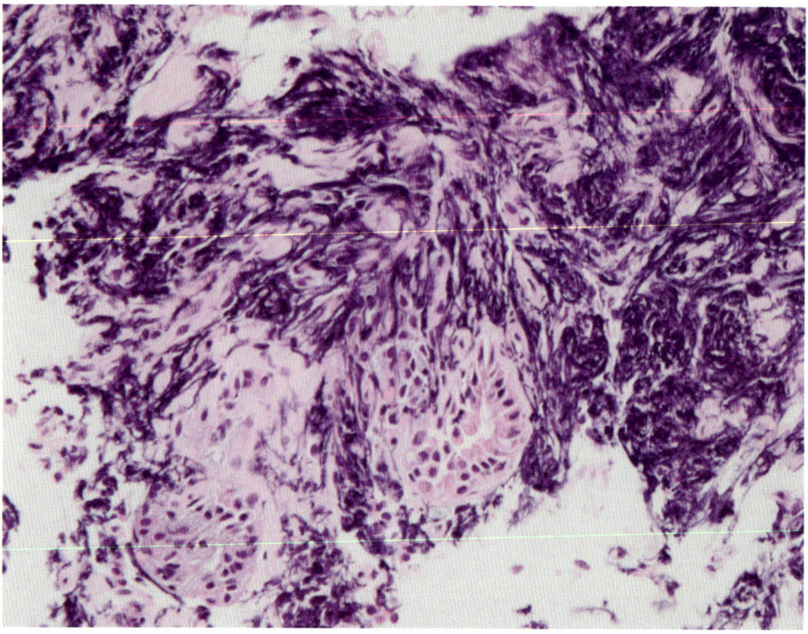

FIGURE 11.14 Endoscopic biopsy in DLBCL shows prominent crush artifact. Such cases can be mistaken for small cell lung carcinoma. Use of special stains may be of aid in the correct diagnosis by highlighting the crushed lymphocytes with CD20 and CD45.

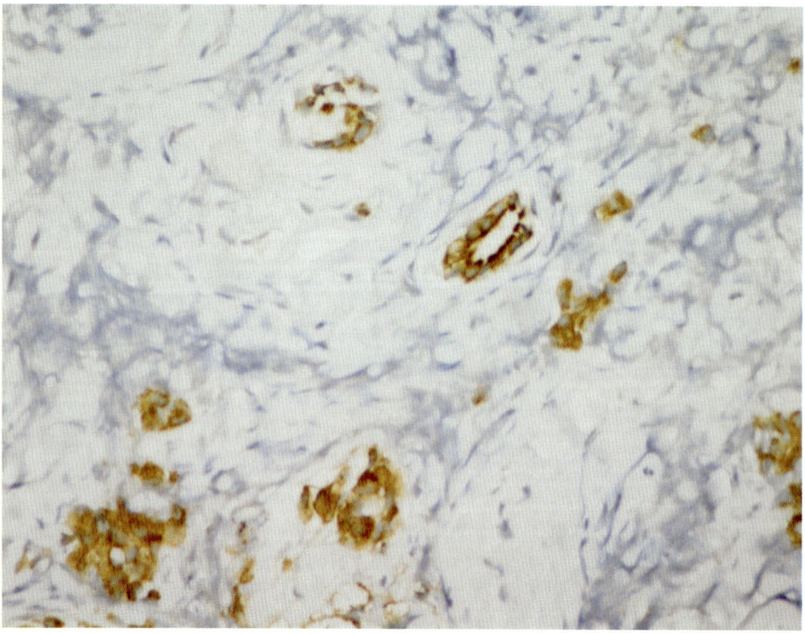

FIGURE 11.15 Immunohistochemical staining for cytokeratin is also of help in the diagnosis of diffuse large cell lymphoma with crush artifact by highlighting the entrapped residual bronchial glands although the crushed cells that surround them are negative.

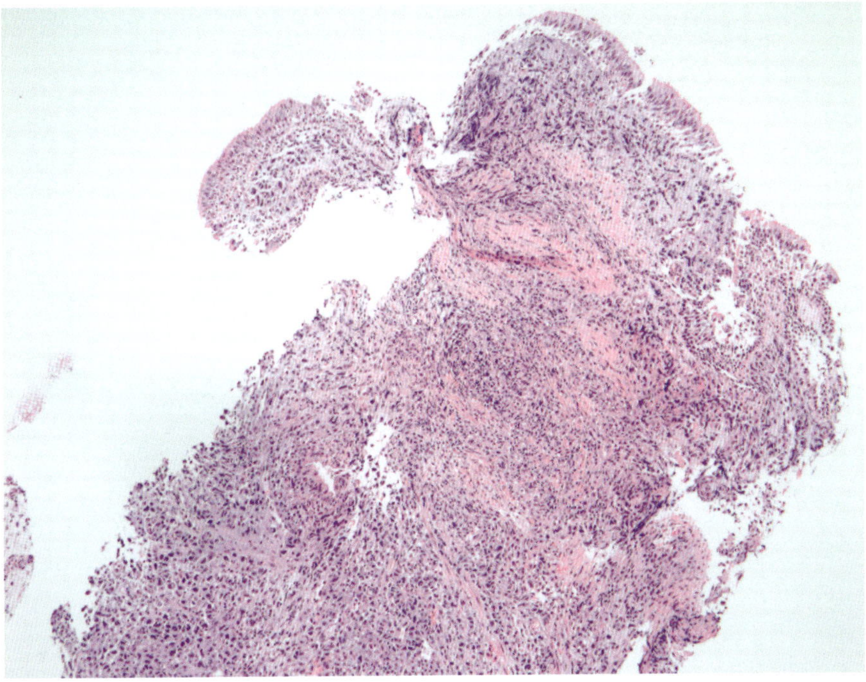

FIGURE 11.16 Core needle biopsy of the lung in patient with ALCL shows confluent sheets of large tumor cells underneath the bronchial epithelium. Even at this low magnification it is possible to appreciate the large size of many of the tumor cells.

tumor cells with pleomorphic nuclei and abundant cytoplasm (Fig. 11.16). Multinucleated tumors cells with a wreath-like arrangement of nuclei and prominent eosinophilic nucleoli resembling Reed–Sternberg cells are often present. Cells with horseshoe or kidney-shaped nuclei (so-called hallmark cells) are characteristic for this condition (Fig. 11.17). Cells showing invaginations of the nuclear membrane resembling nuclear inclusions can also be seen ("doughnut" cells). Occasional tumors can show a prominent component of background epithelioid histiocytes. The anaplastic tumor cells have a tendency to display a cohesive growth pattern that can closely mimic a carcinoma. Mitotic figures, including abnormal mitoses, are frequently encountered. Eosinophils can sometimes be prominent. Rarely, signet-ring cell forms can also be seen. Some lesions may be accompanied by a prominent stromal response comprising fascicles of spindle cells adopting a vague storiform pattern that can resemble a sarcoma. The tumors are characterized by the strong immunohistochemical expression of CD30. The pattern of staining is membranous and cytoplasmic, with prominent paranuclear dot-like positivity in the Golgi zone (Fig. 11.18). The tumor cells usually express one or more T-cell markers, although some cases may display a "null" phenotype. CD3 the most common pan-T cell marker, and CD8 are often negative in the tumor cells, but stains for CD2, CD4, and CD5 are usually positive in a significant number of cases (>70%). Most

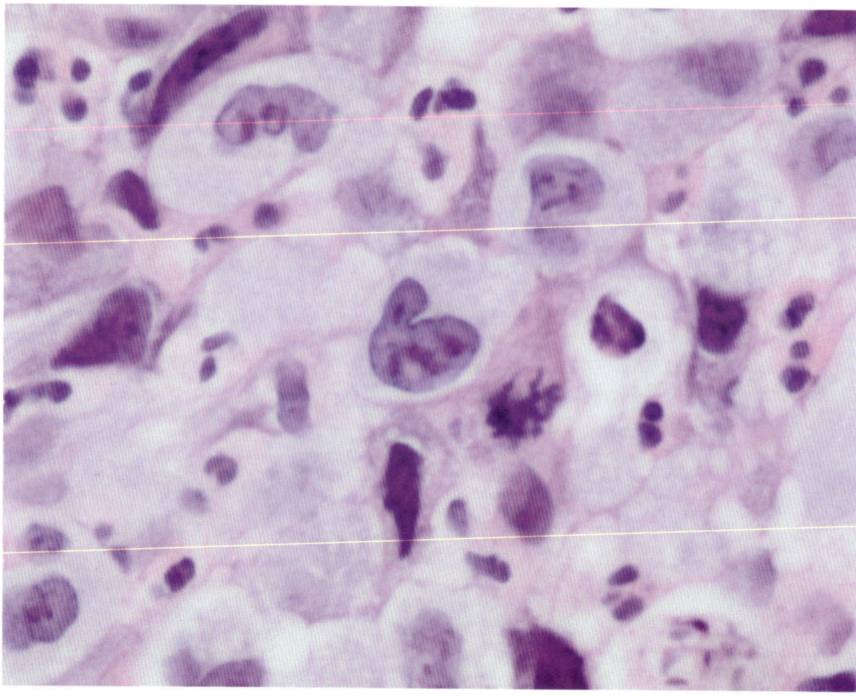

FIGURE 11.17 Higher magnification of core biopsy in ALCL shows pleomorphic population of cells containing large, irregular nuclei with prominent nucleoli. Some of the cells show a horseshoe or kidney-shaped configuration (so-called hallmark cells).

cases also show positivity for cytotoxicity associated antigens such as TIA1, granzyme B, and perforin. The tumor cells are usually positive for CD45 and CD45RO. ALCL can express the ALK1 nuclear and cytoplasmic protein in a number of cases; such cases are associated with a more favorable prognosis than ALK1-negative ALCL. The ALK1+ cases usually stain positively for EMA also. The *ALK* gene in ALCL can be involved in various chromosomal translocations that will lead to the formation of chimeric fusion proteins. The most frequent genetic alteration is a translocation between the *ALK* gene on chromosome 2 and the nucleophosmin (*NPM*) gene on chromosome 5, t(2;5)(p23;q35), but more than 10 variant forms have been identified. For this reason, immunohistochemistry is more reliable, in the appropriate morphological context, for making a definitive diagnosis as molecular testing by PCR for the more common *ALK/NPM* translocation may be negative in a significant percentage of patients.[25,26] More than 90% of cases show clonal rearrangement of the T-cell receptor (*TCR*) genes irrespective of whether or not the cells express T-cell antigens. The latter test can be of value in cases that are negative for all T-cell markers tested. ALCL may be difficult to diagnose on small endoscopic biopsies and can be easily mistaken for poorly differentiated carcinoma or sarcoma. Immunostaining for CD30 should always be considered in small biopsy

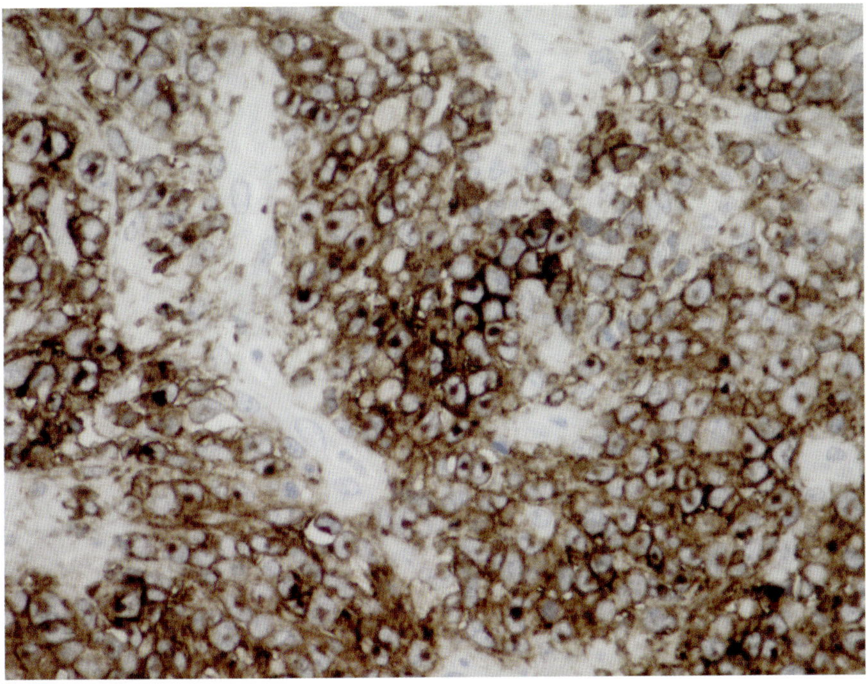

FIGURE 11.18 Immunohistochemical staining for CD30 in ALCL of the lung shows strong membrane and cytoplasmic staining for this marker. Notice the dot-like paranuclear positivity in the Golgi region in association with the membrane staining. CD15 and ALK-1 can show a similar pattern of staining in these lesions.

samples showing a mixed population containing pleomorphic tumor cells. Open lung wedge biopsy or VATS biopsies are the most reliable way for establishing a definitive diagnosis. Peripheral tumors are amenable to diagnosis through percutaneous core biopsies.

Lymphomatoid Granulomatosis

LYG represents a neoplastic clonal proliferation of EBV-infected B-cells that are associated with a heavy population of reactive T-lymphocytes. The condition was initially described by Liebow et al.[27] More recently, the term "angiocentric immunoproliferative lesion" has been proposed for this condition.[1] Most cases have been associated with immunodeficiency states, including AIDS, organ transplant, and the Wiskott–Aldrich syndrome.[28] The process can involve several organs, including skin, central nervous system, and kidney, but more than 70% of patients present with pulmonary involvement. Patients will show bilateral lung nodules that can measure more than 6 cm in diameter and frequently undergo cavitation.[29,30] The patients can also present with diffuse reticulonodular infiltrates or a solitary lesion. Histologically, the lesions are characterized by a mixed lymphoid infiltrate predominantly comprising small lymphocytes admixed with variable numbers of larger, atypical mononuclear lymphoid cells that can be admixed with histiocytes and plasma cells. The large cells can resemble immunoblasts; some of the large cells may also display double nuclei reminiscent of Reed–Sternberg cells. The term "granulomatosis" is misleading; epithelioid granulomas and multinucleated giant cells are not a feature of these lesions. The lymphoid infiltrate characteristically shows prominent angiocentrism, a distinctive feature of this process. The lymphoid cells will tend to surround the wall of pulmonary arteries and veins in a concentric distribution (Fig. 11.19) (eFigs. 11.9 and 11.10). Necrosis is a common feature in LYG and can range from focal and minimal to extensive and diffuse. A histologic grading system has been established that is based on the proportion of the atypical large cells to the background T-lymphocytes.[31] Grade 1 lesions are polymorphous and contain few EBV-infected B-cells (<5 per 10 high power fields); grade 2 lesions contain an increased number of EBV-infected atypical B-cells as well as foci of necrosis and still show marked cellular polymorphism; and grade 3 lesions contain sheets of large, atypical EBV-infected B-cells with abundant necrosis, essentially resembling DLBCL. By immunohistochemistry, LYG shows abundance of polyclonal CD3+ small T-lymphocytes against a background of scattered larger CD20+ B-cells (Fig. 11.20). The enlarged, atypical B-cells will show strong positivity for EBV by in situ hybridization (i.e., EBER) (Fig. 11.21).[32] The atypical cells can also react with CD30. Diagnosis

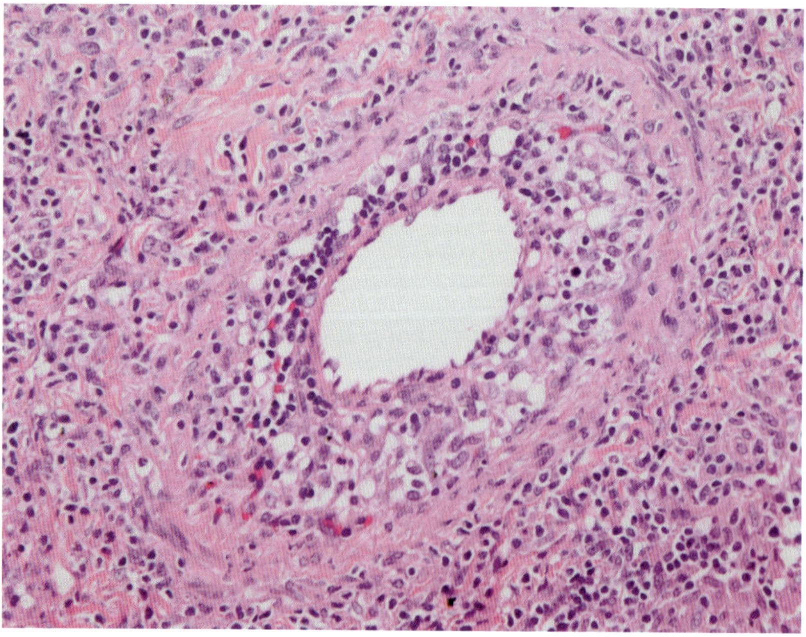

FIGURE 11.19 Lung biopsy in LYG shows a polymorphous lymphoid cell infiltrate surrounding a midcaliber vessel. Notice the extensive infiltration of the vessel wall by atypical lymphoid cells in a concentric distribution.

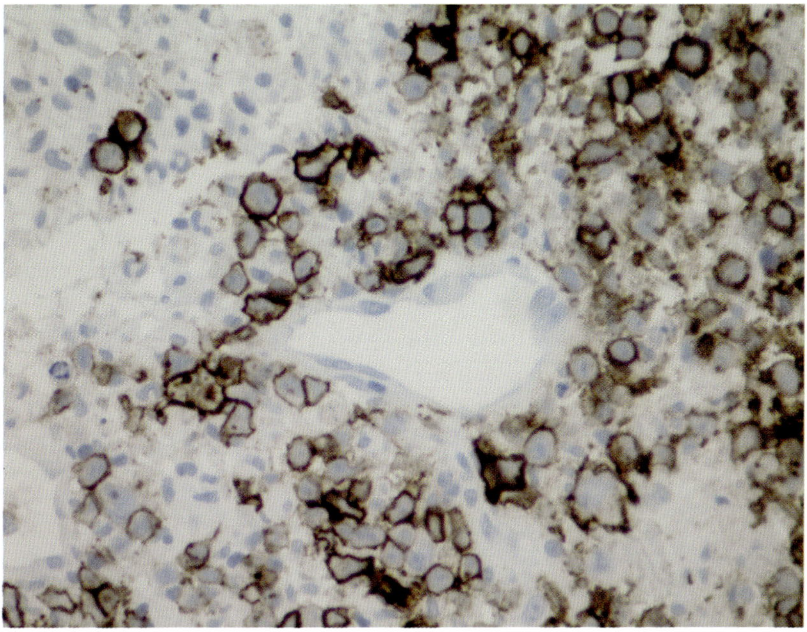

FIGURE 11.20 Immunohistochemical staining for CD20 highlights enlarged, atypical lymphocytes surrounding the wall of a vessel in LYG.

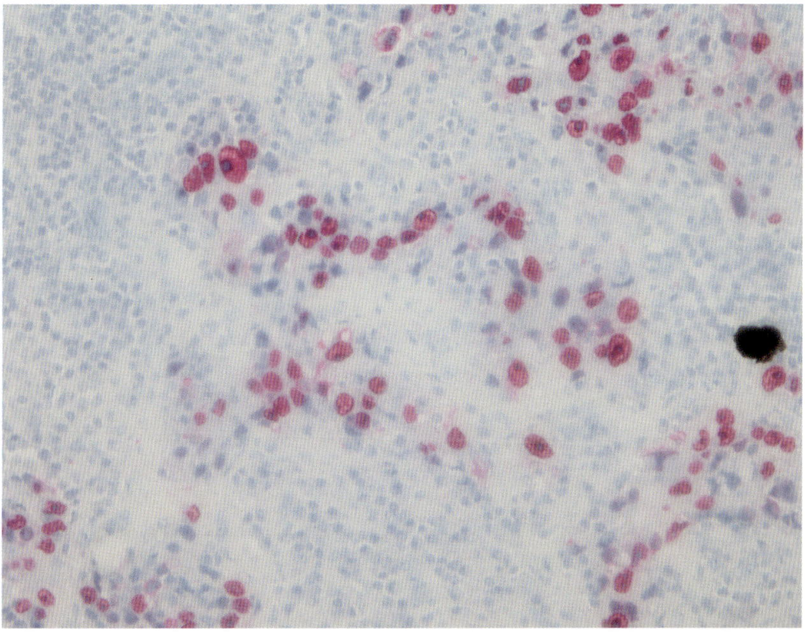

FIGURE 11.21 DNA in situ hybridization shows strong positivity (red signal) for Epstein–Barr virus (EBER) in the enlarged lymphocytes surrounding a vessel wall in pulmonary LYG.

of LYG may be very difficult on small transbronchial biopsies. Less than 30% of cases are successfully diagnosed on endoscopic biopsies. Sometimes the biopsy will yield only necrotic debris, or the cellular infiltrate in grade I lesions may appear quite banal disguising the underlying process. Because of the heavy small T-cell component, it may also be quite difficult to distinguish this process from a T-cell-rich large B-cell lymphoma. Identification of the characteristic angiocentric pattern of involvement of large and midcaliber vessels can be very helpful, although a similar finding can be observed rarely in pulmonary involvement by peripheral T-cell lymphoma. The clinical presentation of multiple, necrotizing nodules in an immunosuppressed patient should also raise the index of suspicion when confronted with a negative yield on an endoscopic biopsy. Open lung biopsy is the most reliable method for making a definitive diagnosis.

Hodgkin Lymphoma

Most cases of HL involving the lung represent secondary involvement of regional or systemic disease, and the diagnosis is generally established on lymph node biopsy. In rare instances, however, HL can be localized to the lung and presents as a primary lesion.[33] Presenting symptoms in such cases include fever, night sweats, weight loss, and cough. The disease has a bimodal age distribution, with peaks between 20 to 30 and 60 to 80 years of age, although it can also occur in children.[34] Chest X-rays or CT scans typically reveal single or multiple, sometimes bilateral nodules that may occasionally show cavitation secondary to necrosis. The tumors may also present as endobronchial lesions.[35] In lymph nodes, two forms of the disease are described, "classical" HL and lymphocyte-predominant HL; however, in the lung, only cases of "classical" HL have been described so far. "Classical" HL is characterized by a mixed lymphoid cell population that is remarkable for the presence of multinucleated Reed–Sternberg cells and mononuclear Hodgkin cells (collectively known as Hodgkin–Reed–Sternberg or HRS cells) (Figs. 11.22 and 11.23). The background infiltrate can comprise a population of small, bland-appearing small T-lymphocytes or a mixture of small lymphocytes with plasma cells, histiocytes, eosinophils, and neutrophils. Four histologic subtypes have been identified: lymphocyte-rich, nodular sclerosis, mixed cellularity, and lymphocyte-depleted type (Table 11.2). The nodular sclerosis and mixed cellularity subtypes are the ones most commonly encountered in the lung (Figs. 11.24 and 11.25).[36] The classical or diagnostic Reed–Sternberg cell is usually large, with abundant slightly basophilic cytoplasm, and at least two nuclear lobes or nuclei (Fig. 11.26). The nuclei are large and contain prominent eosinophilic nucleoli. The cells may contain multiple nuclei and adopt bizarre forms similar to the tumor cells in ALCL. The prototype of the Reed–Sternberg cell is characterized by an "owl-eyed" configuration, whereby two large nuclei sit in parallel next to each other, each displaying a prominent eosinophilic nucleolus. Mononuclear variants are designated Hodgkin cells and show identical features to

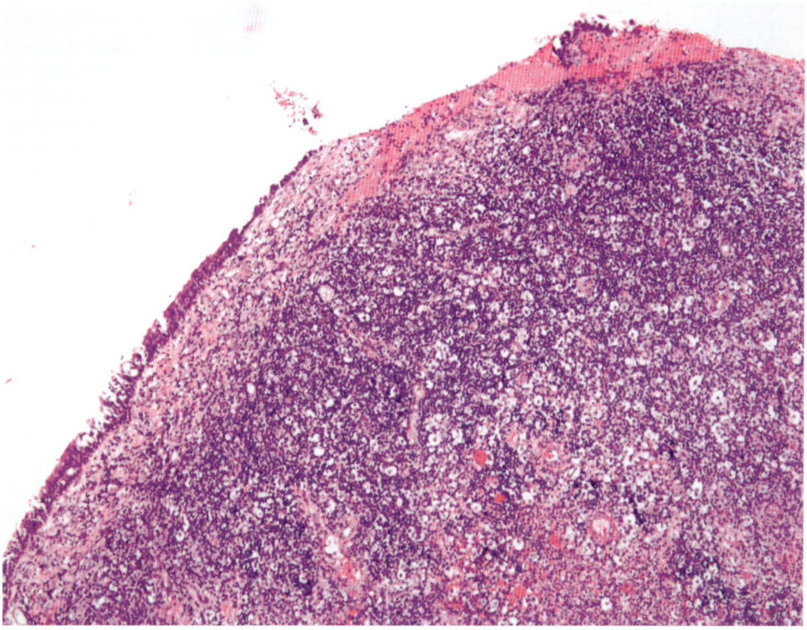

FIGURE 11.22 Endobronchial biopsy in patient with pulmonary HL shows dense lymphoid cell population underlying the bronchial mucosa. Endobronchial cases of pulmonary HL are extremely rare, and the diagnosis may be extremely difficult to establish on endoscopic biopsies.

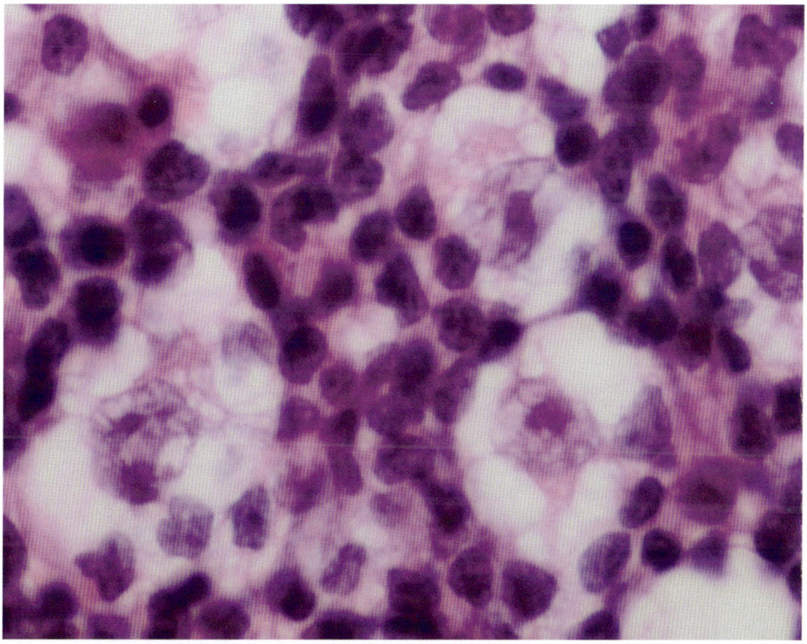

FIGURE 11.23 Higher magnification from endobronchial HL shows multiple lacunar Reed–Sternberg cells displaying large, vesicular nuclei with prominent eosinophilic nucleoli and marked retraction artifact from the surrounding stroma.

TABLE 11.2 Comparison of Types of Hodgkin Lymphomas

Histologic Type	Histology	Type of HRS Cells	Immunophenotype
Nodular lymphocyte-predominant HL (Nonclassical)	Nodular or nodular and diffuse Background: small lymphocytes and epithelioid histiocytes	LP cells ("popcorn" cells) (mononuclear cells with folded or multilobated nuclei and small nucleoli)	CD20+, CD45+, bcl-6+, CD79a+, OCT-2+, Bob-1+EMA+ (in up to 50%) CD15/CD30–
Classical lymphocyte-rich HL	Nodular (or rarely) diffuse Background: small lymphocytes; no eosinophils or neutrophils Small regressed germinal centers	Classical HRS cells (the cells are found within the nodules but not in the germinal centers)	CD30+, CD15+, PAX-5+ CD20/CD45- CD21 highlights regressed germinal centers
Classical nodular sclerosis HL	Nodules separated by dense collagen bands Background: eosinophils, histiocytes, and neutrophils	Lacunar cells (classical HRS with retraction artifact)	CD30+, CD15+, PAX-5+ EBER/LMP EBV+ (10%–40%) CD20/CD45–
Classical mixed cellularity HL	Diffuse growth pattern Background: eosinophils, plasma cells, histiocytes, and neutrophils, may have small granulomas	Classical HRS cells	CD30+, CD15+, PAX-5+ EBER/LMP EBV+ (75%) CD20/CD45–
Classical lymphocyte-depleted HL	Diffuse with predominance of HRS cells over the other elements	Classical HRS cells	CD30+, CD15+ CD20/CD45– T-cell markers negative

HL, Hodgkin lymphoma; LP, lymphocyte-predominant; HRS, Hodgkin–Reed–Sternberg cells.

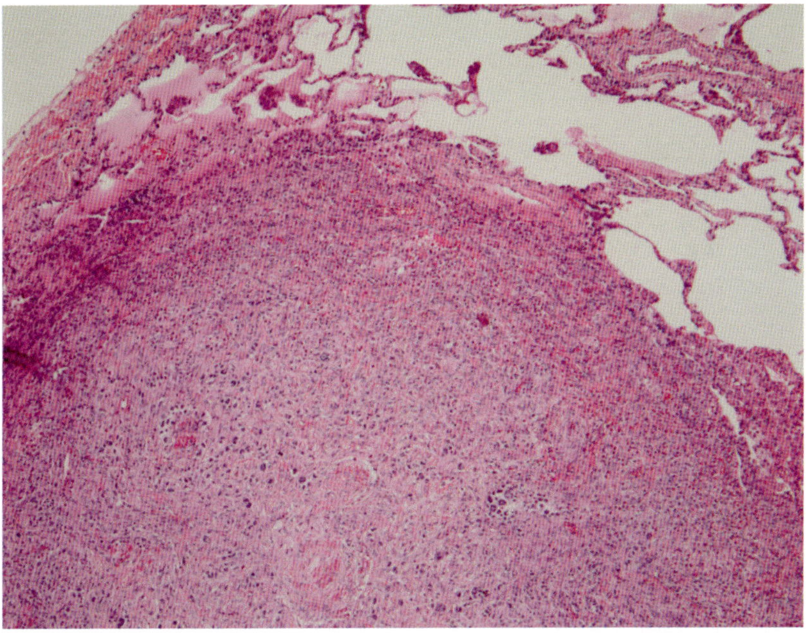

FIGURE 11.24 Wedge biopsy of pulmonary nodule with HL, nodular sclerosis, shows well-circumscribed subpleural nodule containing large cell population admixed with fibrotic stroma.

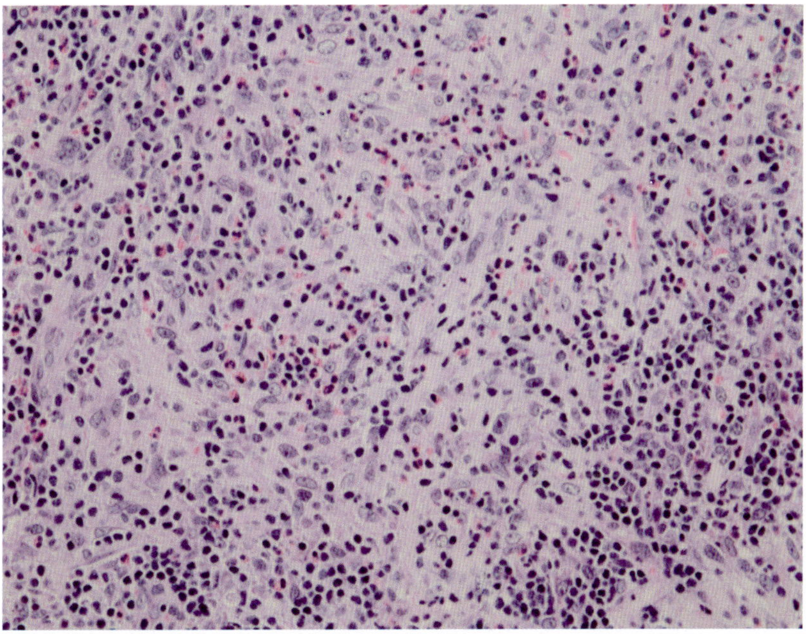

FIGURE 11.25 HL of the lung, mixed cellularity, shows a mixed population of cells comprising small lymphocytes, plasma cells, eosinophils, plasma cells, and scattered larger, atypical mononuclear and multinucleated Reed–Sternberg cells. The presence of a predominant mixed cellular background is an important clue to the diagnosis in these cases.

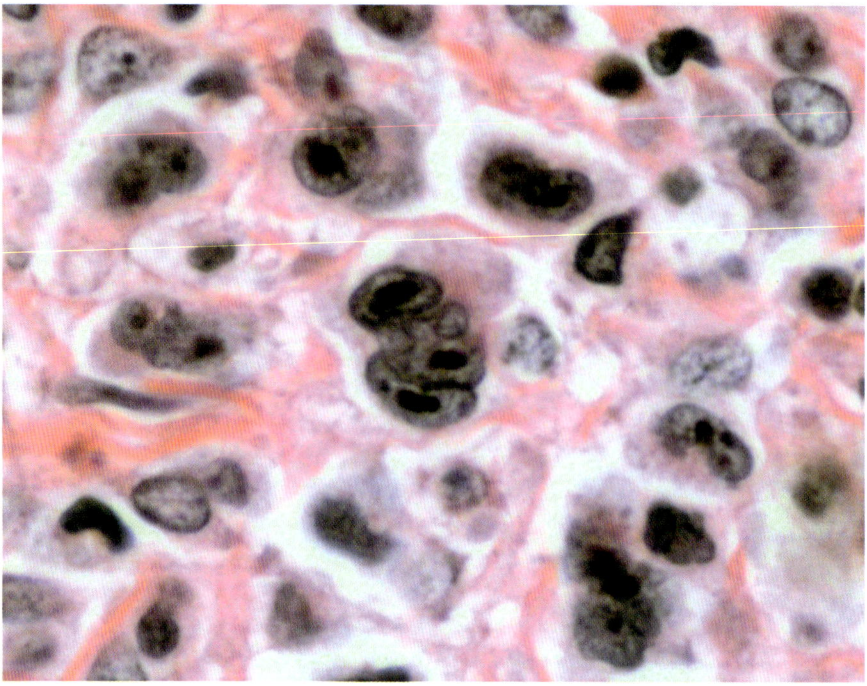

FIGURE 11.26 Classical HRS cell in pulmonary HL shows three large nuclei with prominent eosinophilic nucleoli surrounded by clear perinuclear halos.

the multinucleated types. HRS cells in the nodular sclerosis subtype are characterized by a retraction artifact and are termed "lacunar" cells. HRS cells can undergo apoptosis and appear as a dense, hyperchromatic body ("mummy" cells). Except for the rare lymphocyte-depleted variant, HRS cells are usually few and widely scattered and generally overshadowed by the reactive mixed infiltrate in the background. Pulmonary lesions of HL may undergo extensive necrosis and cavitation. Some cases will form noninfectious epithelioid granulomas; the granulomas can sometimes be observed surrounding the areas of necrosis. The tumors can invade the bronchial wall with destruction of the cartilaginous plate or can infiltrate the pleura. The cellular infiltrate can also involve the walls of arteries and pulmonary veins.

Classical HL has been shown to represent a monoclonal B-cell neoplasm derived from B-cells.[37] HRS cells are characterized by a distinctive immunophenotype; the cells are positive for CD30 (Fig. 11.27) and CD15 and negative for CD45 and, in the majority of instances, for CD20.[1] They also do not stain for the transcription factor OCT-2 and its coactivator, BOB-1. It is postulated that HRS cells are derived from germinal center B-cells that have lost the B-cell-specific expression program and have acquired inappropriate gene products. A strong association between EBV

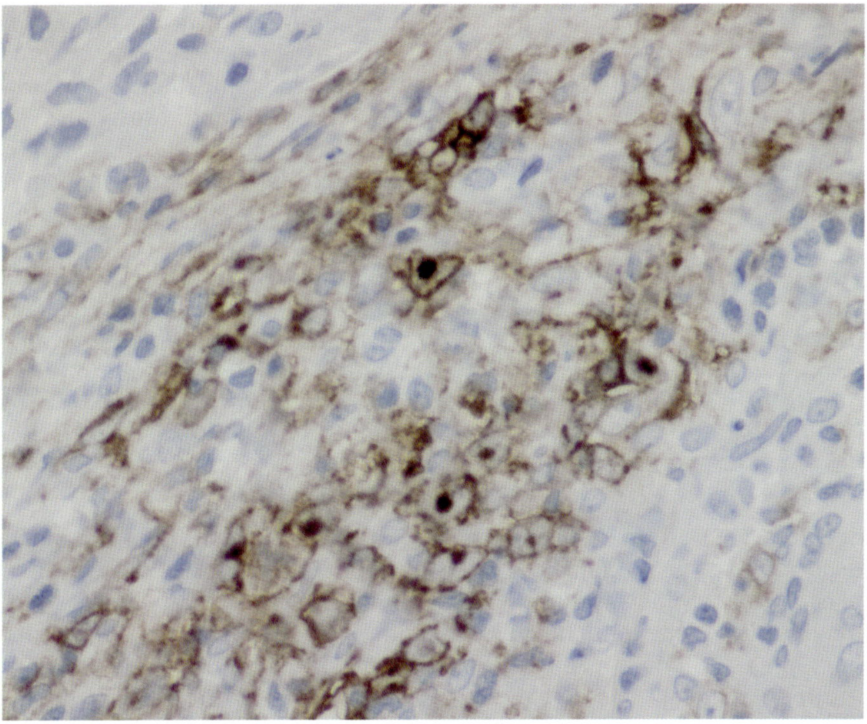

FIGURE 11.27 Immunohistochemical staining for CD30 in HL shows scattered positive cells admixed with nonreactive lymphocytes and other elements. Notice the strong cytoplasmic and dot-like paranuclear positivity in the HRS cells.

infections has also been demonstrated for classical Hodgkin lymphoma (CHL), particularly in cases of mixed cellularity and, to a lesser extent, nodular sclerosis subtypes. The HRS cells in such cases strongly express EBV-encoded latent membrane protein (LMP) by immunohistochemistry, and strongly label for the EBV-encoded RNA (EBER) by in situ hybridization. Clonal IG gene rearrangements can be demonstrated in the majority of microdissected HRS cells, supporting the germinal center derivation. Another marker that can also be of aid for the diagnosis is PAX-5, a B-cell-specific activator protein. The immunostaining of HRS cells in CHL is usually weaker than in reactive B-cells, a feature that makes the PAX-5+ HRS cells more easily identifiable. HRS cells will typically display a peculiar "rosetting" effect owing to their being surrounded by a peripheral ring of small T-lymphocytes. Both CD30 and CD15 are characterized by membrane and paranuclear (dot-like Golgi zone) cytoplasmic positivity. CD30 strongly stains the majority of HRS cells, but CD15 may stain only a few tumor cells or may be absent altogether in some cases. EMA, ALK, and T-cell markers are usually negative in the HRS cells.

The main differential diagnosis for pulmonary HL is with ALCL and CD30+ DLBCL. CD30+ DLBCL, in particular, can pose serious difficulties for diagnosis with CHL, and some have postulated the existence of a continuum or overlap between the two conditions. Because the identification of HRS cells necessary for the diagnosis of CHL can be difficult in small biopsy samples, definitive diagnosis may not be possible in endoscopic or transthoracic core biopsies of the lung. Furthermore, because HRS-like cells may be observed in other conditions, such as small lymphocytic lymphoma/CLL and acute infectious mononucleosis, care must be taken in not overinterpreting such cells out of context. Attention to the background will be indispensable for appropriate interpretation. Small biopsies in which the background infiltrates cannot be adequately assessed may require deferral of the diagnosis to an open biopsy.

Plasmacytoma

Secondary involvement of the lung in multiple myeloma is an infrequent occurrence; primary pulmonary plasmacytoma in the absence of systemic plasma cell dyscrasia is rarer.[38,39] The tumors affect adult patients between the fifth and the seventh decades. Symptoms include cough, dyspnea, and hemoptysis. The tumors most often present as well-circumscribed, solitary intraparenchymal masses but can also occur in hilar location or associated with a prominent endobronchial component.[40] Tumors that harbor a peribronchial component or involve at least partially a major bronchus are amenable to endoscopic biopsy diagnosis. Serum monoclonal gammopathy can be identified in a minority of cases; most patients with pulmonary plasmacytoma present with nonsecretory tumors. Histologically, the tumors are characterized by monotonous sheets of plasma cells with few other intervening cellular elements (Fig. 11.28). Germinal centers are usually absent, a feature that facilitates differentiation from MALT lymphoma with plasmacytic differentiation. The plasma cells are usually mature and indistinguishable from benign plasma cells (Fig. 11.29); some cases, however, may show progressive cytologic atypia and loss of plasmacytic differentiation resembling immunoblastic lymphoma. Mature plasma cells will generally display uniform, round, eccentrically located nuclei with dispersed chromatin. The cytoplasm is brightly eosinophilic and abundant. Stromal amyloid deposits may be seen in some cases and rare cases have been reported in association with epithelioid granulomas. Russell bodies can also be frequently observed. Well-differentiated plasmacytomas comprise terminally differentiated B-cells and, as such, will usually be negative for B-cell markers such as CD45 (LCA), CD19, CD20, and PAX-5. In the majority of instances, however, they will demonstrate cytoplasmic light chain restriction for κ or λ by paraffin-section immunohistochemistry or by DNA in situ hybridization (Fig. 11.30). CD138 (syndecan-1) is another useful marker that will help identify

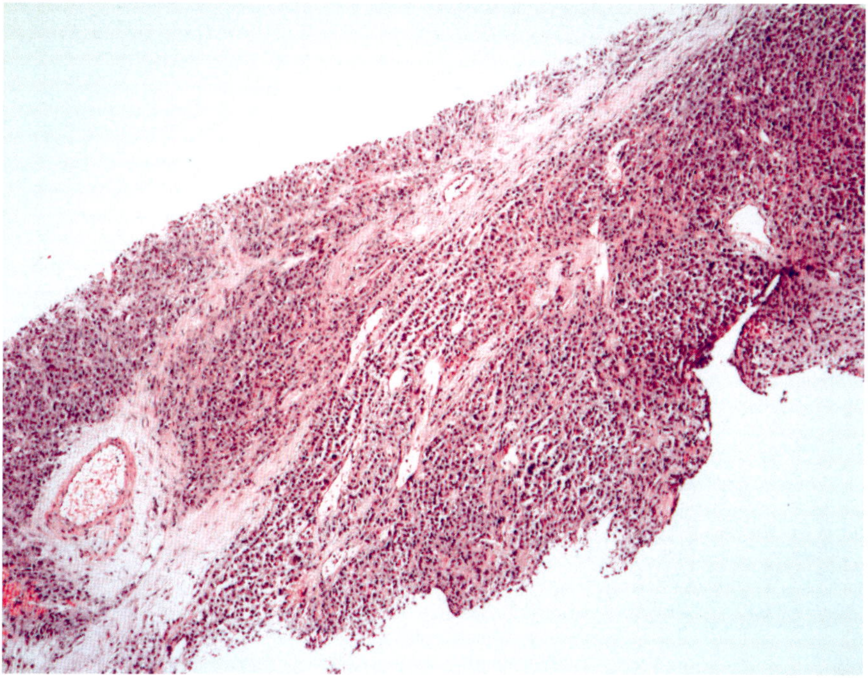

FIGURE 11.28 Needle core biopsy of pulmonary plasmacytoma shows sheets of monotonous small plasmacytoid cells without any intervening lymphoid follicles or germinal centers.

plasma cells on routine immunohistochemistry. Plasma cells may also be positive for EMA and CD56. IG light and heavy chain genes will show clonal rearrangements. The diagnosis is usually straightforward on wedge resection or open lung biopsy specimens but may be occasionally difficult in small endoscopic biopsies. In particular, distinction from small lymphocytic lymphoma with plasmacytic differentiation or marginal zone lymphoma (MALToma) with abundant plasmacytoid small lymphocytes may be quite difficult. Presence of more than 20% of nonplasmacytic lymphocytes in the biopsy sample should raise the possibility of these alterative diagnoses. Immunohistochemical analysis showing strong positivity for surface IG, CD20, and CD45 will support a diagnosis of lymphoma over plasmacytoma. Inflammatory plasma cell pseudotumor may also pose difficulties for diagnosis, but the latter will show a polyclonal pattern of light chain expression and will contain a significant stromal fibroblastic cell population. Another condition that deserves consideration in the differential diagnosis is IgG4-related sclerosing disease. The sheets of plasma cells in IgG4-related disease, however, are polyclonal, and the process is characterized by an increased number of IgG4+ plasma cells, in addition to displaying significant stromal sclerosis.[41]

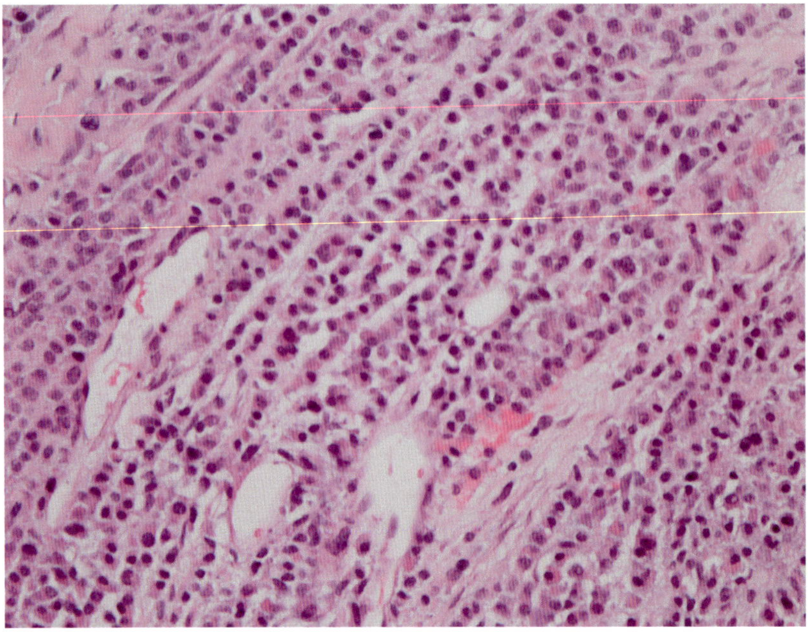

FIGURE 11.29 Higher magnification from core biopsy of pulmonary plasmacytoma shows sheets of small, mature plasma cells adopting a linear configuration.

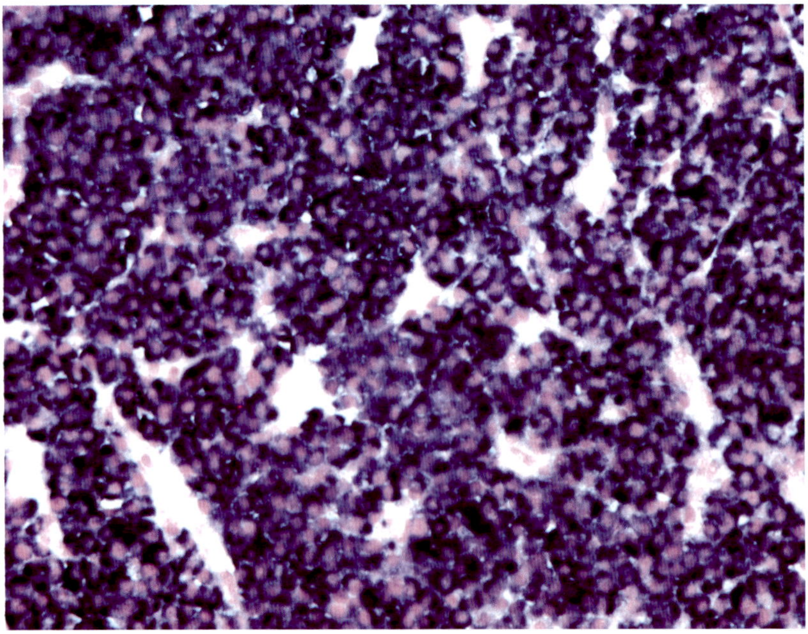

FIGURE 11.30 DNA in situ hybridization of pulmonary plasmacytoma shows κ light chain restriction. Notice the intense signal *(blue)* is present in virtually every cell.

REFERENCES

1. Swerdlow SH, Campo E, Harris NL, et al. *WHO Classification of Tumors of Hematopoietic and Lymphoid Tissue*. Lyon, France: IARC; 2008.
2. Liebow AA. Definition and classification of interstitial pneumonias in human pathology. *Prog Resp Dis*. 1975;8:1–33.
3. Nicholson AG, Wotherspoon AC, Diss TC, et al. Reactive pulmonary lymphoid disorders. *Histopathology*. 1995;26:405–412.
4. Yousem SA, Colby TV, Carrington CB. Follicular bronchitis–bronchiolitis. *Hum Pathol*. 1990;16:700–706.
5. Kinnane BT, Mansell AL, Zwerdling RG, et al. Follicular bronchitis in the pediatric population. *Chest*. 1993;104:1183–1186.
6. Kobzik L. Benign pulmonary lesions that may be misdiagnosed as malignant. *Semin Diagn Pathol*. 1990;7:129–138.
7. Koss M, Hochholzer L, Nichols PW, et al. Primary non-Hodgkin's lymphoma and pseudolymphoma of the lung: a study of 161 patients. *Hum Pathol*. 1983;14:1024–1038.
8. Abbondanzo SL, Rush W, Bijwaard KE, et al. Nodular lymphoid hyperplasia of the lung: a clinicopathologic study of 14 cases. *Am J Surg Pathol*. 2000;24:587–597.
9. Marchevsky A, Rosen MJ, Crystal G, et al. Pulmonary complications of the acquired immunodeficiency syndrome: a clinicopathologic study of 70 cases. *Hum Pathol*. 1985;16:659–670.
10. Joshi VV, Oleske JM, Minnefor AB, et al. Pathologic pulmonary findings in children with the acquired immunodeficiency syndrome: a study of 10 cases. *Hum Pathol*. 1985;16:241–246.
11. Nicholson AG, Kim H, Corrin B, et al. The value of classifying interstitial pneumonitis in childhood according to defined histological patterns. *Histopathology*. 1998;33:203–211.
12. Fiche M, Capron F, Berger F, et al. Primary pulmonary non-Hodgkin's lymphomas. *Histopathology*. 1995;26:529–537.
13. Habermann TM, Ryu JH, Inwards DJ, et al. Primary pulmonary lymphoma. *Sem Oncol*. 1999;26:307–315.
14. Nicholson AG, Wotherspoon AC, Diss TC, et al. Pulmonary B-cell non-Hodgkin's lymphomas. The value of immunohistochemistry and gene analysis in diagnosis. *Histopathology*. 1995;26:395–403.
15. Adis BJ, Hyjek E, Isaacson PG. Primary pulmonary lymphoma: a reappraisal of its histogenesis and its relationship to pseudolymphoma and lymphoid interstitial pneumonia. *Histopathology*. 1998;13:1–17.
16. Li G, Hansmann ML, Zwingers T, et al. Primary lymphomas of the lung: morphological, immunohistochemical and clinical features. *Histopathology*. 1990;16:519–531.
17. Boric R, Wislez G, Antoine M, et al. Clinical characteristics and prognostic factors of pulmonary MALT lymphoma. *Eur Respir J*. 2009;34:1408–1416.
18. Stefanovic A, Morgenstern D, Fong T, et al. Pulmonary marginal zone lymphoma: a single center experience and review of SEER database. *Leuk Lymphoma*. 2008;49:1311–1320.
19. Kurtin RJ, Myers JL, Adlakha H, et al. Pathologic and clinical features of primary pulmonary extranodal marginal zone B-cell lymphoma of MALT type. *Am J Surg Pathol*. 2001;25:997–1008.
20. Okabe M, Inagaki H, Oshima K, et al. API2-MALT1 fusion defines a distinctive clinico-pathologic subtype in pulmonary extranodal marginal zone lymphoma of mucosa-associated lymphoid tissue. *Am J Surg Pathol*. 2003;162:1113–1122.
21. Rush WL, Andriko JA, Taubenberger JK, et al. Primary anaplastic large cell lymphoma of the lung: a clinicopathologic study of five patients. *Mod Pathol*. 2002;13:1285–1292.
22. Yang HB, Li J, Shen T. Primary anaplastic large cell lymphoma of the lung: report of two cases. *Acta Haematol*. 2007;118:188–191.

23. Chott A, Kaserer K, Augustin I, et al. Ki-1-positive large cell lymphoma: a clinicopathologic study of 41 cases. *Am J Surg Pathol.* 1998;14:439–448.

24. Guerra J, Echeverria M, Barrio N, et al. Primary endobronchial anaplastic large cell lymphoma in a pediatric patient. *P R Health Sci J.* 2006;25:159–161.

25. Lamant L, Maggetto F, al Saati T, et al. High incidence of the t(2;5)(p23;q35) translocation in anaplastic large cell lymphoma and its lack of detection in Hodgkin's disease. *Blood.* 1996;87:284–291.

26. Morris SW, Kirstein MN, Valentine MB, et al. Fusion of a kinase gene, ALK, to a nucleolar protein gene, NPM, in non-Hodgkin's lymphoma. *Science.* 1994;263:1281–1284.

27. Liebow A, Carrington CR, Friedman PJ. Lymphomatoid granulomatosis. *Hum Pathol.* 1972;3:457–558.

28. Haque AK, Myers JL, Hudnall SD, et al. Pulmonary lymphomatoid granulomatosis in acquired immunodeficiency syndrome: lesions with Epstein–Barr virus infection. *Mod Pathol.* 1998;11:347–356.

29. Koss MN, Hocholzer L, Nichols PW. Lymphomatoid granulomatosis: a clinicopathologic study of 42 patients. *Pathology.* 1986;18:283–288.

30. Katzenstein AL, Carrington CB, Liebow AA. Lymphomatoid granulomatosis: a clinicopathologic study of 152 cases. *Cancer.* 1979;43:360–373.

31. Lipford EH Jr, Margolick JB, Longo DL, et al. Angiocentric immunoproliferative lesions: a clinicopathologic spectrum of post-thymic T-cell proliferations. *Blood.* 1988;72:1674–1681.

32. Guinee D Jr, Jafee ES, Kingma D, et al. Pulmonary lymphomatoid granulomatosis: evidence for a proliferation of Epstein–Barr virus infected B-lymphocytes with a prominent T-cell component and vasculitis. *Am J Surg Pathol.* 1994;18:753–764.

33. Yousem SA, Weiss LM, Colby TV. Primary pulmonary Hodgkin's disease: a clinicopathologic study of 15 cases. *Cancer.* 1986;57:1217–1224.

34. Urasinski T, Kamienska E, Gawlikowska-Sroka A, et al. Pediatric pulmonary Hodgkin lymphoma: analysis of 10 years data from a single center. *Eur J Med Res.* 2010;15(S):206–210.

35. Harper PG, Fisher C, McLennan K, et al. Presentation of Hodgkin's disease as an endobronchial lesion. *Cancer.* 1984;53:147–150.

36. Rodriguez J, Tirabosco R, Pizzolito S, et al. Hodgkin lymphoma presenting with exclusive or preponderant pulmonary involvement: a clionicopathologic study of 5 new cases. *Ann Diagn Pathol.* 2006;10:83–88.

37. Marafioti T, Hummel M, Foss HD, et al. Hodgkin and Reed–Sternberg cells represent an expansion of a single clone originating from a germinal center B-cell with functional immunoglobulin gene rearrangements but defective immunoglobulin transcription. *Blood.* 2000;95:1443–1450.

38. Koss MN, Hochholzer L, Moran CA, Frizerra G. Pulmonary plasmacytomas: a clinicopathologic and immunohistochemical study of five cases. *Ann Diagn Pathol.* 1998;2:1–11.

39. Morinaga S, Watanabe H, Gemma A, et al. Plasmacytoma of the lung associated with nodular deposits of immunoglobulins. *Am J Surg Pathol.* 1987;11:989–995.

40. Edelstein E, Gal AA, Mann KP, et al. Primary solitary endobronchial plasmacytoma. *Ann Thorac Surg.* 2004;78:1448–1449.

41. Zen Y, Inoue D, Kitao A, et al. IgG4-related lung and pleural disease: a clinicopathologic study of 21 cases. *Am J Surg Pathol.* 2009;33:1886–1893.

12

EPITHELIAL LUNG NEOPLASMS

Epithelial lung neoplasms are the most common type of lung cancer and may be amenable to sampling by several techniques. Core needle and open biopsies are indicated for peripheral tumors located away from the main bronchi; endoscopic biopsies will usually yield adequate diagnostic material in majority of central lesions. Because many lung tumors are found in advanced stages precluding surgical removal, the initial biopsy is often the only tissue diagnosis done and the one on which all future management of the patient will rest. Carcinoma of the lung can arise from the squamous epithelium lining the main bronchi, from respiratory epithelium, including the lining of the alveoli and bronchial adnexa, and from specialized cells within the walls of the bronchial tree such as neuroendocrine cells. There exist several classification schemes for lung carcinoma, including the WHO classification (2004) of tumors of the lung, pleura, thymus and heart,[1] and the International Association for Lung Cancer Study/American Thoracic Society/European Respiratory Society (IALCS/ATS/ERS) international multidisciplinary classification of lung adenocarcinoma.[2] Because the histologic classification of lung cancer continues to evolve constantly, we will use here a more simplified approach (Table 12.1). Although neuroendocrine carcinomas (NECAs) are acknowledged to be derived from neuroepithelial elements and, as such, belong in the family of epithelial neoplasms, they will be dealt with separately in another chapter owing to the highly specialized nature of their particular line of differentiation.[3,4]

The diagnosis of lung carcinoma, in particular for tumors that are not very well differentiated, can be fraught with difficulties in small biopsy samples. In small biopsy specimens, 10% to 30% of cases continue to be diagnosed generically as nonsmall cell lung carcinoma (NSCLC), not otherwise specified (NOS).[5] In clinical practice, diagnosis of NSCLC versus small cell carcinoma may be all that the physician submitting the biopsy sample is interested in. The latter approach was widely favored in the prepersonalized medicine era where patients were stratified for treatment based solely on this distinction. With the advent of targeted therapies, establishing a specific histopathologic diagnosis has gained increasing importance. Thus, great efforts are currently being expended

TABLE 12.1 Classification of Lung Epithelial Neoplasms

Bronchogenic carcinoma	Squamous cell carcinoma (SCC) – *Variants*: Small cell type/basaloid Polypoid endophytic Spindle cell (sarcomatoid) Clear cell Lymphoepithelioma-like Adenocarcinoma – *Variants*: Acinar Solid Papillary, micropapillary Fetal-type (monophasic pulmonary blastoma), bronchioloalveolar type (lepidic growth) Endometrioid-like Clear cell Mucinous (colloid) Signet-ring cell type Hepatoid Spindle cell (sarcomatoid) Large cell carcinoma – *Variants*: Sarcomatoid Anaplastic Pleomorphic Inflammatory Rhabdoid Clear cell Mixed Adenosquamous carcinoma Other
Neuroendocrine carcinoma (NECA)	Well-differentiated NECA (so-called carcinoid tumor) Moderately differentiated NECA (so-called atypical carcinoid) Poorly differentiated NECA – Small cell neuroendocrine carcinoma – Large cell neuroendocrine carcinoma – Mixed small/large cell neuroendocrine carcinoma

TABLE 12.1 (*Continued*)

Salivary gland type tumors	Mucoepidermoid carcinoma
	Adenoid cystic carcinoma
	Epimyoepithelial carcinoma
	Salivary gland-type mixed tumor
	Acinic cell carcinoma
	Oncocytoma
Biphasic neoplasms	Carcinosarcoma
	Biphasic pulmonary blastoma

for increasing the accuracy of histologic diagnosis and subclassification of lung tumors, particularly in small biopsy samples.[6] Some basic principles, however, need to be first acknowledged when dealing with limited biopsy sample material for the diagnosis of lung cancer: (1) The diagnosis rendered on a limited biopsy sample cannot accurately predict what the remainder of the tumor will look like or its exact cellular composition; variations in degrees of differentiation or tumors with mixed histology cannot be predicted from the findings in a small biopsy; (2) lung cancer, in particular NSCLC, is notorious for its cellular heterogeneity and a precise and definitive diagnosis may not be possible on a limited small biopsy sample; (3) poorly differentiated malignancies may be difficult to precisely categorize on small tissue samples, even with special techniques, and such cases may not be amenable to definitive classification; (4) tumors of mixed histogenesis containing combined elements (i.e., carcinosarcoma, biphasic pulmonary blastoma) may not show all of its components in a small biopsy and a higher grade or more aggressive component could be missed; (5) endoscopic and core biopsies may be prone to artifactual distortion that can be extensive and preclude a definitive diagnosis; (6) small biopsy samples may not be adequate for counting mitoses per 10 high-power fields, thus limiting the use of such criterion for precise subclassification of certain types of neoplasms based on current diagnostic standards (i.e., neuroendocrine tumors); and (7) certain ancillary diagnostic techniques may not be applicable on small biopsy samples (i.e., flow cytometry, electron microscopy), limiting further the ability for full workup in some cases.

Despite the above limitations, the discovery in recent years of the biologic and therapeutic importance of acquired genetic alterations in genes that encode pharmacologically targetable tyrosine kinases involved in growth factor receptor signaling (such as *EGFR* and *ALK*) has ushered in the era of molecular testing in lung cancer.[7] The most important abnormality currently being investigated in lung cancer is the presence of *EGFR* mutations in NSCLC. The majority of lung tumors with *EGFR* mutations are adenocarcinomas or mixed carcinomas with an adenocarcinoma component.[8] The evidence also suggests that *EGFR* mutations are infrequent in patients with SCC and have not been detected in small cell lung cancer either. The histologic distinction between squamous and adenocarcinoma, thus, becomes critical for the selection of cases for mutational analysis. Another important genetic alteration in lung cancer with therapeutic implications is the *EML4–ALK* fusion, which also predicts response to targeted therapy with tyrosine kinase inhibitors.[9] Although present in only about 5% of all NSCLC patients, targeted therapy for this gene has resulted in improved survival for patients with adenocarcinoma of the lung that harbors the translocation. Testing for *EGFR* and *ALK* is recommended for patients with NSCLC that show adenocarcinoma histology as well as for patients with large cell carcinoma and in small biopsies where the histologic type is difficult to classify. In the latter setting, use of a combination of immunohistochemical stains has been recommended to better define the histologic tumor type. Testing for these translocations, however, is not recommended for SCCs, small cell carcinoma, or neuroendocrine malignancies. Another molecular alteration that is of interest in this setting is the *KRAS* mutation, present in 25% to 35% of cases of lung adenocarcinoma and is used as a negative predictor of response to anti-EGFR therapy.[10] Finally, bevacizumab, an angiogenesis inhibitor, has been used for the treatment of advanced lung cancer but is contraindicated in patients with SCC owing to its association with pulmonary hemorrhage.[11] As additional targeted therapies and new potential molecular targets are developed in lung cancer, accurate distinction of the specific histologic subtypes in small endoscopic biopsies has become an issue of increasing relevance. For the time being, the impact of molecular targeting in lung cancer lies in the fact that detecting *EGFR* mutations is critical for predicting response to treatment with tyrosine kinase inhibitors in patients with advanced lung adenocarcinoma; that tumors with *EGFR* mutations have been associated with a more indolent behavior; that *EGFR* and *KRAS* are virtually exclusive events; and that cases that are negative for *EGFR* and *KRAS* mutations may have detectable fusion of *EML4–ALK*. Identifying morphologic features or immunohistochemical markers that may permit stratification of cases for molecular testing thus acquires increasing importance. Based on the above, it should be noted that the term "NSCLC" is bound to become increasingly less acceptable as a pathologic diagnosis or as a valid diagnostic category for the clinical management of lung cancer patients as we gain additional insights into the molecular mechanisms of lung cancer.

Several immunohistochemical panels have been proposed for the evaluation of small biopsies and for making the distinction between adenocarcinoma and SCC.[12–14] The search for the elusive optimal panel is made more difficult by the lack of strict specificity of most of the markers currently in use for either lines of differentiation or for their capability for distinguishing between a primary tumor of lung origin and a metastasis from an extrapulmonary carcinoma. Most studies, however, appear to recommend a mixture of p63 and CK5/6 as markers of squamous differentiation, and thyroid transcription factor-1 (TTF-1) and napsin A as adenocarcinoma markers. It is important to point out a few caveats: p63 has been shown to react with lung adenocarcinoma in a significant percentage of cases.[15] Another limitation of p63 is its strong expression in large cell lymphomas that can be confused morphologically for anaplastic or poorly differentiated NSCLC, a finding observed in approximately 50% of pulmonary lymphoma cases.[16] More recent studies, however, have shown that a p63 isoform—p40 (ΔNp63) shows much higher specificity and sensitivity for SCC and does not appear to react with adenocarcinoma cells and other tumors, thus representing a much better choice for immunohistochemical evaluation of squamous differentiation in lung cancer biopsies.[17] TTF-1—a transcription factor expressed in lung epithelial cells and thyroid follicular epithelium—has been acknowledged as a helpful and sensitive marker for the diagnosis of lung adenocarcinoma. However, its specificity is not restricted to primary lung adenocarcinoma, and a few studies have reported reactivity in SCCs.[18] Likewise, napsin A—an epithelial marker commonly expressed in up to 80% of lung adenocarcinomas—has also been claimed to be positive in up to 26% of lung SCC.[19] Caution, therefore, should be exercised in making purely "immunohistochemical" diagnoses based on the results of these stains in isolation of the morphologic and clinical context.

BRONCHOGENIC CARCINOMA

The term "bronchogenic carcinoma" is understood generically as any tumor that arises from the bronchial tree and its branches, including the terminal respiratory unit (alveolar ducts and alveoli) and epithelial cells located along the walls of the entire bronchial tree. Bronchogenic carcinoma represents the commonest form of lung cancer.

Squamous Cell Carcinoma

SCC is a malignant neoplasm that arises from bronchial epithelium and can show varying degrees of squamous differentiation. More than 90% of SCCs of the lung are associated with a history of cigarette smoking. The majority of pulmonary SCC arise from the mainstem bronchi or segmental bronchi and are readily accessible to biopsy on endoscopy. SCC is thus the most frequently diagnosed cancer in endobronchial biopsy material. SCC may also arise in the periphery of the lung and form an expansile nodule that can secondarily infiltrate the pleura and chest wall. Some tumors may be cavitated and show extensive central areas of necrosis. Occasionally the tumor can show an endobronchial polypoid, exophytic growth pattern; such tumors can display a papillary architecture. SCC is often associated with an in situ or high-grade dysplastic component. The dysplastic, in situ lesion, most often, is seen in continuity with normal respiratory epithelium and will display lack of maturation, nucleomegaly, cytologic atypia, and abnormal mitotic figures (Fig. 12.1); it may or may not show evidence of an endophytic or superficially invasive component. Occasionally the in situ component may extend into and replace the bronchial glands resembling

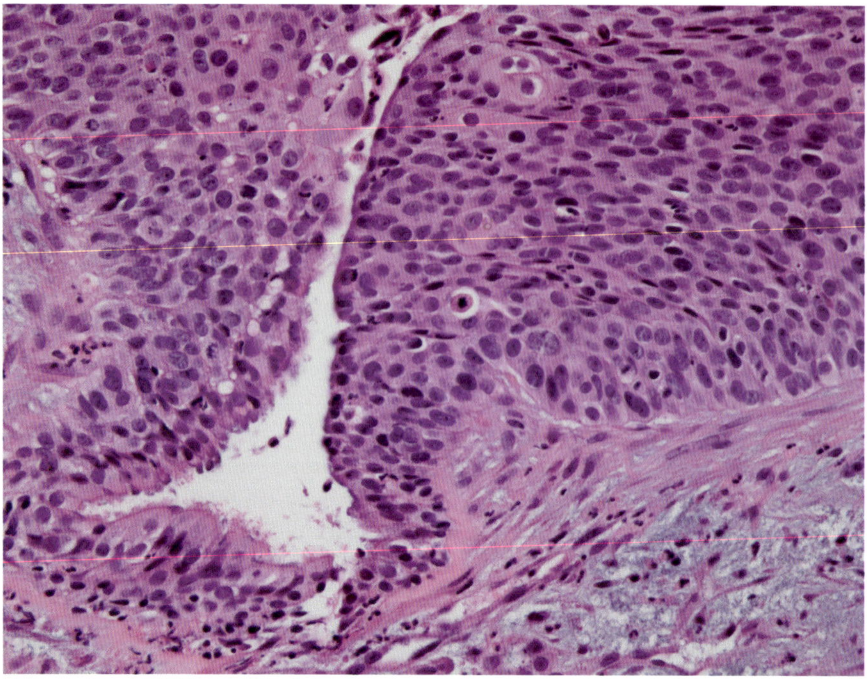

FIGURE 12.1 Endobronchial SCC in situ. There is full-thickness atypia with lack of maturation, nucleomegaly , and scattered mitoses in the in situ component. Notice a focus of residual normal respiratory mucosa showing tall ciliated columnar cells **(lower left)** in continuity with the in situ carcinoma.

invasive carcinoma. It may also be difficult to confirm the presence of an invasive component in a small endoscopic biopsy, thus requiring a disclaimer in the report that an invasive component cannot be ruled out. The presence of an in situ carcinoma component in any endoscopic biopsy sample from a patient with an abnormal lung imaging study will require strict clinicopathologic correlation. In clinically equivocal cases, it will most likely represent an indication for surgical excision as it invariably heralds the existence of an invasive component.

Histologically, SCC of the lung may be well, moderately, or poorly differentiated. The most distinctive features of well-differentiated squamous carcinoma are keratinization with keratin pearl formation and intercellular bridges. The tumor cells show enlarged nuclei and are surrounded by abundant eosinophilic cytoplasm displaying sharp cell borders (eFigs. 12.1 and 12.2). The nuclei will show increased chromatin and one or multiple nucleoli. Mitotic figures can be easily identified. The cells usually have a tendency to form small, cohesive groups that adopt a pavement-like architecture and are attached to each other by intercellular bridges. Foci of central keratinization with concentric islands of keratin "pearl" formation are frequently identified (Fig. 12.2). Moderately differentiated neoplasms show a tendency to display a less obvious pavement-like

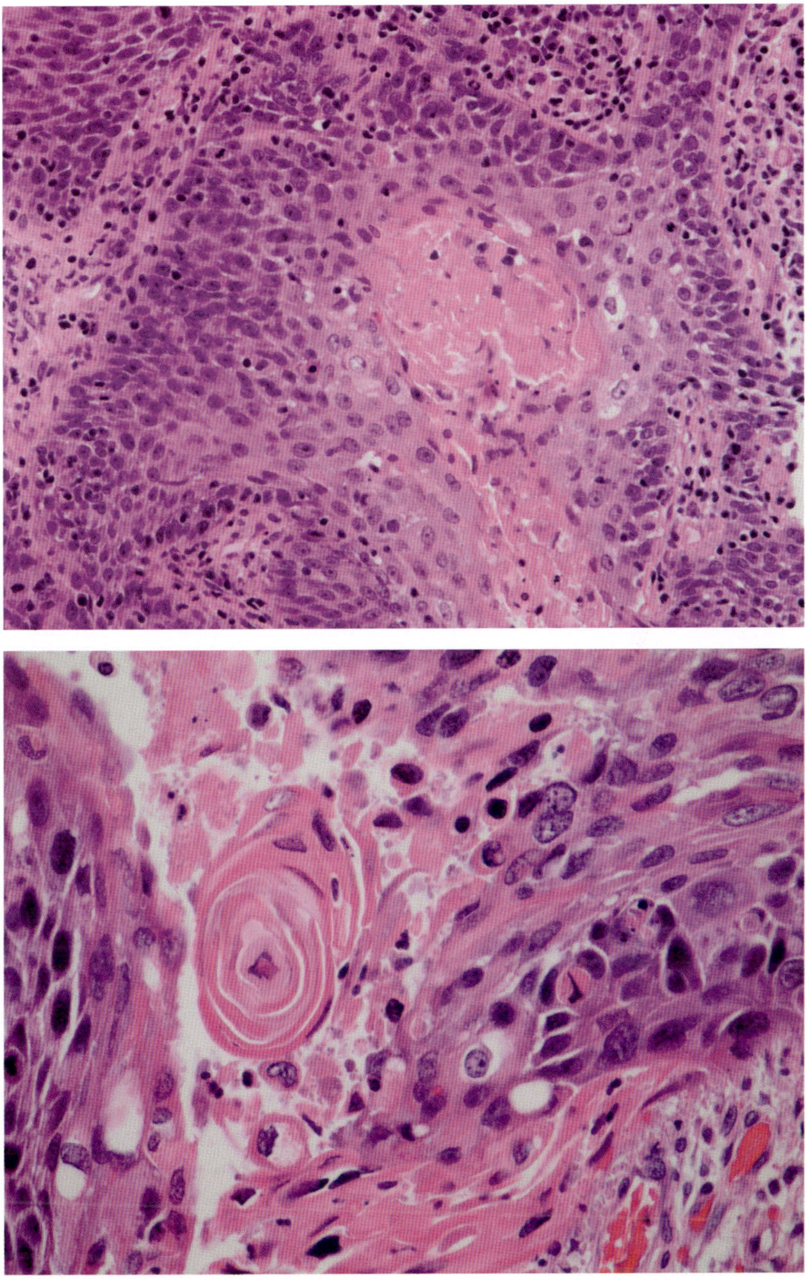

A

B

FIGURE 12.2 **A:** Well-differentiated SCC shows cohesive tumor cells with pavement-like architecture and central areas of keratinization. **B:** Higher magnification of well-differentiated SCC shows atypical tumor cells and a focus of keratin pearl formation.

architecture, with only occasional or no intercellular bridges, increased size of the nuclei with more prominent nucleoli, and foci of single-cell keratinization. Poorly differentiated tumors show a more advanced degree of loss of keratinization; the cells may adopt bizarre shapes with nucleomegaly and nucleolar prominence and abundant, often abnormal mitoses. Extensive tumor cell necrosis is often a prominent feature in these tumors (Fig. 12.3). Islands of poorly differentiated SCC will show a tendency to display central, comedo-like areas of necrosis with prominent peripheral palisading of the tumor cells (eFig. 12.3).

Unusual morphologic appearances in SCC of the lung include tumors displaying clear cell features with abundant, optically clear cytoplasm filled with glycogen; tumors with prominent spindling of the cells that can closely resemble a spindle cell sarcoma; and tumors comprising relatively small cells with scant cytoplasm that may resemble small cell NECA (the so-called small cell variant of poorly differentiated SCC; Fig. 12.4). Such cases may be extremely difficult to diagnose with confidence on small endoscopic biopsies unless more conventional, better-differentiated areas are present in the sample. Tumors with ample clear cytoplasm may be confused with metastases of clear cell carcinoma, such as metastatic renal cell carcinoma. Spindle (sarcomatoid) SCC may be confused with various spindle cell sarcomas, in particular monophasic synovial sarcoma, which can also express cytokeratin positivity. Molecular testing for the *SYT* fusion product of the x;18 translocation associated with synovial sarcoma may be of assistance in such instances for making that distinction. In cases of the small cell variant of SCC, absence of reactivity for chromogranin, synaptophysin, and CD56 coupled with nuclear positivity for p63 may be of aid in arriving at the correct diagnosis. A "basaloid" variant of NSCLC has also been described, that may show some morphologic overlap with several entities, including NECA and the small cell variant of SCC. We believe basaloid carcinoma corresponds to the same condition as the small cell variant of SCC; distinction from large cell NECA or moderately differentiated NECA (atypical carcinoid) can generally be achieved using immunohistochemical stains for neuroendocrine markers. Another unusual type of lung tumor is the lymphoepithelioma-like carcinoma of the lung, which essentially corresponds to a nonkeratinizing, poorly differentiated SCC containing a heavy lymphoplasmacytic cell infiltrate in the stroma. The tumors resemble poorly differentiated nasopharyngeal carcinomas and "lymphoepithelioma-like" carcinomas at other locations and are associated with an aggressive behavior. Some of these tumors have been found to be related to Epstein–Barr virus (EBV) infection and may contain EBV latent membrane protein. The cells in these tumors are large, round to oval, with vesicular nuclei and prominent, usually centrally placed nucleoli, and are surrounded by a scant rim of amphophilic cytoplasm with indistinct cell borders.

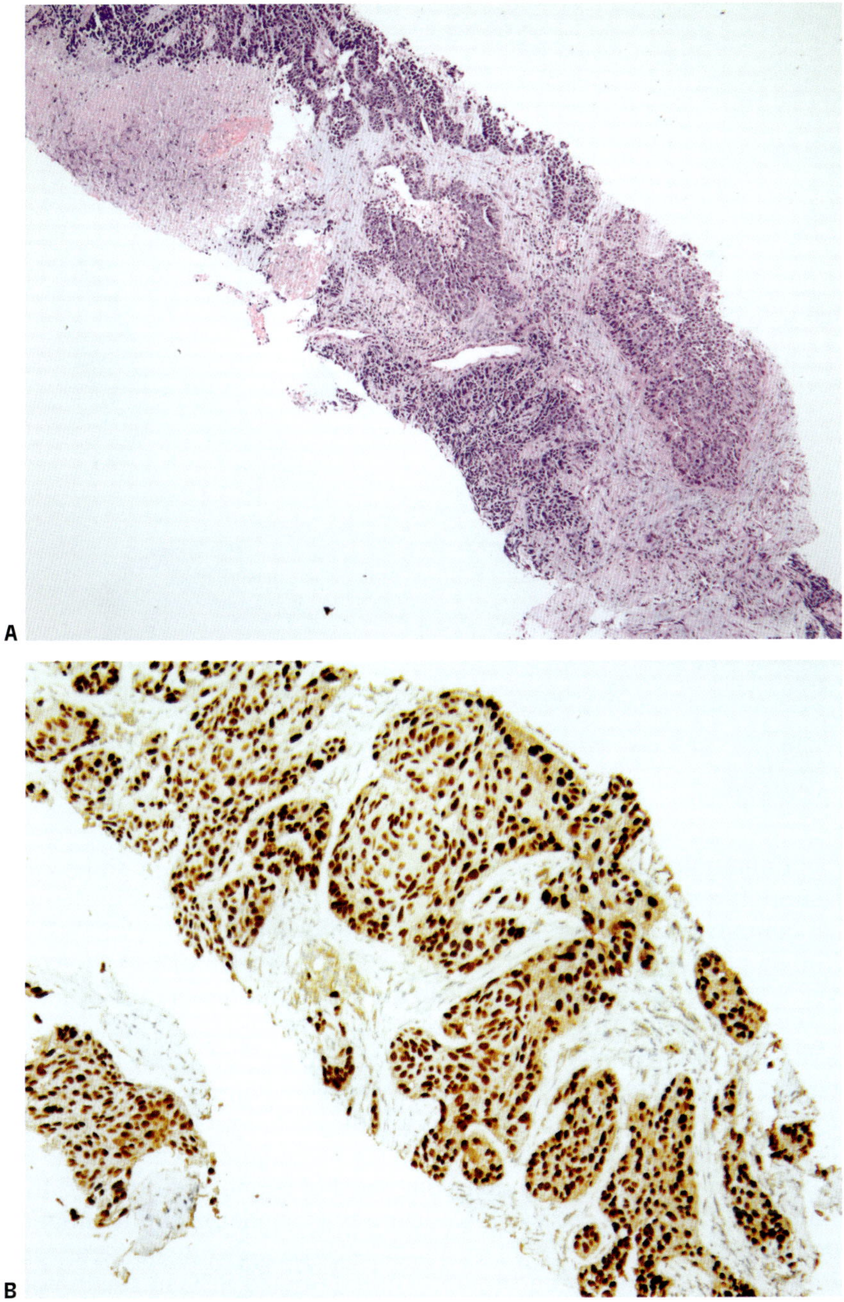

FIGURE 12.3 **A**: Core biopsy shows poorly differentiated SCC with clusters of large cells with pleomorphic and hyperchromatic nuclei and areas of necrosis. **B:** P63 stain in poorly differentiated SCC shows strong nuclear positivity in the tumor cells.

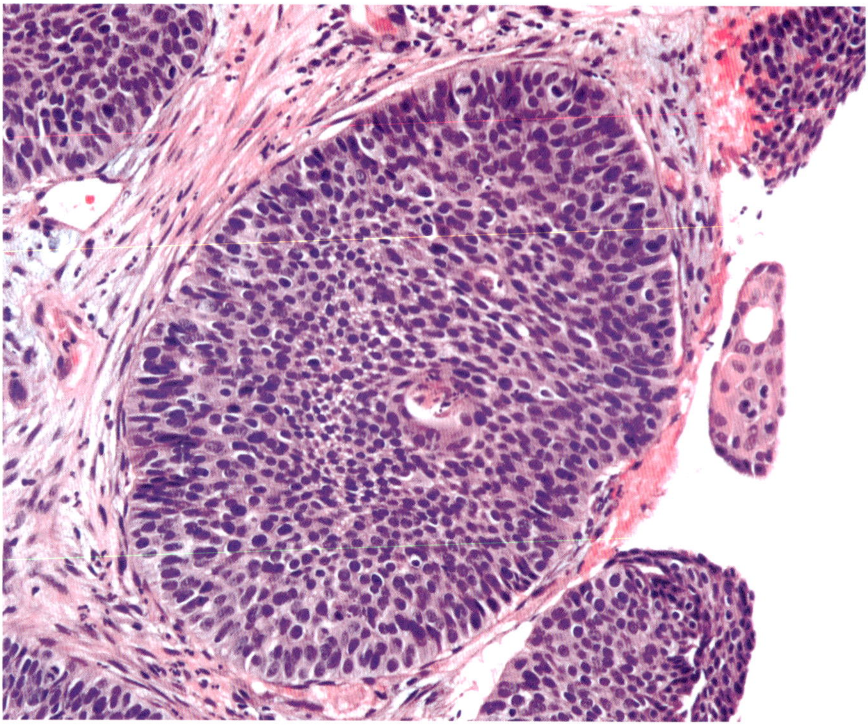

FIGURE 12.4 Small cell variant of SCC is characterized by the relatively smaller size of the tumor cells, which are monotonous, contain scant cytoplasm, and show striking peripheral palisading of nuclei.

Immunohistochemistry can be successfully applied in some cases to support a diagnosis of SCC on small endoscopic biopsies of the lung that contain poorly differentiated tumors. In general, CK5/6 and p63 are strongly positive in most SCCs (Fig. 12.5). Expression of p63, however, may be lost or significantly diminished in poorly differentiated examples of SCC, and some cases may express only low-molecular weight cytokeratins and vimentin. P40, an isoform of p63, may be more specific as a marker of squamous differentiation but may show diminished expression in poorly differentiated tumors, thus limiting its utility for distinguishing poorly differentiated SCC from anaplastic or large cell carcinoma. P63 expression can also occur in up to one-third of adenocarcinomas[20]; thus, in a tumor that lacks morphologic features of squamous differentiation, coexpression of p63 and TTF-1 is more likely to indicate an adenocarcinoma. Exact categorization of poorly differentiated SCC in small biopsy samples may not always be feasible, and a noncommittal diagnosis of "poorly differentiated, nonsmall cell carcinoma" may be more appropriate in such instances than attempting to categorize the tumor based on equivocal or new potentially misleading results of immunohistochemistry. It has been stated that excluding squamous differentiation in poorly

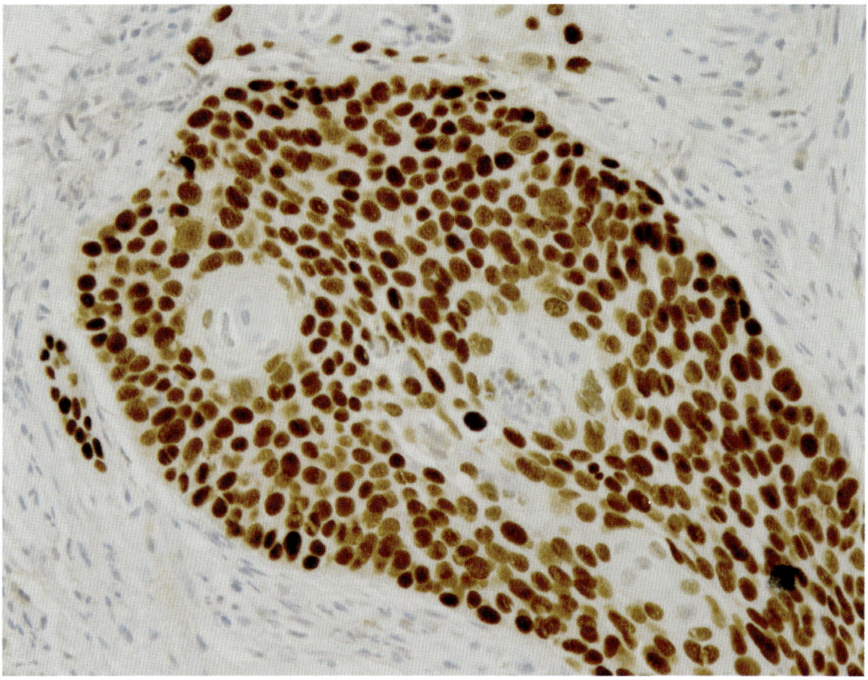

FIGURE 12.5 A small island of SCC of the lung shows strong nuclear staining for p63.

differentiated tumors is of importance to determine eligibility of patients for treatment with pemetrexed (because of increased efficacy)[21] or bevacizumab (because of increased toxicity).[22] Additional studies are needed, however, to determine whether this also applies to poorly differentiated tumors or only to those that can be readily identified as squamous by routine histology alone.

Adenocarcinoma

Adenocarcinoma of the lung represents a malignant glandular proliferation that most commonly originates in the peripheral airways. Lung adenocarcinoma is the most common form of epithelial malignancy of this organ. Its peripheral location makes this tumor less likely to be diagnosed through endoscopic biopsy. Nonetheless, large tumors may invade extensively and be present in the vicinity of large airways where they will be accessible to endoscopic biopsies. Lung adenocarcinoma is subclassified by the WHO[1] into four histologic subtypes: acinar, papillary, solid with mucin, and mixed. It has been increasingly acknowledged that lung adenocarcinoma is characterized by marked morphologic heterogeneity, and that a large proportion of these tumors (>90%) display a mixed pattern (Fig. 12.6).[2,23,24] Because of perceived shortcomings in the 2004 WHO histologic classification of lung adenocarcinoma, a new proposal for the classification of lung adenocarcinoma has been presented by the IASLC/ATS/ERS.[2] The proposal

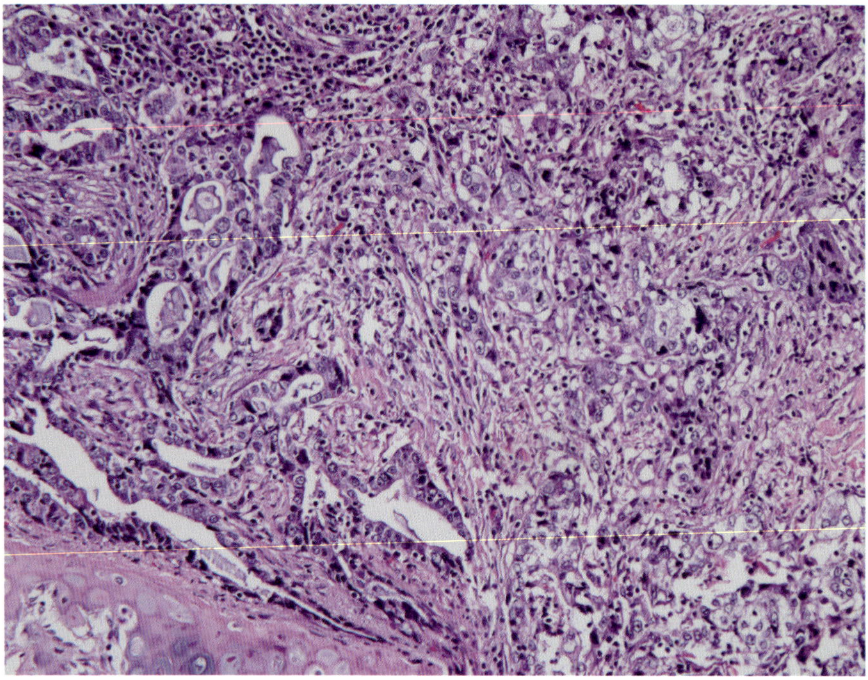

FIGURE 12.6 Transbronchial biopsy showing mixed adenocarcinoma, with areas containing well- to moderately differentiated adenocarcinoma with acinar pattern **(left)** and areas containing a more poorly differentiated, solid adenocarcinoma pattern **(right)**.

includes changes to the reporting and classification of resected lung cancer specimens as well as for small biopsy/cytology specimens (Table 12.2).

The need for this proposal stemmed in part from difficulties encountered with the diagnostic criteria and definition of bronchioloalveolar carcinoma as proposed in the 2004 WHO classification, which permitted only accurate classification of this tumor type in resected specimens, thus, essentially, eliminating this diagnostic option in small biopsy samples or cytology specimens, and because of the recognition of additional histologic variants of lung adenocarcinoma, such as the micropapillary type, which had not been included in the 2004 WHO schema.[2] The 2004 WHO definition of bronchioloalveolar carcinoma was that of a tumor showing growth of neoplastic cells along preexisting alveolar structures (lepidic growth pattern) without evidence of stromal, vascular, or pleural invasion.[1] The latter features can be properly evaluated only in completely resected specimens. Moreover, many mixed type adenocarcinomas will often show a lepidic growth pattern in part of the tumor, whereas other areas may harbor conventional adenocarcinoma with acinar, papillary, or solid features. It is also important to point out that metastases to the lung from adenocarcinoma from other organs can also display a prominent bronchioloalveolar growth pattern. Equally important, atypical adenomatous hyperplasia, a premalignant lesion that is histologically indistinguishable from bronchioloalveolar carcinoma, can be separated from the latter based only on its size (<0.5 cm), a feature that cannot be assessed in a small biopsy sample. The newly proposed IASLC/ATS/ESP classification of lung adenocarcinoma has essentially

TABLE 12.2 IASLC/ATS/ERS Proposal for the Classification of Lung Adenocarcinoma (2011)

Classification of Lung Adenocarcinoma in Resection Specimens	Classification of Lung Adenocarcinoma in Small Biopsy/ Cytology Specimens
Preinvasive lesions: Atypical adenomatous hyperplasia Adenocarcinoma in situ (<3 cm; formerly BAC) Mucinous Nonmucinous Mixed	Morphologic adenocarcinoma patterns clearly present: Adenocarcinoma: describe identifiable patterns present (including micropapillary pattern not included in 2004 WHO). Adenocarcinoma with lepidic pattern (if pure, add note that invasive component cannot be excluded) Mucinous adenocarcinoma Adenocarcinoma with fetal pattern Adenocarcinoma with colloid pattern Adenocarcinoma with (describe pattern) and signet-ring features Adenocarcinoma with (describe pattern) and clear cell features
Minimally invasive carcinoma (<3 cm, lepidic predominant tumor with <5 mm invasion) Mucinous Nonmucinous Mixed Invasive adenocarcinoma Lepidic predominant (formerly nonmucinous BAC with >5 mm invasion) Acinar predominant Papillary predominant Micropapillary predominant Solid predominant with mucin production	Morphologic adenocarcinoma patterns not present but supported by special stains: Nonsmall cell carcinoma, favor adenocarcinoma

(Continued)

TABLE 12.2 *(Continued)*

Variants of invasive adenocarcinoma
Invasive mucinous adenocarcinoma (formerly mucinous BAC)
Colloid
Fetal
Enteric

BAC, bronchioloalveolar carcinoma.

Adapted from Travis WD, Brambilla E, Noguchi M, et al. International Association for the Study of Lung Cancer/American Thoracic Society/European Respiratory Society international multidisciplinary classification of lung adenocarcinoma. *J Thorac Oncol.* 2011;6:244–285, with permission.

eliminated the category of bronchioloalveolar carcinoma, and introduced the concept of "adenocarcinoma in situ" and "minimally invasive adenocarcinoma."[2] Adenocarcinoma in situ is defined as a well-differentiated tumor with a bronchioloalveolar growth pattern that is less than 3 cm in greatest diameter and does not show evidence of invasion. Minimally invasive adenocarcinoma is defined as a tumor with bronchioloalveolar growth pattern that measures less than 3 cm and shows areas of invasion that are less than 5 mm. Because neither of these features can be demonstrated in small endoscopic biopsies, the diagnosis of "in situ adenocarcinoma" or "minimally invasive adenocarcinoma" cannot be rendered on endoscopic biopsy material. For these reasons, the IASLC/ATS/ESP panel recommended that the interpretation of small biopsies harboring adenocarcinoma be reported as (1) "adenocarcinoma," followed by the description of the specific growth patterns identified, (2) "adenocarcinoma with lepidic growth pattern admixed with other growth pattern," and (3) "adenocarcinoma with pure lepidic growth pattern," in which case a disclaimer to the effect that an invasive component cannot be excluded should be appended (Fig. 12.7).[2] It is worth emphasizing that the diagnosis of "bronchioloalveolar cell carcinoma" is no longer a valid diagnostic category in endoscopic biopsy material, and the term should no longer be used when interpreting endoscopic lung biopsies. It is, however, of importance to state whether a bronchioloalveolar growth *pattern* (i.e., lepidic growth along the alveolar septae) is present, as recommended by the IASLC/ATS/ESP because such tumors are associated with an increased probability of favorable response to *EGFR*-targeted tyrosine kinase inhibitor therapy (eFigs. 12.4 and 12.5).

In clinical practice, identification of adenocarcinoma on a biopsy sample is not usually difficult, except when dealing with poorly differentiated tumors or adenocarcinoma with solid pattern, or when the biopsy is

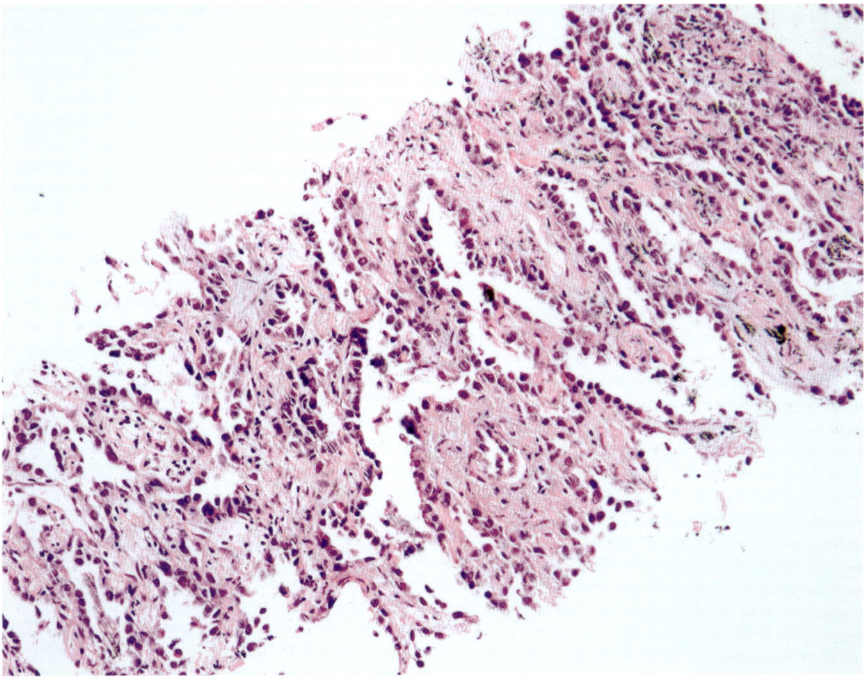

FIGURE 12.7 Percutaneous core biopsy of pulmonary adenocarcinoma with lepidic growth pattern (bronchioloalveolar pattern). Notice growth of atypical cells lining alveolar spaces. In the past these biopsies were diagnosed as "bronchioloalveolar carcinoma." Current recommendations are to diagnose "adenocarcinoma with lepidic pattern," with a comment that an invasive component cannot be excluded from this biopsy.

inadequate and does not contain sufficient viable tumor. More problematic is making a distinction between a primary adenocarcinoma of the lung and a metastasis to the lung from another organ. Metastases to the lung from adenocarcinomas originating from other organs are a frequent occurrence. Although most metastatic adenocarcinomas to the lung present as multiple lesions with a history of a primary tumor elsewhere, solitary metastases can be observed in up to 10% of cases.[3,4] Furthermore, an appropriate clinical history may have not been provided at the time of histologic examination that would allow the pathologist to properly identify the tumor as primary versus metastatic. Clinical correlation is therefore an indispensable step when evaluating a small lung biopsy containing adenocarcinoma. When in doubt, immunohistochemical stains may be of value. Most lung adenocarcinomas (approximately 80%) express nuclear positivity for TTF-1 and cytoplasmic reactivity for napsin A (Fig. 12.8).[13] Although these markers display high sensitivity for the diagnosis of pulmonary adenocarcinoma, they lack specificity and may also be expressed in other types of tumors capable of metastasizing to the lung, including renal cell carcinoma and thyroid papillary carcinoma.[25,26] Napsin A, a proteinase involved in the maturation of surfactant protein B, has paradoxically been found to be

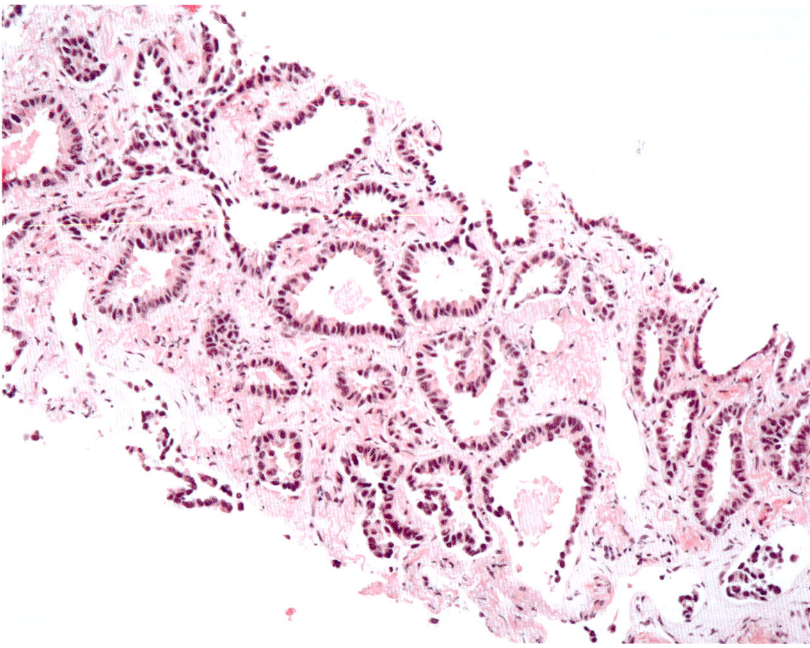

A

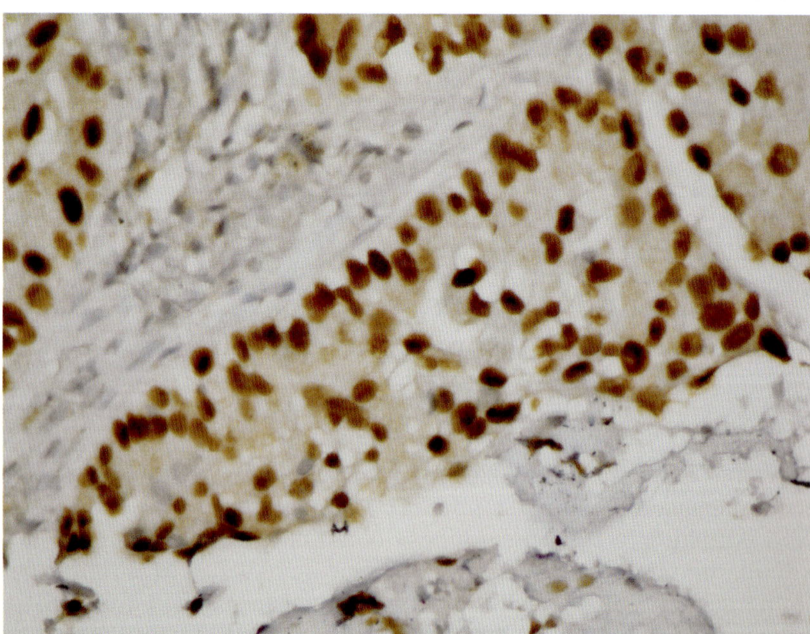

B

FIGURE 12.8 **A:** Endoscopic biopsy of well-differentiated pulmonary adenocarcinoma shows regular, evenly distributed glands separated by a desmoplastic stroma. **B:** Immunohistochemical staining shows strong nuclear positivity for TTF-1 in the tumor cells.

strongly expressed in a significant number of cases of renal cell carcinoma of both papillary and clear cell types.[25] TTF-1, a transcription factor expressed in thyroid and lung epithelial cells, on the other hand, has been consistently absent in renal cell carcinomas. TTF-1, however, is not entirely specific for lung adenocarcinoma and is strongly expressed in most types of thyroid cancer, and has shown variable expression in a number of other tumors, such as breast carcinoma,[27] colorectal adenocarcinoma,[28] and endometrial and endocervical adenocarcinomas.[29] For this reason, it has been postulated that double labeling of napsin A and TTF-1 can increase the specificity for the diagnosis of lung adenocarcinoma, which has led to the proposal that the combination of both stains should be utilized when evaluating lung biopsies of adenocarcinoma to increase the yield for an accurate diagnosis.[26] It should also be kept in mind that results of immunostaining for TTF-1 in adenocarcinoma with bronchioloalveolar pattern of the lung may yield different results depending on its subtype. One study found that more than 90% of nonmucinous lung adenocarcinomas of bronchioloalveolar type were positive for TTF-1, whereas only 20% of cases of the mucinous variant showed weak and focal positivity.[30] TTF-1 may, therefore, not be a reliable or sensitive marker for evaluating lung biopsies of adenocarcinoma with mucinous features. Conventional histochemical stains for mucin, in particular mucicarmine, also play a role in the diagnosis of adenocarcinoma, particularly of the solid type or in poorly differentiated cases. Care must be taken, however, not to overinterpret focal positive staining for mucin in poorly differentiated tumors because SCCs can also harbor occasional foci of aberrant mucin-secreting cells as an expression of tumor heterogeneity.

Once a diagnosis of primary lung adenocarcinoma has been established, it may also be of importance to specify the degree of differentiation, cytologic grade of the tumor, and any other specific morphologic features pertinent for the prognosis or treatment of the patient. Well-differentiated adenocarcinoma is characterized by well-formed glands with mild-to-moderate cytologic atypia that may or may not be accompanied by a prominent desmoplastic stromal response. Moderately differentiated adenocarcinoma is characterized by imperfectly formed glands, usually displaying a more marked degree of cytologic atypia and often containing small or imperfectly formed lumens. Poorly differentiated adenocarcinoma is characterized by solid clusters of tumor cells with very minimal gland formation, often growing in sheets without readily identifiable lumens and displaying marked cytologic atypia (Fig. 12.9A) (eFigs. 12.6 and 12.7). These tumors overlap with the growth pattern described as solid adenocarcinoma with mucin in the WHO classification, which display scattered mucinous cells on higher magnification. The latter type must be distinguished from large cell carcinoma of the lung, and the diagnosis can be confirmed using mucicarmine or other histochemical stains for mucin (Fig. 12.9B). Other unusual patterns of growth that are less frequently observed in primary lung adenocarcinoma include papillary, micropapillary,

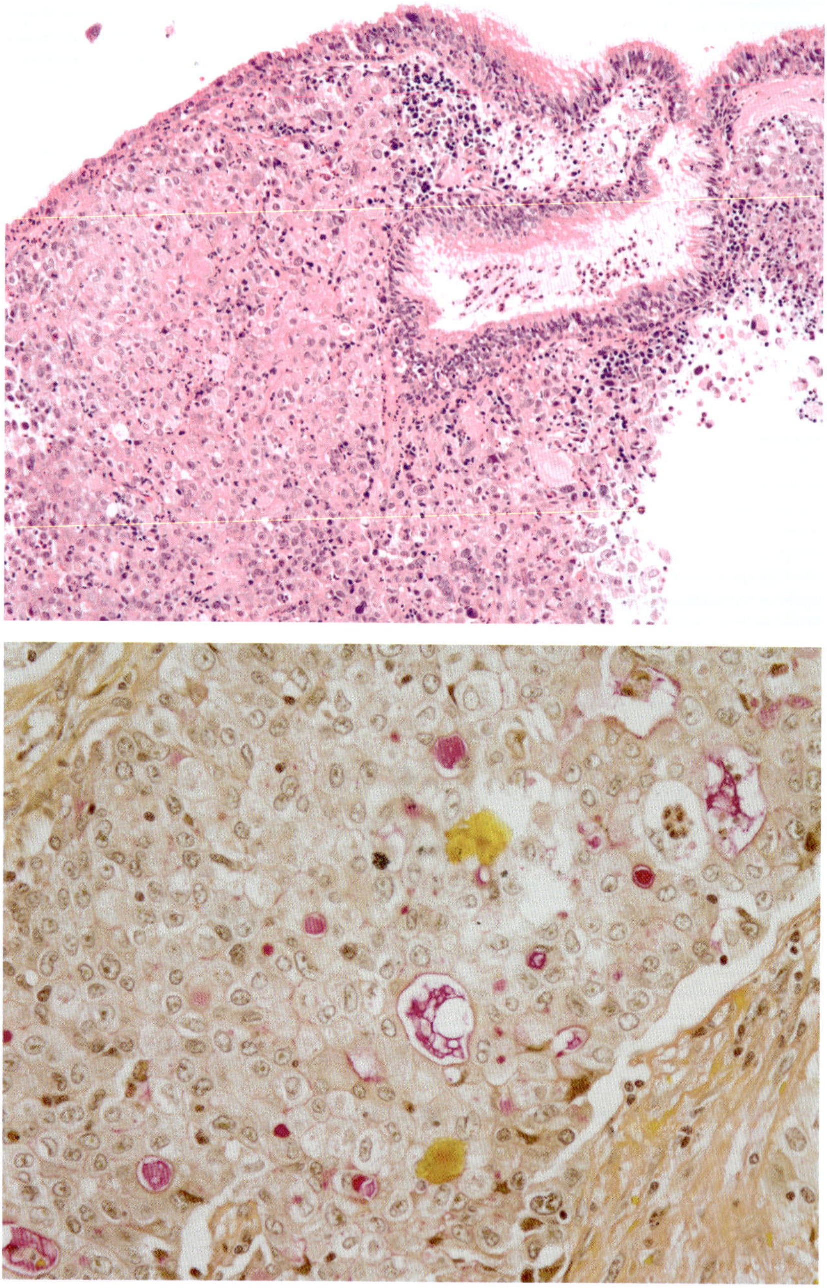

FIGURE 12.9 **A:** Endoscopic biopsy of the lung shows a solid sheet of tumor cells replacing the submucosa without any gland formation. **B:** Mucicarmine stains highlight scattered single cells containing intracellular mucin, establishing a diagnosis of adenocarcinoma, solid pattern with mucin. An arbitrary requirement of five or more mucin positive cells per high-power field has been set by the WHO to establish this diagnosis.

cribriform, signet-ring cell, mucinous ("colloid"), clear cell, fetal type (monophasic pulmonary blastoma), endometrioid-like, and hepatoid. The current recommendation by the IASLC/ATS/ERS[2] for small biopsy sample reporting is that when an adenocarcinoma pattern is identified, any specific or unusual pattern of growth observed be also recorded in the diagnosis. *Papillary adenocarcinoma* of the lung is characterized by a complex proliferation of papillary structures with secondary and tertiary branches that contain well-developed fibrovascular cores (Fig. 12.10). The cytology in such tumors is usually high grade, with frequent mitotic figures and foci of necrosis. In small biopsies the tumors need to be distinguished from metastases from papillary thyroid carcinoma; stains for napsin A or PE-10 (surfactant protein) and thyroglobulin may be of help in this setting as TTF-1 will be positive in both. Occasionally, pulmonary adenocarcinoma with lepidic growth pattern may display prominent intranuclear cytoplasmic inclusions resembling metastases from the follicular variant of papillary thyroid carcinoma (Fig. 12.11A). Stains for CK7/TTF-1 will also be of no assistance in such instances as both lung and thyroid adenocarcinomas will be positive for these markers; use of thyroglobulin or a surfactant protein-associated marker will aid in the distinction between the two (Fig. 12.11B). The *micropapillary* variant of pulmonary adenocarcinoma is a more recently described type of tumor characterized by small, abortive

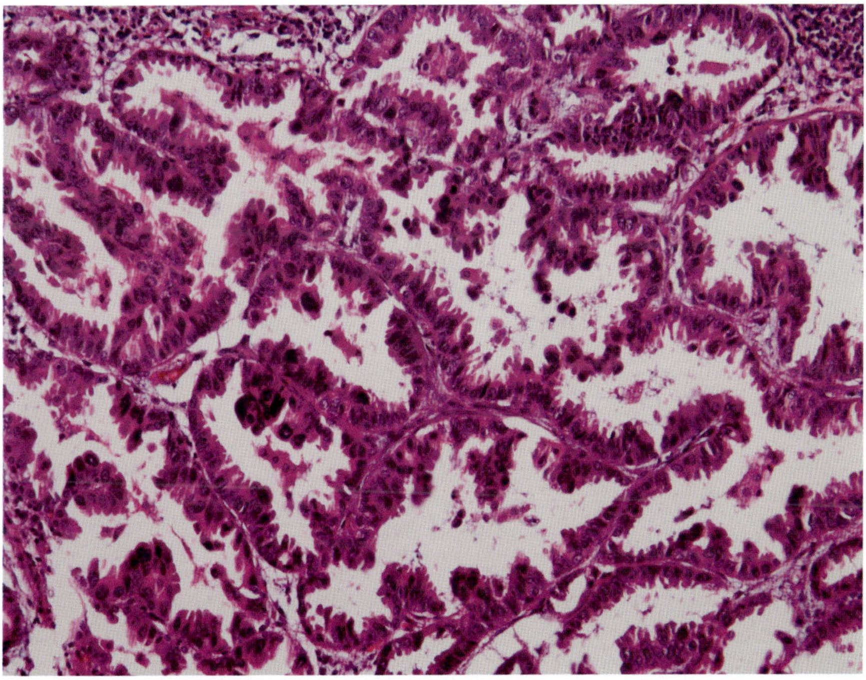

FIGURE 12.10 Papillary carcinoma of the lung shows complex branching of papillary structures lined by cells with marked cytologic atypia.

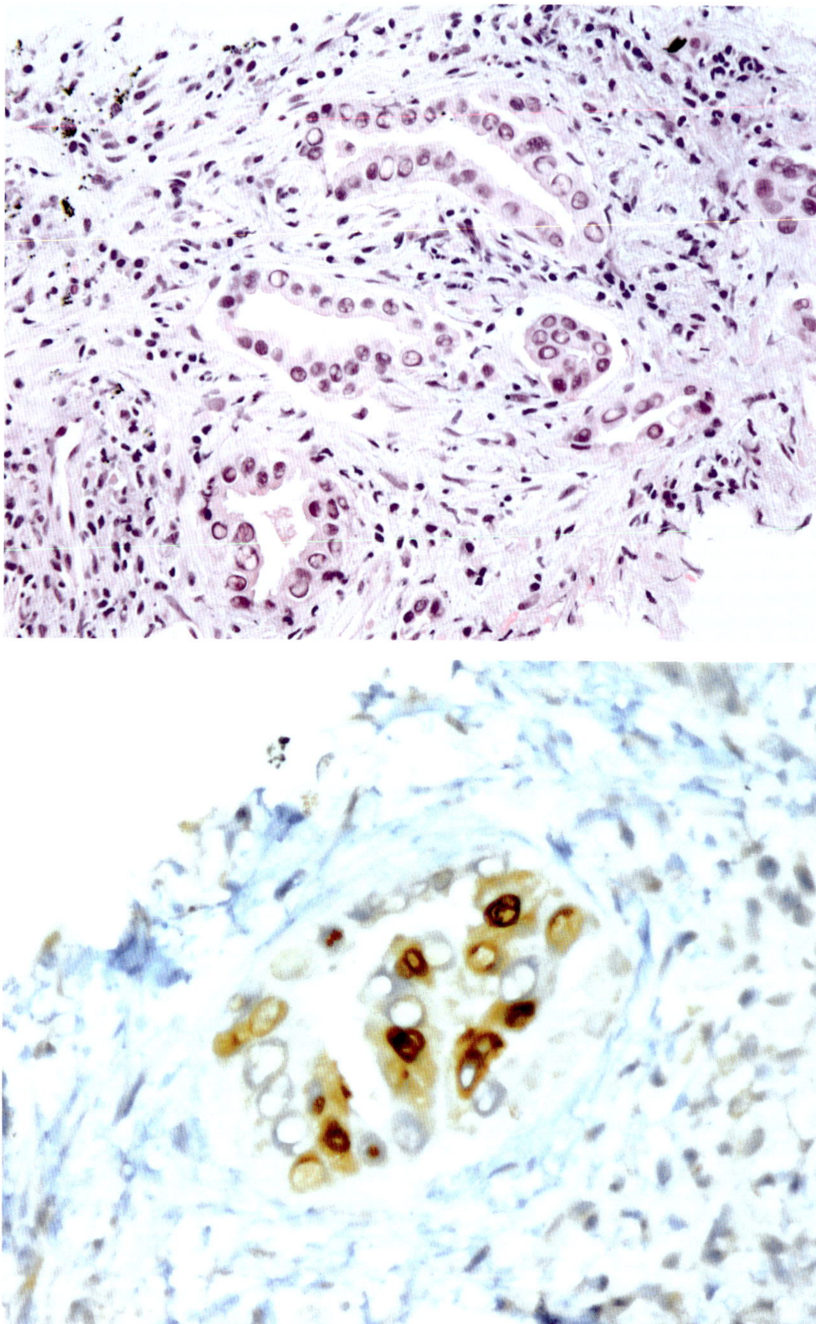

A

B

FIGURE 12.11 **A:** Transbronchial biopsy shows well-differentiated adenocarcinoma displaying prominent intranuclear cytoplasmic inclusions mimicking metastatic papillary thyroid carcinoma of follicular variant. **B:** Immunohistochemical stain for napsin A shows strong cytoplasmic reactivity in the tumor cells, indicating a primary lung origin.

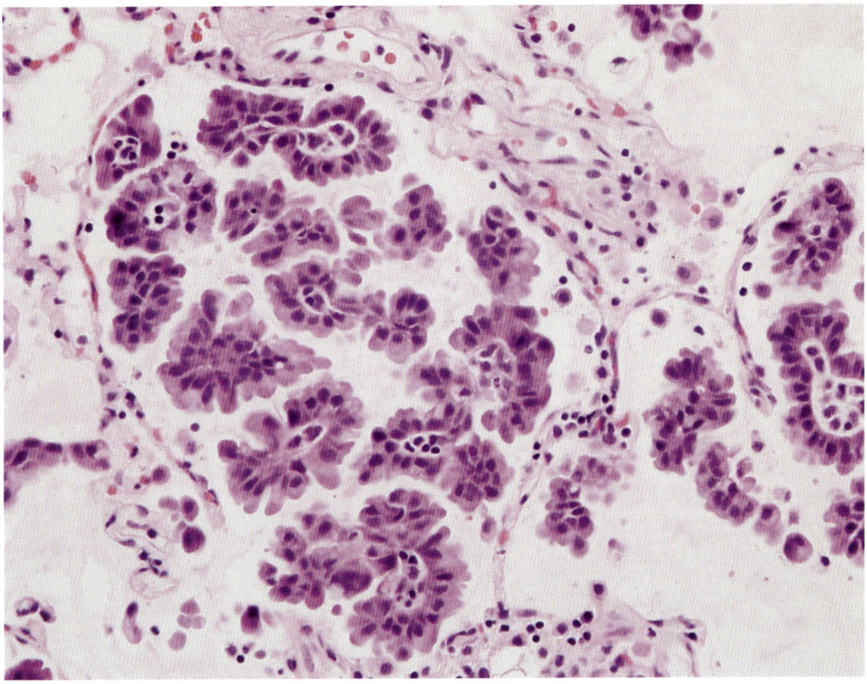

FIGURE 12.12 Micropapillary carcinoma of the lung is characterized by small papillary structures floating within the alveolar lumen. The cells lining the papillae have a hobnail appearance.

papillae devoid of fibrovascular cores that appear to be lying within an empty space caused by retraction artifact simulating lymphatics plugged by tumor or within the air sacs (Fig. 12.12).[31] The tumors are a highly aggressive variant of lung adenocarcinoma associated with a higher incidence of regional lymph node and distant metastases. They need to be differentiated from metastases of breast micropapillary adenocarcinoma and from metastases from other papillary tumors, such as endometrial and ovarian serous carcinoma. *Cribriform adenocarcinoma* of the lung is an unusual variant characterized by glandular structures with regular, punched-out luminal spaces that resemble in situ ductal carcinoma of the breast or high-grade cribriform adenocarcinoma of the prostate (Fig. 12.13). The cribriform pattern has been commonly observed in primary lung adenocarcinoma of enteric type (or with enteric differentiation) but may also be seen in tumors that more closely resemble metastases from the breast, prostate, uterus, ovaries, and salivary glands.[32] Although the cribriform architecture most often suggests the possibility of a metastasis, primary cribriform adenocarcinomas of the lung are strongly positive for CK7 and TTF-1 and will be negative for other specific differentiation markers. *Colloid adenocarcinoma* of the lung is a tumor characterized by pools of extracellular mucin containing small clusters or single mucin-secreting tumor cells floating in

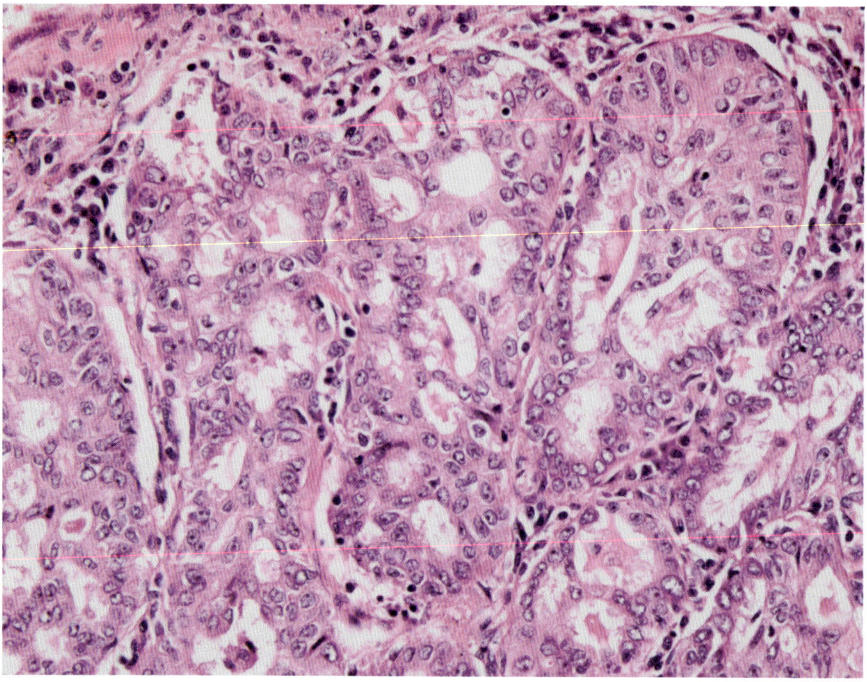

FIGURE 12.13 Cribriform adenocarcinoma of the lung is characterized by a glandular proliferation containing regular, evenly spaced punched-out lumens; these tumors can resemble metastases of breast or prostate carcinoma. The tumors are characterized by strong CK7/TTF-1 positivity and are negative for breast or prostate-associated markers.

the mucin.[33] The tumor cells are usually of goblet cell type but may be simple mucin-secreting cells. These tumors can often undergo cystic changes, in which case they are designated as mucinous cystadenocarcinoma. They can be identified in endoscopic biopsies by the presence of single atypical cells or small clusters of cells floating in pools of mucin (Fig. 12.14). The tumors are most often TTF-1/CK7+ but may also show a TTF-1/CK7-, CDX2/CK20+ immunophenotype. It may be very difficult to distinguish the latter cases from metastases from a colorectal or other primary types; clinicopathologic correlation is always necessary for establishing the correct diagnosis. It is important to distinguish colloid carcinoma from mucinous carcinoma displaying a bronchioloalveolar (lepidic) growth pattern (Fig. 12.15). The latter have been reclassified, depending on their size and invasive properties, into mucinous adenocarcinoma in situ, minimally invasive mucinous adenocarcinoma, or invasive mucinous adenocarcinoma (see Table 12.2).[2] These distinctions, however, cannot be made on small endoscopic biopsies; a generic diagnosis of mucinous adenocarcinoma with bronchioloalveolar pattern should be rendered on small biopsy samples with a note indicating that the findings need to be correlated with the imaging studies and that an invasive component cannot be ruled out. *Signet-ring cell adenocarcinoma* of lung is another rare variant that is characterized by the presence of signet-ring cells; these may be only

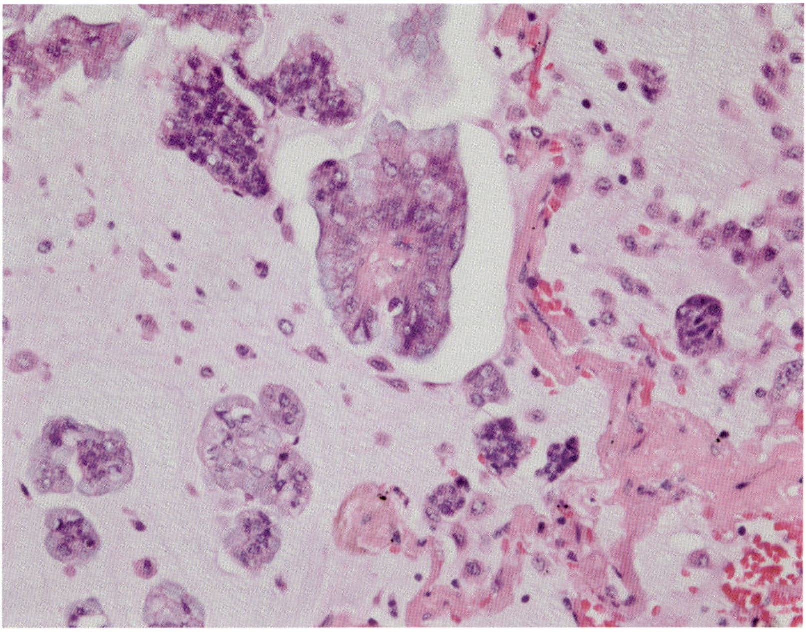

FIGURE 12.14 Colloid carcinoma of the lung showing clusters of mucinous epithelium as well as single atypical cells floating in mucin within the distended alveolar spaces.

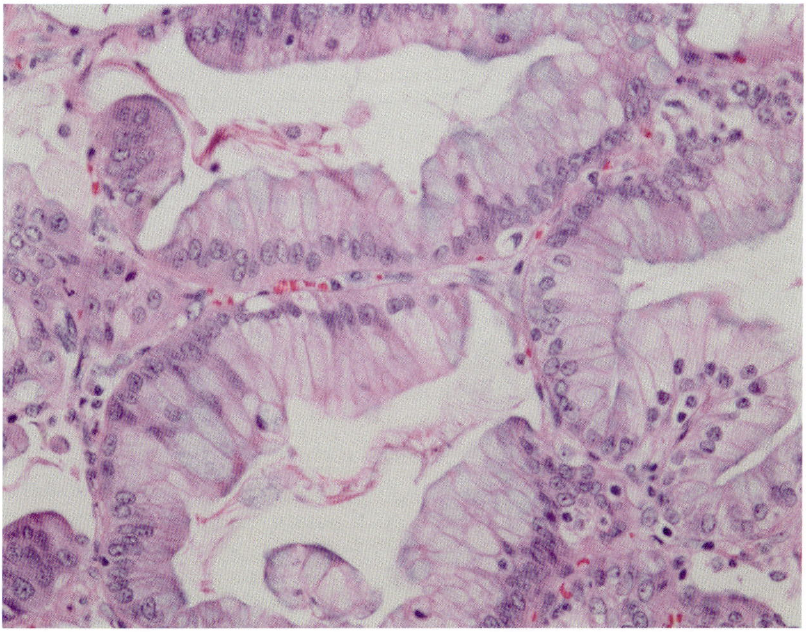

FIGURE 12.15 Mucinous carcinoma with lepidic growth pattern shows replacement of the lining of the alveoli by tall columnar, mucin-secreting cells admixed with occasional goblet cells. Tumors with these features were classified in the past as "bronchioloalveolar carcinoma, mucinous type."

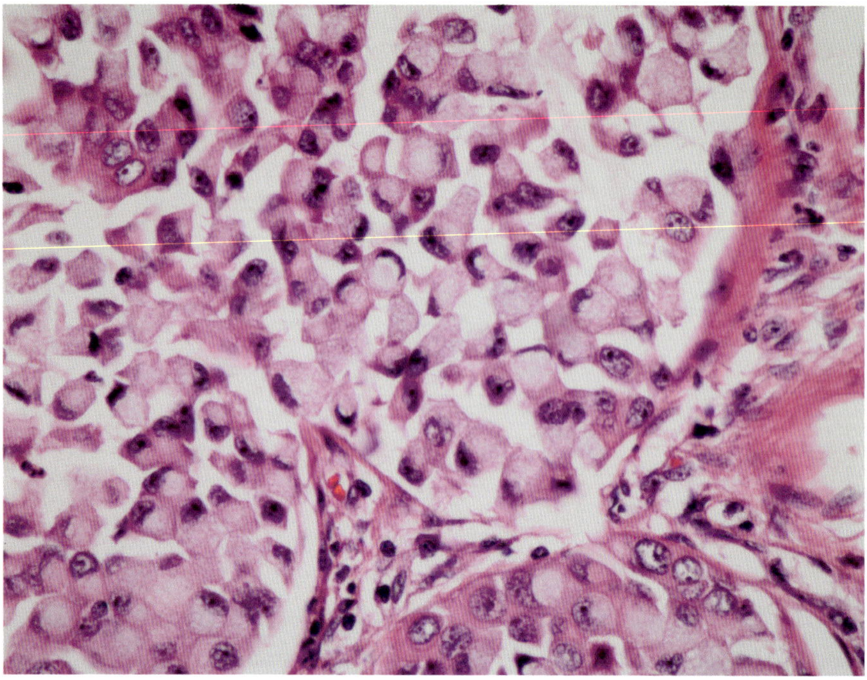

FIGURE 12.16 Signet-ring cell adenocarcinoma of the lung is characterized by cells displaying abundant intracytoplasmic mucin displacing the nuclei toward the periphery.

focally identified and admixed with other growth patterns (Fig. 12.16). The tumor cells are negative for CK20 and strongly positive for TTF-1, an important feature that distinguishes them from metastatic signet-ring cell adenocarcinoma from the gastrointestinal tract.[34] A *secretory endometrioid-like adenocarcinoma* of the lung has also been described by Steinhauer et al.[35] which is characterized by complex glandular structures that are lined by columnar cells with clear cytoplasm resembling secretory endometrium. The tumor cells are positive for CK7 and TTF-1 but do not stain with CK20, WT1, chromogranin, and estrogen and progesterone receptors, helping to facilitate the distinction between a metastasis from the uterus, ovary, or from the fetal-type adenocarcinoma (monophasic pulmonary blastoma), which it may closely resemble. The *fetal-type adenocarcinoma* of the lung is a rare tumor, regarded by some as a monophasic variant of pulmonary blastoma characterized by glandular structures with a striking cribriform appearance that are lined by columnar cells containing abundant clear vacuoles in the cytoplasm and basally oriented nuclei resembling fetal lung tubules (Fig. 12.17). A common finding is the presence of squamoid "morules" at the base of the glands. The tumor cells contain abundant diastase-resistant periodic acid–Schiff (PAS) material in the cytoplasm and are positive for TTF-1 and CK7. A distinctive feature is reactivity for chromogranin and for ß-catenin in both nuclear and

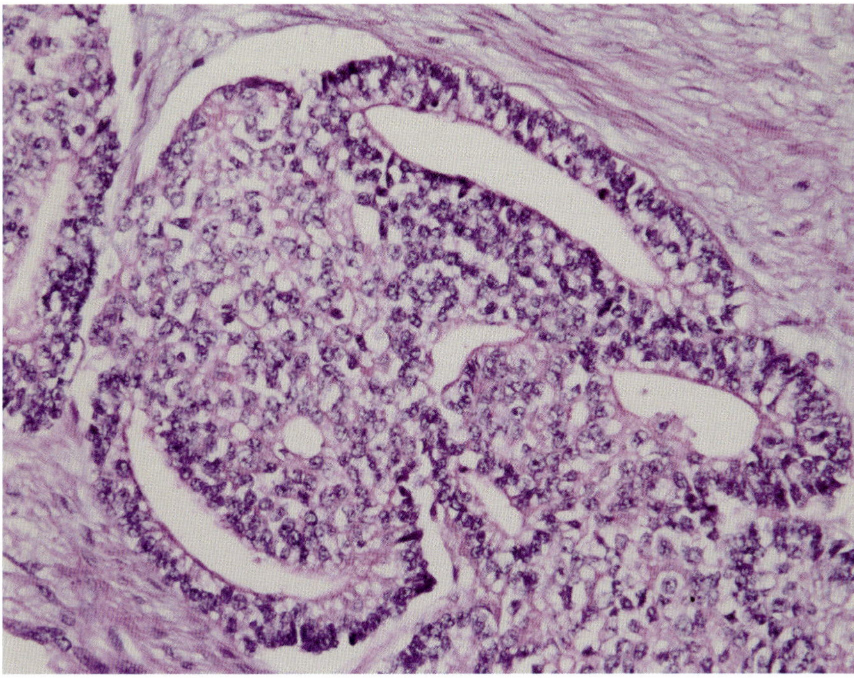

FIGURE 12.17 Fetal-type adenocarcinoma is characterized by glandular structures with a cribriform architecture that are lined by columnar cells with clear cytoplasmic vacuoles and basally oriented nuclei that resemble fetal lung. The glandular structures usually contain a solid proliferation of squamoid cells located at the base of the glands ("morules").

cytoplasmic distribution within cell clusters in the morular structures.[36] The cribriform architecture may cause confusion with cribriform adenocarcinoma of the lung, a tumor with a more aggressive behavior. *Hepatoid adenocarcinoma* of the lung is a rare variant characterized by sheets of monotonous round to polygonal tumor cells with abundant eosinophilic cytoplasm admixed with scattered small empty vacuoles resembling hepatic parenchyma. The tumor cells show cytoplasmic positivity for α-fetoprotein but are often negative for the Hepar-1 antibody.[37] They need to be distinguished from metastases of hepatocellular carcinoma to the lung. *Sarcomatoid adenocarcinoma* is an unusual histologic variant that shows extensive overlap with large cell carcinoma and SCC with spindle cell features and can be appropriately diagnosed only on resection specimens in which ample sampling may allow proper identification of better-differentiated areas. In small endoscopic biopsies, it may not be possible to state more than "spindle cell carcinoma" based on results of immunohistochemical stains (cytokeratin positivity), but further subcategorization may be impossible. It is important to distinguish these tumors from monophasic synovial sarcoma, which is also cytokeratin positive but will show a more uniform and monotonous cell population devoid of nuclear pleomorphism and strongly react with bcl-2, TLE-1, and CD99. *Clear cell adenocarcinoma* of the lung is characterized by cells with abundant clear cytoplasm; the tumors need to be distinguished from metastases to the lung from renal cell carcinoma, adrenal carcinoma, and other clear cell tumors. Special stains and close clinicopathologic correlation are indispensable in such cases.

Features that can introduce difficulties for the diagnosis in small endoscopic biopsies include artifactual distortion of the cells owing to mechanical crushing by the forceps or secondary to prominent desmoplastic reaction, obscuring of the tumors cells by heavy inflammatory stromal infiltrates, and subtle infiltration by cancer cells underneath an intact respiratory mucosa. Artifactual distortion of tumor cells owing to a prominent desmoplastic reaction is a common source of diagnostic difficulty; the desmoplastic stroma can almost completely obliterate the underlying tumor cells making them very difficult to recognize as such (Fig. 12.18). Mechanical distortion from the forceps can also damage the tumor cells to a degree that it may be very difficult to recognize them or make a proper histologic characterization of the tumor (Fig. 12.19). Some tumors may be accompanied by a very heavy lymphoplasmacytic inflammatory stromal infiltrate; the tumor cells in such instances may be overshadowed by the inflammation. Attention to the irregular architecture of the glands and the increased cytologic atypia may be of help in identifying an underlying adenocarcinoma (Fig. 12.20). Endoscopic biopsies may often display a normal intact mucosa lining the bronchus but will contain cancerous elements in the submucosa that sometimes may be quite subtle (Fig. 12.21). A careful search for atypical cells or abnormal glands should always be undertaken in small endoscopic biopsies; deeper sections and special stains for cytokeratin may be helpful in cases with a strong clinical suspicion of malignancy.

Large Cell Carcinoma

Large cell carcinoma has traditionally been defined as a malignant epithelial neoplasm of the lung characterized by large cell morphology lacking features of squamous or glandular differentiation (Fig. 12.22). The term essentially overlaps with poorly differentiated NSCLC. A large number of subtypes have been described under the umbrella of the "large cell" category, including clear cell, pleomorphic, anaplastic, sarcomatoid, and giant cell carcinoma. A distinctive subtype frequently encountered in the lung is the anaplastic carcinoma variant with prominent inflammatory component. Such tumors are characterized by discohesive sheets of large, anaplastic tumor cells admixed with prominent inflammatory elements, including small lymphocytes, neutrophils, eosinophils, plasma cells, and histiocytes (Fig. 12.23). Another distinctive variant is one characterized by cells containing prominent "rhabdoid" cytoplasmic inclusions that displace the nuclei toward the periphery (Fig. 12.24). Large cell carcinoma of the lung is characterized by large, pleomorphic and bizarre cells with enlarged nuclei containing very large and prominent eosinophilic nucleoli

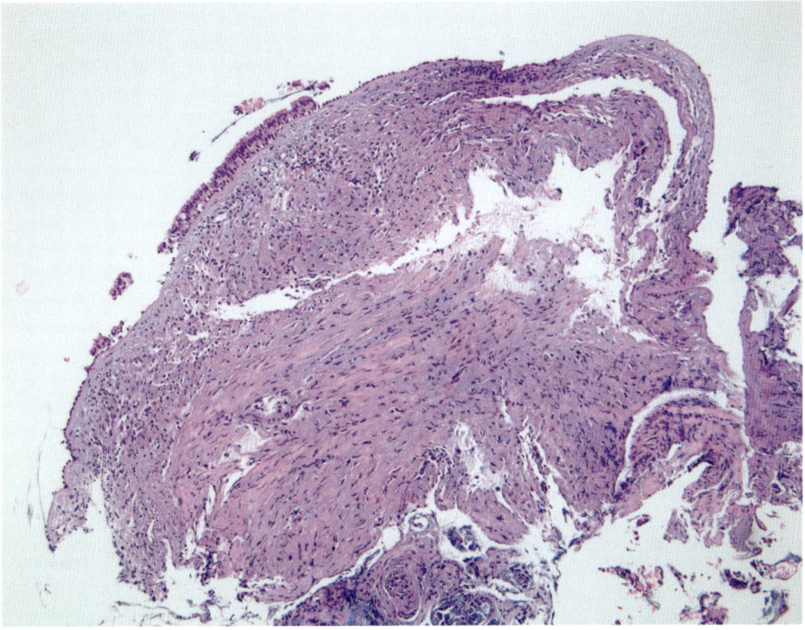

A

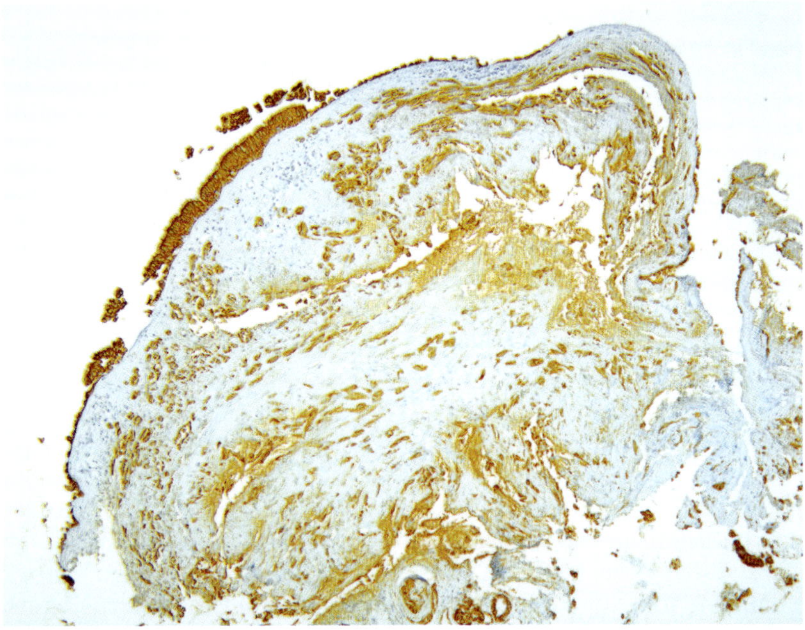

B

FIGURE 12.18 **A:** Transbronchial biopsy showing an intact layer of bronchial mucosa with thickening of the submucosa by dense fibrous connective tissue. Scattered cells are seen embedded in the connective tissue. **B:** Broad-spectrum cytokeratin stain highlights entrapped tumor cells within the connective tissue.

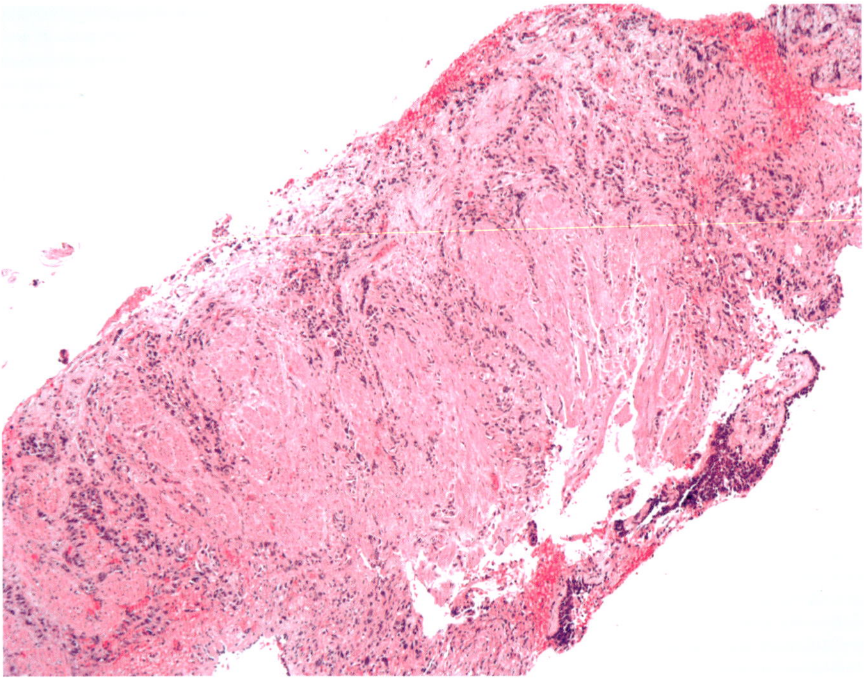

FIGURE 12.19 Transbronchial biopsy shows extensive mechanical distortion of tumor cells in the submucosa by compression due to the forceps. It may be difficult in such instances to determine the exact type of tumor contained in this biopsy without the aid of special stains.

(eFigs. 12.8 to 12.10). Multinucleated, trophoblastic-type giant cells can also be seen, and in some cases they may stain positive for human chorionic gonadotrophic hormone (ß-HCG). Tumors showing combinations of atypical spindle cells and multinucleated atypical giant cells are also included in this category under the designation of "pleomorphic" carcinoma. What all these tumors have in common is the absence of features of either squamous or glandular differentiation at the light microscopic level and nonsmall cell morphology (i.e., large size of the tumor cells). A recent recommendation by the IASLC/ATS/ERS[2] for small biopsy sample reporting is that the term "large cell carcinoma" be avoided in small biopsy or cytology specimens because of the possibility that better differentiated areas might be present in a resected specimen. They also recommend the use of a very limited immunohistochemical panel on such tumors to attempt to define whether there is evidence of squamous or glandular differentiation, including TTF-1 for the diagnosis of adenocarcinoma, and p63 or CK5/6 for SCC, as well as mucin stains (such as mucicarmine) for the identification of intracellular mucin. To conserve tissue for molecular studies, they recommend the use of cocktails of nuclear and cytoplasmic antigens, such as TTF-1/CK5/6 or p63/napsin A.

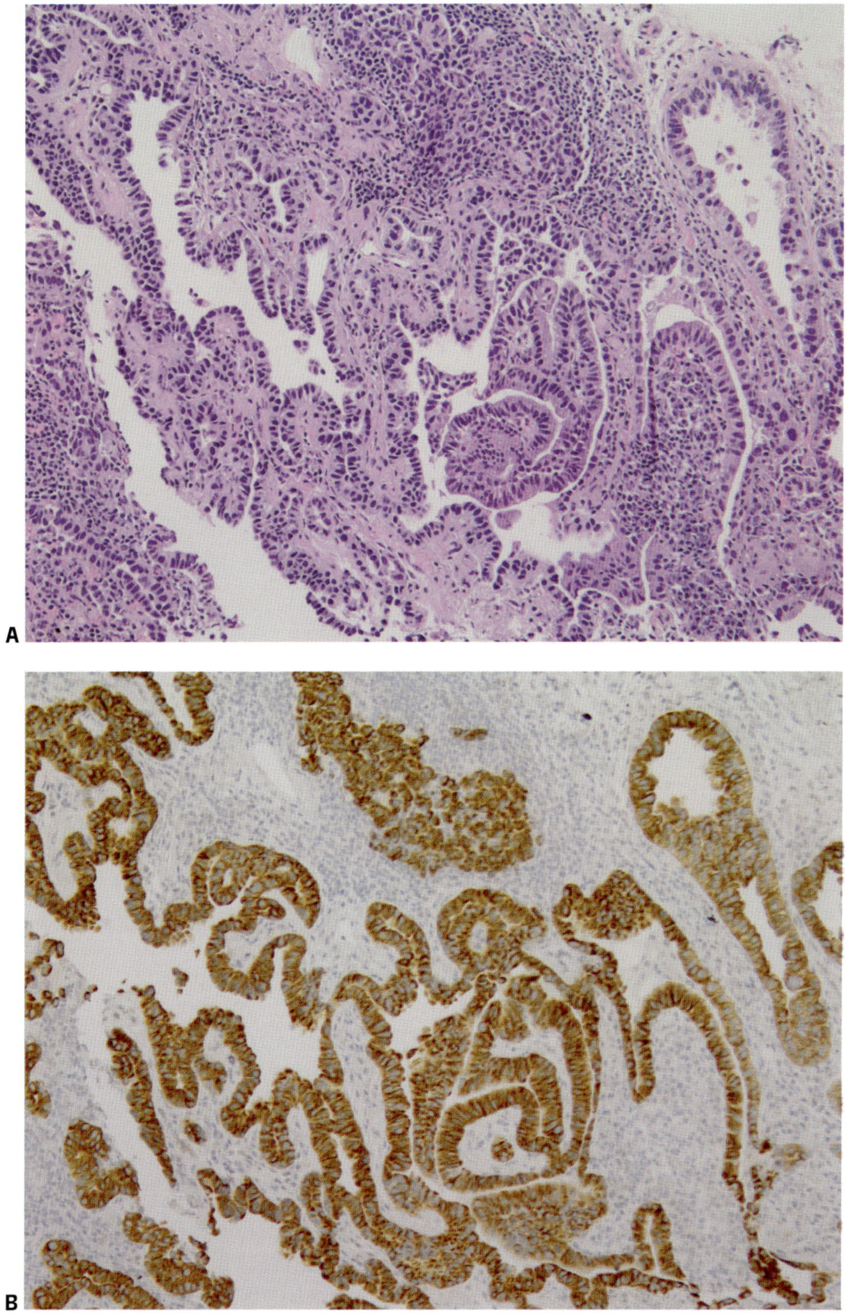

FIGURE 12.20 **A:** Core needle biopsy of peripheral lung mass shows dense lymphoid stromal infiltrates overshadowing the glandular elements. The tortuous character of the glands, complex branching, and atypia of the tumor cells serve to distinguish them from entrapped normal alveolar structures. **B:** Cytokeratin stain (CK7) serves to highlight the complex glandular component in this biopsy.

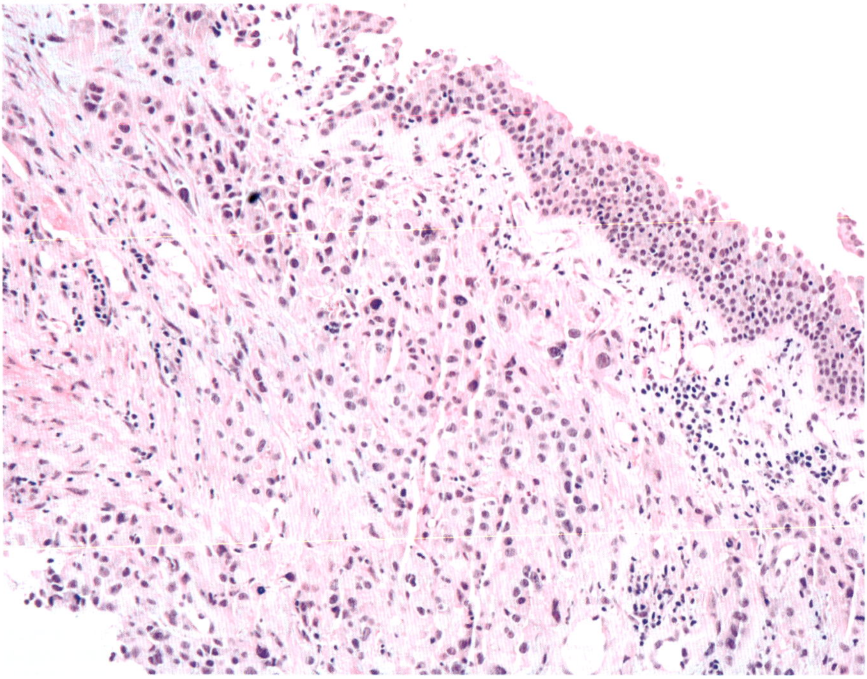

FIGURE 12.21 Transbronchial biopsy shows unremarkable bronchial mucosa lining the lumen; notice, however, scattered atypical cells in the submucosa with subtle, abortive gland formation in this poorly differentiated adenocarcinoma of then lung.

It was proposed that cases positive for an adenocarcinoma marker and/or mucin stains with a negative squamous marker be classified as "NSCLC favor adenocarcinoma," and those positive for a squamous marker and a negative adenocarcinoma and/or mucin marker be classified as "NSCLC favor SCC." Unfortunately, this formula is not foolproof and there exists much overlap in the expression patterns of these antibodies as well as aberrant expression of markers that may lead to incorrect assumptions by clinicians. In a significant number of cases, it may be impossible and impractical to attempt to force a given sample into a defined diagnostic category. Such cases are best reported as NSCLC, NOS, poorly differentiated NSCLC, or NSCLC, large cell type. This is particularly true when equivocal or conflicting results are obtained using immunohistochemical markers (i.e., positivity for both adenocarcinoma and SCC-associated markers; or negative staining for both). The IASLC/ATS/ERS[2] recommendation, however, is that all large cell carcinomas be reported either as "NSCLC, favor adenocarcinoma (or SCC)" or as "NSCLC, NOS."

Perhaps a more important issue is to separate poorly differentiated, large cell carcinoma (NSCLC, NOS) from other large cell malignancies of nonepithelial origin, such as epithelioid or pleomorphic sarcomas, large cell lymphomas, and metastases from germ cell tumors or other poorly differentiated large cell neoplasms. A short battery of immunohistochemical stains may

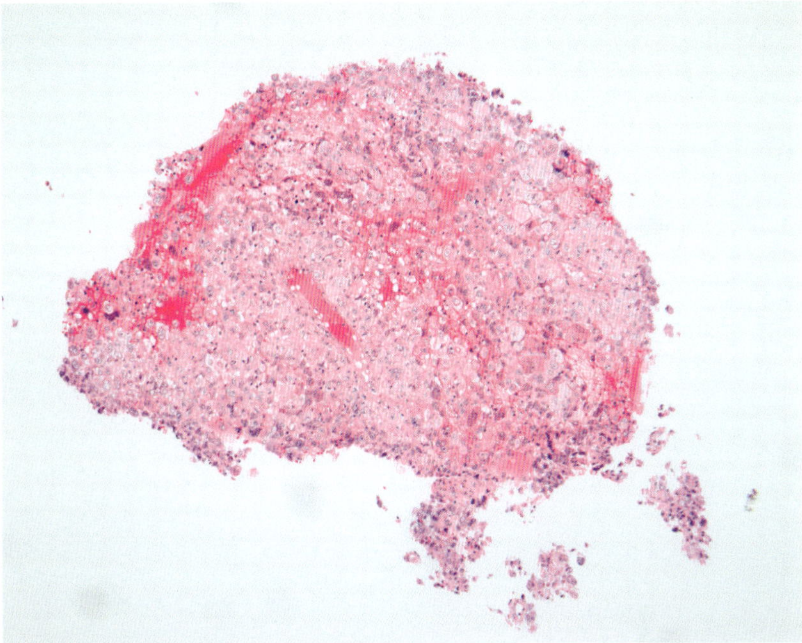

A

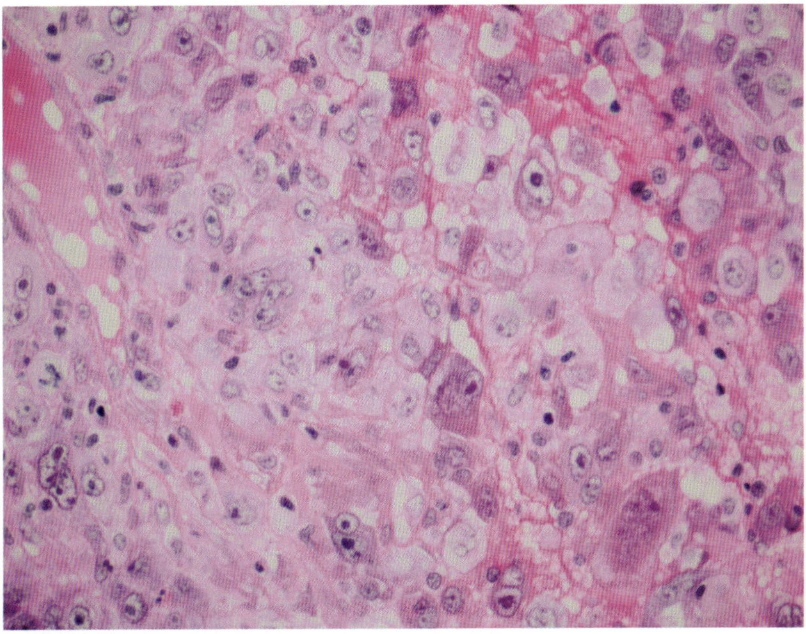

B

FIGURE 12.22 **A:** Endobronchial biopsy shows replacement of the wall of the bronchus by sheets of large, atypical cells without evidence of gland formation or keratinization. **B:** Higher magnification of large cell carcinoma of the lung shows large tumor cells with pleomorphic nuclei containing prominent eosinophilic nucleoli.

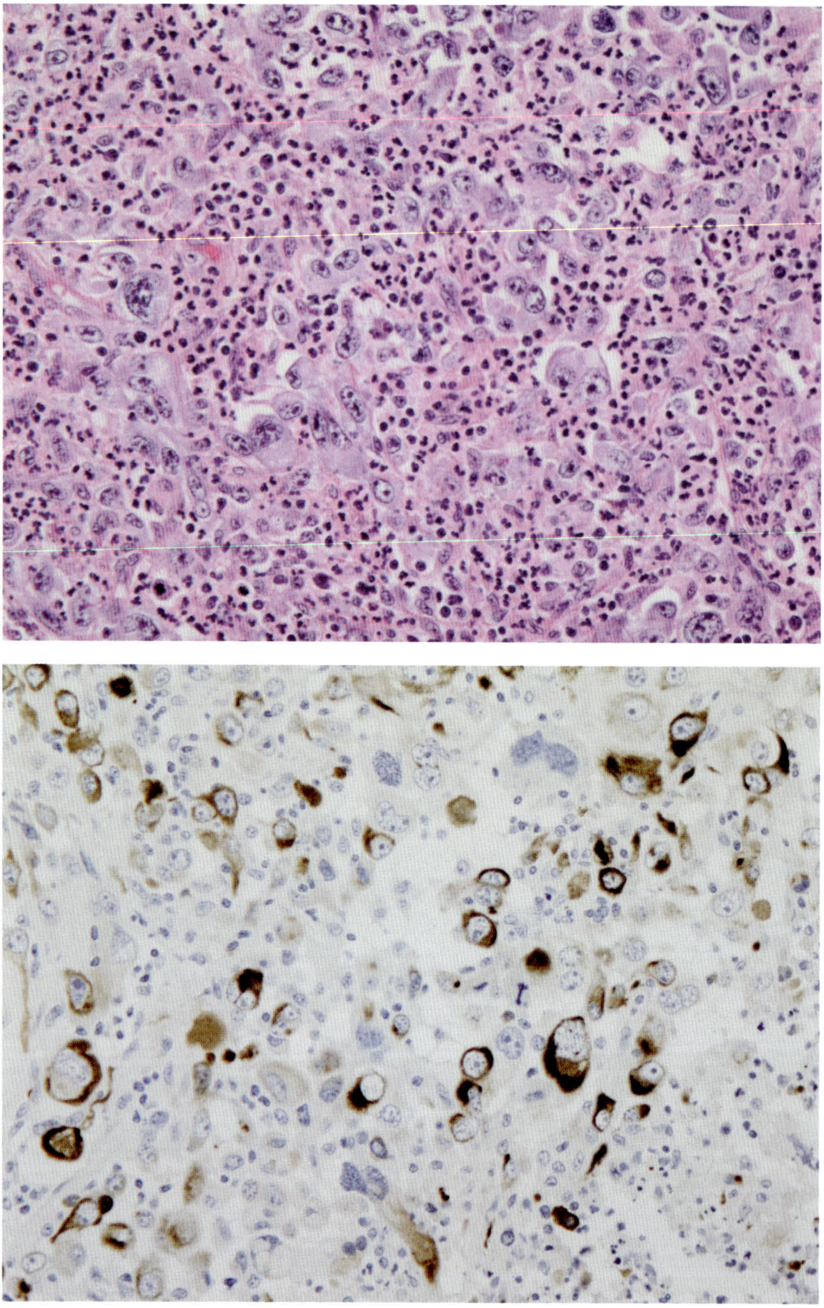

A

B

FIGURE 12.23 **A:** Large cell carcinoma of the lung, "inflammatory" type, shows abundant singly scattered, large, pleomorphic tumor cells with bizarre nuclei and prominent nucleoli, surrounded by dense inflammatory infiltrate. **B:** Low-molecular weight cytokeratin (CAM5.2) shows positivity in the scattered atypical epithelial cells.

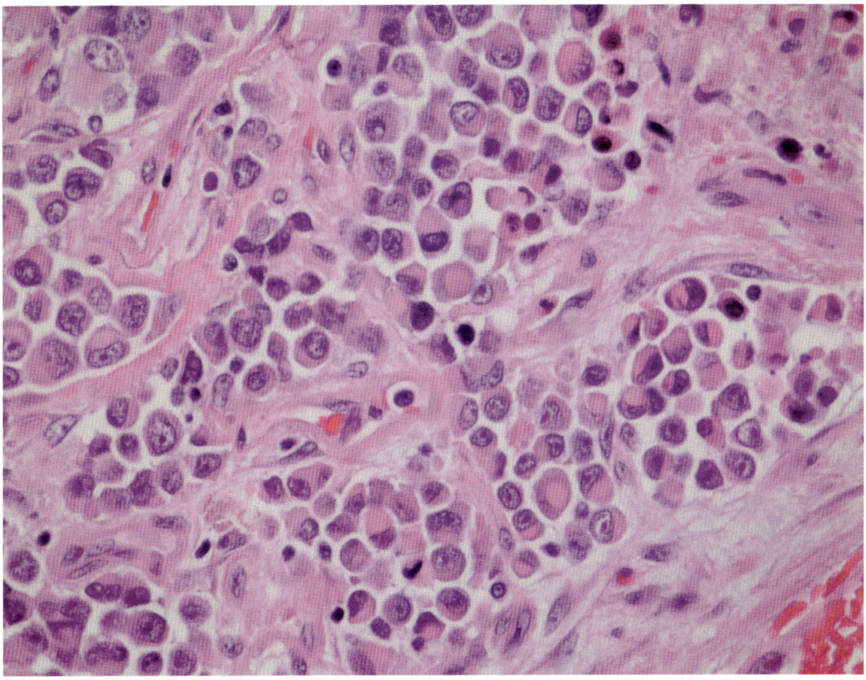

FIGURE 12.24 Anaplastic carcinoma of the lung with "rhabdoid" features shows a population of cells with large atypical nuclei that are displaced to the periphery by densely eosinophilic cytoplasmic inclusions containing intermediate filaments.

be of value in such instances to verify that the tumor is, indeed, of epithelial origin. In particular, broad spectrum cytokeratin and low-molecular weight cytokeratins (such as AE1/AE3 and CAM5.2.) at a minimum, are indicated to demonstrate epithelial origin. Pleomorphic high-grade sarcoma (malignant fibrous histiocytoma), epithelioid sarcoma, epithelioid angiosarcoma, epithelioid malignant peripheral nerve sheath tumors, epithelioid fibrosarcoma, and various other nonepithelial neoplasms with large cell morphology may arise as primary tumors in the lung or can metastasize to the lung from other primary sites. Use of appropriate immunohistochemical stains is indicated in such instances to better define the phenotype; clinicopathologic correlation is required in all cases of poorly differentiated large cell malignancies in the lung to rule out the possibility of a metastasis from another source. Diffuse large cell lymphoma, as mentioned previously, may also express p63 in a significant number of cases[16]; use of appropriate lymphoid markers such as CD3, CD20, CD30, CD45, and ALK-1 are indicated if there is a suspicion of lymphoma. Finally, large cell or anaplastic carcinomas arising from other organs, including the thyroid, breast, gastrointestinal tract, pancreas, biliary tract, and urinary bladder may also metastasize to the lung; clinicopathologic correlation and a proper history are indispensable for arriving at the correct diagnosis.

SALIVARY GLAND-TYPE TUMORS OF LUNG

Tumors recapitulating the features of salivary gland neoplasms can infrequently arise in the lung. Such tumors are felt to originate from bronchial glands located along the bronchial tree and because of their close relationship to the bronchus will often present as endobronchial masses, leading to early symptoms of bronchial obstruction. Some cases can also rarely present as well-circumscribed, peripheral lung nodules. Because of their predilection for the central airways they are easily amenable to diagnosis through endoscopic biopsies. Clinicopathologic correlation and careful clinical history are indispensable to rule out a late or occult metastasis from a primary lesion in the salivary glands.

Mucoepidermoid Carcinoma

Mucoepidermoid carcinoma is one of the most frequent endobronchial tumors to occur in the pediatric age population, although they can also affect older individuals. Histologically they resemble their salivary gland counterpart and are characterized by a proliferation of squamous cells admixed with mucin-secreting cells and cells showing intermediate features. The tumors can be either of low- or high-grade histology, based on the degree of cytologic atypia, mitotic activity, necrosis, and degree of differentiation of the tumor cells.[38] Low-grade tumors often display cystic changes and contain sheets of epidermoid cells with intercellular bridges and foci of keratinization alongside "intermediate" cells with less-developed squamous features. Admixed with the squamoid elements are small glands, tubules, and cysts lined by cytologically bland goblet or columnar cells showing secretion of abundant mucin into the lumens (Fig. 12.25). High-grade tumors show sheets and islands of less well-differentiated squamous cells with an inconspicuous mucinous component. The cells usually display more pronounced nuclear atypia with high mitotic activity, foci of necrosis, and extensive infiltration of surrounding pulmonary parenchyma. Mucicarmine stains are helpful for highlighting the isolated mucocytes admixed with the squamous elements. Distinction between high-grade mucoepidermoid carcinoma and adenosquamous carcinoma is not possible on endoscopic biopsies. Although in general, an intimate admixture of the squamous and mucinous elements favors mucoepidermoid carcinoma (as opposed to areas that clearly comprise only squamous elements alongside areas that purely comprise mucinous elements), the requirement by the 2004 WHO that one of the components comprise at least 10% of the tumor can only be assessed in resected specimens. Such cases are, therefore, best reported as "high-grade NSCLC with predominantly squamous differentiation and foci of adenocarcinomatous differentiation," with a comment that the tumor is consistent with a high-grade mucoepidermoid carcinoma and that an adenosquamous carcinoma cannot be ruled out from the limited biopsy sample (Fig. 12.26).

Low-grade mucoepidermoid carcinoma of the bronchus is associated with an excellent prognosis, with an extremely low rate of metastases to

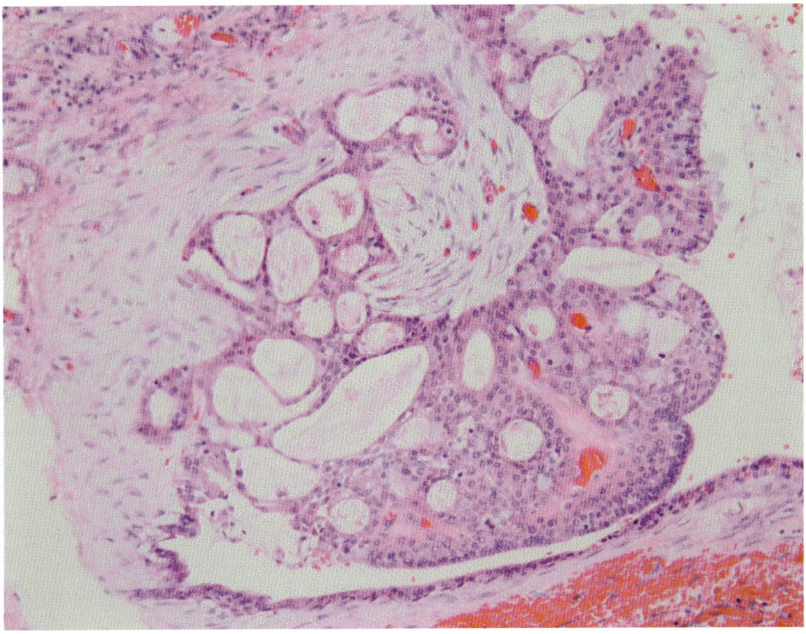

FIGURE 12.25 Mucoepidermoid carcinoma of bronchus shows sheets of monotonous squamoid cells admixed with luminal spaces containing PAS/mucicarmine-positive mucinous secretions.

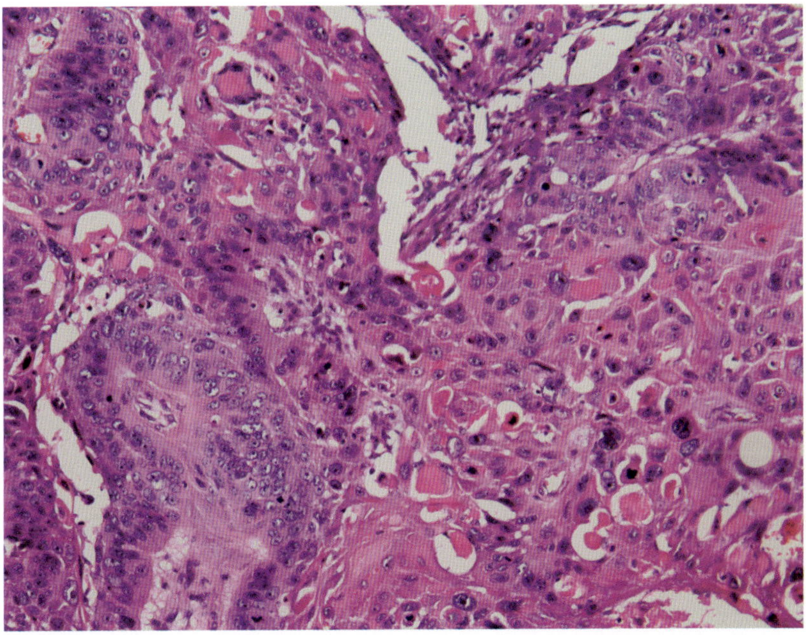

FIGURE 12.26 Endobronchial biopsy of tumor showing mixed features of squamous and glandular differentiation. It may not be possible on such limited material to distinguish a poorly differentiated mucoepidermoid carcinoma from an adenosquamous carcinoma.

regional lymph nodes. Children have a particularly indolent clinical course. The high-grade tumors are associated with aggressive behavior and in general are treated as other NSCLC, depending on their clinical stage at the time of diagnosis.

Adenoid Cystic Carcinoma

Adenoid cystic carcinoma of the bronchus is a distinctive tumor comprising tubular structures with a prominent cribriform architecture that are surrounded by abundant deposits of extracellular eosinophilic basement membrane material along the periphery as well as in the lumens of the tubular structures.[39] The tubular structures are usually embedded in a hyalinized or myxoid matrix and are surrounded by a layer of myoepithelial cells that stain positive for myoepithelial markers (i.e., a combination of SMA/calponin/SMMS with various epithelium-associated markers, including cytokeratins and p63) (Fig. 12.27). The myoepithelial cells can also be immunoreactive for S-100 protein and GFAP. The cells lining the tubules are usually small, with scant cytoplasm and hyperchromatic nuclei with rare mitotic figures. The tumors can sometimes show a tubular growth pattern devoid of a cribriform architecture comprising single, discrete

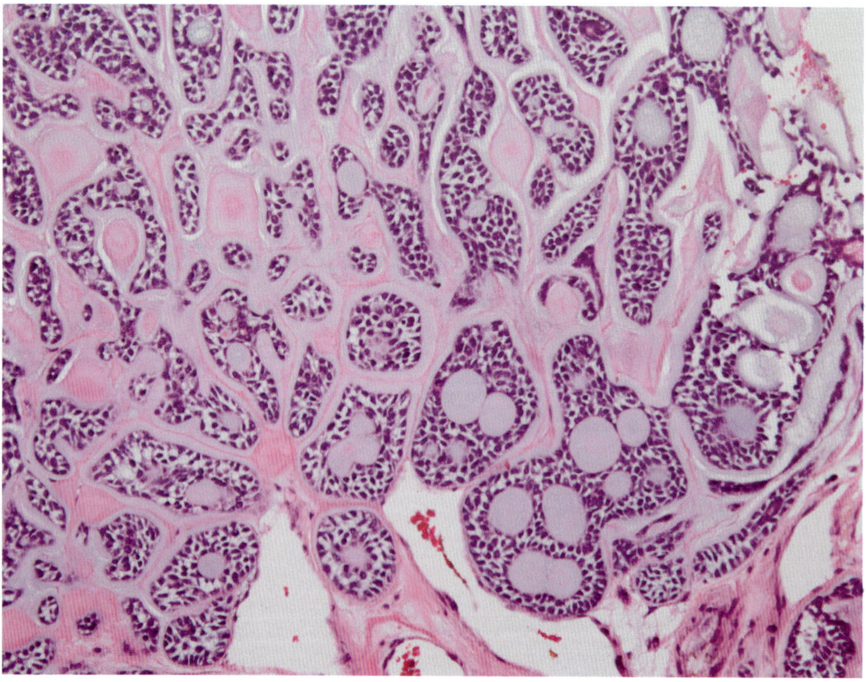

FIGURE 12.27 Adenoid cystic carcinoma of the bronchus shows tumor islands with cribriform architecture as well as individual acinar structures lined by a double layer of cells and displaying deposits of dense, eosinophilic hyaline material within the lumens and surrounding the tubules.

tubular structures surrounded by basement membrane material or may adopt a solid growth pattern characterized by sheets or islands of monotonous small tumor cells that will contain focally small abortive tubular structures. Adenoid cystic carcinoma of the bronchus almost always grows as an endobronchial, polypoid tumor that occludes the bronchial lumen. Perineurial invasion is a common feature, and the tumor frequently extends along the bronchi and bronchioles as well as along lymphatics at the edges of the lesion accounting for the high incidence of recurrence owing to incomplete excision. The tumors have a predilection for men in their fifth decade. They are, for the most part, slow-growing malignancies that may give rise to multiple recurrences and late metastases. Clinical stage at the time of initial diagnosis is the best predictor of prognosis.[39]

Other Types of Salivary Gland-Type Tumors of the Lung

Other types of salivary gland-type tumors of the lung include acinic cell carcinoma, mixed tumor, epimyoepithelial carcinoma, and oncocytoma. *Acinic cell carcinoma (Fechner tumor)* is rare and can present either as a central or as a peripheral lung lesion.[40] It is histologically characterized by islands of monotonous tumor cells that can sometimes grow forming cords or acinar structures or may adopt a papillocystic architecture. The tumor cells are large and contain abundant granular eosinophilic cytoplasm with small nuclei. The tumor cells can sometimes adopt a signet-ring cell appearance with the nuclei displaced toward the periphery. The tumor cells can be positive for amylase and α-1-antichymotrypsin, but a negative reaction does not exclude the diagnosis. PAS histochemical stain will strongly stain the cytoplasm of the tumor cells; the reaction will not be abolished by treatment with diastase. The most distinctive and sensitive marker for diagnosis is the demonstration of dense zymogen granules at the ultrastructural level. The tumors generally behave as low-grade neoplasms and are often cured by simple excision. Diagnosis of acinic cell carcinoma may be difficult to make on small endoscopic biopsies when the signet-ring cell features predominate as it may not be possible to distinguish this tumor from a signet-ring cell adenocarcinoma. *Mixed tumor (pleomorphic adenoma)* of the lung is another rare salivary gland-type tumor that occurs predominantly in adults without any gender predilection and can present in central or peripheral location. Central lesions generally grow as endobronchial polypoid masses filling the bronchial lumen and causing obstruction. Histologically, the tumors are indistinguishable from mixed tumors of salivary glands and comprise an admixture of epithelial and mesenchymal elements (Fig. 12.28).[41] The epithelial component comprises tubular or cystic structures lined by a double layer of cells, with the luminal cells showing low cuboidal epithelium and the peripheral cells comprising a layer of myoepithelial cells. The intervening stroma is dense, collagenous, and with prominent myxoid matrix. Cartilaginous differentiation, a common occurrence in the salivary gland tumors, is seldom a feature seen in the bronchial lesions.[41] Malignant forms have also been described, in which the malignant component is widely invasive, shows marked cytologic atypia

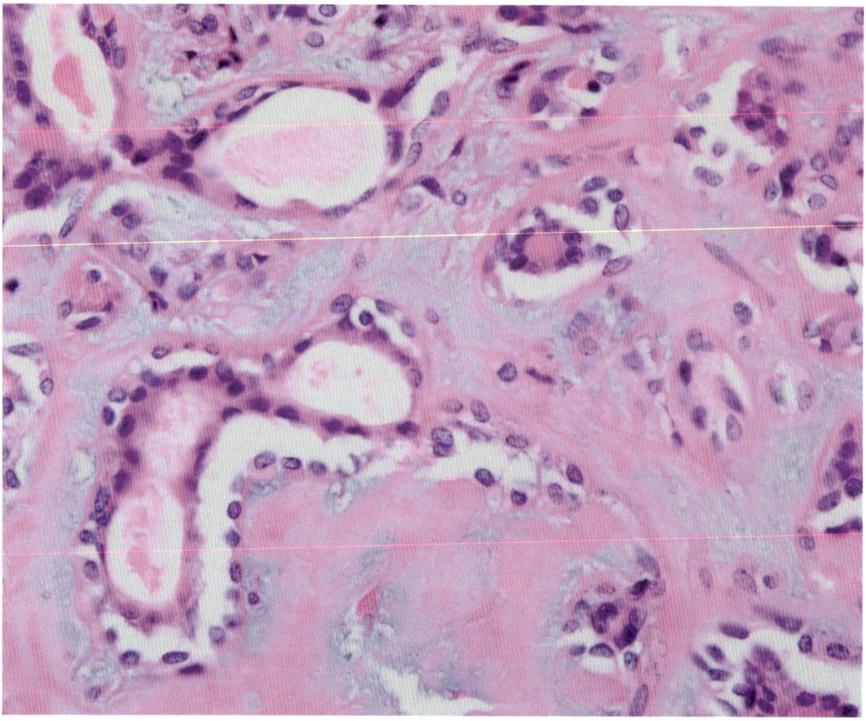

FIGURE 12.28 Endobronchial biopsy shows tubular structures lined by bland-appearing epithelial cells surrounded by abundant connective tissue comprising hyaline matrix with myxoid changes, characteristic of salivary gland-type mixed tumor of the lung.

with high mitotic activity, and may show transitions with preexisting areas of conventional mixed tumor.[41] Because of the myoepithelial cell component, the outer layer of tumor cells will stain for conventional myoepithelium-associated markers (see adenoid cystic carcinoma). In small biopsy samples, it may be impossible to distinguish a mixed tumor from some of the tubular variants of adenoid cystic carcinoma or from an epimyoepithelial carcinoma. *Epimyoepithelial carcinoma* is one of the most unusual salivary gland-type lung tumors. The majority of the reported cases have occurred in adults in central location. The tumors are usually endobronchial, well circumscribed, and present with symptoms of bronchial obstruction; they are histologically characterized by a proliferation of small acinar structures containing a dual cell population.[42] There is an inner cell population surrounding the lumen comprising small, basaloid cells with hyperchromatic nuclei and scant cytoplasm, surrounded by a peripheral cell layer of myoepithelial cells with abundant clear cytoplasm (Fig. 12.29). As with mixed tumors and adenoid cystic carcinoma, the myoepithelial component will stain with myoepithelium-associated markers (see adenoid cystic carcinoma). In a small endoscopic biopsy, it may be extremely difficult to distinguish an epimyoepithelial carcinoma of the lung from a mixed tumor or an adenoid cystic carcinoma. *Oncocytoma*

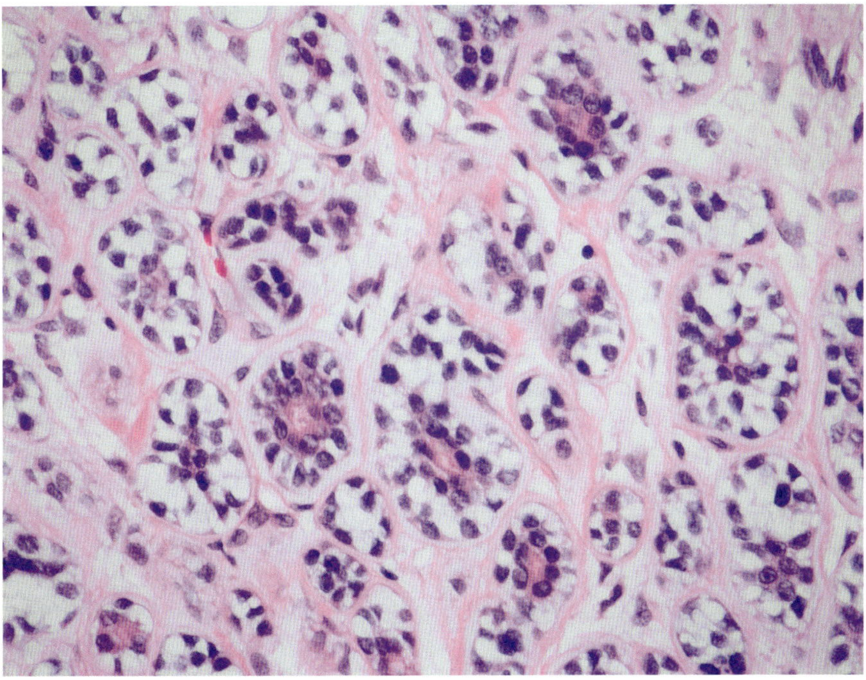

FIGURE 12.29 Epithelial–myoepithelial carcinoma of the lung is characterized by small ductular structures lined by a double layer of cells; an inner layer comprising small cuboidal epithelium and an outer layer comprising myoepithelial cells with prominent clearing of the cytoplasm.

is a rare lung tumor, with only a handful of case reports in the literature. The tumors are characterized by a monotonous population of large cells with abundant granular eosinophilic cytoplasm and small centrally placed nuclei. Their histologic appearance is indistinguishable from that of oncocytomas arising in other locations. These tumors need to be distinguished from other primary lung tumors showing oncocytic features, including oncocytic NECA of the lung, adenocarcinoma with oncocytic changes, and metastases from oncocytic tumors from other organs to the lung.

BIPHASIC EPITHELIAL/MESENCHYMAL NEOPLASMS

Rare tumors showing a combination of both mesenchymal and epithelial neoplastic components within the same tumor mass have been described in the lung. These include mainly biphasic pulmonary blastoma and carcinosarcoma. Because of the variability in cellular composition of these tumors, it may not be possible to render a reliable and definitive diagnosis on small endoscopic or core needle biopsies except under very specific conditions. Such tumors, therefore, require a completely excised surgical specimen with adequate sampling for definitive diagnosis. A specific diagnosis can be suggested in cases where the features fulfill some of the requirements for this diagnosis.

Biphasic Pulmonary Blastoma

Biphasic pulmonary blastoma is characterized by a primitive epithelial component that can be very similar to that observed in fetal-type adenocarcinoma (monophasic pulmonary blastoma), admixed with a malignant mesenchymal component characterized by primitive atypical spindle cells that seldom harbors osteosarcomatous, chondrosarcomatous, or rhabdomyosarcomatous elements.[43] The primitive spindle cell component in pulmonary blastoma often resembles the primitive blastema-like spindle cells seen in Wilm tumor (Fig. 12.30). The epithelial elements comprise glandular structures or tubules that are lined by glycogen-rich, tall cylindrical cells with basally oriented nuclei and abundant clear cytoplasm that resemble fetal lung at the pseudoglandular stage of development (between 10 and 16 weeks of gestation). The glandular structures can also be lined by pseudostratified, nonciliated columnar cells with large oval, hyperchromatic nuclei displaying brisk mitotic activity. The glandular structures sometimes contain solid aggregates of squamoid cells ("morules") at the base of the glands. These morules will stain positively for neuroendocrine markers and ß-catenin (see fetal-type adenocarcinoma). Biphasic pulmonary blastoma is a highly aggressive tumor associated with a poor prognosis. As mentioned above, it may be extremely difficult to establish a definitive diagnosis of

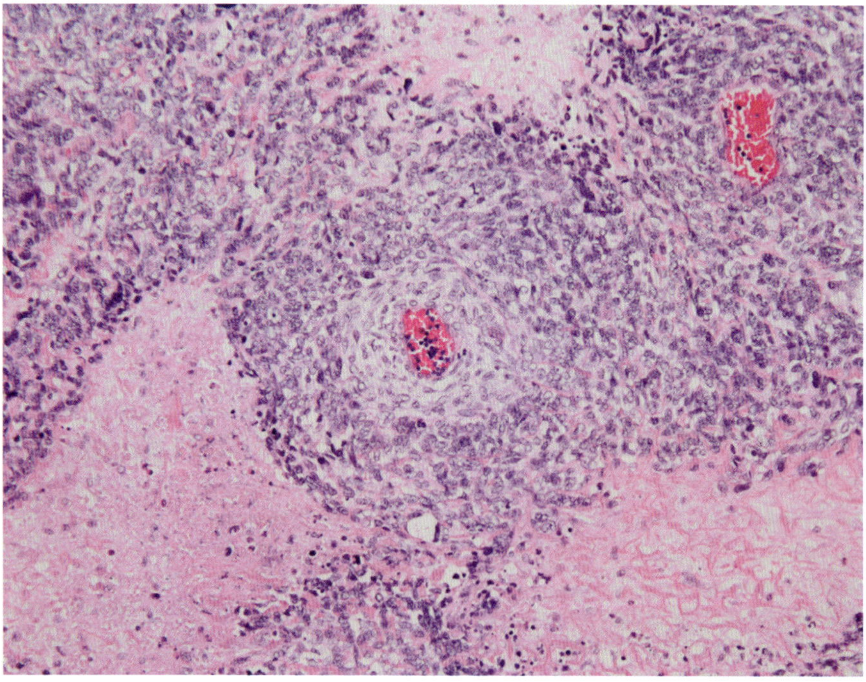

FIGURE 12.30 Mesenchymal component in a biphasic pulmonary blastoma shows primitive population of atypical spindle cells embedded in a lightly myxoid stroma reminiscent of blastemal elements in Wilm tumor.

biphasic pulmonary blastoma on a small biopsy sample, unless both the epithelial and mesenchymal components are clearly present in the biopsy. Cases in which only the mesenchymal component is present may be confused for spindle cell carcinoma or for different spindle cell sarcomas, including monophasic synovial sarcoma, fibrosarcoma, and solitary fibrous tumors. Cases in which only the epithelial component is present may be confused for metastasis of endometrial carcinoma or for a monophasic pulmonary blastoma (fetal-type adenocarcinoma). The latter, in particular, is an extremely important distinction with significant prognostic connotations because monophasic pulmonary blastoma (fetal-type adenocarcinoma) is associated with a much better prognosis than biphasic pulmonary blastoma.

Carcinosarcoma

Carcinosarcoma represents a rare lung tumor. Carcinosarcoma is defined as a biphasic lung neoplasm comprising intimately admixed and clearly identifiable malignant epithelial and malignant mesenchymal elements within the same tumor mass (Fig. 12.31).[43] The epithelial component in carcinosarcoma may be made up of adenocarcinoma, SCC, large cell carcinoma, and small cell NECA. The mesenchymal component is generally made up of a well-defined and clearly recognizable sarcoma such

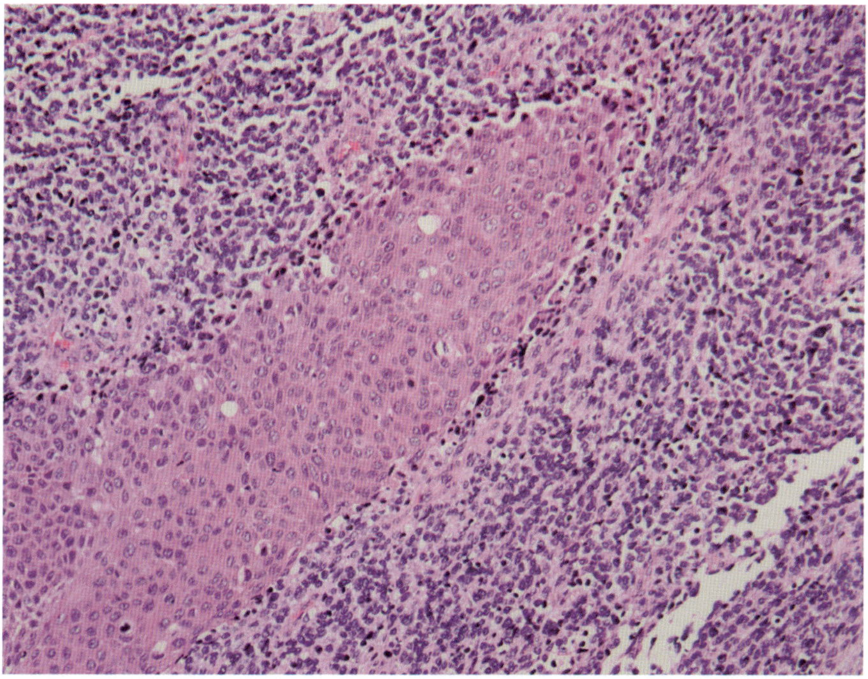

FIGURE 12.31 Pulmonary carcinosarcoma showing island of SCC surrounded by primitive spindle cell sarcomatous elements. Immunohistochemical stains in this case did not identify any epithelial markers within the spindle cell component.

as rhabdomyosarcoma, leiomyosarcoma, chondrosarcoma, or osteosarcoma. In some instances, the mesenchymal component will consist of only a primitive atypical spindle cell proliferation without any particular line of differentiation. Immunohistochemical stains may be of help in identifying the line of differentiation in the malignant mesenchymal component. The malignant epithelial component is usually pretty evident and straightforward, although cytokeratin stains may highlight small, entrapped poorly differentiated epithelial elements entrapped within the sarcomatous components. The malignant epithelial component is often overshadowed by the sarcomatous elements. Tumors showing small cell NECA components tend to be endobronchial and polypoid and may be amenable to adequate sampling by endoscopy. Attention needs to be paid in such instances not to miss the atypical spindle stromal component so that a proper diagnosis of carcinosarcoma can be rendered. The main differential diagnosis for these tumors is with spindle cell (sarcomatoid) carcinoma. In the latter, both the well-differentiated (squamous or adenocarcinomatous) epithelial elements as well as the atypical spindle (sarcomatoid) cells in the stroma should be positive for epithelial markers (cytokeratins, in particular low-molecular weight cytokeratin); whereas in carcinosarcoma, the atypical spindle cells should be negative for epithelium-associated markers and show instead staining for mesenchymal markers, depending on their specific line of differentiation. In small biopsies in which both components are not clearly evident, a noncommittal descriptive diagnosis of "high-grade spindle cell sarcoma" or "high-grade spindle cell malignant neoplasm" may be warranted with a comment that carcinosarcoma or a high-grade NSCLC cannot be ruled out.

REFERENCES

1. Travis WD, Brambilla E, Muller-Hermelink HK, et al. *World Health Organization Classification of Tumors: Pathology and Genetics. Tumors of the Lung, Pleura, Thymus and Heart*. Lyon, France: IARC Press; 2004.
2. Travis WD, Brambilla E, Noguchi M, et al. International Association for the Study of Lung Cancer/American Thoracic Society/European Respiratory Society international multidisciplinary classification of lung adenocarcinoma. *J Thorac Oncol*. 2011;6:244–285.
3. Suster S, Moran CA. The lung. In: Weidner N, Cote R, Suster S, et al, eds. *Modern Pathology*. 2nd ed. Vol I. Philadelphia, PA: WB Saunders; 2009:365–433.
4. Suster S, Moran CA. Tumors of the lung and pleura. In: Fletcher CDM, ed. *Diagnostic Histopathology of Tumors*. 4th ed. London Edinburgh, New York: Churchill-Livingston. In press.
5. Edwards SI, Roberts C, McKean ME, et al. Preoperative histological classification of primary lung cancer: accuracy of diagnosis and use of the non-small cell category. *J Clin Pathol*. 2000;53:537–540; Cataluna JJ, Perpina M, Greses JV, et al. Cell type accuracy of bronchial biopsy specimens in primary lung cancer. *Chest*. 1996;109:1199–1203.
6. Travis WD, Rekhtman N, Riley GJ, et al. Pathologic diagnosis of advanced lung cancer based on small biopsies and cytology: a paradigm shift. *J Thorac Oncol*. 2010;5:411–414.

7. Moran CA. Importance of molecular features of non-small cell lung cancer for choice of treatment. *Am J Pathol.* 2011;178:1940–1948.

8. Shigematsu H, Lin L, Takahashi T, et al. Clinical and biological features associated with epidermal growth factor receptor gene mutations in lung cancers. *J Natl Cancer Inst.* 2005;97:339–346.

9. Takahashi T, Sonobe M, Kobayashi M, et al. Clinicopathologic features of non-small cell lung cancer with EML4-ALK fusion gene. *Ann Surg Oncol.* 2010;17:889–897.

10. Girard N, Deshpande C, Azzoli CG, et al. Use of EGFR/KRAS mutation testing to define clonal relationships among multiple lung adenocarcinomas: comparison with clinical guidelines. *Chest.* 2010;137:46–52.

11. Johnson DH, Fehrenbacher L, Novotny WF, et al. Randomized phase II trial comparing bevacizumab plus carboplatin and paclitaxel with carboplatin and paclitaxel alone in previously untreated, locally advanced or metastatic non-small cell lung cancer. *J Clin Oncol.* 2004;22:2184–2191.

12. Mukhopadhyay S, Katzenstein AL. Subclassification of non-small cell lung carcinomas lacking morphologic differentiation on biopsy specimens: utility of an immunohistochemical panel containing TTF1, napsin A, p63, and CK5/6. *Am J Surg Pathol.* 2011;35:15–25.

13. Terry J, Leung S, Laskin J, et al. Optimal immunohistochemical markers for distinguishing lung adenocarcinomas from squamous cell carcinomas in small tumor samples. *Am J Surg Pathol.* 2010;34:1805–1811.

14. Loo PS, Thomas SC, Nicolson MC, et al. Subtyping of undifferentiated non-small cell carcinomas in bronchial biopsy specimens. *J Thorac Oncol.* 2010;5:436–441.

15. Yoshida A, Tsuta K, Watanabe S, et al. Frequent ALK rearrangement and TTF1/p63 coexpression in lung adenocarcinoma with signet ring cell component. *Lung Cancer.* 2011;72:309–315.

16. Hallack Neto AE, Siqueira SA, Dulley FL, et al. p63 protein expression in high risk diffuse large B-cell lymphoma. *J Clin Pathol.* 2009;62:77–79.

17. Rhigi L, Graziano P, Fornari A, et al. Immunohistochemical subtyping of nonsmall cell lung cancer not otherwise specified in fine needle aspiration cytology: a retrospective study of 103 cases with surgical correlation. *Cancer.* 2011;117:3416–3423.

18. Matoso A, Singh K, Jacob R, et al. Comparison of thyroid transcription factor 1 expression by 2 monoclonal antibodies in pulmonary and nonpulmonary primary tumors. *Appl Immunohistochem Mol Morphol.* 2010;18:142–149.

19. Pereira TC, Share SM, Magalhaes AV, et al. Can we tell the site of origin of metastatic squamous cell carcinoma? An immunohistochemical tissue microarray study of 194 cases. *Appl Immunohistochem Mol Morphol.* 2011;19:10–14.

20. Au NH, Gown AM, Cheang M, et al. p63 expression in lung carcinoma: a tissue microarray study of 408 cases. *Appl Immunhistochem Mol Morphol.* 2004;12:240–247.

21. Seagliotti GV, Parikh P, von Pawel J, et al. The differential efficacy of pemetrexed according to NSCLC histology: a review of two phase III studies. *Oncologist.* 2009;14:253–263.

22. Cohen MH, Gootemberg J, Keegan P, et al. FDA drug approval summary: bevacizumab (Avastin) plus carboplatin and paclitaxel as first-line treatment of advanced/metastatic recurrent nonsquamous non-small cell lung cancer. *Oncologist.* 2007;12:713–718.

23. Kerr KM. Pulmonary adenocarcinomas: classification and reporting. *Histopathology.* 2009;54:12–27.

24. Motoi N, Szoke J, Riley GJ, et al. Lung adenocarcinoma: modification of the 2004 WHO mixed subtype to include the major histologic subtype suggests correlations between papillary and micropapillary adenocarcinoma subtypes, *EGFR* mutations and gene expression analysis. *Am J Surg Pathol.* 2008;32:810–827.

25. Bishop JA, Sharma R, Illei PB. Napsin A and thyroid transcription factor-1 expression in carcinomas of the lung, breast, pancreas, colon, kidney, thyroid, and malignant mesothelioma. *Hum Pathol.* 41:20-25, 2010.
26. Ye J, Findeis-Hossey JJ, Yang Q, et al. Combination of napsin-A and TTF-1 immunohistochemistry help in differentiating primary lung adenocarcinoma from metastatic carcinoma in the lung. *Appl Immunohistochem Mol Morphol.* 2011;19:313–317.
27. Robens J, Goldstein L, Gown AM, et al. Thyroid transcription factor—1 expression in breast carcinoma. *Am J Surg Pathol.* 2010;34:1881–1885.
28. Compcrat E, Zhang F, Perrotin C, et al. Variable sensitivity and specificity of TTF1 antibodies in lung metastatatic adenocarcinoma of colorectal origin. *Mod Pathol.* 2005;18:1371–1376.
29. Siami K, McCluggage WG, Ordoñez NG, et al. Thyroid transcription factor-1 expression in endometrial and endocervical adenocarcinoma. *Am J Surg Pathol.* 2007;31:1759–1763.
30. Goldstein NS, Thomas M. Mucinous and nonmucinous bronchioloalveolar adenocarcinomas have distinct staining patterns with thyroid transcription factor and cytokeratin 20 antibodies. *Am J Clin Pathol.* 2001;116:319–325.
31. Kamiya K, Hayashi Y, Douguchi J, et al. Histopathological features and prognostic significance of the micropapillary pattern in lung adenocarcinoma. *Mod Pathol.* 2008;l21:992–1001.
32. Luevano A, Rao N, MacKinnon A, et al. Cribriform adenocarcinoma of the lung: clinicopathologic, immunohistochemical and molecular study of 15 cases. *Mod Pathol.* 2012;25:483A.
33. Moran CA, Hochholzer L, Fishback N, et al. Mucinous (so-called Colloid) carcinomas of the lung. *Mod Pathol.* 1992;5:634–638.
34. Castro CY, Moran CA, Flieder DG, et al. Primary signet ring cell adenocarcinoma of the lung: a clinicopathologic study of 15 cases. *Histopathology.* 2001;39:397–401.
35. Steinhauer JR, Moran CA, Suster S. "secretory endometrioid-like" adenocarcinoma of the lung. *Histopathology.* 2005;47:219–220.
36. Sekine S, Shibata T, Matsuno Y, et al. Beta-catenin mutations in pulmonary blastomas: association with morule formation. *J Pathol.* 2003;200:214–221.
37. Terracciano LM, Glatz K, Mhawech P, et al. Hepatoid adenocarcinoma with liver metastases mimicking hepatocellular carcinoma: an immunohistochemical and molecular study of eight cases. *Am J Surg Pathol.* 2003;27:1302–1312.
38. Moran CA. Primary salivary gland type tumors of the lung. *Semin Diagn Pathol.* 1995;12:106–122.
39. Moran CA, Suster S, Koss MN. Primary adenoid cystic carcinoma of the lung: a clinicopathologic and immunohistochemical study of 16 cases. *Cancer.* 1994;73:1390–1397.
40. Moran CA, Suster S, Koss MN. Acinic cell carcinoma of the lung ("Fechner tumor"): a clinicopathologic, immuinohistochemical and ultrastructural study of five cases. *Am J Surg Pathol.* 1992;16:1039–1050.
41. Moran CA, Suster S, Askin FB, et al. Benign and malignant salivary gland type tumors of the lung: clinicopathologic and immunohistochemical study of 8 cases. *Cancer.* 1994;73:2481–2490.
42. Nguyen CV, Suster S, Moran CA. Pulmonary epithelial–myoepithelial carcinoma: a clinicopathologic and immunohistochemical study of 5 cases. *Human Pathology.* 2009;40:366–374.
43. Berho M, Moran CA, Suster S. Mixed malignant epithelial/mesenchymal lung neoplasms. *Semin Diagn Pathol.* 1995;12:123–139.

13

NEUROENDOCRINE LUNG NEOPLASMS

Neuroendocrine lung tumors are relatively rare neoplasms that have undergone a number of revisions in the past several years in their nomenclature and diagnostic approach. In particular, the terminology applied to these tumors has been a topic of much debate and controversy in the literature.[1] Most authors today seem to accept the concept that neuroendocrine tumors form part of a family of neoplasms that can show a wide spectrum of differentiation and morphologic appearances. In previous years, the term "carcinoid tumor" was applied to tumors belonging in the more benign end of the spectrum. The majority of poorly differentiated tumors were designated as "small cell carcinoma." Eventually, the realization that intermediate forms also existed led to the creation of the category designated as "atypical carcinoid." The general trend today is to include all these tumors under the umbrella of "neuroendocrine carcinoma" and to subdivide them according to their morphologic features and potential behavior into well-differentiated, moderately differentiated, and poorly differentiated tumors, or by grade into low-, intermediate-, and high-grade tumors.[2–4] It is unfortunate that the WHO classification of tumors of the lung continues to retain the terms "carcinoid tumor" and "atypical carcinoid" for designating these lesions, as such terms are generally acknowledged to be outdated and imprecise.[5] The terminology we use divides these tumors into a three-tiered system based on degrees of differentiation: well-differentiated, moderately differentiated, and poorly differentiated neuroendocrine carcinoma PDNEC (roughly equivalent to the terms carcinoid, atypical carcinoid, and small cell carcinoma from the older literature) (Table 13.1).

The diagnosis of neuroendocrine tumors of the lung continues to be a problem area for pathologists. Although there have been many attempts over the years at refining our criteria for the diagnosis of these tumors, reproducibility in diagnosis remains poor, even among expert pulmonary pathologists. In a study by Travis et al.,[6] a unanimous agreement among five experienced pulmonary pathologists could only be achieved in 58% of carcinoid tumors, 50% of atypical carcinoids, and 40% of large cell neuroendocrine carcinomas (LCNECs). Morphometric studies carried out on surgically resected tissues in patients with poorly differentiated lung cancers have underscored the difficulties inherent in separating these tumors based on morphology by demonstrating considerable overlap in nuclear

TABLE 13.1 Neuroendocrine Neoplasms of the Lung

Tumor	Older Nomenclature	Features
Well-differentiated neuroendocrine carcinoma	Bronchial adenoma Carcinoid tumor Kulchistky cell tumor Typical carcinoid	Prominent "neuroendocrine" (organoid) growth pattern No cytologic atypia Stippled chromatin ("salt and pepper") Low mitotic activity Absence of tumor cell necrosis Strong expression of neuroendocrine markers by immunohistochemistry
Moderately differentiated neuroendocrine carcinoma	Atypical carcinoid	Preservation of neuro endocrine growth pattern Increased cytologic atypia Prominent nucleoli Moderately increased mitotic activity Frequent areas of comedonecrosis Retained expression of neuroendocrine immuno histochemical markers
Poorly differentiated neuroendocrine carcinoma	Small cell carcinoma Oat cell carcinoma Kulchistky cell carcinoma Large cell neuroendocrine carcinoma Undifferentiated small cell carcinoma	Poorly developed neuro endocrine growth pattern Marked cytologic atypia Small cell or large cell morphology High mitotic activity (>10 per 10 HPF) Extensive areas of necrosis Reduced expression of neuroendocrine immuno histochemical markers

size between "small cells" and "large cells" in examples of small cell lung cancer (SCLC) and LCNECs.[7] It, thus, follows that making a specific diagnosis based on cells size and cytologic features can be extremely problematic and sometimes unreliable when applied to these tumors, especially in small biopsy samples. Another factor, in addition to the difficulties involved in evaluating cell size, has been the emphasis placed by many experts on mitotic activity as a means for distinguishing among the various categories. Mitotic activity, although consistently high in the poorly differentiated tumors and consistently low in the well-differentiated tumors, can show significant variability in the tumors between the two extremes, making strict separation based on this criterion alone very difficult and sometimes arbitrary. Moreover, the requirement for assessing mitotic counts on 10 high power fields (HPF) has been based on review of resection specimens and may not be applicable to small biopsies in all instances, thus limiting the use of this parameter further for the evaluation of small lung biopsies. An additional aspect that has been either neglected or underemphasized in most of the current classification schemes is the tumor's architecture and growth pattern. Well-differentiated tumors are generally characterized by a well-developed "endocrine" or "organoid" pattern of growth (nests, ribbons, trabeculae, peripheral palisading of tumor cells, etc.), whereas poorly differentiated neuroendocrine neoplasms are characterized by loss of the organotypical architecture (i.e., sheets of tumor cells without any particular organization). Tumors that show a combination of well-preserved features of endocrine growth pattern in combination with high histologic grade are likely to be located along the middle of the spectrum of this family of tumors (i.e., moderately differentiated neuroendocrine carcinoma or atypical carcinoid), rather than at the extremes. Lack of inclusion of the assessment of the growth pattern for these tumors, thus, detracts from our ability to properly evaluate their degree of differentiation and biologic potential.

An additional difficulty that is commonly encountered in clinical practice is to distinguish between moderately differentiated neuroendocrine carcinoma (atypical carcinoid) and the recently created category of LCNEC (currently regarded as belonging in the high-grade, poorly differentiated end of the spectrum of neuroendocrine carcinomas). In fact, critical reading of the criteria and features that distinguish such tumors shows significant overlap, to the point of suggesting that these two categories may be one and the same. The main diagnostic features that permit separation of "LCNEC" from other types of nonneuroendocrine large cell carcinomas are precisely the well-developed "neuroendocrine" growth pattern (i.e., architecture) in the former.[8] In the setting of an endoscopic biopsy, in particular, it may be nearly impossible to separate these two categories with absolute certainty, regardless of the results of special markers or morphologic features.

WELL-DIFFERENTIATED NEUROENDOCRINE CARCINOMA ("CARCINOID" TUMOR)

Well-differentiated neuroendocrine carcinoma (or "carcinoid tumor" of the older literature) has traditionally been regarded as the prototype of neuroendocrine tumors of the lung. Because up to 15% of conventional "carcinoids" of the lung can metastasize to regional lymph nodes, these tumors are now generally regarded as low-grade malignant neoplasms.[9] The tumors occur predominantly in adults and are more often centrally located within the lung, although some tumors can also be present in peripheral

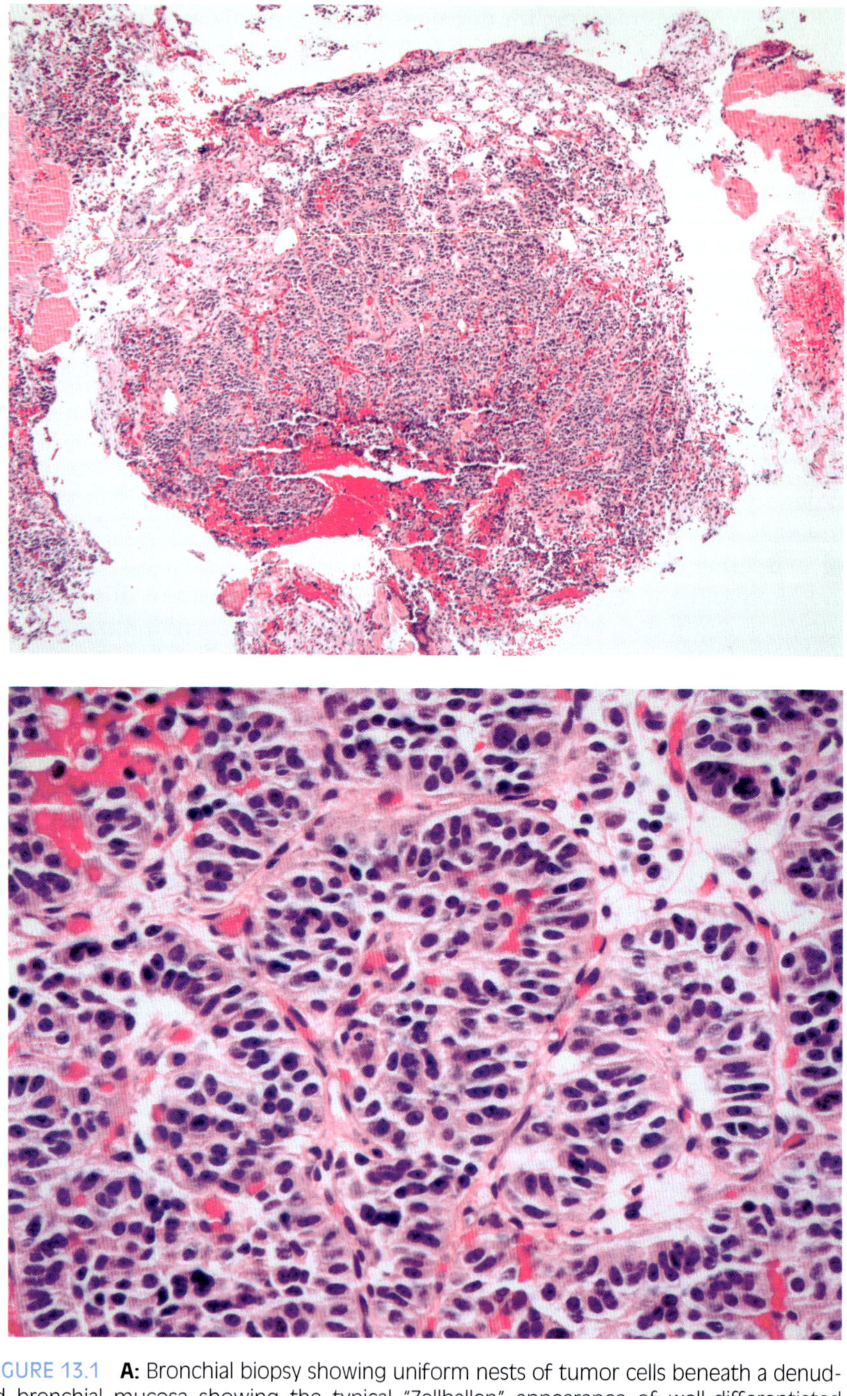

A

B

FIGURE 13.1 **A:** Bronchial biopsy showing uniform nests of tumor cells beneath a denuded bronchial mucosa showing the typical "Zellballen" appearance of well-differentiated neuroendocrine carcinoma of the lung (bronchial carcinoid). **B:** Higher magnification showing monotonous population of tumor cells with stippled chromatin pattern and rim of eosinophilic cytoplasm.

locations away from cartilage-bearing airways. The tumors may be rarely associated with paraneoplastic syndromes (such as Cushing syndrome) owing to aberrant synthesis of peptic hormones and can give rise to the carcinoid syndrome when they develop liver metastases.[10] The majority of the tumors are characterized by endobronchial growth into the bronchial lumen and are thus readily amenable to sampling by endoscopic biopsies. They usually present as tan, polypoid, and smooth endobronchial lesions that cause obstruction and hemoptysis. Bleeding is a common complication of the endoscopic biopsy procedure. The histologic diagnosis of well-differentiated neuroendocrine carcinoma on endoscopic biopsy is generally straightforward (eFigs. 13.1 to 13.3). The tumors are characterized by their striking neuroendocrine ("organoid") growth pattern, comprising nests of monotonous tumor cells separated by thin fibrovascular septa (Zellballen), serpiginous trabeculae, or ribbons of tumor cells, and epithelial pseudorosettes (Fig. 13.1). The tumor cells are round to oval, with round, centrally located nuclei showing a characteristically stippled ("salt and pepper") chromatin pattern and devoid of significant cytologic atypia. The nuclei are surrounded by an ample rim of eosinophilic cytoplasm, with a normal nuclear-to-cytoplasmic ratio. The cells can also be spindled, pigmented (owing to melanin granules), or contain abundant granular eosinophilic cytoplasm (oncocytic variant). Tumors comprising spindle cells show a tendency to present as peripheral, subpleural lesions and for that reason are seldom encountered in endoscopic biopsies (Fig. 13.2). Rare mitoses can

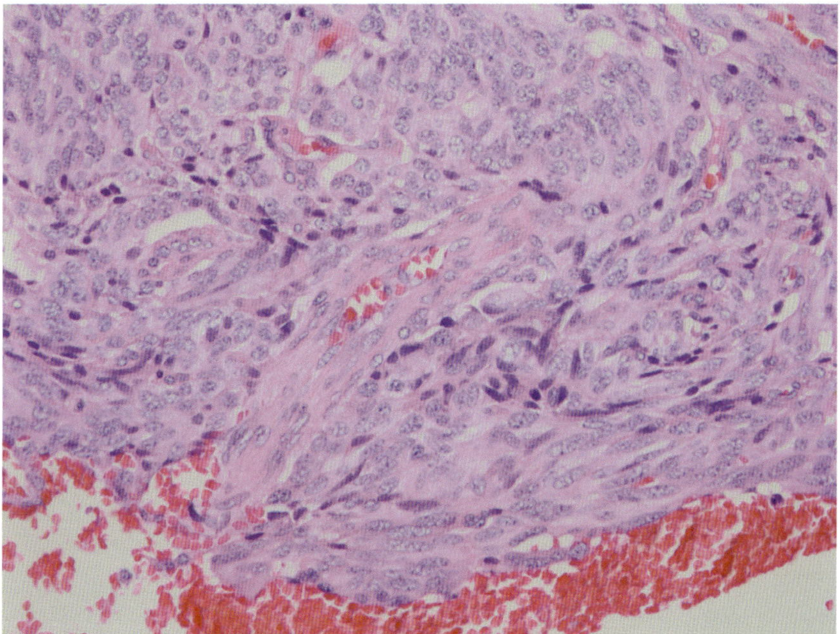

FIGURE 13.2 Well-differentiated neuroendocrine carcinoma of the lung showing spindling of the tumor cells ***(lower right)***.

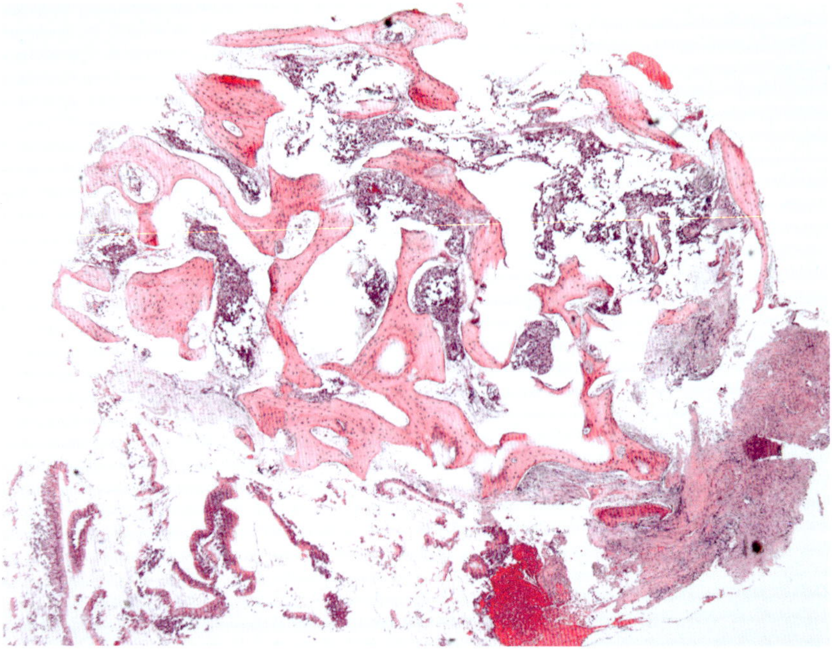

A

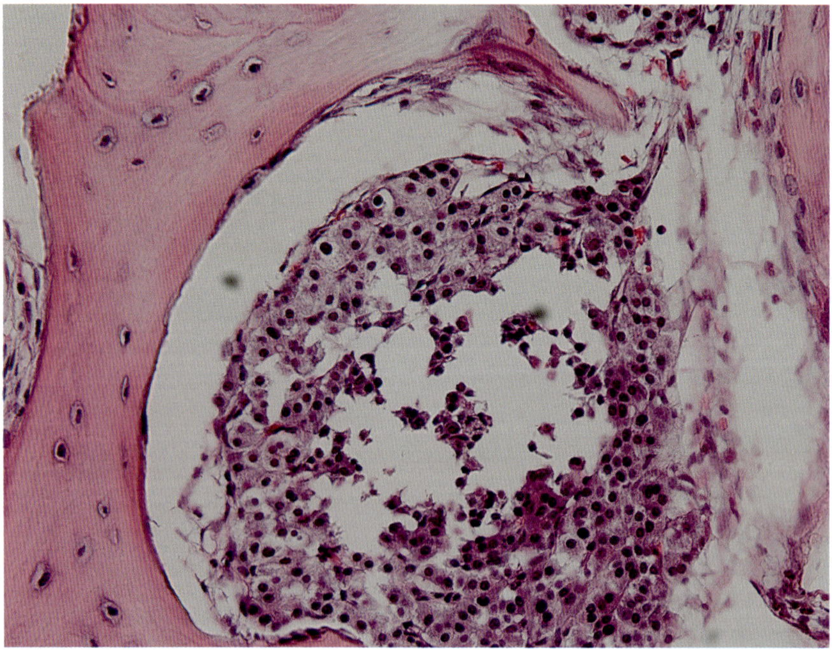

B

FIGURE 13.3 **A:** Bronchial biopsy showing extensive bony deposition circumscribing small cellular islands of tumor cells. **B:** Higher magnification showing monotonous population of bland-appearing tumor cells surrounded by bone in well-differentiated neuroendocrine carcinoma of the lung with extensive osseous metaplasia.

be observed, but they should normally not exceed 2 mitoses per 10 HPF. An accurate count of mitoses can often be difficult to establish in small endoscopic biopsies where there may not be 10 HPF available for a proper assessment, making this criterion difficult to apply in endoscopic biopsy material. However, the finding of more than one mitosis in a small endoscopic biopsy, coupled with mild or moderate cytologic atypia, should raise the possibility of a moderately differentiated neuroendocrine carcinoma. Some unusual morphologic variants of well-differentiated neuroendocrine carcinoma have been observed that may pose difficulties for interpretation, including tumors with metaplastic cartilage or bone formation (Fig. 13.3), tumors containing abundant mucinous stroma that may be confused for mucinous bronchogenic carcinomas or metastasis from other organs (Fig. 13.4), tumors with prominent angiectatic features that may resemble vascular neoplasms, tumors with prominent cystic changes, tumors with a glandular arrangement resembling adenocarcinoma (Fig. 13.5), and tumors with amyloid-like or sclerotic stroma (Fig. 13.6).[11–15] In small biopsies, the tumors may often display a solid, sheet-like pattern of growth with bland-appearing, monotonous small tumor cells without any particular architectural organization that can resemble a lymphoma or sometimes raise the suggestion of a higher-grade neoplasm (Fig. 13.7). Attention to the bland nuclear morphology, ample rim of eosinophilic cytoplasm, and absence of mitotic activity should prompt investigation with neuroendocrine markers to confirm the diagnosis. Another potential pitfall for diagnosis is artifactual distortion of the tumor cells in small biopsy samples leading to spindling or crushing of the tumor cells, making recognition of the underlying process very difficult (Fig. 13.8A, B). Use of immunohistochemical stains in such instances can facilitate the diagnosis (Fig. 13.8C). An important distinction to make for well-differentiated neuroendocrine carcinoma is with so-called pulmonary tumorlet. The latter is generally an incidental finding generally seen away from cartilage-bearing airways in lung resection specimens and, therefore, usually not amenable to sampling by endoscopic techniques. The pulmonary tumorlet is histologically indistinguishable from well-differentiated neuroendocrine carcinoma and is separated from it by an arbitrary size criterion (<0.5 cm). The diagnosis of pulmonary tumorlet should not be made on endoscopic biopsy specimens and should be reserved only for the incidental finding of this lesion in lung resected specimens.

Immunohistochemistry plays an important role in the diagnosis of neuroendocrine carcinomas of the lung. Well-differentiated neuroendocrine carcinoma is characterized by the strong expression of neuroendocrine markers, including chromogranin A, synaptophysin, neuron-specific enolase (NSE), and CD56. The staining pattern is cytoplasmic and diffuse (Fig. 13.9). These tumors are also strongly positive for cytokeratins, in particular CK7 and low-molecular weight cytokeratins.[16] The tumors can also express specific peptide hormones, including gastrin, somatostatin, and bombesin. A subpopulation of S-100 protein-positive sustentacular cells can sometimes also be identified in some of these tumors. It is of interest

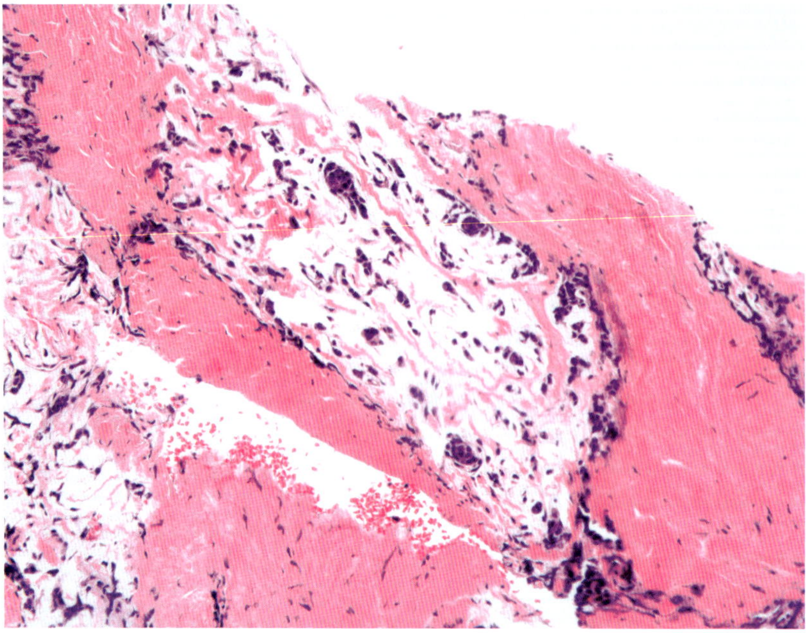

A

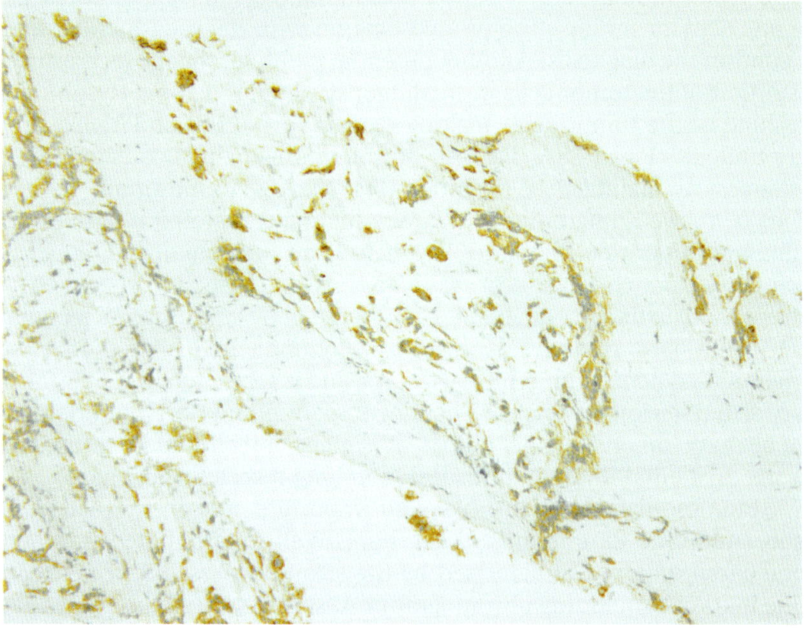

B

FIGURE 13.4 **A:** Core biopsy of well-differentiated neuroendocrine carcinoma of the lung shows small clusters and cords of small, monotonous tumor cells embedded in a mucinous stroma simulating metastatic mucin secreting (colloid) carcinoma. **B:** Immunohistochemical staining for synaptophysin demonstrates cytoplasmic positivity of the tumor cells, indicating a diagnosis of well-differentiated neuroendocrine carcinoma with abundant mucinous stroma. Such tumors must be distinguished from metastases from breast and gastrointestinal tract carcinomas.

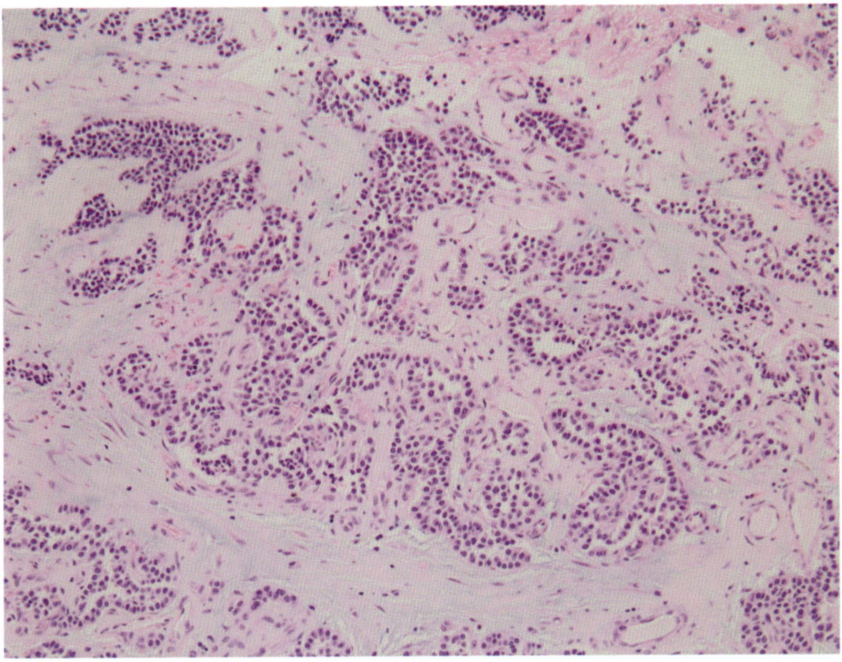

A

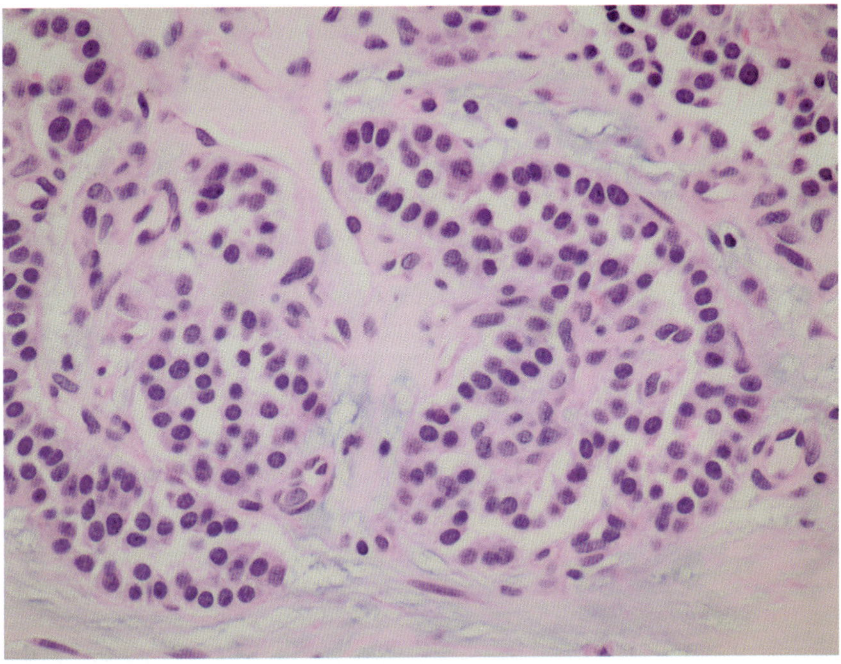

B

FIGURE 13.5 **A:** Endoscopic biopsy of well-differentiated neuroendocrine carcinoma with pseudoglandular pattern simulating well-differentiated adenocarcinoma. **B:** Higher magnification showing monotonous population of small tumor cells lining the pseudoglandular structures; these cells reacted strongly with chromogranin and synaptophysin.

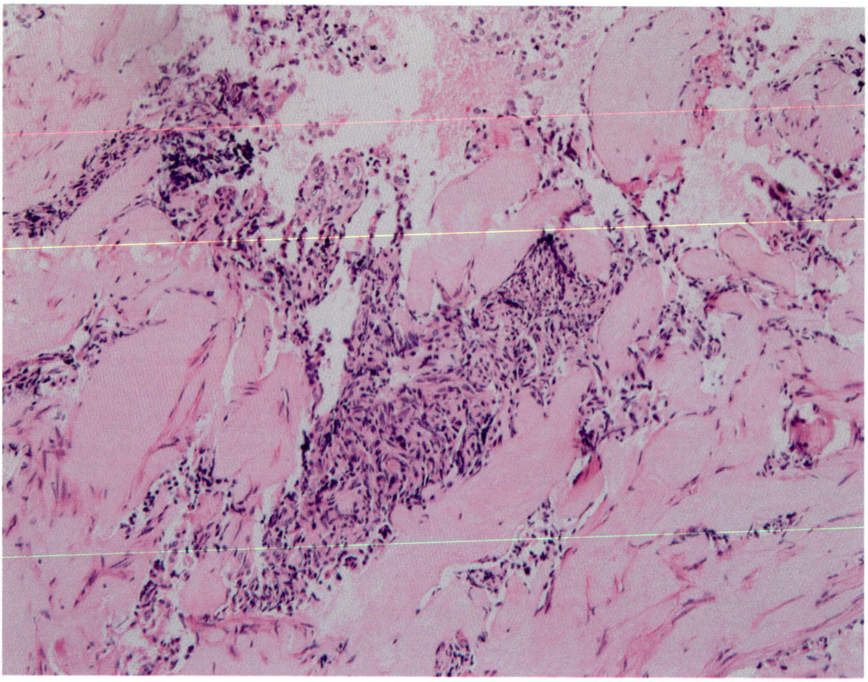

FIGURE 13.6 Well-differentiated neuroendocrine carcinoma of the lung with abundant stromal sclerosis; notice bland-appearing population of tumor cells with focal crushing artifact. These tumors need to be distinguished from metastases or desmoplastic carcinomas.

to note, thyroid transcription factor-1 (TTF-1), an intranuclear transcription factor expressed in poorly differentiated neuroendocrine carcinomas PDNECs of the lung, is only weakly expressed or absent in well-differentiated neuroendocrine carcinoma.[17] Demonstration of numerous dense-core, membrane-bound neurosecretory granules by electron microscopy is another way to establish the diagnosis in equivocal cases, but this methodology has largely fallen in disuse owing to the broad availability of immunohistochemical markers in routine practice.

MODERATELY DIFFERENTIATED NEUROENDOCRINE CARCINOMA (ATYPICAL CARCINOID)

The first recognition of this intermediate category of tumors was in a study by Arrigoni et al.[18] who introduced the term "atypical carcinoid" for tumors that closely resembled histologically carcinoid tumors but showed increased nuclear pleomorphism and cytologic atypia, with increased mitotic activity and foci of necrosis. Unlike conventional "carcinoid" tumors, moderately differentiated neuroendocrine carcinomas are associated with cigarette smoking and are more often peripheral in location. They are usually unassociated with a bronchus and present as a well-circumscribed intraparenchymatous

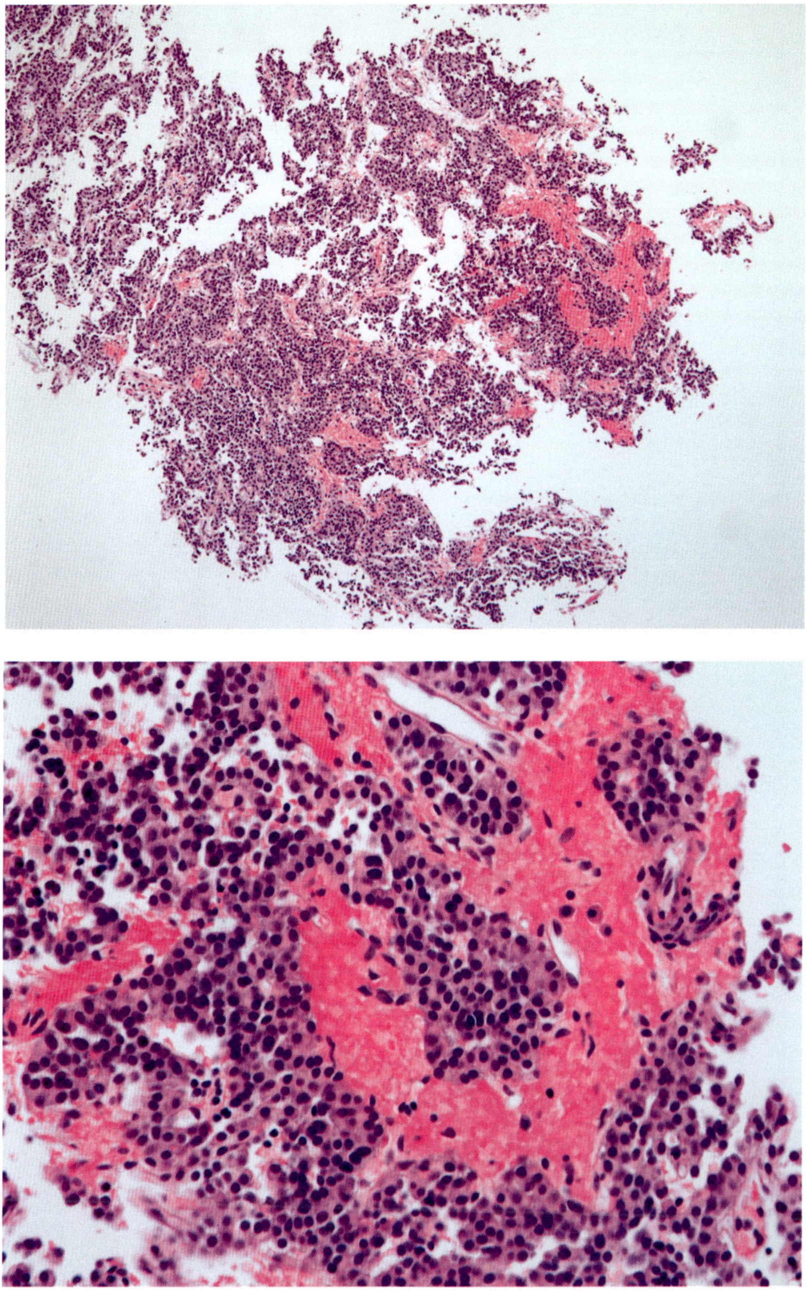
A
B

FIGURE 13.7 **A:** Bronchial biopsy of well-differentiated neuroendocrine carcinoma of the lung shows a solid proliferation of uniform small cells without any particular organization or distinctive growth pattern. This is a frequently encountered presentation for these tumors in small endoscopic biopsies. **B:** Higher magnification shows monotonous tumor cell population with no evidence of cytologic atypia or mitotic activity. This finding should prompt ordering of stains for neuroendocrine markers to confirm the diagnosis.

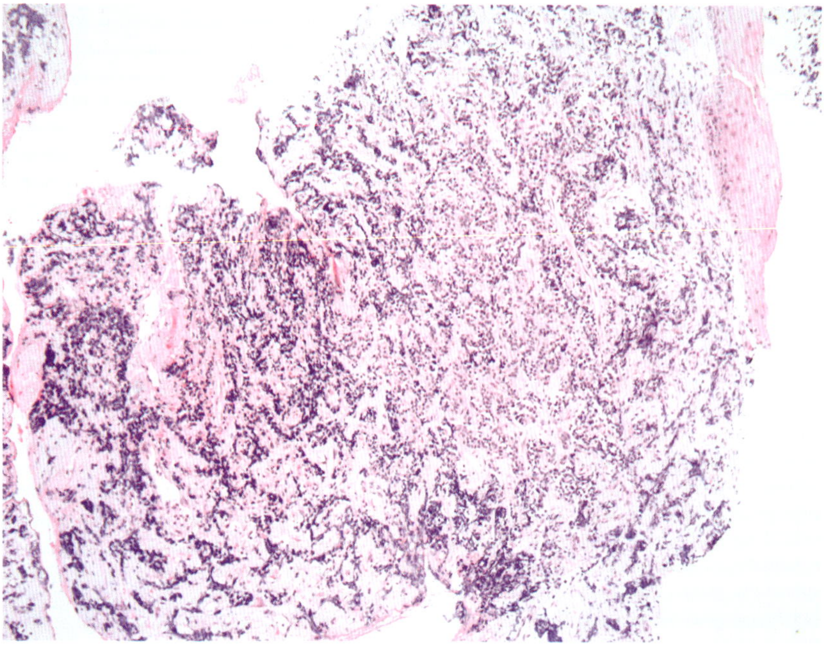
A

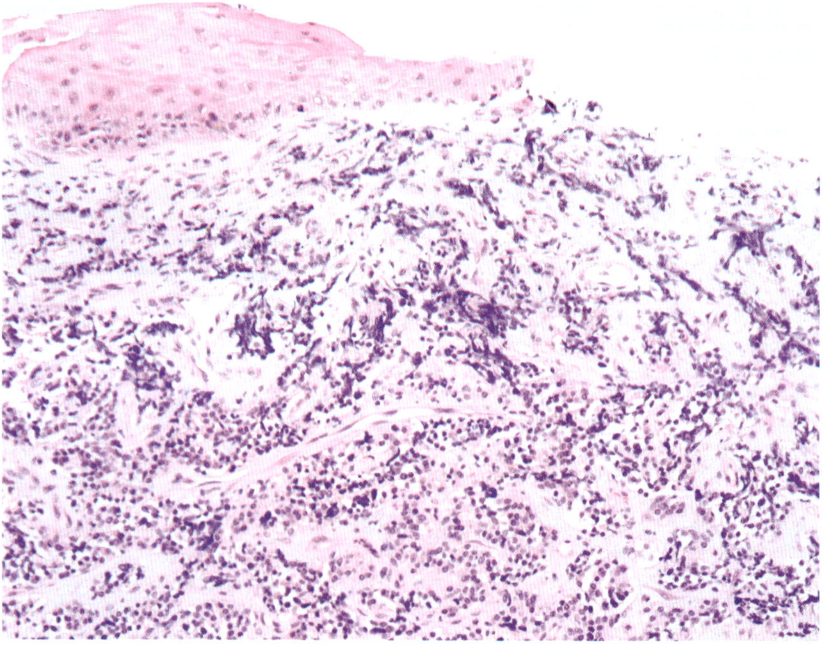
B

FIGURE 13.8 **A:** Bronchial biopsy of well-differentiated neuroendocrine carcinoma showing monotonous population of tumor cells lying beneath the squamous bronchial epithelium and showing focal crush artifact. **B:** Higher magnification shows clusters of cells with prominent crush artifact underlying the squamous mucosa with more well-preserved round, uniform tumor cells lying underneath.

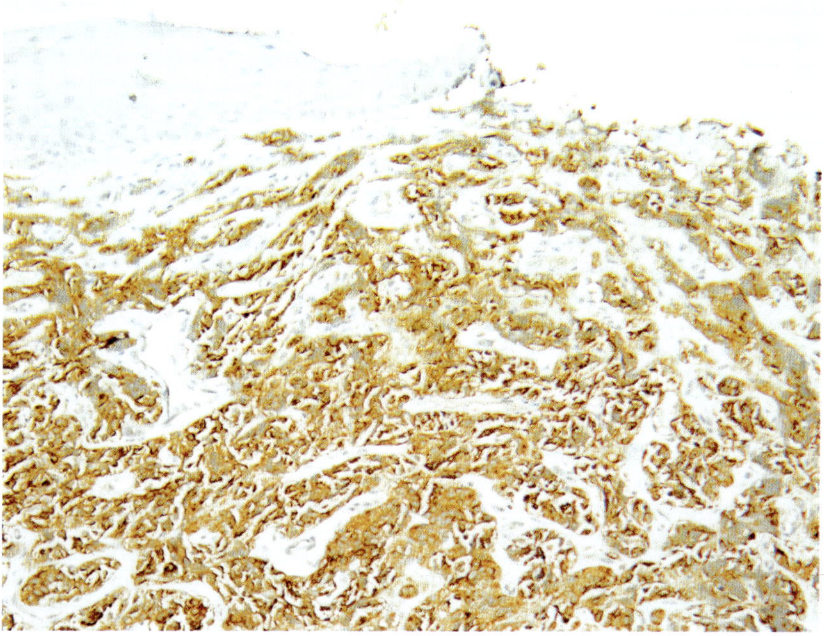

C

FIGURE 13.8 (*continued*) **C:** Immunohistochemical stain for synaptophysin shows strong cytoplasmic positivity in both the crushed and viable tumor cells.

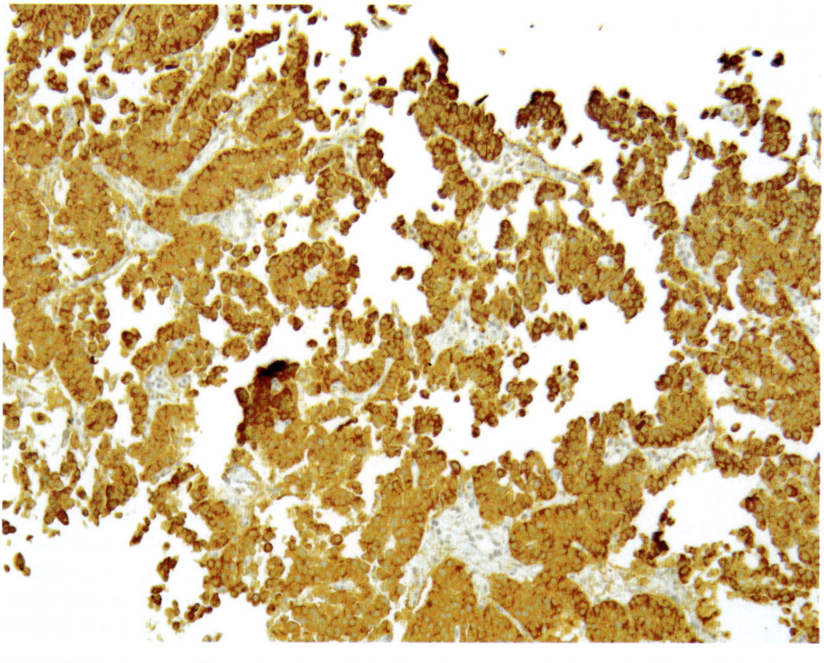

FIGURE 13.9 Immunohistochemical stain for chromogranin in well-differentiated neuroendocrine carcinoma of the lung shows strong cytoplasmic positivity in the majority of the tumor cells.

lung mass. The criteria for the histologic diagnosis of "atypical carcinoid" have remained controversial over the years and have varied widely depending on the investigator.[9,19] In general terms, we reserve the designation of moderately differentiated neuroendocrine carcinoma for tumors that still retain a recognizable neuroendocrine architectural growth pattern; however, the tumor cells show marked cytologic atypia, including enlargement of nuclei and hyperchromasia, prominent nucleoli, decreased nuclear-to-cytoplasmic ratio, and increased mitotic activity (Fig. 13.10) (eFigs. 13.4 to 13.6).[3] A coarse stippled chromatin pattern is usually still retained by these tumors, similar to that seen in well-differentiated neuroendocrine carcinoma, but they differ from the latter by harboring prominent nucleoli. Another important discriminating feature for these tumors is the presence of tumor cell necrosis. This is characteristically seen as central, comedo-like areas of necrosis within large islands of tumor cells (Fig. 13.11). The cells in moderately differentiated neuroendocrine carcinomas can be round or polygonal, but they can also adopt an oval or spindle configuration. Peripheral palisading of tumor cells within large tumor cell islands is also seen in many cases. The main criterion adopted by the WHO for the definition of atypical carcinoid is mitotic activity; tumors containing from 3 to 9 mitoses per 10 HPF are considered to fall within this category. In practice, this criterion may be very difficult to apply, as mitotic activity in these tumors can vary widely, and some tumors may have low-mitotic activity in the presence of necrosis and nuclear atypia, whereas others may have high-mitotic counts (>10 per 10 HPF) despite being well circumscribed and displaying a perfectly well-developed organoid architecture. Review of the literature reveals that mitotic activity in "atypical carcinoid" has ranged from 2 to 80 per 10 HPF, depending on the study quoted.[18,20–23] Mitotic counts can thus be a poor discriminating factor for making this diagnosis. This is particularly true in small endoscopic biopsies where an adequate mitotic count may not be possible owing to the limited amount of the specimen. In our opinion, architectural features and growth pattern play a more important role in the diagnosis of these tumors as they constitute the most important parameters for assessing the degree of differentiation of the tumor. PDNEC seldom displays a well-developed "organoid" growth pattern. The identification of a recognizable endocrine pattern of growth in a tumor with cytologic atypia and positive neuroendocrine markers should prompt consideration of a diagnosis of moderately differentiated neuroendocrine carcinoma ("atypical carcinoid").

The lack of clearly defined criteria for diagnosis in this group of tumors has also led to considerable confusion and overlap with the group of tumors known as "LCNEC" (see Poorly Differentiated Neuroendocrine Carcinoma). Making a diagnosis of moderately differentiated neuroendocrine carcinoma versus LCNEC on endoscopic biopsies can, thus, be highly problematic in most instances. A diagnosis of moderately differentiated neuroendocrine carcinoma is favored in small biopsy samples when the cytologic features of the tumor display marked atypia, with prominent nucleoli, tumor cell necrosis, and more than two mitoses in a

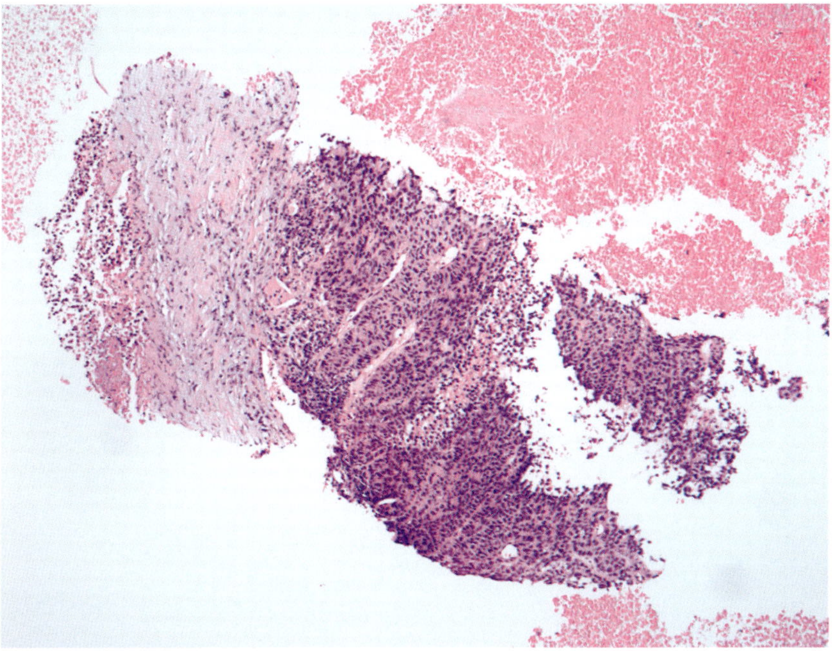

A

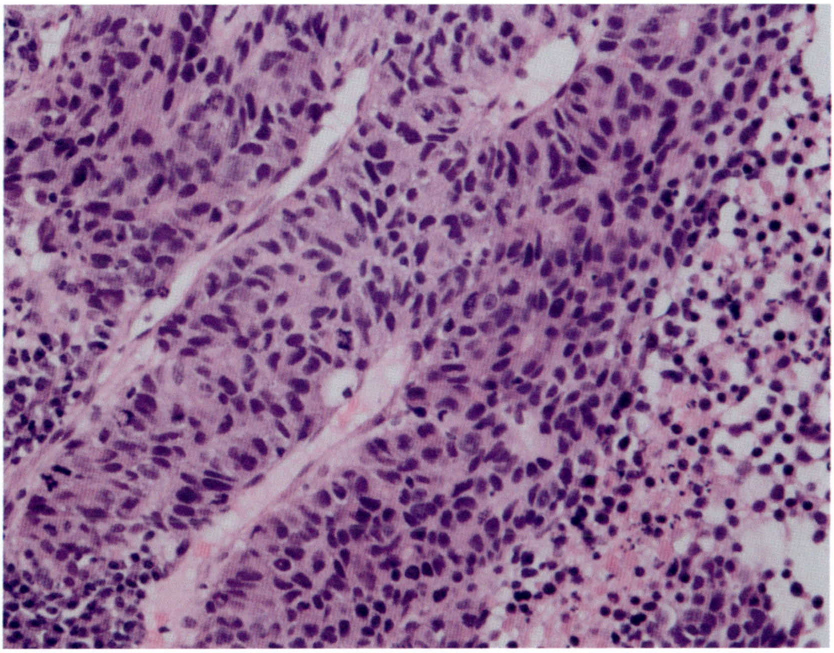

B

FIGURE 13.10 **A:** Core biopsy of moderately differentiated neuroendocrine carcinoma of the lung (atypical carcinoid) shows cords of large tumor cells with focal pinpoint areas of necrosis within the tumor and abundant necrotic debris in the vicinity. **B:** Higher magnification shows a population of atypical cells with marked nuclear pleomorphism and frequent mitoses.

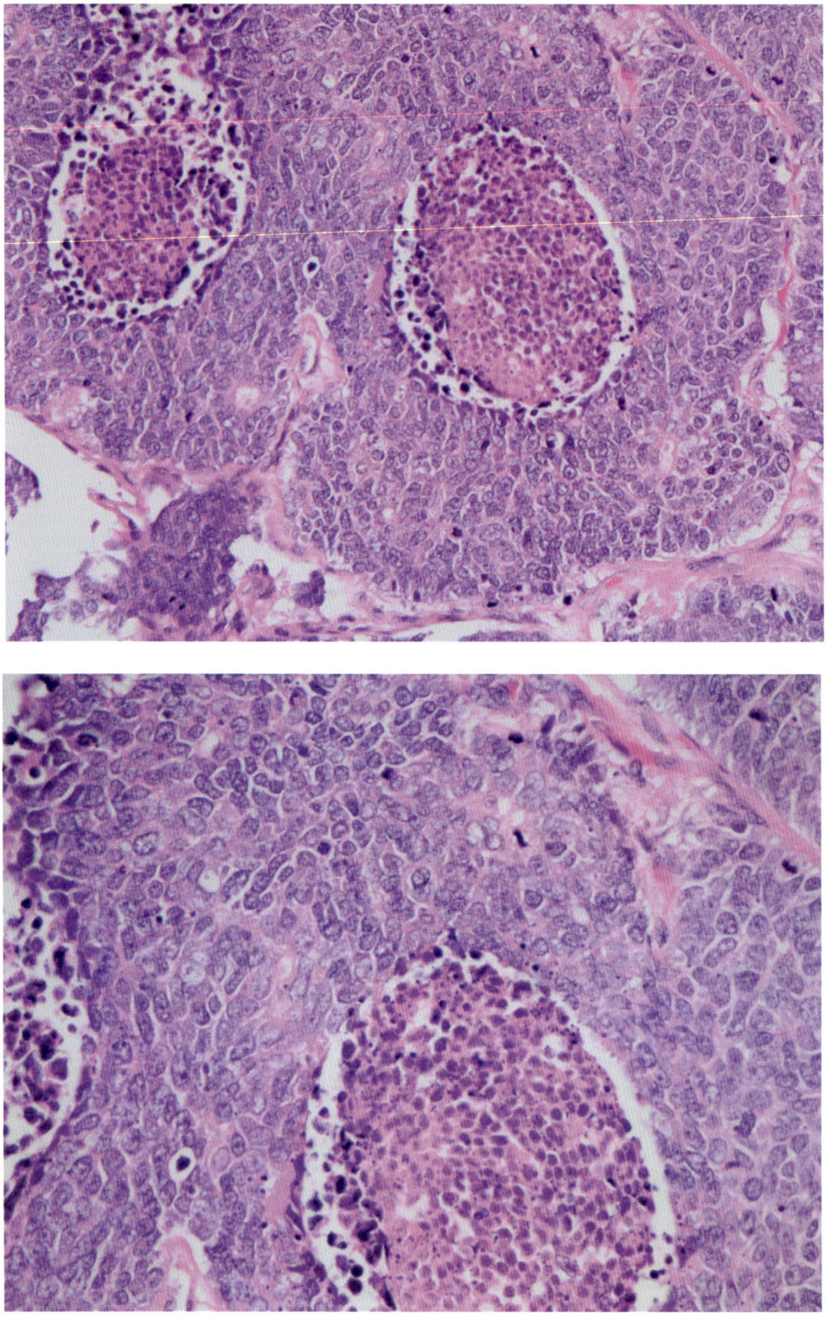

A

B

FIGURE 13.11 **A:** Moderately differentiated neuroendocrine carcinoma shows areas with central comedo-like foci of necrosis surrounded by atypical population of cells with large nuclei, visible nucleoli, and ample rim of cytoplasm. **B:** Higher magnification showing cytologic atypia of the tumor cells and abundant mitoses.

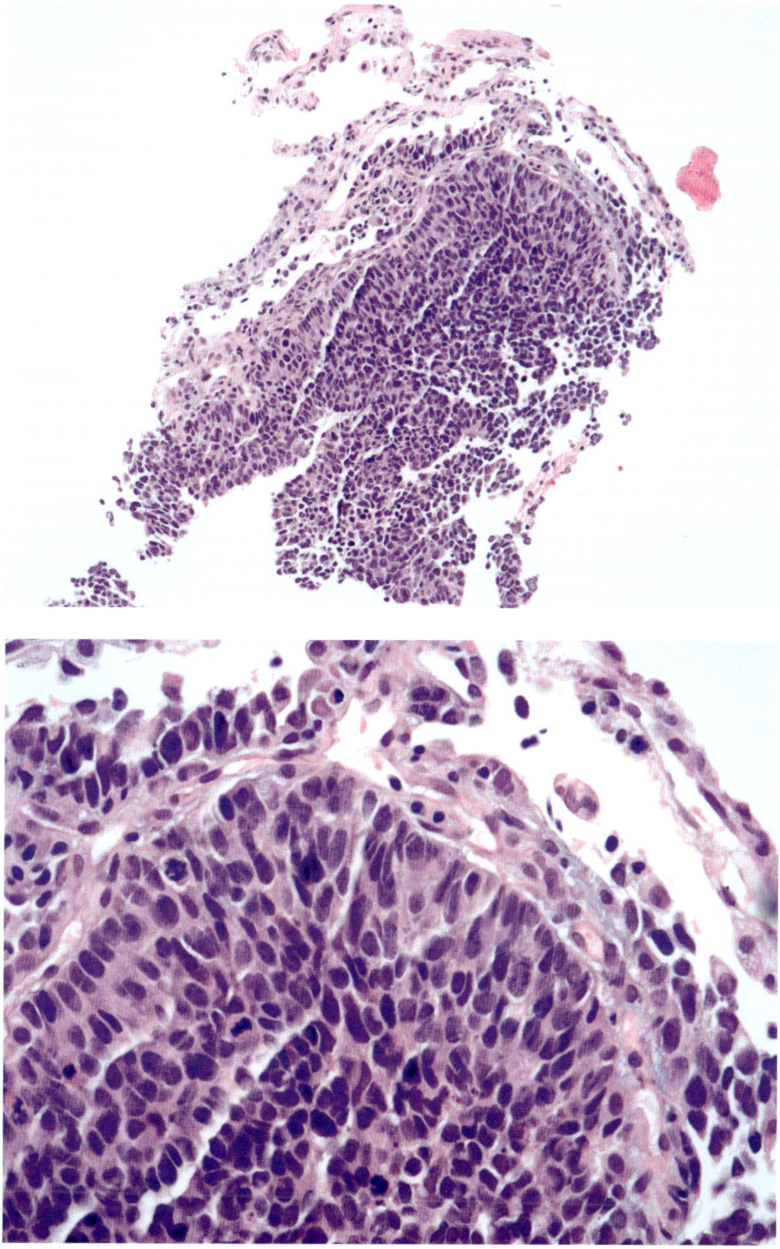

A

B

FIGURE 13.12 **A:** Endoscopic biopsy of neuroendocrine carcinoma with borderline features between atypical carcinoid and LCNEC. The tumor shows sheets of large tumor cells with abundant cytoplasm displaying a vague organoid pattern. **B:** Higher magnification shows large cells with speckled chromatin pattern, a hint of peripheral palisading of nuclei, and frequent mitotic figures. The tumor cells showed positivity for neuroendocrine markers. Tumors like this may be best categorized as "moderate to PDNEC, NOS."

tumor that is still showing a well-preserved neuroendocrine architectural growth pattern. In many instances, it may not be possible to distinguish a moderately differentiated neuroendocrine carcinoma from a PDNEC of large cell type. This situation must be acknowledged in the report, and a generic diagnosis of neuroendocrine carcinoma can be rendered with a note indicating the diagnostic possibilities and recommending complete excision and further sampling for a more definitive diagnosis (Fig. 13.12).

The immunohistochemical features of moderately differentiated neuroendocrine carcinoma are similar to those of well-differentiated neuroendocrine carcinoma, except that the extent of immunoreactivity for neuroendocrine markers may be somewhat diminished and not as intense as in well-differentiated neuroendocrine carcinoma.[24] Because these tumors occupy a central position in the spectrum of neuroendocrine lung tumors, their biologic behavior may vary depending on whether they are closer in the spectrum to well-differentiated neuroendocrine carcinoma or to poorly differentiated lesions. In general, however, the majority of published studies have demonstrated that moderately differentiated neuroendocrine carcinoma follows an aggressive behavior with a high incidence of distant metastases and tumor-associated deaths in up to 50% of patients. As with most other forms of lung cancer, clinical stage will also play a significant role in the outcome of these patients.

POORLY DIFFERENTIATED NEUROENDOCRINE CARCINOMA (SMALL CELL CARCINOMA AND LARGE CELL NEUROENDOCRINE CARCINOMA)

This designation refers to primary lung neoplasms located at the far end of the spectrum of neuroendocrine carcinomas. The prototype of poorly differentiated ("undifferentiated," in the old literature) neuroendocrine carcinoma over the years has been the small cell or oat cell type of lung carcinoma. In recent years, however, an additional category of tumors termed "LCNEC" has been added to this group.

Small cell neuroendocrine carcinoma (SCNEC) or SCLC is characterized by a close association with cigarette smoking and highly aggressive behavior; it accounts for approximately 25% of all lung carcinomas.[25] The tumors can be associated with paraneoplastic syndromes, including hypercalcemia, hyponatremia, or Cushing syndrome owing to ectopic production of peptide hormones. Symptoms include cough, hemoptysis, weight loss, hypertrophic osteoarthropathy, and fatigue. The commonest location is central in association with a proximal bronchus, although they can originate in peripheral locations in rare instances. Peribronchial or mediastinal adenopathy is a prominent finding and can be massive. Pleural involvement with pleural effusion is a common complication. Small cell carcinoma is characterized clinically by early dissemination and by being highly sensitive to chemotherapy. The tumors are thus not generally regarded as candidates for surgical excision (with the exception of early, limited disease in peripheral locations).[26] The endoscopic biopsy is therefore the only tissue that will be available for final diagnosis in the majority of patients. A diagnosis of small cell carcinoma rendered on an endoscopic biopsy usually precludes surgery as a therapeutic option. Unfortunately, the limited size of the sample and frequent artifactual distortion caused by the forceps can sometimes make the diagnosis quite difficult. In general, the majority of authors are in agreement that the diagnosis of SCNEC is a straightforward morphologic diagnosis, largely based on the histologic features as observed by the examination of hematoxylin and eosin (H&E)-stained sections. Immunohistochemical stains, however, can be of help in problematic or equivocal cases.

SCNEC can exhibit a spectrum of microscopic features (eFigs. 13.7 to 13.10). The most common form is characterized by cells that are two to three times the size of a small lymphocyte. The cell nuclei are large, hyperchromatic, with stippled or smudged chromatin, and absent or inconspicuous nucleoli imparting the cells with a "primitive" or undifferentiated appearance. The latter feature, that is, absent or inconspicuous nucleoli, is a particularly important feature to remember in the evaluation of small endoscopic biopsies to avoid making a mistaken diagnosis of SCNEC in tumors comprising sheets of "small" cells that, however, exhibit prominent or easily discernible nucleoli. This feature is of particular importance for the distinction between SCNEC and the small cell or "basaloid" variant of squamous cell carcinoma. In well-preserved samples, the cells often show a tendency for molding. The nuclei are surrounded by an indistinct, scant rim of cytoplasm (Fig. 13.13). The tumors often contain numerous apoptotic bodies and are characterized by high mitotic activity (>10 mitoses per 10 HPF). Tumor cell necrosis is a frequent finding and the necrosis is irregular and "geographic" (with jagged, irregular borders, as opposed to the comedo-like areas seen in moderately differentiated neuroendocrine carcinoma). A well-developed neuroendocrine growth pattern is usually not observed in PDNEC, although resected specimens can sometimes demonstrate focally a vague "organoid" growth pattern. Identification of a neuroendocrine growth pattern is even harder in small endoscopic biopsies and is rarely seen under such circumstances. Incrustation of basophilic nucleic acid material around vessel walls (Azzopardi phenomenon) is another frequent occurrence. Crush artifact, with distortion of the nuclei, is a common event that is frequently encountered in small endoscopic biopsies owing to the scant connective tissue stroma of these tumors. The distortion of the tumor cells may be massive and affect virtually the entire sample making definitive interpretation difficult (Fig. 13.14). Close correlation with the clinical history and radiographic findings is important in such instances before making a final diagnosis. Endoscopic biopsies can often present challenges for diagnosis not only on account of the extensive crush artifact but also owing to the paucity of well-preserved tumor cells making reliable interpretation of nuclear features difficult. The cells in SCNEC can sometimes be very small and round and closely resemble lymphocytes, thus simulating a lymphoma (Fig. 13.15). Attention to the nuclear detail

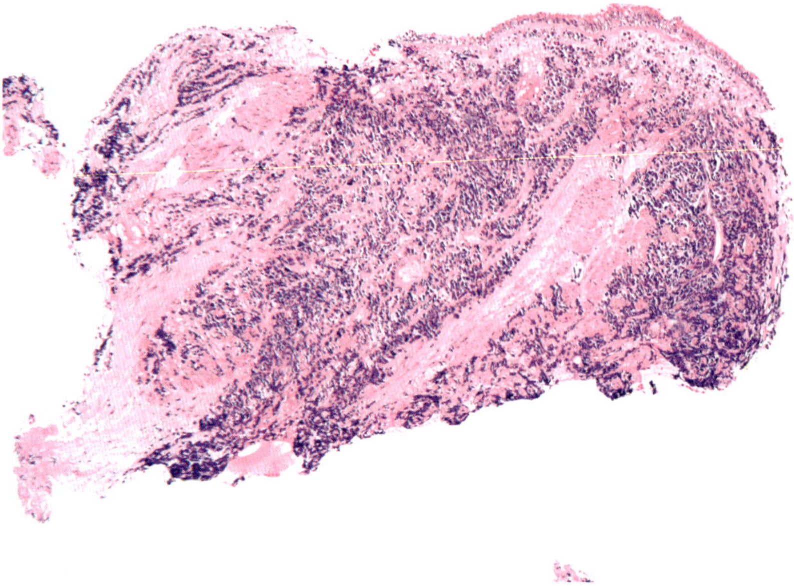

A

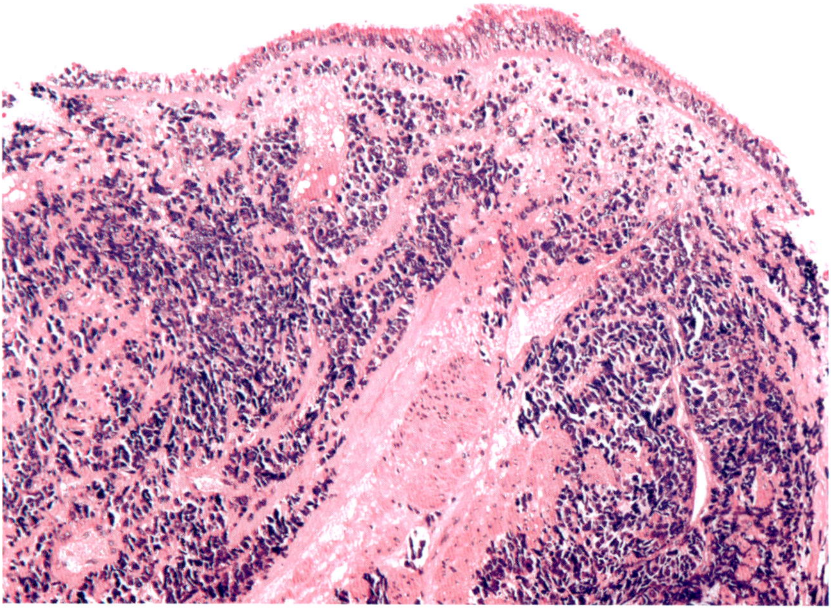

B

FIGURE 13.13 **A:** Endoscopic biopsy of SCNEC showing an overlying intact respiratory mucosa with a population of small tumor cells infiltrating the connective tissue in the submucosa. **B:** Higher magnification shows preserved small islands and clusters of primitive small tumor cells typical of small cell carcinoma.

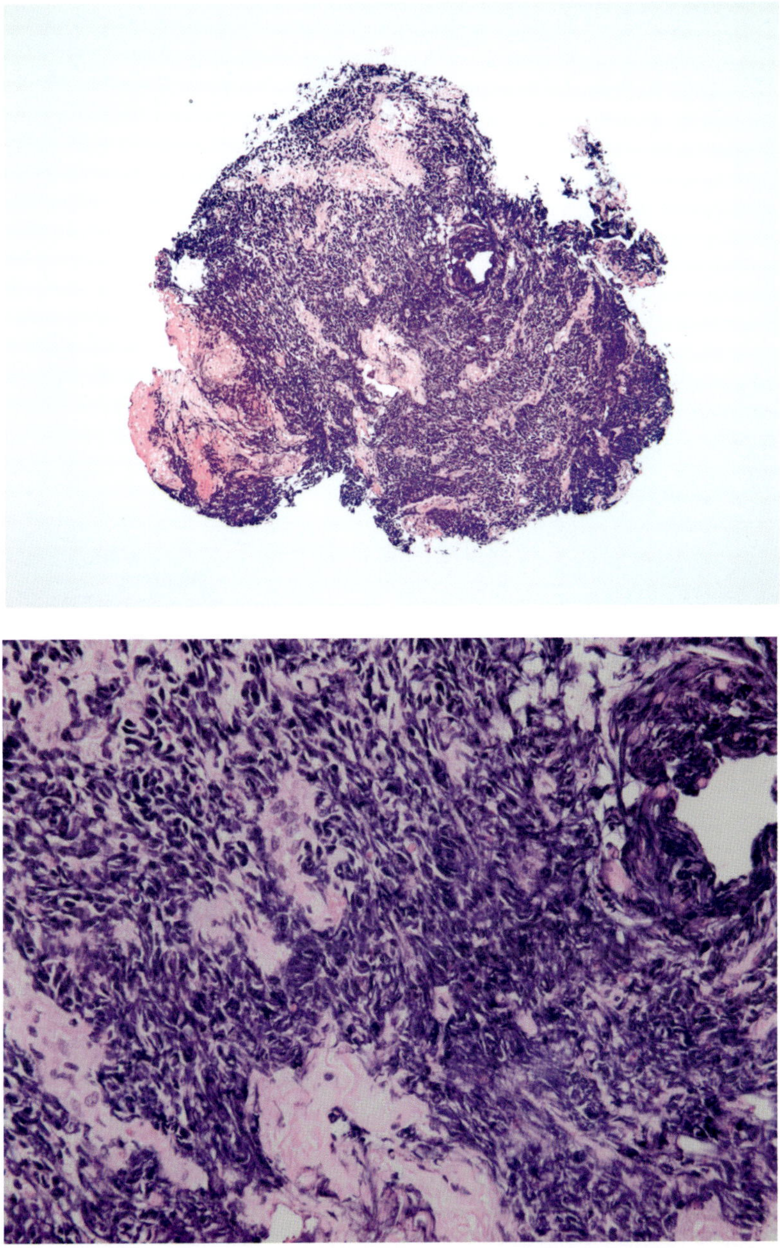

A

B

FIGURE 13.14 **A:** Small endoscopic biopsy shows sheets of small, hyperchromatic tumor cells in a haphazard arrangement with total absence of recognizable structures; this is a very common presentation of SCNEC in endoscopic biopsies. **B:** Higher magnification shows extensive distortion of the tumor cells by crushing artifact, making assessment of the cytology of the tumor impossible. Use of immunohistochemical stains may be of assistance in such cases to support a diagnosis of SCNEC.

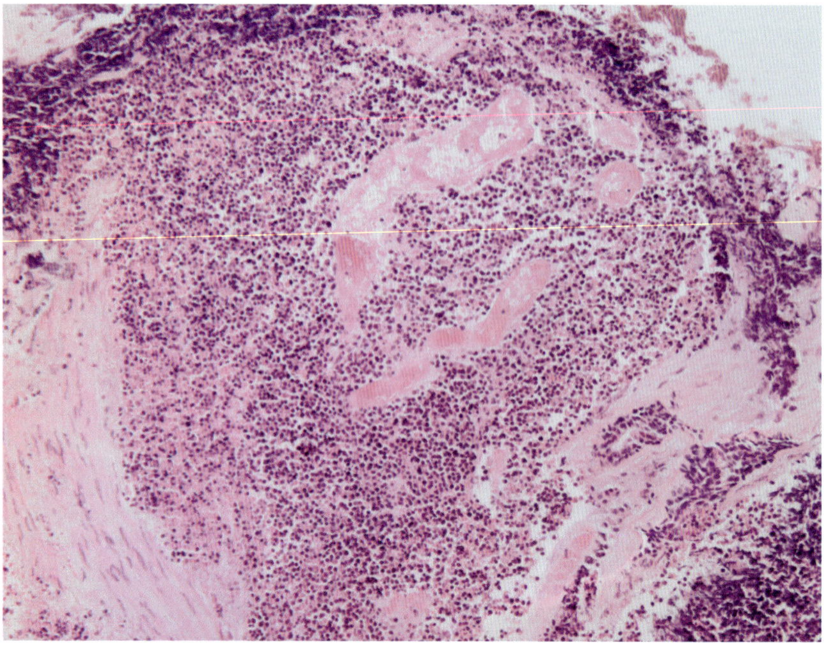

A

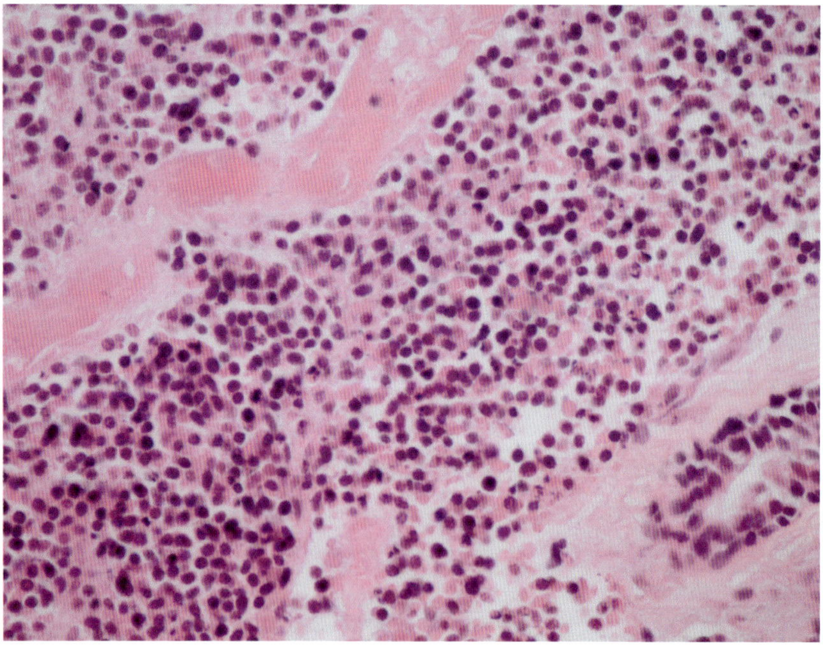

B

FIGURE 13.15 **A:** Bronchial biopsy of SCNEC, lymphocyte-like type, shows monotonous population of small round cells with peripheral areas of necrosis; tumors like this may be mistaken for lymphomas. **B:** Higher magnification shows monotonous round blue cell population with no nuclear detail and scant mitotic activity.

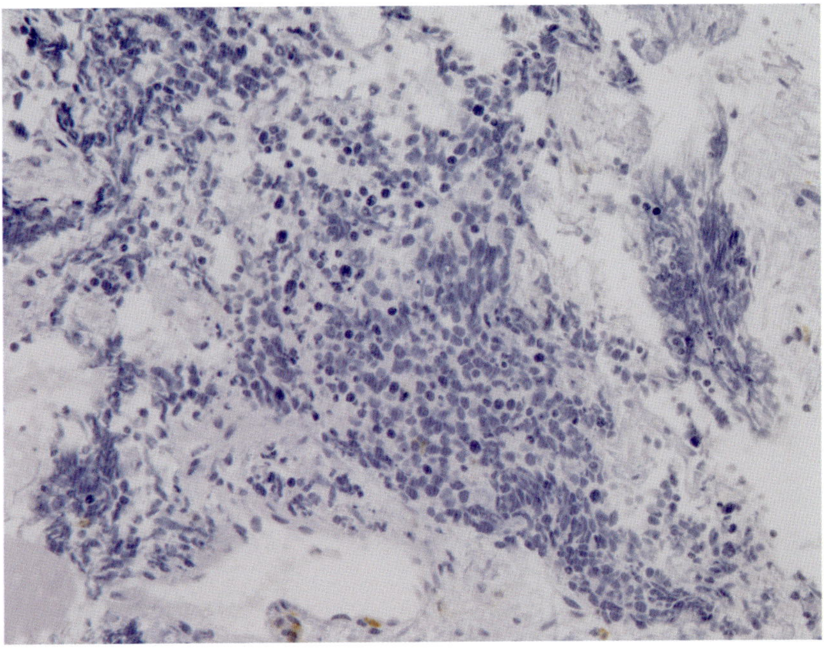

C

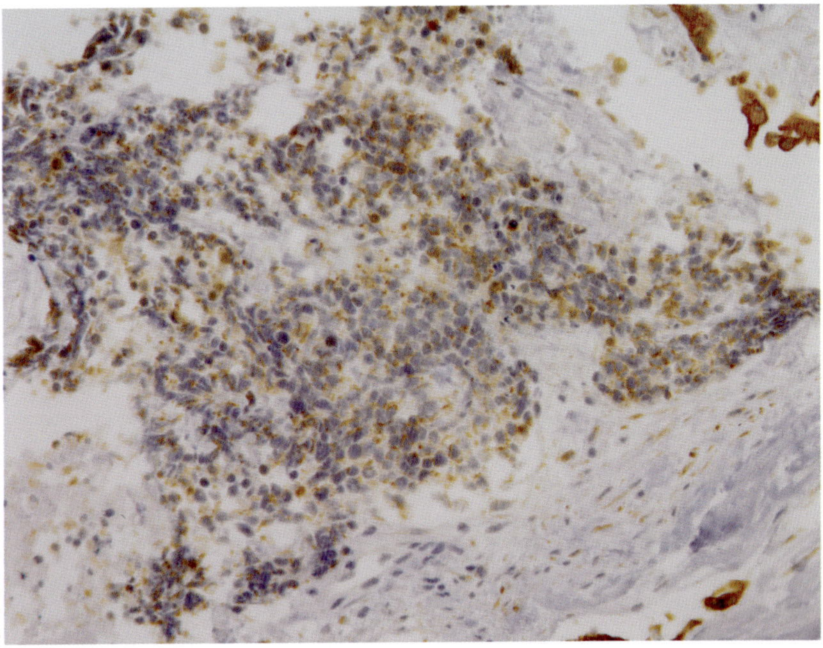

D

FIGURE 13.15 (*continued*) **C:** Immunohistochemical stain for LCA (i.e., CD45) shows negative reaction in the tumor cells. **D:** Immunohistochemical stain for CK7 shows dot-like, paranuclear positivity in the tumor cells supporting the diagnosis of PDNEC.

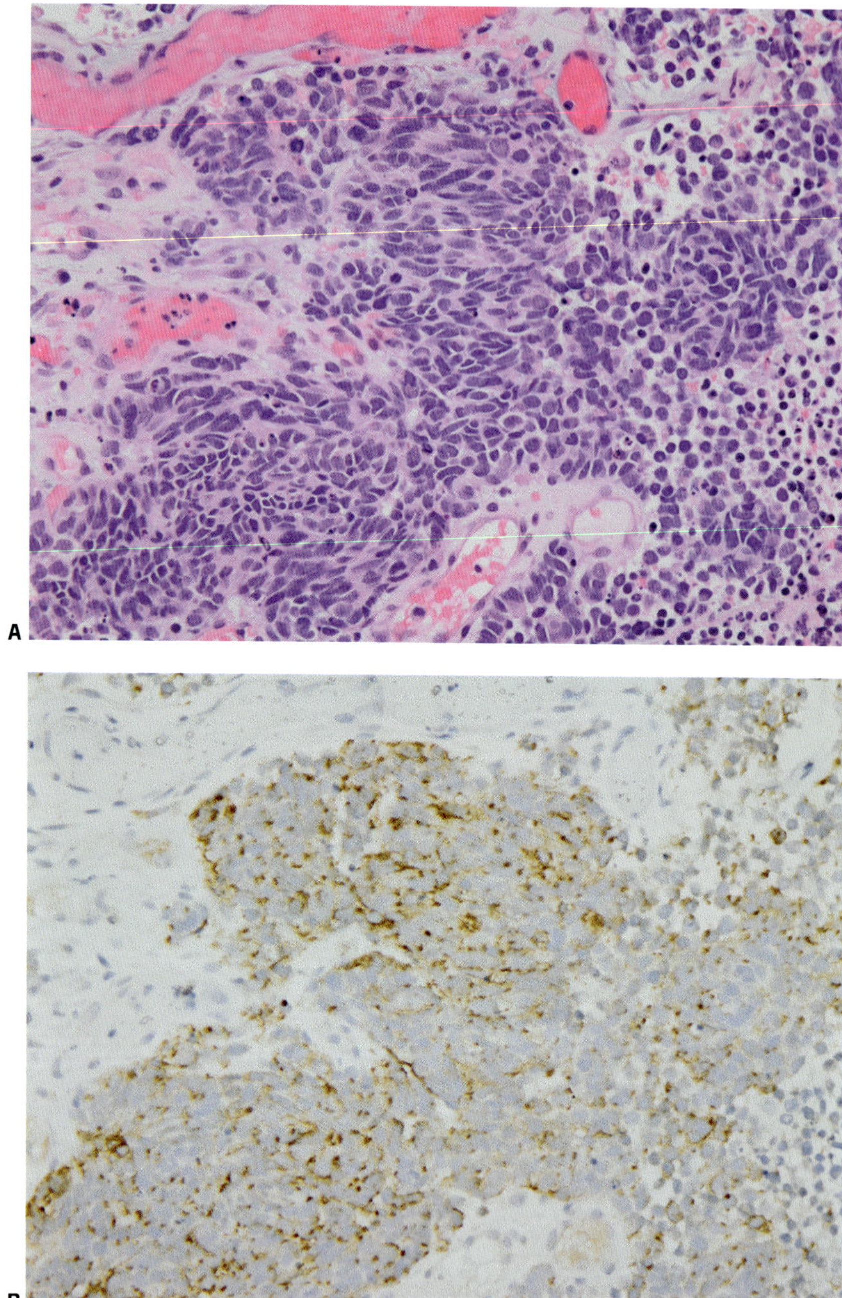

FIGURE 13.16 **A:** SCNEC showing admixture of small round cells with a prominent spindle cell component containing elongated nuclei with scant cytoplasm and distinct molding. **B:** Immunohistochemical stain for chromogranin shows cytoplasmic staining in many of the tumor cells.

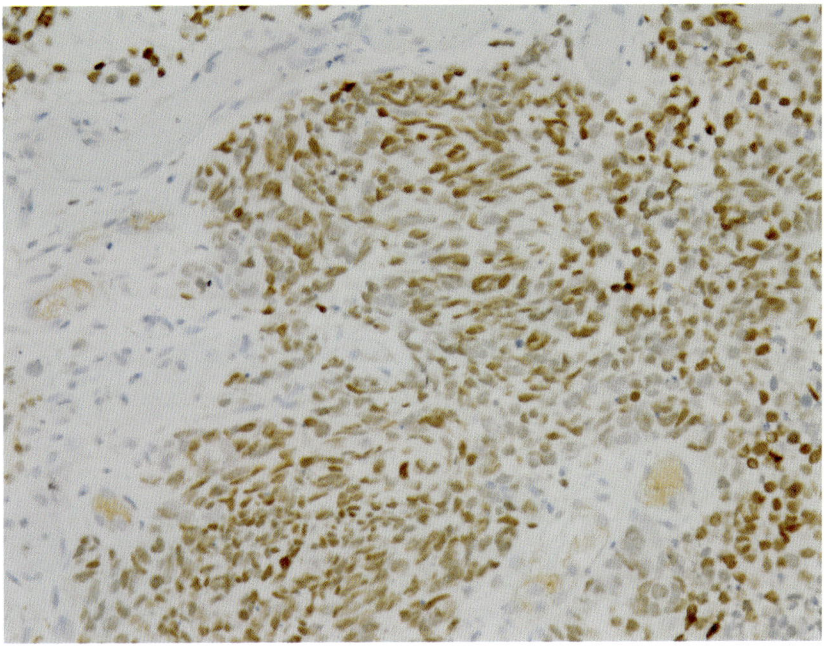

C

FIGURE 13.16 (*continued*) **C:** Immunohistochemical stain for TTF-1 shows strong nuclear positivity of the tumor cells.

will be of importance for correct diagnosis; use of immunohistochemical stains can also be of help in separating the two conditions. Another morphologic variant of SCNEC is one characterized by prominent spindling of the tumor cells. Such cases can be confused for a sarcomatous lesion in small biopsy samples; immunohistochemical stains may also be of help in separating them from its mimics (Fig. 13.16). Some other unusual morphologic variants include mixed small cell/LCNEC and combined small cell-adenocarcinoma or small cell-squamous cell carcinoma. In previous classification schemes, a *polygonal cell type* or *intermediate cell type* of small cell carcinoma was also recognized. These have been merged in the current WHO schema with the conventional small cell type and are no longer regarded as clinically significant histologic variants of these tumors. Many of the cases diagnosed as polygonal or intermediate cell type in the past most likely corresponded to moderately differentiated neuroendocrine carcinoma or LCNEC.[7] The cells in the latter type were described as being larger, oval to polygonal in shape, with sharp cell membranes, prominent nucleoli and abundant rim of cytoplasm. The description of this cell type thus significantly overlaps with that of "atypical carcinoid" and "LCNEC." It follows that distinction of these three types of tumors can be a veritable challenge in small endoscopic biopsies.

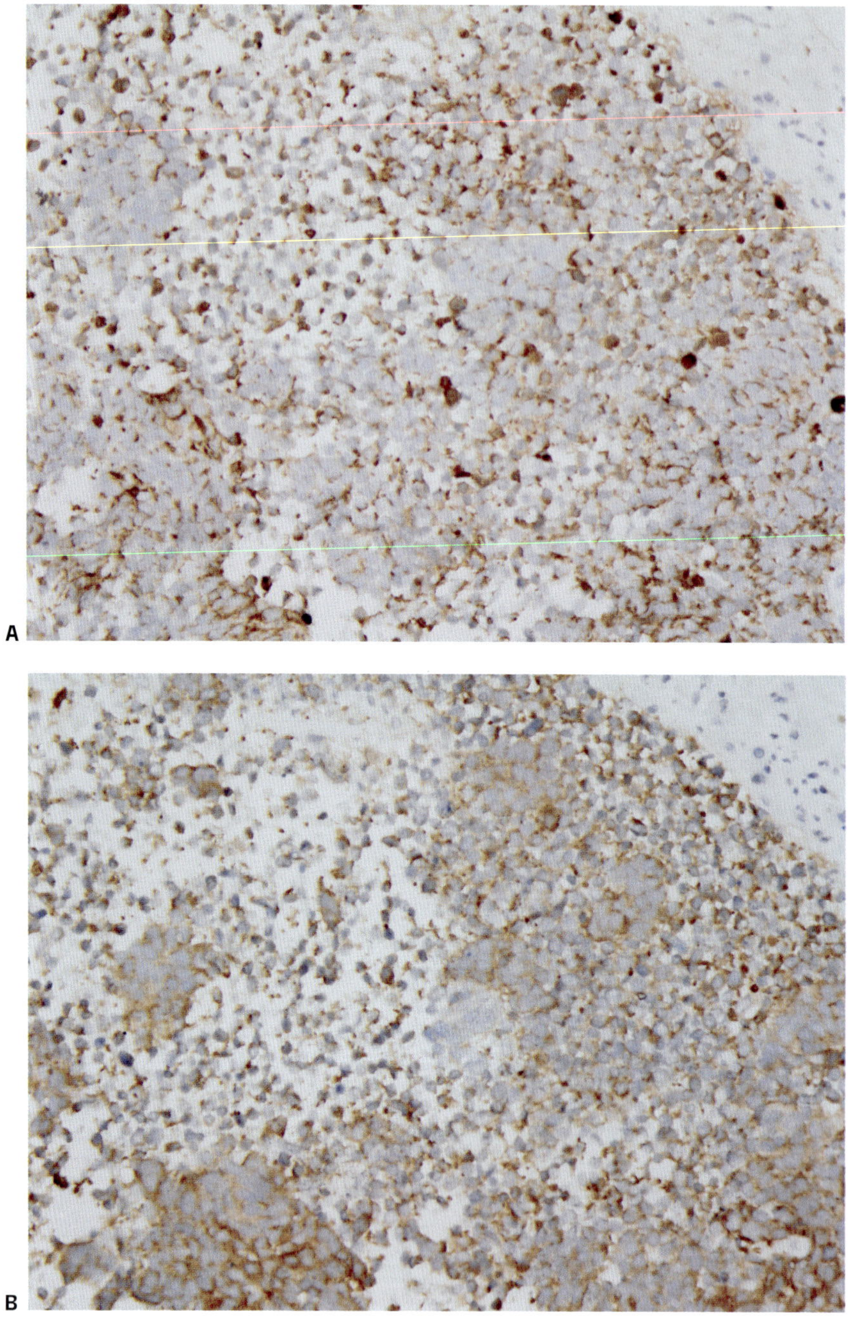

FIGURE 13.17 Immunohistochemical reactions in SCNEC of the lung. **A:** Immunohistochemical stain for CK7 shows faint cytoplasmic positivity in this small cell carcinoma, with dot-like paranuclear accentuation in many of the cells. **B:** Immunostaining for chromogranin also shows faint cytoplasmic positivity in the tumor cells.

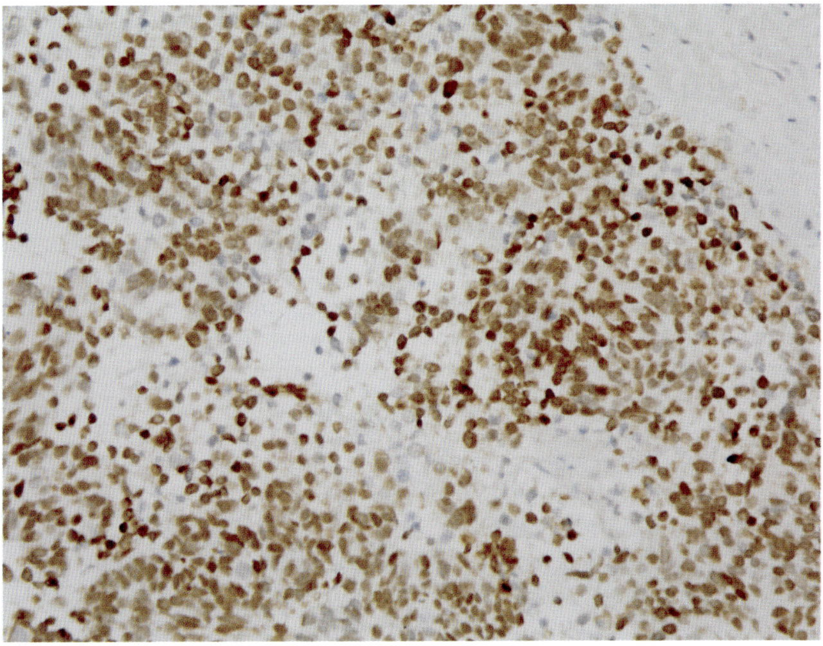

C

FIGURE 13.17 *(continued)* **C:** A TTF-1 stain shows strong nuclear positivity in the majority of the tumor cells.

The role of ancillary techniques in the diagnosis of PDNEC varies depending on the specific type of tumor examined. SCNEC consistently labels with keratin antibodies but may show variable and inconsistent expression of neuroendocrine markers. An immunohistochemical study of small cell carcinoma showed reactivity for chromogranin in transbronchial biopsy specimens in only 47% of cases and for synaptophysin in only 19%.[27] Pan-cytokeratin antibodies and low-molecular weight cytokeratins are particularly useful for the diagnosis of small cell carcinoma, and in many instances, when the cells are well preserved, they will show a characteristic dot-like paranuclear staining pattern. Another marker that has been found to be of utility, particularly for the evaluation of skin metastases, is CK7 (Fig. 13.17A), which is strongly expressed in SCNEC of the lung as opposed to primary small cell carcinoma of the skin (Merkel cell tumor), which preferentially expresses CK20 and is usually negative for CK7. Neuroendocrine markers may show variable degrees of positivity in small cell carcinoma and can be a source of confusion in small biopsy samples when they are negative. Stains such as chromogranin A, synaptophysin, NSE, and CD56 can all be positive in small cell carcinoma (Fig. 13.17B), but in tumors with extensive crush artifact or poorly preserved samples, the results of these stains may be quite difficult to evaluate. Absence of reactivity for any particular neuroendocrine marker should, therefore, not be regarded as an indication that the tumor is not an SCNEC; in fact, negative staining for neuroendocrine markers should not be used as a criterion for eliminating the diagnosis of SCNEC. The final interpretation should rely heavily on the H&E and can be supported by strong cytokeratin positivity. Another marker that may be of utility for making the diagnosis of SCNEC is TTF-1, a nuclear transcription factor, strongly expressed in the majority of SCNEC (Fig. 13.17C). Because TTF-1 is a nuclear protein, it may be very helpful in instances where the biopsy is poorly preserved or shows extensive crush artifact with loss of cytoplasmic contents. In cases showing a lymphocyte-like morphology (comprising small round cells that resemble a lymphoma), addition of a stain for leukocyte common antigen (LCA such as CD45) or other lymphoid marker (such as CD3, CD45RO, or CD20) may be of help to separate SCNEC from lymphoma. In small biopsies with extensive crush artifact, it is a good practice to add a LCA stain to the panel to ensure that the crushed cells are not lymphocytes, which are also subject to the same type of artifact. Surprisingly, strong extracellular reactivity for either LCA or keratin can be observed in between the cells in extensively crushed biopsies, pointing the pathologist in the direction of a lymphoid or epithelial neoplasm. Electron microscopy can also be utilized in cases of PDNEC to demonstrate cytoplasmic membrane-bound dense-core granules; however, this is often feasible only in resection specimens and will be of very limited utility in endoscopic biopsy samples.

LCNEC is a newly introduced category of PDNEC that has also been the subject of much confusion and debate.[8] It has been noted across most organ systems that aberrant neuroendocrine differentiation is a common occurrence in poorly differentiated neoplasms arising in epithelial organs. The lines that separate large cell carcinoma of the lung with aberrant neuroendocrine differentiation from LCNEC have not yet been clearly defined. Current recommendations by the International Association for Lung Cancer Study/American Thoracic Society/European Respiratory Society classification for small biopsy samples are that tumors showing morphologic features that are consistent with LCNEC be reported as (1) "nonsmall cell carcinoma with neuroendocrine morphology and positive neuroendocrine markers, possible LCNEC" or (2) "nonsmall cell carcinoma with neuroendocrine morphology and negative neuroendocrine markers, LCNEC suspected," thus betraying a bias to force consideration of this diagnosis in such instances.[28] Unfortunately, the situation is not that simple, and currently at least three categories of tumors that may share similar features have been recognized: (1) LCNEC, for tumors characterized by a neuroendocrine histologic growth pattern plus positivity for neuroendocrine markers; (2) large cell carcinoma with neuroendocrine morphology, for tumors characterized by a neuroendocrine histologic growth pattern but without positive neuroendocrine immunohistochemical markers; and (3) large cell carcinoma with neuroendocrine differentiation, which refers to tumors with large cell morphology but without histologic neuroendocrine growth pattern that display positivity for neuroendocrine markers.[11,29–32]

The current definition of LCNEC is that of a lung neoplasm comprising large, atypical cells (five times larger than a small lymphocyte) displaying a "neuroendocrine" light microscopic growth pattern and demonstrating evidence of neuroendocrine differentiation at the immunohistochemical or ultrastructural level (Fig. 13.18). The "organoid" or neuroendocrine growth pattern in LCNEC has been described as comprising islands or cords of tumor cells with central areas of comedonecrosis and with peripheral palisading of nuclei. Such features are said to be best appreciated in resection specimens and may be often difficult to discern in small endoscopic biopsies. Moreover, these features are not distinctive or specific for neuroendocrine tumors and may be observed in several other lung neoplasms that do not have immunohistochemical or ultrastructural evidence of neuroendocrine differentiation. The only reliable criterion for neuroendocrine differentiation in these tumors is, therefore, the demonstration of neuroendocrine features by immunohistochemistry or electron microscopy. As noted earlier, it may be very difficult, sometimes bordering on arbitrary, to determine whether the aforesaid features are the result of aberrant expression of neuroendocrine markers in an otherwise poorly differentiated adeno- or squamous cell carcinoma, or whether they truly represent evidence of primary neuroendocrine differentiation. The diagnosis of LCNEC should, thus, always be made with caution in small endoscopic biopsies. It may be preferable to make a generic diagnosis of "poorly differentiated large cell carcinoma" of the lung with a comment that the differential diagnosis includes a LCNEC and to wait for the examination of the resected specimen before a final diagnosis is rendered in equivocal cases.

Clinically, LCNEC presents with similar signs and symptoms as other conventional lung cancers and are closely associated with cigarette smoking.[33–35] The tumors may occur in central location but are more often located in the periphery or subpleural portions of the lung. They are therefore more often sampled by core needle biopsy or open lung biopsy than through the endoscope. The biologic behavior of these tumors has varied depending on the study cited, but most studies are in agreement that the tumors behave aggressively and have a similar outcome as large cell carcinoma of the lung.

The role of immunohistochemical markers is more critical in the diagnosis of LCNEC than in the small cell carcinoma type. The demonstration of unequivocal evidence of neuroendocrine differentiation is part of the requirements for the current definition of this entity and, therefore,

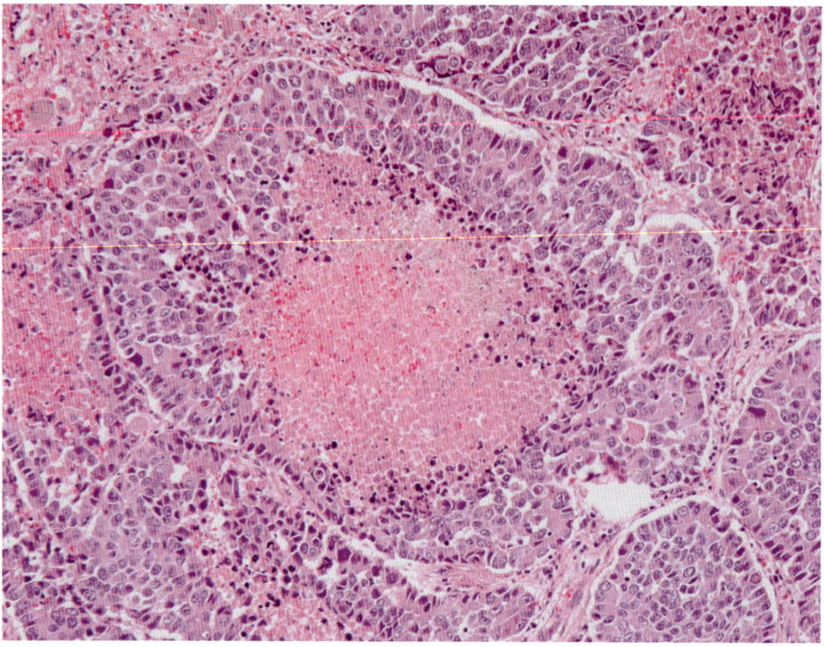
A

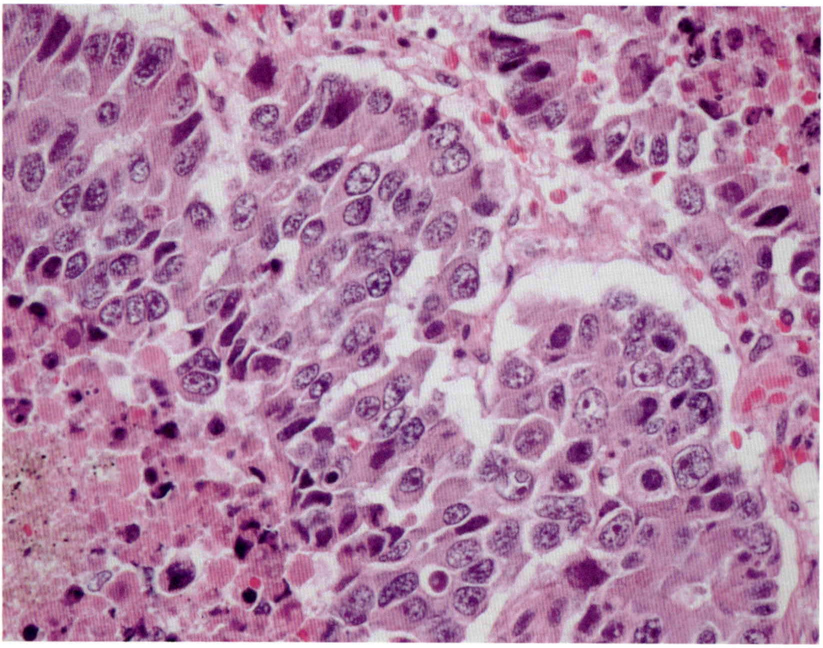
B

FIGURE 13.18 **A:** LCNEC of the lung shows islands of large tumor cells with central comedonecrosis and peripheral palisading of nuclei; notice close similarity with moderately differentiated neuroendocrine carcinoma of the lung (atypical carcinoid). **B:** Higher magnification of LCNEC shows cells with enlarged nuclei and prominent nucleoli.

C 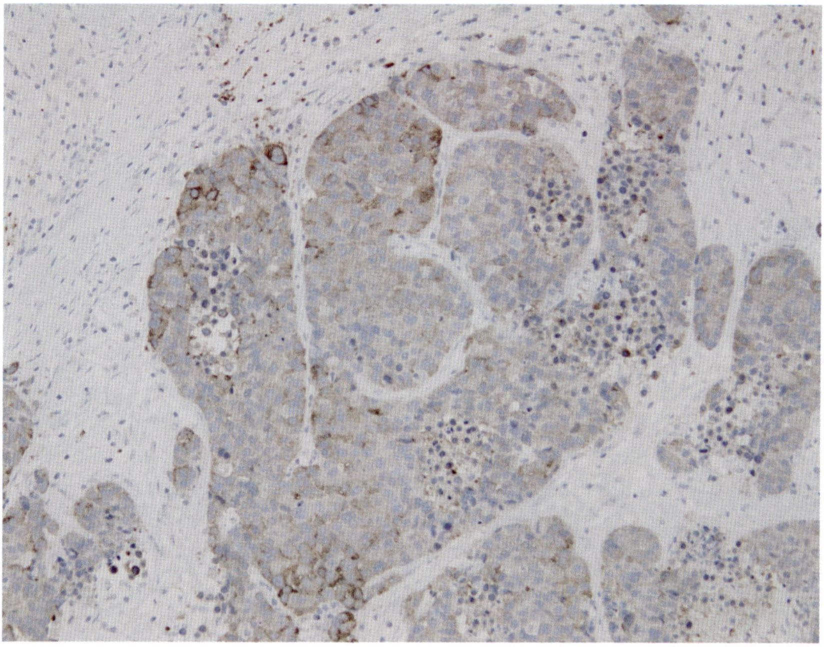

FIGURE 13.18 (*continued*) **C:** Immunohistochemical staining for chromogranin in LCNEC shows cytoplasmic positivity of the tumor cells. Positive staining for neuroendocrine markers is an indispensable requirement for making this diagnosis.

must be applied in every case. All cases of LCNEC should demonstrate cytokeratin positivity and virtually all will react with antibodies to NSE. Chromogranin A is the most consistently detected specific neuroendocrine marker; synaptophysin and CD56 are less frequently observed.[36] The extent or intensity of labeling that is necessary to separate LCNEC from large cell carcinoma with aberrant neuroendocrine differentiation has not been determined. Electron microscopy has also been claimed to demonstrate dense core neurosecretory granules in the cytoplasm of the tumor cells in all cases and can be used as alternative evidence of neuroendocrine differentiation in cases where adequately fixed material is available for that study. For the time being, LCNEC remains a controversial diagnosis because of the difficulties in separating this condition from large cell carcinoma with aberrant (or spurious) neuroendocrine differentiation, large cell carcinoma with an architectural growth pattern that may be suggestive of neuroendocrine differentiation, and moderately differentiated neuroendocrine carcinoma (atypical carcinoid), from which precise criteria for distinction do not exist. It is possible that in coming years, the category of LCNEC may be eliminated altogether and merged with moderately differentiated neuroendocrine carcinoma, with which it closely shares morphologic, immunohistochemical, and biologic features.

OTHER NEUROENDOCRINE LUNG TUMORS

Neuroendocrine tumors of the lung of nonepithelial origin are quite rare and include primary intrapulmonary paraganglioma and primary PNETs of the lung.

Pulmonary Paraganglioma

The existence of this tumor has been controversial for many years, with some authors claiming that primary tumors of this type do not exist in the lung and represent either metastases or misdiagnosed carcinoid tumors and others who support their existence. We have observed a few rare examples of primary lung tumors that exhibited all the features of paraganglioma in whom an extrapulmonary source of the tumor could not be detected on thorough clinical and radiographic examination.[11] The majority of patients reported in the literature have been middle-aged adults with a slight male predominance. Some patients have been associated with the MEN-II syndrome. Many of the tumors were clinically characterized by the active production of neuropeptides leading to clinical manifestations of Cushing syndrome Verner–Morrison syndrome, or episodes of sustained hypertension. Nonfunctional tumors usually come to the attention of the physician owing to symptoms caused by the growing intrapulmonary mass lesion. The tumors can be central and close to major airways, or they can be peripheral; the latter is most commonly found incidentally on chest X-rays. Histologically, the tumors are characterized by their prominent nested neuroendocrine growth pattern (Zellballen) separated by thin fibrovascular septa.[37] Unlike well-differentiated neuroendocrine carcinoma ("carcinoid" tumors), ribbons, trabeculae, festoons, and rosettes are not a feature of paragangliomas. The tumor cells are usually large, round to oval with centrally placed nuclei, and often show nucleomegaly with bizarre nuclear forms, large hyperchromatic nuclei, and intranuclear pseudoinclusions owing to cytoplasmic invaginations. Despite the marked nuclear pleomorphism and atypia, however, mitotic activity and tumor cell necrosis are minimal or absent. The presence of mitotic activity is not a very reliable indicator of malignancy as it may be seen in both benign and malignant forms. By immunohistochemistry, paragangliomas uniformly react with neuroendocrine markers, particularly chromogranin A and synaptophysin. A distinctive feature of paragangliomas that is very useful for separating them from other epithelial neuroendocrine neoplasms is the absence of reactivity for cytokeratins. Because of the positivity for neuroendocrine markers and the frequent presence of focal cytologic atypia, the lesions must be distinguished from LCNEC. This is best accomplished by the demonstration of the absence of cytokeratin reactivity and by noting the absence of brisk mitotic activity in paraganglioma. The most important differential diagnosis of paraganglioma is with well-differentiated neuroendocrine carcinoma ("carcinoid tumor"), particularly in small biopsy samples or when the characteristic nucleomegaly is not evident. Absence of cytokeratin reactivity will also be critical for making this distinction, as carcinoids are almost universally positive for cytokeratin. In previous years, the presence of a rich network of S-100 protein sustentacular cells surrounding the tumor cell islands was regarded as a valuable criterion for establishing the above distinction, but more recent studies have demonstrated that these sustentacular cells can also be seen in carcinoid tumors, thus severely limiting their value for making this diagnosis.

Pulmonary PNET

Pulmonary PNETs are rare neoplasms of the lung. Only three cases have been reported so far in literature.[38,39] The tumors essentially show features of small blue cell tumors at other locations with strong membrane positivity for CD99 and harbor a t(11;22) chromosomal translocation typical of this family of tumors. The differential diagnosis involves other small round cell tumors of the lung, including lymphoma/leukemia and small cell carcinoma, and metastases to the lung from PNET arising in other organs.

REFERENCES

1. Moran CA, Suster S, Coppola D, et al. Neuroendocrine carcinomas of the lung: a critical analysis. *Am J Clin Pathol.* 2009;131:206–221.
2. Suster S, Moran CA. Tumors of the lung and pleura. In: Fletcher CDM, ed. *Diagnostic Histopathology of Tumors.* 4th ed. London: Churchill Livingstone. In press.
3. Suster S, Moran CA. The lung. In: Weidner N, Cote R, Suster S, et al, eds. *Modern Surgical Pathology.* 2nd ed. Philadelphia, PA: WB Saunders; 2009.
4. Wick MR, Ritter JH. Neuroendocrine neoplasia of the lung. *Ann Thorac Surg.* 2000; 69:307–308.
5. Travis WD, Brambilla E, Muller-Hermelink HK, et al. *World Health Organization Classification of Tumors. Pathology & Genetics, Tumors of the Lung, Pleura, Mediastinum and Heart.* Lyon, France: IARC Press; 2004.
6. Travis WD, Gal AA, Colby TV, et al. Reproducibility of neuroendocrine lung tumor classification. *Hum Pathol.* 1998;29:272–279.
7. Marchevsky AM, Gal AA, Shah S, et al. Morphometry confirms the presence of considerable nuclear size overlap between "small cells" and "large cells" in high-grade pulmonary neuroendocrine neoplasms. *Am J Clin Pathol.* 2001;116:466–472.
8. Travis WD, Linnoila RI, Tsokos MG, et al. Neuroendocrine tumors of the lung with proposed criteria for large-cell neuroendocrine carcinoma: an ultrastructural, immunohistochemical, and flow cytometric study of 35 cases. *Am J Surg Pathol.* 1991;15:529–553.
9. Travis WD, Rush W, Flieder DB, et al. Survival analysis of 200 pulmonary neuroendocrine tumors with clarification of criteria for atypical carcinoid and its separation from typical carcinoid. *Am J Surg Pathol.* 1998;22:934–944.
10. Fink G, Krelbaum T, Yellin A, et al. Pulmonary carcinoid: presentation, diagnosis, and outcome in 142 cases in Israel and review of 640 cases from the literature. *Chest.* 2001; 119:1647–1651.
11. Moran CA, Suster S. *Tumors and Tumor-Like Conditions of the Lung and Pleura.* Philadelphia, PA: WB Saunders; 2010:137–164.

12. Kalhor N, Suster S, Moran CA. Primary sclerosing neuroendocrine carcinomas of the lung: a clinicopathologic and immunohistochemical study of 10 cases. *Am J Clin Pathol.* 2010;133:618–622.
13. Moran CA, Suster S. Cystic well-differentiated neuroendocrine carcinoma (carcinoid tumor): a clinicopathologic and immunohistochemical study of two cases. *Am J Clin Pathol.* 2006;126:377–380.
14. Sklar JL, Churg A, Bensch KG. Oncocytic carcinoid tumor of the lung. *Am J Surg Pathol.* 1980;4:287–292.
15. Gal AA, Koss MN, Hochholzer L, et al. Pigmented pulmonary carcinoid tumor. *Arch Pathol Lab Med.* 1993;117:832–836.
16. Cai YC, Banner B, Glickman J, et al. Cytokeratin 7 and 20 and thyroid transcription factor 1 can help distinguish pulmonary from gastrointestinal carcinoid and pancreatic endocrine tumors. *Hum Pathol.* 2001;32:1087–1093.
17. Sturm N, Rossi G, Lantuejoul S, et al. Expression of thyroid transcription factor-1 in the spectrum of neuroendocrine cell lung proliferations with special interest in carcinoids. *Hum Pathol.* 2002;33:175–182.
18. Arrigoni MG, Woolner LB, Bernatz PE. Atypical carcinoid tumors of the lung. *J Thorac Cardiovasc Surg.* 1972;64:413–421.
19. Soga J, Yakuwa Y. Bronchopulmonary carcinoids: An analysis of 1875 reported cases with special reference to a comparison between typical carcinoids and atypical varieties. *Ann Thorac Cardiovasc Surg.* 1999;5:211–219.
20. Gould VE, Linnoila RI, Memoli VA, et al. Neuroendocrine cells and neuroendocrine neoplasms of the lung. *Pathol Annu.* 1983;18:287–330.
21. Paladugu RR, Benfield JR, Pak HY, et al. Bronchopulmonary Kulchitzky cell carcinoma: a new classification scheme for typical and atypical carcinoids. *Cancer.* 1985;55:1303–1311.
22. Valli M, Fabris GA, Dewar A, et al. Atypical carcinoid tumors of the lung: a study of 33 cases with prognostic features. *Histopathology.* 1994;24:363–369.
23. Mills SE, Cooper PH, Walker AN, et al. Atypical carcinoid tumor of the lung. *Am J Surg Pathol.* 1982;6:643–654.
24. Wick MR. Immunohistology of neuroendocrine and neuroectodermal tumors. *Semin Diagn Pathol.* 2000;17:194–203.
25. Leslie KO, Colby TV. Pathology of lung cancer. *Curr Opin Pulm Med.* 1997;3:252–256.
26. Johnson DH. Management of small cell lung cancer: current state of the art. *Chest.* 1999;116(6 suppl):525S–530S.
27. Guinee DG Jr, Fishback NF, Koss MN, et al. The spectrum of immunohistochemical staining of small-cell lung carcinoma in specimens from transbronchial and open-lung biopsies. *Am J Clin Pathol.* 1994;102:406–414.
28. Travis WD, Brambilla E, Noguchi M, et al. International Association for the Study of Lung Cancer/American Thoracic Society/European Respiratory Society international multidisciplinary classification of lung adenocarcinoma. *J Thorac Oncol.* 2011;6:244–285.
29. Iyoda A, Hiroshima K, Baba M, et al. Pulmonary large cell carcinomas with neuroendocrine features are high-grade neuroendocrine tumors. *Ann Thorac Surg.* 2002;73:1049–1054.
30. Howe MC, Chapman A, Kerr K, et al. Neuroendocrine differentiation in non-small cell lung cancer and its relation to prognosis and therapy. *Histopathology.* 2004;46:195–201.
31. Ionescu DN, Treaba D, Gilks CB, et al. Nonsmall cell lung carcinoma with neuroendocrine differentiation—an entity of no clinical or prognostic significance. *Am J Surg Pathol.* 2007;31:26–32.

32. Iyoda A, Hiroshima K, Toyozaki T, et al. Clinical characterization of pulmonary large cell neuroendocrine carcinoma and large cell carcinoma with neuroendocrine morphology. *Cancer*. 2001;91:1992–2000.
33. Dresler CM, Ritter JH, Patterson GA, et al. Clinical–pathologic analysis of 40 patients with large cell neuroendocrine carcinoma of the lung. *Ann Thorac Surg*. 1997;63: 180–185.
34. Takei H, Asamura H, Maeshima A, et al. Large cell neuroendocrine carcinoma of the lung: a clinicopathologic study of eighty-seven cases. *J Thorac Cardiovasc Surg*. 2002;124:285–292.
35. Paci M, Cavazza A, Annessi V, et al. Large cell neuroendocrine carcinoma of the lung: a 10-year clinicopathologic retrospective study. *Ann Thorac Surg*. 2004;77:1163–1167.
36. Jiang SX, Kameya T, Shoji M, et al. Large cell neuroendocrine carcinoma of the lung: a histologic and immunohistochemical study of 22 cases. *Am J Surg Pathol*. 1998;22: 526–537.
37. Aubertine CL, Flieder DB. Primary paraganglioma of the lung. *Ann Diagn Pathol*. 2004;8:237–241.
38. Imamura F, Funakoshi T, Nakamura S, et al. Primary primitive neuroectodermal tumor of the lung: report of two cases. *Lung Cancer*. 2000;27:55–60.
39. Mikami Y, Nakajima M, Hashimoto H, et al. Primary pulmonary primitive neuroectodermal tumor (PNET): a case report. *Pathol Res Pract*. 2001;197:113–119.

14

UNUSUAL LUNG TUMORS AND TUMOR-LIKE CONDITIONS

A series of unusual lung tumors and tumor-like conditions can be occasionally encountered in lung biopsies. These include primary and metastatic sarcomas, lung tumors derived from presumed ectopic tissues, various lung tumors of uncertain histogenesis, and a few rare benign tumors and tumor-like conditions.

MESENCHYMAL NEOPLASMS

Varied mesenchymal neoplasms can arise in the lung, although the presence of a sarcoma in the lung, most often, is the result of a metastasis from a distant soft tissue site.[1] Clinicopathologic correlation and a thorough clinical history are, therefore, essential for a correct interpretation.

Benign Mesenchymal Neoplasms

Benign mesenchymal neoplasms that can originate in the lung include cartilaginous hamartoma, pulmonary adenofibroma, endobronchial lipoma, leiomyoma, schwannoma, neurofibroma, and intrapulmonary solitary fibrous tumor.

Cartilaginous hamartoma is probably the most common benign mesenchymal neoplasm of the lung. The term "hamartoma" was coined because of the presence of an admixture of mature cartilage with mature adipose tissue, myxoid stroma, or a fibroblastic spindle cell component. Recent studies have demonstrated a high frequency of mutations in these tumors, more suggestive of a neoplastic process.[2] The majority of these lesions present as a solitary "coin lesion" within lung parenchyma, but they may also present as endobronchial tumors causing bronchial obstruction. Histologically, they are characterized by lobules comprising mature hyaline cartilage surrounded by other mesenchymal elements such as fat, bone, smooth muscle, and occasional myxoid matrix with sparse fibroblastic spindle cells (Fig. 14.1). A characteristic feature is the entrapment of benign respiratory epithelium from the surrounding lung parenchyma inside the cartilaginous lesion. The latter feature serves to separate them from bronchopulmonary chondromas, which tend to be multiple when seen as part of Carney triad. *Pulmonary adenofibroma* is a rare lesion of disputed histogenesis that is characterized

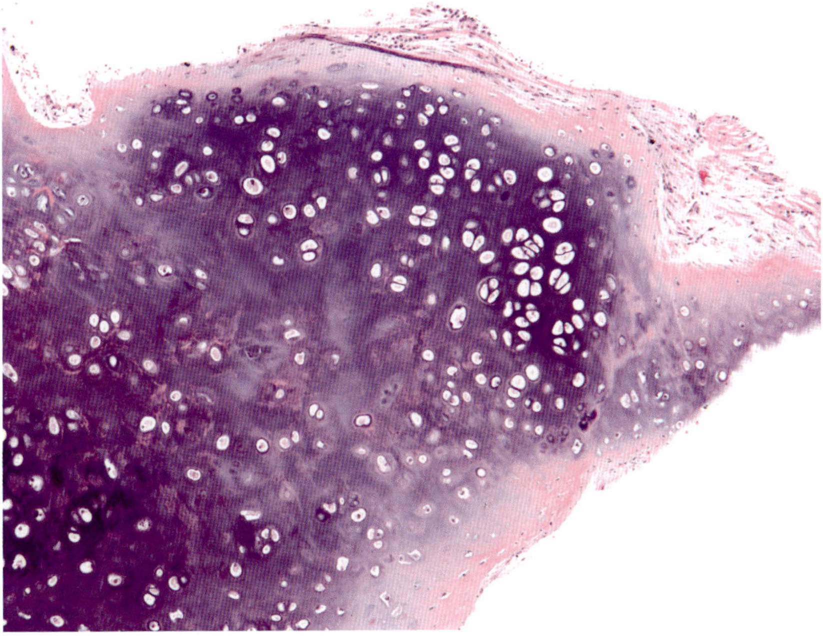

FIGURE 14.1 Endoscopic biopsy of cartilaginous hamartoma shows mature hyaline cartilage surrounded by fibroconnective tissue.

by club-like papillae lined by cuboidal or columnar cells that contain a bland fibroblastic spindle cell proliferation in the cores of the papillae.[3] The histologic appearance of the lesion is reminiscent of Mullerian adenofibromas of the female genital tract and ovary. The lesions are usually small (1 to 2 cm) and intraparenchymatous, without relationship to the bronchial tree. The spindle cells stain only with vimentin and are negative for all other specific markers such as smooth muscle actin (SMA), desmin, S-100 protein, and CD34. Similar tumors can also show expression of smooth muscle-associated markers, such as SMA, H-caldesmon, and desmin and have been designated as adenomyomas. It has been postulated that they may represent hamartomatous lesions, similar to cartilaginous hamartoma but lacking the cartilaginous component. *Endobronchial lipomas* affect adult patients in their fifth or sixth decade of life and present with clinical signs and symptoms of bronchial obstruction.[4] The tumors can range in size from 1 to 5 cm in greatest diameter and are soft, yellow, and well circumscribed (Fig. 14.2). They are histologically characterized by mature adipose tissue without any evidence of cytologic atypia. Tumors characterized by a prominent vascular component associated with a perivascular epithelioid smooth muscle proliferation, in addition to adipose tissue, are diagnostic of *angiomyolipoma*.[5] Such tumors are most often seen in the background of tuberous sclerosis and are characterized by coexpression of melanocytic (HMB45) and smooth muscle markers (SMA) in the epithelioid perivascular cells. *Pulmonary leiomyoma* is a rare tumor that has been

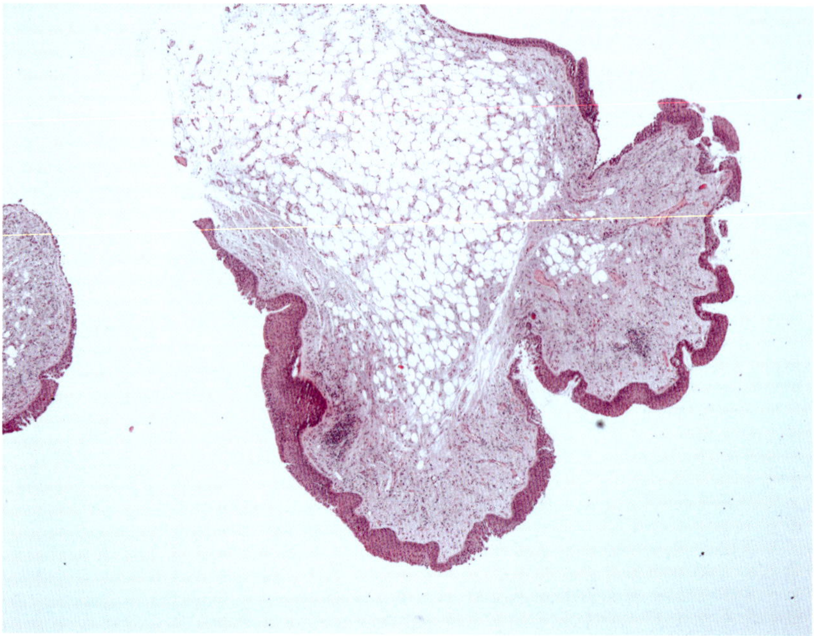

FIGURE 14.2 Endoscopic biopsy of endobronchial lipoma shows an intact overlying squamous mucosa overlying a well-circumscribed proliferation of mature adipose tissue.

the subject only of case reports. Care must be taken not to confuse them for *benign metastasizing leiomyoma*, a condition that occurs mainly in young women with a history of prior hysterectomy for uterine leiomyomas and presents as multifocal lesions (see Chapter 15). Intrapulmonary leiomyomas are usually single and can present as endobronchial masses, making them amenable to diagnosis through endoscopic biopsies.[6] The tumor is characterized by a bland-appearing population of spindle cells with large nuclei showing blunted ends and surrounded by a rim of finely fibrillary cytoplasm. The tumor cells are devoid of cytologic atypia or mitotic activity and strongly stain with muscle markers such as SMA, desmin, calponin, and H-caldesmon. *Intrapulmonary schwannomas* are rare tumors that can occur in any age group and usually present as polypoid endobronchial masses or as an intraparenchymal peripheral nodule.[7] They are usually well circumscribed and unencapsulated and measure from 1 to 5 cm in greatest diameter. They comprise a bland spindle cell proliferation with wavy nuclei devoid of nuclear atypia or mitotic activity. Antoni A or Antoni B features may be difficult to identify in small endoscopic or core biopsies. The diagnosis can be made by observing the combination of a bland spindle cell proliferation with wavy nuclei and strong S-100 protein reactivity. *Intrapulmonary solitary fibrous tumor* is characterized by a bland-appearing spindle cell fibroblastic proliferation admixed with prominent sclerotic changes in the stroma, with a particular tendency to show linear deposition of hyalinized collagen alongside the spindle cells (i.e., deposition of rope-like collagen) (Fig. 14.3A).[8]

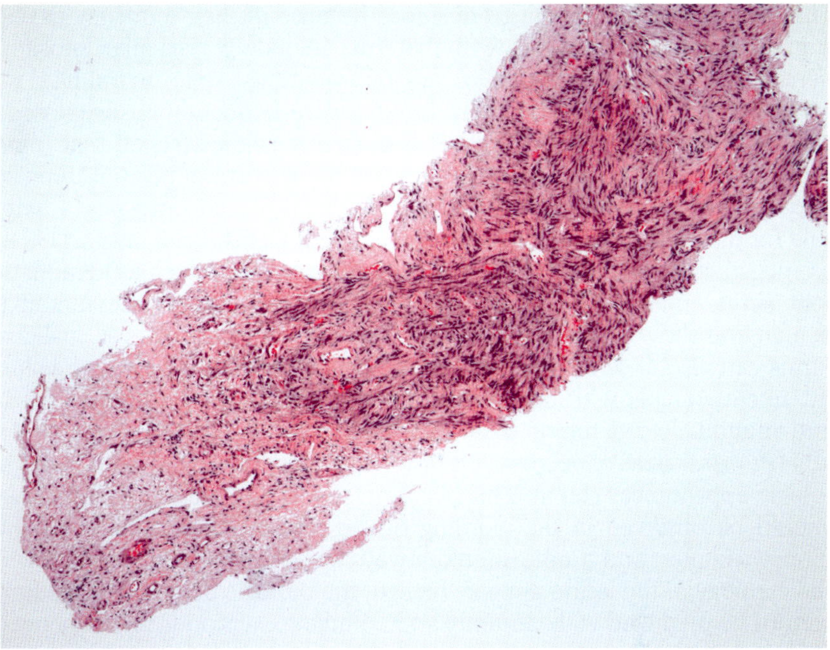

A

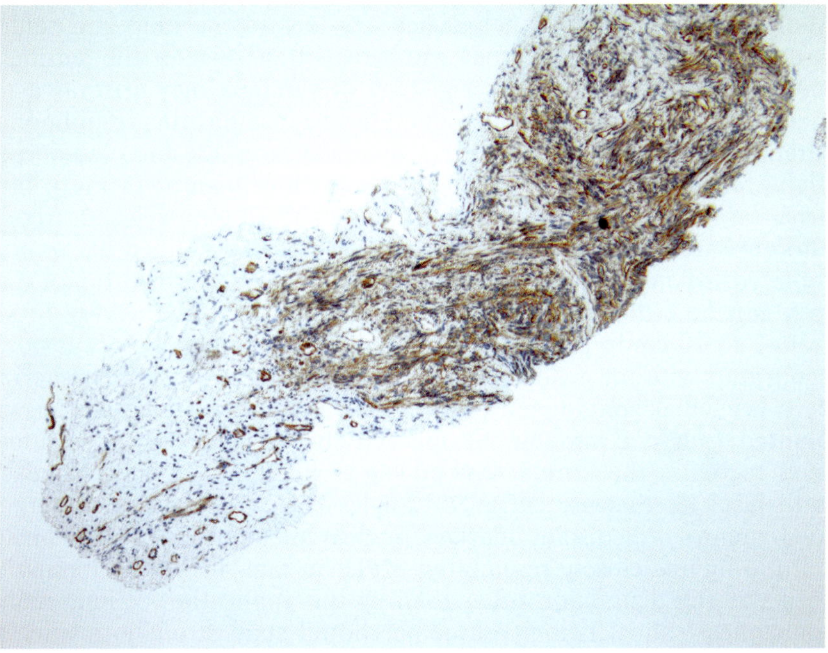

B

FIGURE 14.3 **A:** Core biopsy of peripherally located intrapulmonary solitary fibrous tumor showing a bland-appearing spindle cell proliferation with abundant collagenous stroma. **B:** Immunohistochemical staining for CD34 shows strong cytoplasmic positivity in the tumor cells.

The tumors can be difficult to diagnose because of their tendency to show a great heterogeneity of growth patterns, including fascicular, storiform, herringbone, hemangiopericytic, angiofibromatous, and neural-like with wavy nuclei.[9] In years past, these tumors were frequently misdiagnosed as pulmonary hemangiopericytoma. It is currently acknowledged that tumors reported under the latter designation most likely correspond to intrapulmonary solitary fibrous tumors. Immunohistochemical stains can play a helpful role for diagnosis; the tumors usually react with CD34, bcl-2, and CD99 and are negative for other specific markers of differentiation, such as keratin, desmin, actin, and S-100 protein (Fig. 14.3B). The majority of these tumors are benign and show a very bland morphologic appearance; however, malignant forms can also arise in the lung and are characterized by increased cellularity, nuclear atypia with prominent nucleoli, nuclear pleomorphism, bizarre and multinucleated tumor cells, increased mitotic activity (>3 mitoses per 10 HPF), and areas of necrosis. Occasionally, cases presenting with bland histologic appearances can also behave aggressively and metastasize.[10] Caution should be observed in the wording of the report when interpreting small biopsy samples, and a note should always be added to indicate that even if the cytology of the lesion appears benign, the biologic behavior of the tumor cannot be predicted with certainty and complete excision is recommended.

Malignant Mesenchymal Neoplasms

Malignant mesenchymal neoplasms are rare in the lung and seldom arise as primary tumors; they are most often seen in the setting of metastatic disease. Virtually any type of sarcoma may arise as a primary tumor in the lung.[1] The commonest types of primary pulmonary sarcomas include leiomyosarcoma, synovial sarcoma, and pleomorphic high-grade sarcoma (malignant fibrous histiocytoma or [MFH]); however, cases of malignant peripheral nerve sheath tumor, osteosarcoma, chondrosarcoma, and other types have also been described. *Pulmonary leiomyosarcoma* usually presents as a well-circumscribed tumor mass that can be either endobronchial or peripheral and can vary in size from 1 to 10 cm in greatest diameter.[11] These tumors can occur in any age group without gender predilection. The tumors are characterized by a fascicular spindle cell proliferation that often shows nuclei with blunted ends and variable mitotic activity. Well-differentiated tumors tend to retain the normal low-power architecture of smooth muscle, with fascicles that are cut at 90° angles (Fig. 14.4); poorly differentiated tumors will display marked nuclear pleomorphism with bizarre mitotic figures closely resembling MFH; in fact, it may be impossible to make any distinction other than by the application of immunohistochemical stains. Leiomyosarcoma should stain strongly positive for muscle-associated markers, such as desmin, SMA, smooth muscle myosin, H-caldesmon, and calponin. *Intrapulmonary synovial sarcoma* has become increasingly recognized in recent years as one of the most common primary spindle cell sarcomas to arise in the lung.[12]

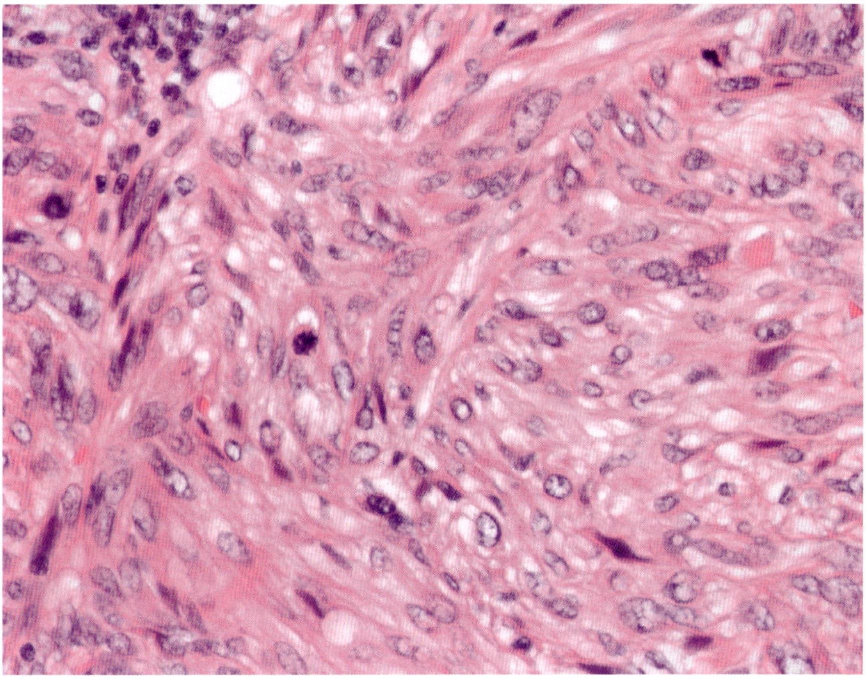

FIGURE 14.4 Low-grade pulmonary leiomyosarcoma shows fascicles of atypical spindle cells that intersect at 90° angles and show scattered mitoses.

The tumors can occur in patients of any age but are more common in young to middle-aged adults (mean age 38 years), with a slight predilection for women. The lesions are usually well circumscribed but unencapsulated and are most often peripheral but may also present as endobronchial masses that are amenable to examination by endoscopy. The majority of synovial sarcomas of the lung are of the monophasic spindle cell type; they are characterized by a monotonous population of atypical spindle cells with scant stroma and variable mitotic activity (1 to 10 mitoses per 10 HPF). The tumors can show varied growth patterns that can sometimes obscure the diagnosis, including herringbone, storiform, hemangiopericytic, and palisading resembling a neural neoplasm (Fig. 14.5A–C). Tumors in central location may show entrapment of residual respiratory structures by the spindle cell proliferation simulating a biphasic malignancy (Fig. 14.6). Some tumors can show prominent myxoid degeneration of the stroma. Another morphologic variant is characterized by round, rather than oval, cells, with an epithelioid appearance; such tumors have been termed "poorly differentiated" synovial sarcoma. Immunohistochemical stains will usually show focal positivity in small clusters of spindle cells for cytokeratin stains or epithelial membrane antigen (EMA), and strong cytoplasmic positivity in the majority of the tumor cells for vimentin and bcl-2.[13] Other

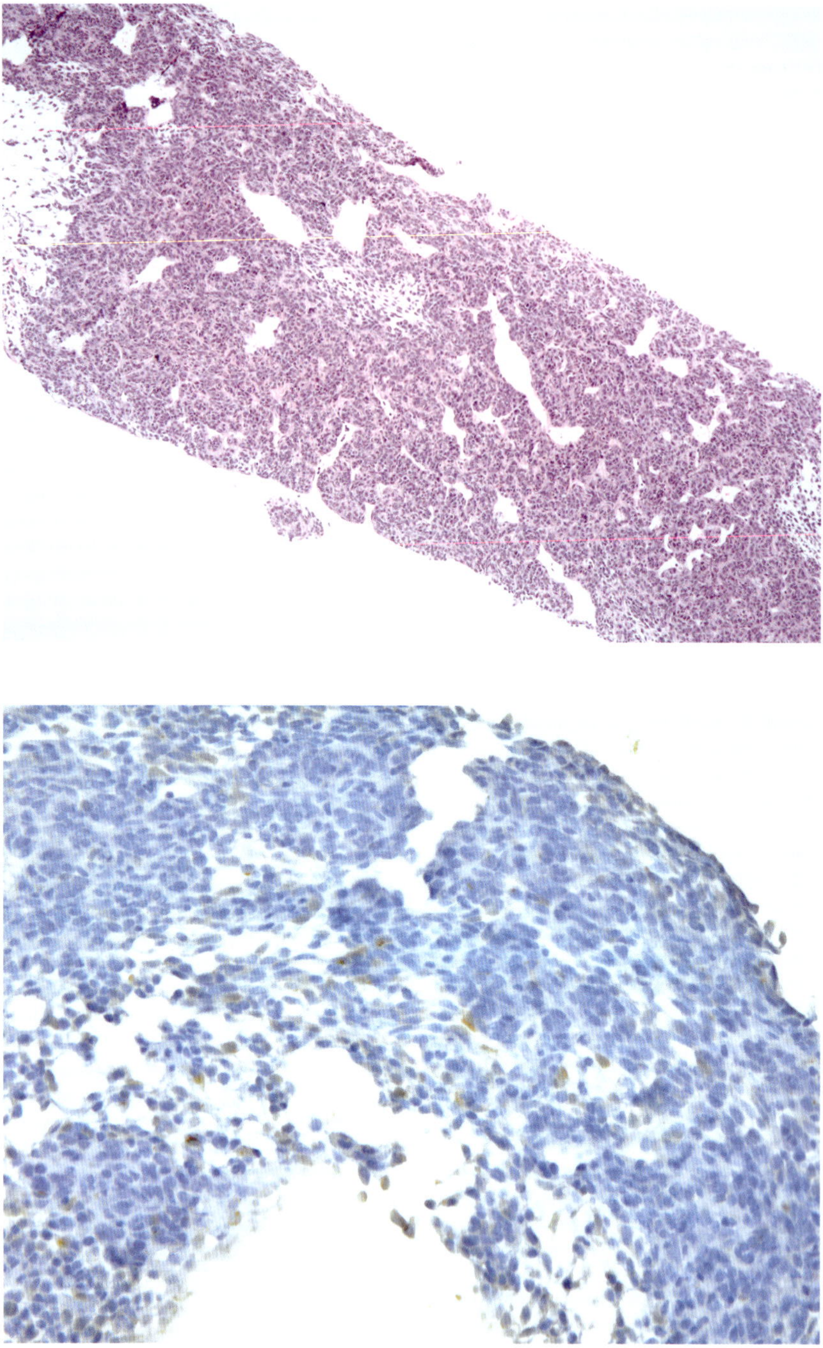

A

B

FIGURE 14.5 **A:** Core biopsy of pulmonary synovial sarcoma showing monotonous small spindle cells with a hemangiopericytic growth pattern. **B:** Immunohistochemical staining of the tumor cells in synovial sarcoma for cytokeratin AE1/AE3; notice the patchy, focal staining in only a few scattered cells.

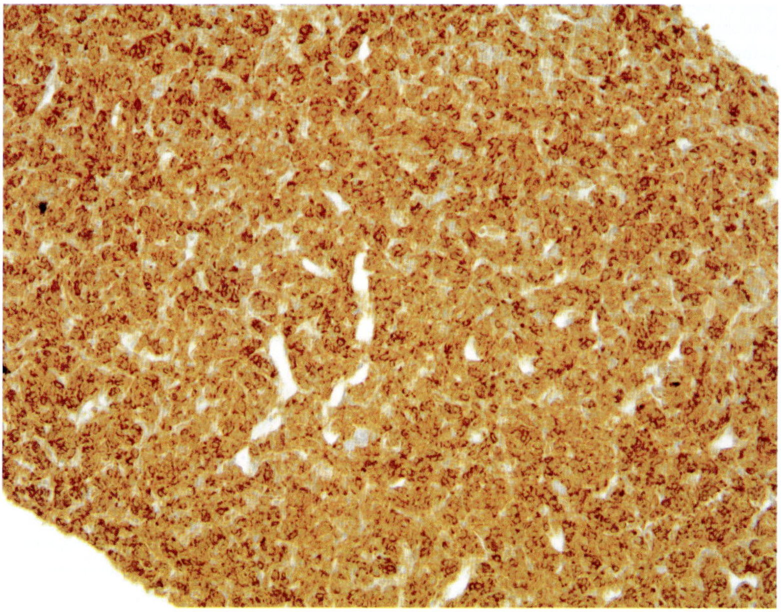

C

FIGURE 14.5 (*continued*) **C:** Immunohistochemical staining of pulmonary synovial sarcoma for bcl-2; notice strong, diffuse cytoplasmic staining in the majority of the tumor cells, a pattern that is quite characteristic for this tumor.

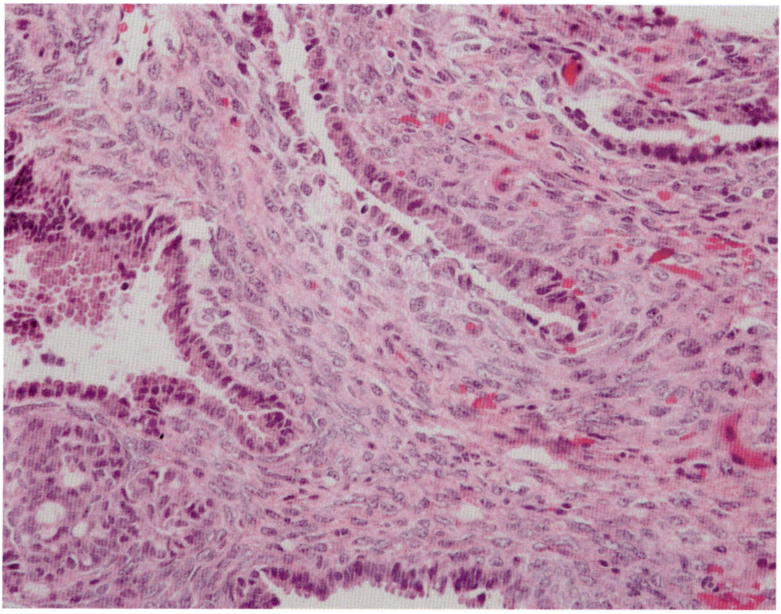

FIGURE 14.6 Endoscopic biopsy of pulmonary synovial sarcoma showing entrapment of respiratory structures by the monotonous spindle cell proliferation resembling a biphasic neoplasm. The bland morphology of the lining of the glands and thyroid transcription factor-1 (TTF-1) positivity serve to identify them as entrapped benign elements.

markers that have been demonstrated in synovial sarcoma include calponin, TLE-1, calretinin, S-100 protein, HBME-1, and CD117. The majority of cases (>80%) show a characteristic X;18 translocation that can be detected on formalin-fixed, paraffin-embedded tissues by fluorescence in situ hybridization (FISH) or PCR techniques.[14] The demonstration of the *SYT–SSX* fusion product by molecular techniques in these tumors is an extremely helpful adjunct for diagnosis in equivocal cases and may be very useful for separating these tumors from sarcomatoid carcinoma or from the spindle cell component of a biphasic pulmonary blastoma, which it may closely resemble. Because the lung is the second most common site of metastasis for synovial sarcoma of soft tissues, ruling out a primary source outside of the lungs is necessary before a diagnosis of primary pulmonary synovial sarcoma can be rendered. *Pleomorphic high-grade sarcoma ("MFH")* arising in the lung has been the subject only of case reports in literature. The tumors are characterized by high cellularity, marked nuclear pleomorphism with bizarre multinucleated tumor cells and frequent abnormal mitotic figures.[15] The tumors can show a prominent storiform pattern or grow as sheets of atypical tumor cells with a haphazard arrangement. Some tumors may display prominent myxoid stromal changes; hemorrhage and necrosis are also a common finding. There are no specific markers associated with MFH; the tumors generally type only for vimentin, although some may show aberrant expression of desmin, keratin, or S-100 protein in isolated tumor cells; they, thus, represent a "wastebasket" category for poorly differentiated sarcomas. The diagnosis of MFH must be made with caution, particularly in small biopsy material, because of the difficulties for separating them from other pleomorphic poorly differentiated tumors of the lung, in particular, large cell anaplastic carcinoma of the lung. Immunohistochemical stains for cytokeratins should be routinely ordered to rule out the possibility of an anaplastic carcinoma of the lung.

In general terms, a definitive diagnosis of primary sarcoma of the lung may be impossible to render on a small biopsy sample because of the difficulties associated on limited biopsy material for determining whether other epithelial components may be present, such as in carcinosarcoma and biphasic pulmonary blastoma. Moreover, metastases from soft tissue sarcomas to the lung greatly outnumber primary lung sarcomas. Clinicopathologic correlation, thorough radiographic studies, and a very detailed clinical history are, therefore, necessary to establish whether the tumor is primary or metastatic, even when dealing with a solitary lesion. Another important consideration when dealing with biopsies of sarcoma-like tumors in the lung is the need to rule out the possibility of a sarcomatoid carcinoma. The latter are generally positive for epithelial markers, such as cytokeratin, p63, or EMA. Some types of sarcoma may also express cytokeratin, either aberrantly or as part of the inherent makeup of the lesion (i.e., epithelioid sarcoma, synovial sarcoma), but the reactivity in such cases is usually spotty and weak, and the tumors will also express other markers that are not normally expressed in carcinomas, such as CD99, bcl-2, and CD34. Unless very specific features associated with a given tumor are identified, or the results of special studies, such as immunohistochemistry and molecular pathology, yield convincing evidence in favor of a specific diagnosis, it is preferable to diagnose the lesion descriptively and generically as a "low-grade (or high-grade) spindle cell sarcoma," with a note detailing the diagnostic possibilities.

Vascular Endothelial Neoplasms

Different kinds of neoplasms of vascular endothelium may arise in the lung, including hemangiomas, epithelioid hemangioendothelioma, Kaposi sarcoma, and angiosarcoma. Of these, epithelioid hemangioendothelioma is the one most frequently encountered as a primary tumor of the lung. Another condition that can be encountered in endoscopic biopsy samples and needs to be distinguished from a malignant vascular neoplasm is capillary hemangiomatosis.

Epithelioid hemangioendothelioma is a malignant vascular neoplasm characterized by a proliferation of large, epithelioid cells with abundant eosinophilic cytoplasm and large, vesicular nuclei with prominent nucleoli. The tumors are most common in young adults but can occur at any age with female predilection.[16] The tumor is usually multifocal and bilateral and presents as multiple pulmonary nodules within lung parenchyma that measure from a few millimeters to a few centimeters in greatest diameter. Some lesions have been known to regress spontaneously.[17] The lesions have a tendency to fill up the lumen of alveolar spaces in a polypoid fashion resembling glomerular structures (Fig. 14.7A). The epithelioid cells are usually found embedded in abundant chondromyxoid matrix and are characterized by prominent cytoplasmic vacuoles. Stromal sclerosis is a common finding and some cases may show foci of calcification or develop a cartilage-like matrix. The tumor cells are positive for vascular endothelium-associated markers, including CD31, CD34, and FVIII-RA (Fig. 14.7B). The cells can also be positive for cytokeratins. The lesions need to be distinguished mainly from metastases of chondrosarcoma, chordoma, or metastatic carcinoma. *Kaposi sarcoma* is a low-grade vascular malignancy that is commonly associated with HIV infection in patients with AIDS and is associated with the human herpes virus 8 (HHV8).[18,19] When it involves the lung, the condition is associated with a poor prognosis. It presents clinically as bilateral interstitial pulmonary infiltrates with ill-defined nodularity in a patient with a history of immunosuppression, in particular transplant patients or intravenous drug abusers. Histologically it is characterized by a fascicular spindle cell proliferation that follows intrapulmonary fibrous septa and lymphatics with a perivascular and peribronchial distribution.[20] The cells show mild-to-moderate atypia with scattered mitoses, and they are admixed with extravasated RBCs and inflammatory cells

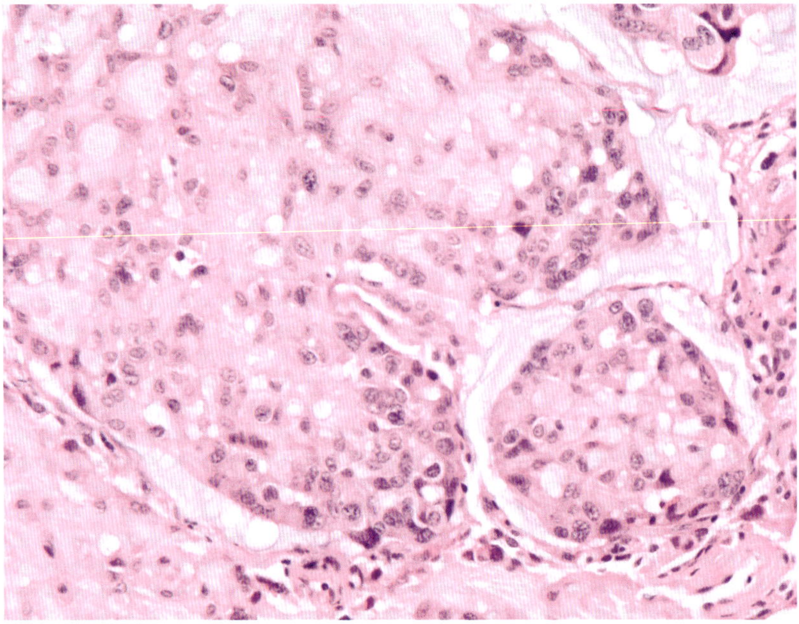

A

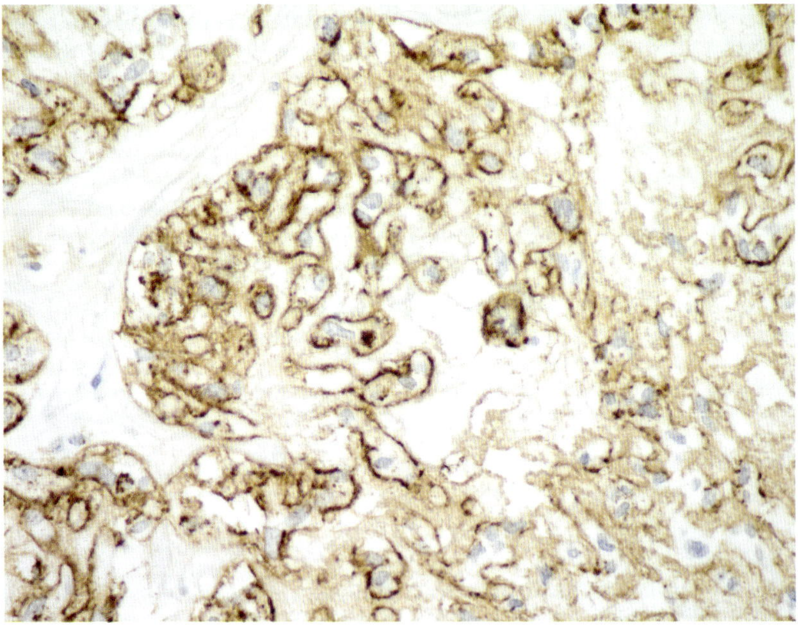

B

FIGURE 14.7 **A:** Epithelioid hemangioendothelioma of lung shows polypoid cellular structures filling the alveoli comprising large epithelioid cells with prominent myxoid stroma and numerous cytoplasmic empty vacuoles. **B:** Immunohistochemical staining of epithelioid hemangioendothelioma with factor VIII-related antigen highlights the positive epithelioid cells embedded in the myxoid stroma.

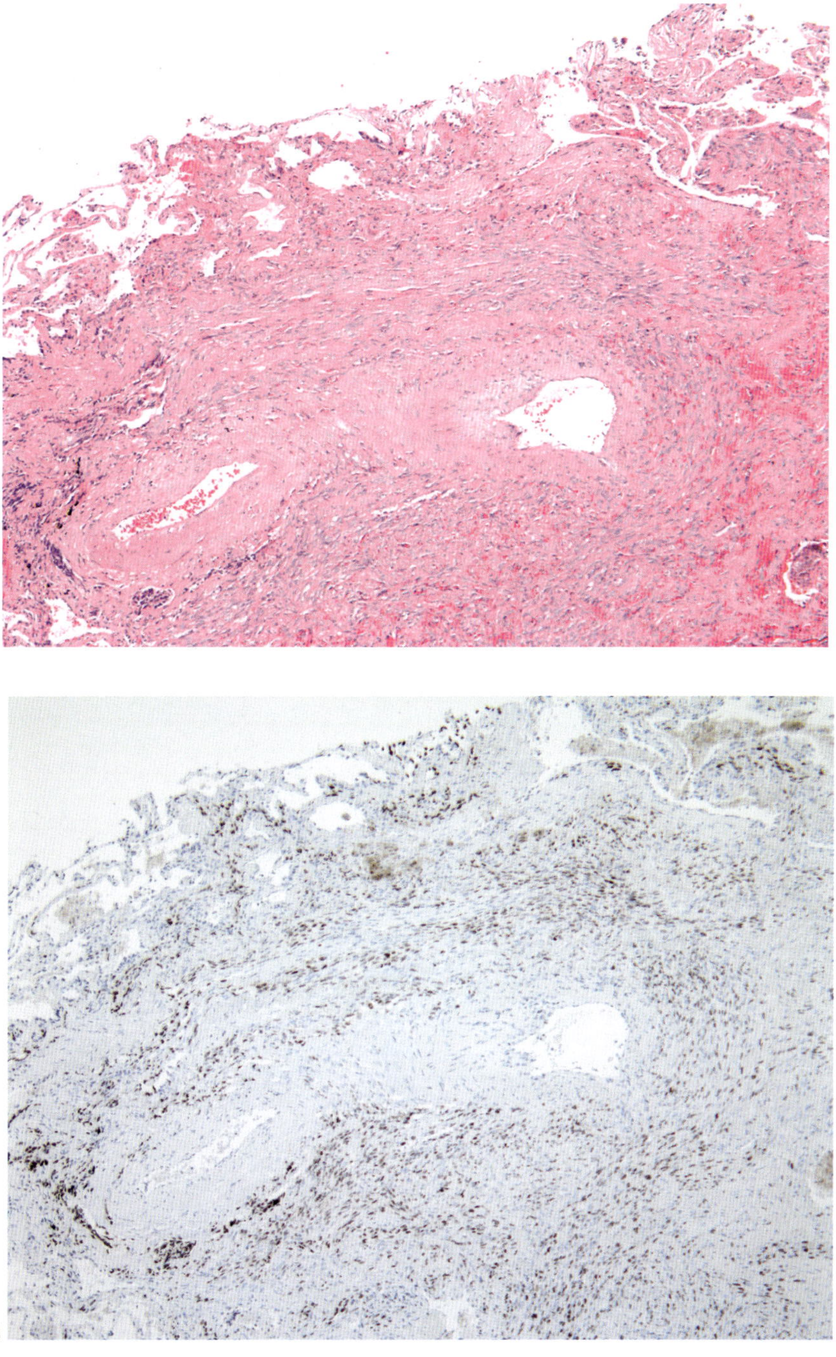

A

B

FIGURE 14.8 **A:** Endobronchial biopsy of pulmonary lesion in Kaposi's sarcoma shows dense spindle cell proliferation in perivascular location admixed with extravasated RBCs. **B:** Immunohistochemical staining for HHV-8 in Kaposi's sarcoma shows strong nuclear staining in the spindle cells.

(Fig. 14.8A). Dense, eosinophilic hyaline globules can also be seen scattered in the interstitium. The spindle cells are positive for CD31 and, to a lesser extent, CD34 and also show strong nuclear staining for HHV8 (Fig. 14.8B). The diagnosis should be suspected in endoscopic biopsies of patients with a history of immunodeficiency with multiple nodules showing a dense spindle cell proliferation surrounding vessels or lymphatics; appropriate stains should always be ordered to support the diagnosis. *Angiosarcoma* of the lung is a rare condition that most often represents a metastasis to the lung rather than a primary tumor. It can present either as a single or as multiple hemorrhagic nodules.[21,22] The tumor can exhibit the whole spectrum of features associated with angiosarcoma in their more common locations, including anastomosing vascular spaces lined by atypical endothelial cells, to an atypical spindle cell proliferation with abortive vasoformative structures, to a highly atypical malignant neoplasms with epithelioid or pleomorphic features with prominent stromal hemorrhage (Fig. 14.9). The tumor cells are usually positive for vascular markers (CD31, CD34) but may show patchy or inconsistent staining for FVIII-RA. The nuclear

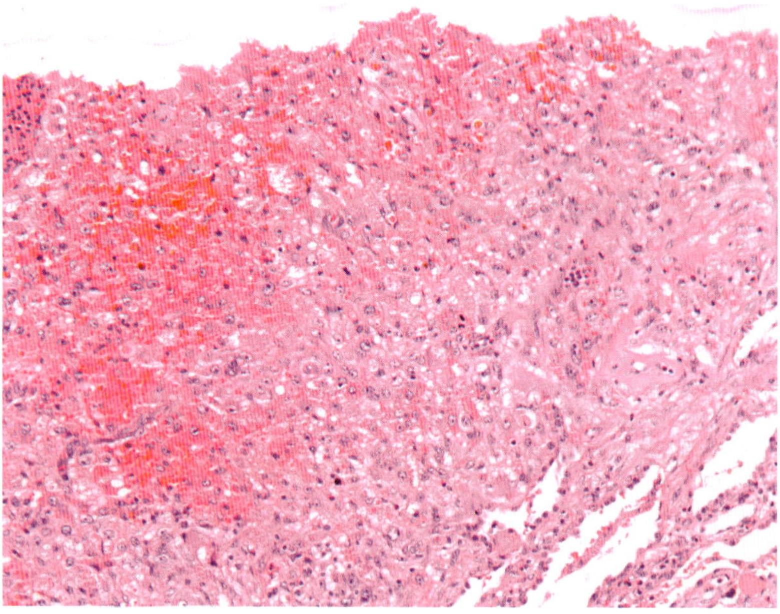

FIGURE 14.9 Endoscopic biopsy in a patient with angiosarcoma of the lung shows an atypical, primitive cell population with extensive stromal hemorrhage and no distinctive growth pattern; such tumors can be diagnosed properly only by the application of immunohistochemical stains for vascular endothelium-associated markers.

transcription factor, FLI-1, although not specific for vascular endothelium, may be an additional helpful positive marker for the diagnosis of these tumors. *Pulmonary capillary hemangiomatosis (PCH)* is a rare cause of pulmonary hypertension characterized by uncontrollable capillary proliferation in the pulmonary interstitium and alveolar walls secondary to postcapillary obstruction.[23] The condition has a peak incidence in the second or third decade of life without any gender predilection and presents clinically with worsening dyspnea on exertion in patients with signs of primary pulmonary hypertension. The process is benign and commonly regarded as nonneoplastic and reactive in nature. Histologically, it is characterized by a striking capillary proliferation infiltrating vascular, bronchial, and interstitial pulmonary structures (Fig. 14.10A, B). Similar findings can be seen in patients with pulmonary veno-occlusive disease, but unlike the latter, PCH is not accompanied by venulitis or infarction, and there is no identifiable cause for the venous obliteration. Some authors, however, have suggested that these two conditions may be closely related.[24]

A

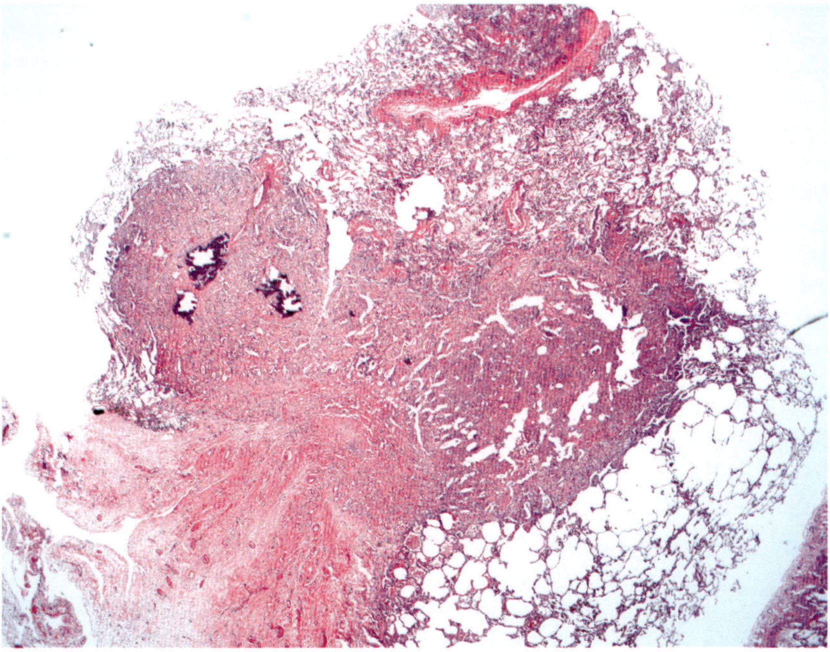

FIGURE 14.10 **A:** Endoscopic biopsy in patient with capillary hemangiomatosis shows focal replacement of lung parenchyma by a dense cellular proliferation causing consolidation of airspaces. *(continued)*

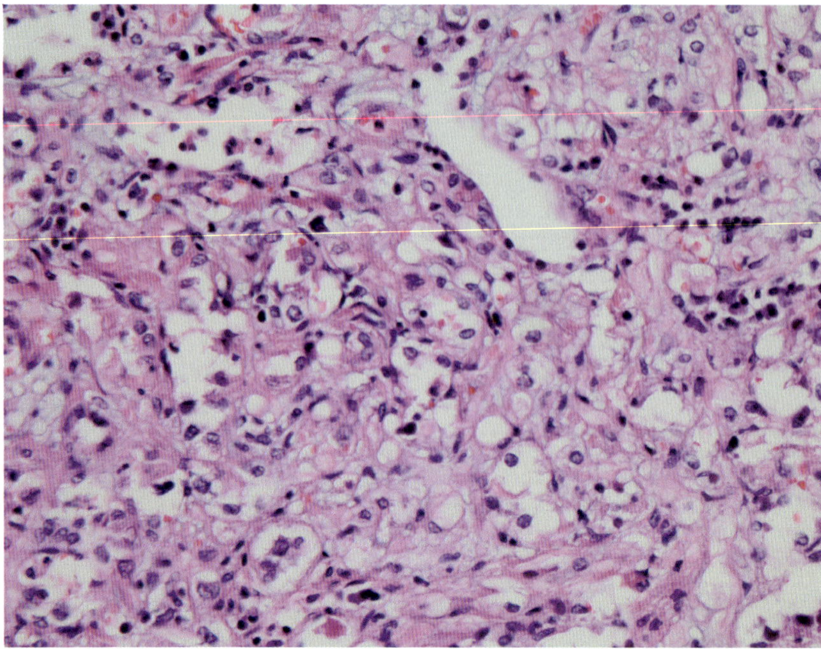

B

FIGURE 14.10 (*continued*) **B:** Higher magnification shows compact proliferation of minute capillary vessels replacing the normal underlying architecture.

TUMORS DERIVED FROM ECTOPIC TISSUES

Different tumors, such as melanocytic, meningothelial, tumors with a thymic phenotype, glomus cell tumors, and teratomas, can occasionally arise in the lung that can display features or evidence of certain lines of differentiation that are not normally present in the lung. Such tumors are presumed to arise from ectopic or embryologically displaced elements.

Bronchial Melanoma

Primary melanoma of the lung is a rare and controversial entity.[25] Because the lung is a common site of metastases from cutaneous melanoma, care must be taken to obtain a very thorough clinical history before a diagnosis of primary melanoma of the bronchus is rendered.[26] The tumors can present as polypoid, endobronchial lesions that obstruct the bronchial lumen, or they may grow as an intraparenchymatous mass. Histologically, the tumors can show an in situ component in the bronchial mucosa that can be confused for squamous carcinoma in small endoscopic biopsies. The lesions, however, extensively infiltrate the bronchial wall and grow as sheets or nests of epithelioid to spindle cells with marked cytologic atypia, prominent nucleoli, and frequent mitotic figures. Melanin pigment may or may not be seen. Identification of the characteristic nested growth pattern is a helpful clue for diagnosis. Immunohistochemical stains will show strong positivity of the tumor cells for melanoma-associated markers, including S-100 protein, HMB45, Melan-A, and tyrosinase. Melanoma may also be positive for epithelial markers, in particular carcinoembryonic antigen (CEA); caution must be exercised in interpreting such results and for adding melanocytic markers in the panel to avoid a misdiagnosis.

Pulmonary Meningioma and Pulmonary Minute Meningothelial Nodules

Cellular proliferations arising from presumed ectopic or misplaced meningothelial elements in the lung are rare but may be the source of confusion on small biopsy samples. *Primary meningioma* of the lung has been described in the absence of any past history or synchronous evidence of intracranial lesions.[27] The possibility of a late metastasis from an intra cranial tumor, in particular, needs to always be ruled out by means of a thorough clinical history; for instance, metastases to the lung from intracranial meningioma have been reported up to 19 years later.[28] Primary meningioma usually occurs in adults between 30 and 72 years of age and are usually discovered incidentally on routine chest X-rays. They present as well-circumscribed, subpleural lesions that measure on average 3 to 4 cm in greatest dimension. Histologically, they resemble their intracranial counterpart and are characterized by a proliferation of spindle-to-oval cells with bland cytologic appearance and occasional intranuclear cytoplasmic inclusions that tend to display focally a marked whorling pattern. Psammoma bodies may be seen scattered throughout the tumor. Mitoses are rare or absent. Immunohistochemical stains show positivity of the tumor cells for EMA and vimentin, and some tumors may stain focally for S-100 protein, cytokeratin, and CD34. Many tumors will also show nuclear positivity for progesterone receptors. The tumors are almost always benign and adequately treated by surgical excision. *Pulmonary minute meningothelial nodules* usually represent an incidental finding at autopsy or in resected lung specimens removed for another condition. They are characterized by minute (1 to 5 mm) cellular aggregates that show all of the histologic and immunophenotypic attributes of meningothelial cells and are located in the pulmonary interstitium, in the vicinity of small-and medium-sized vessels (Fig. 14.11 A, B).[29] Because the lesions are microscopic and asymptomatic, they are often missed when other dominant pathology is present. A rare presentation of this condition, however, has been more recently described, which has been designated as *diffuse pulmonary meningotheliomatosis.*[30] Such lesions are usually multiple and bilateral and can present with symptoms of progressive shortness of breath and bilateral interstitial reticulonodular lung infiltrates on imaging studies. Endoscopic or open lung biopsies performed in such patients will show the meningothelial nodules to be the sole pathology. Correct diagnosis in such instances will be of importance to explain the symptoms and the results of imaging studies.

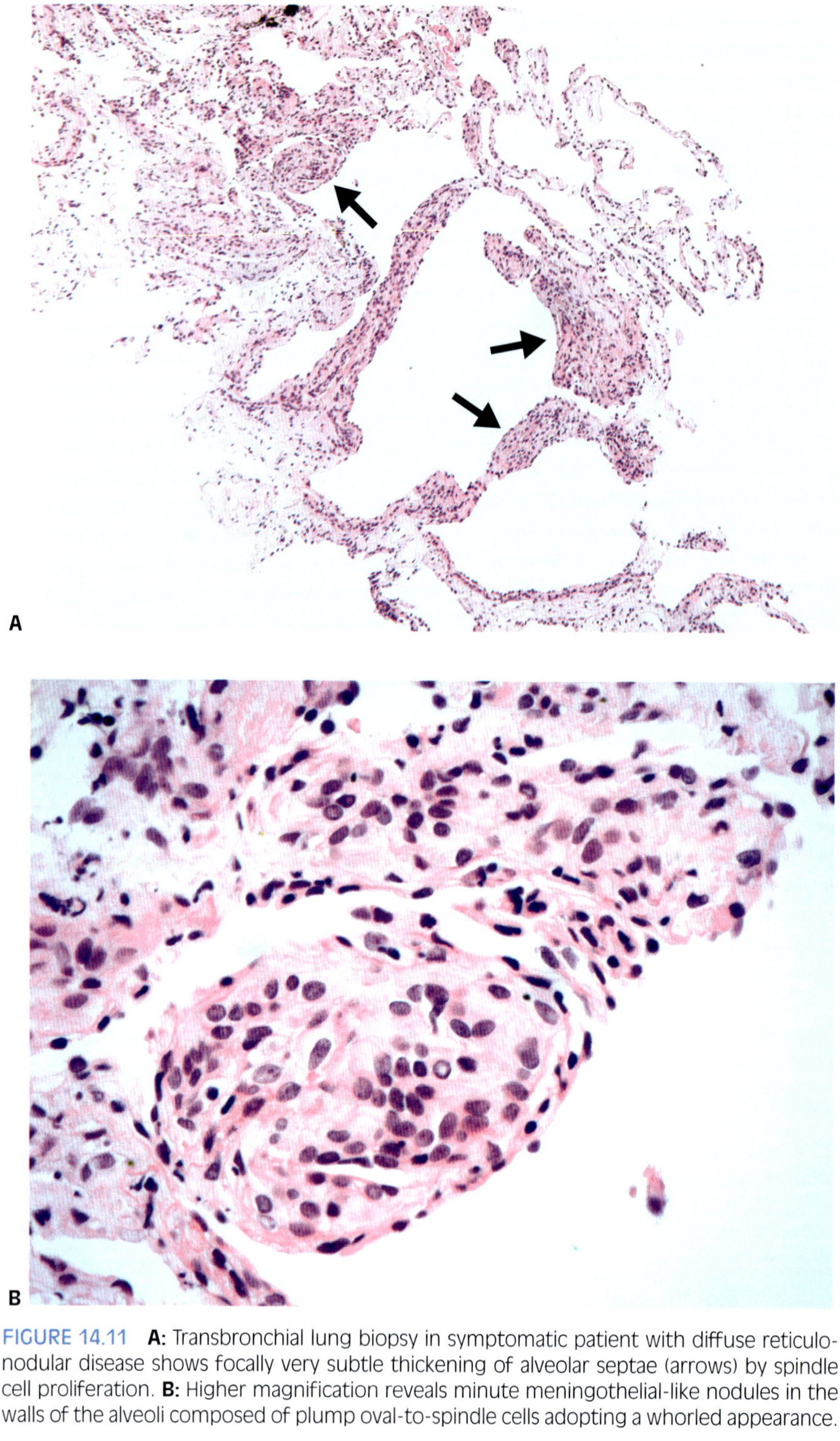

FIGURE 14.11 **A:** Transbronchial lung biopsy in symptomatic patient with diffuse reticulonodular disease shows focally very subtle thickening of alveolar septae (arrows) by spindle cell proliferation. **B:** Higher magnification reveals minute meningothelial-like nodules in the walls of the alveoli composed of plump oval-to-spindle cells adopting a whorled appearance.

Intrapulmonary Thymoma

Intrapulmonary thymoma represents a rare form of presentation for these tumors, which are normally located in the anterior mediastinum. When arising as primary tumors in the lung, they can essentially display the entire gamut of histologic features of mediastinal thymomas.[31] The tumors can be located either in the lung hilum or in the periphery and can range in size from 1 to 10 cm in greatest diameter. They are usually well circumscribed, unencapsulated, and with a rubbery cut surface. Histologically, they can show the features of spindle cell, lymphocyte-rich, mixed lymphoepithelial, or epithelial-rich (atypical) thymoma. The majority of tumors will retain some of the organotypical features of the thymus, including lobulation, dilated perivascular spaces, and admixture of the epithelial cells with immature T-lymphocytes in varying proportions (Fig. 14.12 A, B). The lymphocyte-rich tumors can be confused for lymphoma, particularly in small biopsies in which the lobulation or perivascular spaces are not easily identified. Immunohistochemical stains for cytokeratin or p63 will be indicated to identify the scattered proliferating epithelial cells admixed with the lymphocytes.[32] Epithelial-rich tumors may be confused with well-differentiated squamous cell carcinomas; the lack of small, infiltrative islands of tumor cells and of marked cytologic atypia will be a helpful clue to separate them from the latter. All thymomas react very strongly with cytokeratin and show nuclear positivity in all of the tumor cells with p63; In addition, the lymphocytes will stain strongly with CD1a, TdT and CD99, indicating their immature lymphoblastic phenotype. Use of these markers is therefore recommended when evaluating a bland-appearing spindle or epithelioid cell population of the lung showing an intimate admixture of epithelial cells with scattered small T-lymphocytes.

Benign and Malignant Glomus Tumors

Tumors bearing the morphologic and immunohistochemical features of both benign and malignant glomus tumors have been reported in the lung. Because glomus tumors can sometimes metastasize late in the course of the disease, care must be taken to rule out the possibility of a late metastasis in patients with such lesions. Glomus tumors can encompass a range of morphologic features and biologic behavior that ranges from benign glomangioma to malignant glomus tumor, or glomangiosarcoma.[33] Glomus tumors can present either as a central or as a peripheral solitary lesion located within lung parenchyma. They range in size from 1 to 6 cm in greatest dimension and can occur across a broad age range (20 to 65 years).[34,35] Histologically, pulmonary glomus tumors resemble their soft tissue counterpart and are characterized by a fairly monotonous population of round-to-polygonal cells containing dark, round nuclei and ample eosinophilic or clear cytoplasm. The tumor cells have a tendency to surround vascular spaces, which can often display striking perivascular hyalinization. The malignant variant, glomangiosarcoma, is characterized by more pronounced cytologic atypia with mitotic activity and focal areas of tumor necrosis.

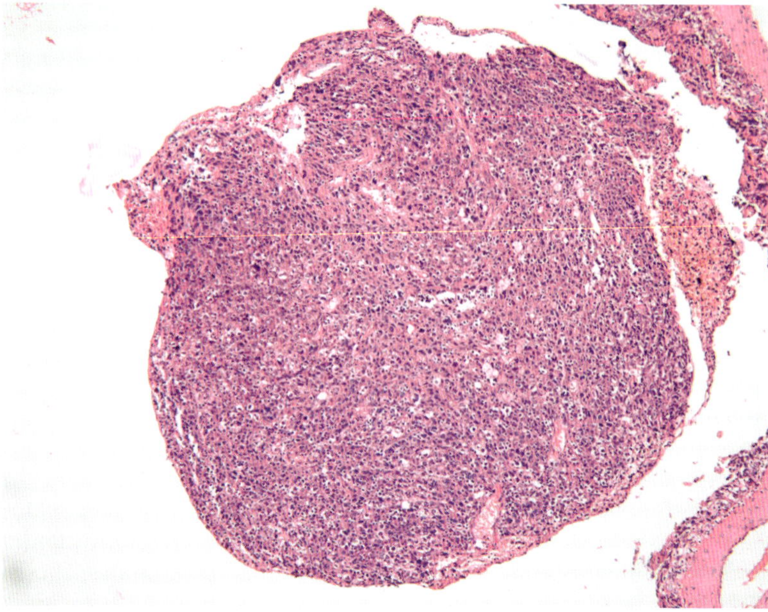

A

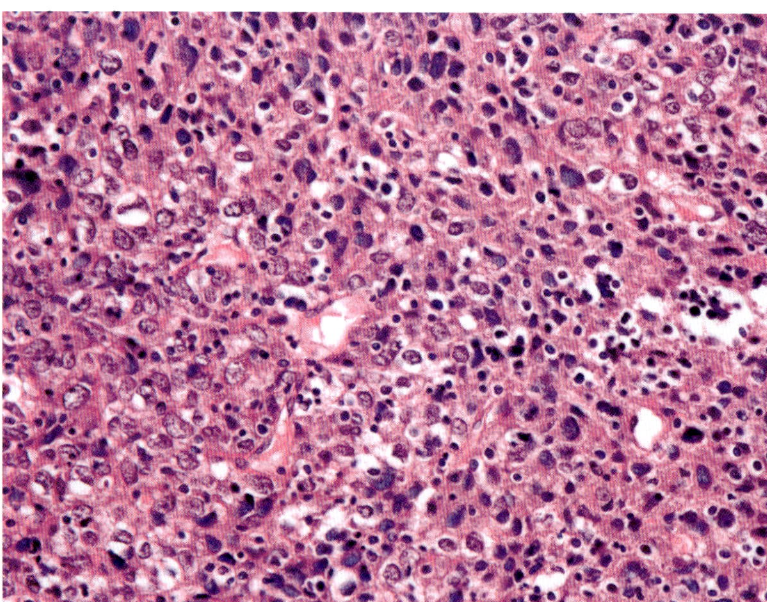

B

FIGURE 14.12 **A:** Endoscopic biopsy of intrapulmonary thymoma shows a cluster of cells showing sheets of small lymphocytes admixed with larger epithelioid cells. **B:** Higher magnification showing admixtures of small lymphocytes with larger cells with vesicular nuclei and indistinct rim of amphophilic cytoplasm. Immunohistochemical stains are necessary to make the correct diagnosis; the large cells with vesicular nuclei should be strongly positive for cytokeratin and p63, and the surrounding lymphocytes should type as immature T-lymphocytes (CD1a+, CD3+, TdT+, CD99+).

The tumor cells are positive for vimentin and muscle-specific actin and do not stain for other differentiation markers such as cytokeratins, EMA, CEA, S-100 protein, HMB45, CD31, CD34, and FVIII-RA.

Teratoma

Teratoma is defined as a germ cell tumor that contains elements derived from all three germ layers. Such tumors are exceedingly rare in the lung and may be present either in endobronchial location or as a solitary intraparenchymatous nodule. In some instances, the diagnosis may become quite evident when hair is found on endoscopic examination.[36] Well-formed teeth can also be sometimes observed on imaging studies. The majority of the tumors are identified as cystic structures on chest X-rays that may vary from a few centimeters to 10 cm in size. The clue to the diagnosis lies in identifying the various normal cellular elements of diverse histogenesis present in the lesion, including glandular and epithelial structures of skin, sebaceous adnexa, enteric or other origin admixed with mature cartilage, neural tissue, bone, and other mesodermal elements. Such lesions will only rarely be sampled endoscopically, and the diagnosis is most often established on completely resected specimens following a high index of suspicion on the imaging studies. Testicular malignant teratomas can also occasionally metastasize to the lung as mature teratomas; care must be taken to obtain a careful clinical history before a diagnosis of primary lung teratomas is rendered.[37]

LUNG TUMORS OF UNCERTAIN HISTOGENESIS

Several lung tumors of uncertain histogenesis can infrequently be encountered in biopsy material. The majority represent benign conditions in which the histogenesis is either disputed or unknown, but they have sufficiently distinctive morphologic and/or immunophenotypic features that will permit accurate diagnosis in the majority of instances.

Sclerosing Hemangioma (Pneumocytoma)

Sclerosing hemangioma (pneumocytoma) is a tumor of unknown histogenesis that tends to occur more frequently in women in their fourth or fifth decade of life. They are usually found incidentally on routine chest X-rays as a solitary coin lesion. The tumors are most often found in peripheral subpleural location with a predilection for the lower lobes and are usually well circumscribed, measuring from 1 to 6 cm in greatest dimension.[38] Rare cases have been found in endobronchial location.[39] The tumors are characterized by varying histologic appearance; four major growth patterns that can be present in varying proportions are identified: solid, papillary, sclerosing, and angiomatous. The solid pattern is characterized by sheets of monotonous round-to-polygonal tumor cells with small, round, bland-appearing nuclei surrounded by abundant, lightly eosinophilic cytoplasm (Fig. 14.13A). The tumor cells in these areas are strongly positive for EMA and TTF-1 and are negative

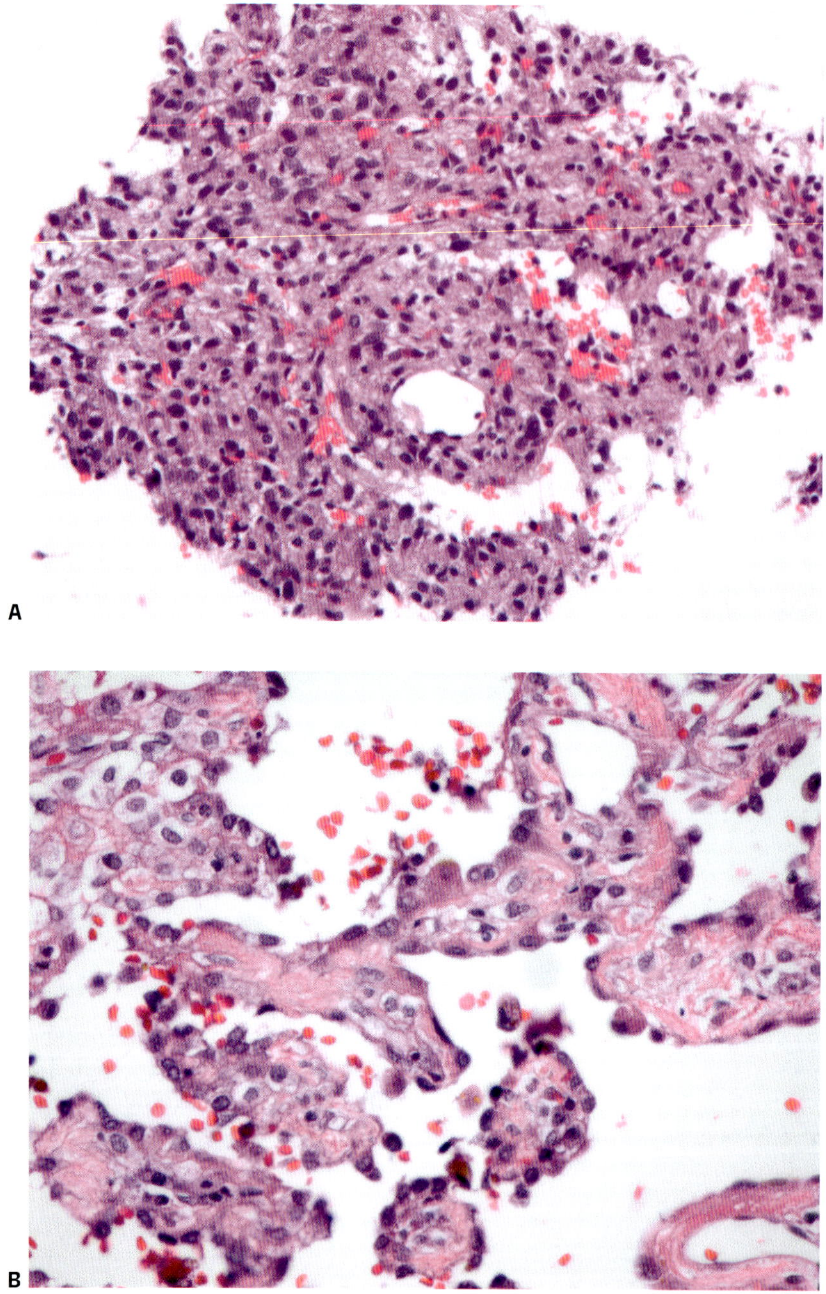

FIGURE 14.13 **A:** Endobronchial biopsy of sclerosing hemangioma shows a small fragment containing solid population of monotonous, bland-appearing, round-to-polygonal tumor cells devoid of cytologic atypia; tumor cells in these areas label with EMA and TTF-1. **B:** Papillary areas in sclerosing hemangioma show characteristic hyperchromatic hobnail cells lining the papilla; notice, however, the distinctive round cells with clear cytoplasm located within the cores of the papillae.

for cytokeratins, vascular endothelium-associated markers, and surfactant apoprotein markers.[40] The papillary pattern is characterized by papillary structures lined by round cells with a hobnail appearance that contain large, hyperchromatic nuclei and scant cytoplasm. These cells are positive for CK7 and TTF-1 and also react with surfactant apoprotein and Clara cell markers, indicating a close kinship with normal alveolar lining epithelial cells—reason why it has been proposed that the tumor be redesignated as a pneumocytoma.[41] The cores of the papillae contain monotonous round or polygonal cells identical to those seen in the solid areas (Fig. 14.13B). The sclerosing pattern is characterized by confluent areas of stromal hyalinization, particularly around vessels, admixed with the solid monotonous round cell population. The angiomatous pattern is characterized by clusters of dilated vascular spaces filled with pools of blood showing a superficial resemblance on scanning magnification to cavernous hemangioma; the stroma surrounding the dilated vascular spaces is occupied by the same type of cells as in the solid pattern. On small biopsy samples, making a diagnosis of sclerosing hemangioma can be quite challenging because it will not be feasible to appreciate the admixture of the various patterns, which is one of the hallmarks of this lesion. A high level of suspicion needs to be observed to make the correct diagnosis. In general, the diagnosis should be suspected when dealing with a bland-appearing cell population comprising monotonous round or polygonal tumor cells with clear cytoplasm and absence of nuclear pleomorphism or mitotic activity. The presence of papillary structures lined by hobnail cells should prompt a search for the characteristic monotonous round cells with clear cytoplasm in the stroma, with application of an appropriate panel of immunohistochemical stains. A tentative diagnosis can be rendered under such circumstances with the recommendation that the tumor be completely excised for further histologic examination and definitive characterization.

Clear Cell "Sugar" Tumor

Clear cell "sugar" tumor is a rare type of tumor that usually presents as a solitary, well-circumscribed intraparenchymatous pulmonary nodule discovered incidentally on routine chest X-rays. The term "sugar" tumor derives from the fact that its cytoplasm is rich in glycogen. Although for many years this tumor was thought to be of unknown histogenesis, it has more recently been demonstrated that they show cytoplasmic expression of HMB45, similar to that observed in tumors in other locations with a similar morphology, leading to the proposal that they may be part of the family of tumors (PEComas) comprising perivascular epithelioid cells (PECs).[42,43] Histologically, the tumors are characterized by a solid, sheet-like proliferation of large round, oval, or polygonal cells with abundant clear to lightly eosinophilic cytoplasm. The tumor cells usually have distinct cytoplasmic borders and contain small, dark nuclei with inconspicuous nucleoli (Fig. 14.14). The tumors often display a

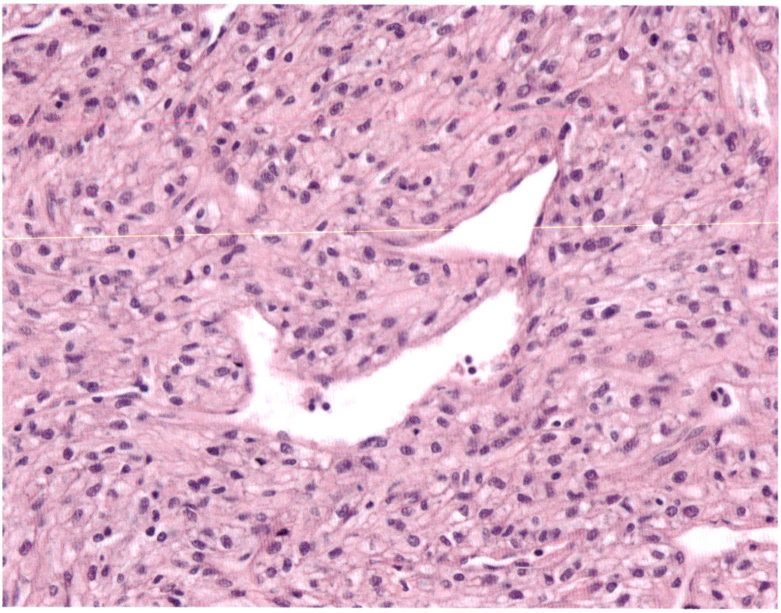

FIGURE 14.14 Clear cell "sugar" tumor of lung shows sheets of round-to-oval cells with small nuclei and abundant clear to lightly eosinophilic cytoplasm. Branching vessels with open lumens are a constant feature of these tumors.

prominent stromal vascular component characterized by large, dilated vessels with branching lumens resulting in a hemangiopericytomatous growth pattern. The tumors are negative for all epithelial markers (keratin, EMA, CEA, etc.), which serve to separate them from metastatic clear cell carcinomas, as well as for other specific differentiation markers. HMB45 is a marker consistently expressed in these tumors; some cases may also show focal positivity for CD34, S-100 protein, synaptophysin, and neuron-specific enolase. The presence of cytoplasmic glycogen can be demonstrated with a periodic acid–Schiff (PAS) stain with diastase.

Granular Cell Tumor

Granular cell tumor is a tumor of middle-aged adults (although they can also occur in children) that characteristically presents as an endobronchial mass in central location.[44] They can measure from 1 to 5 cm in diameter and present as polypoid tumors obstructing the airway. Because of the proximal endobronchial location they are amenable to diagnosis on endoscopic biopsies.[45] The tumors are regarded as of unknown histogenesis; however, many modern authors consider this to merely represent the granular cell variant of schwannoma. Histologically, the tumor shows sheets of large, round-to-polygonal cells with abundant eosinophilic granular cytoplasm and small, centrally placed nuclei devoid of atypia (Fig. 14.15A, B). The tumors are

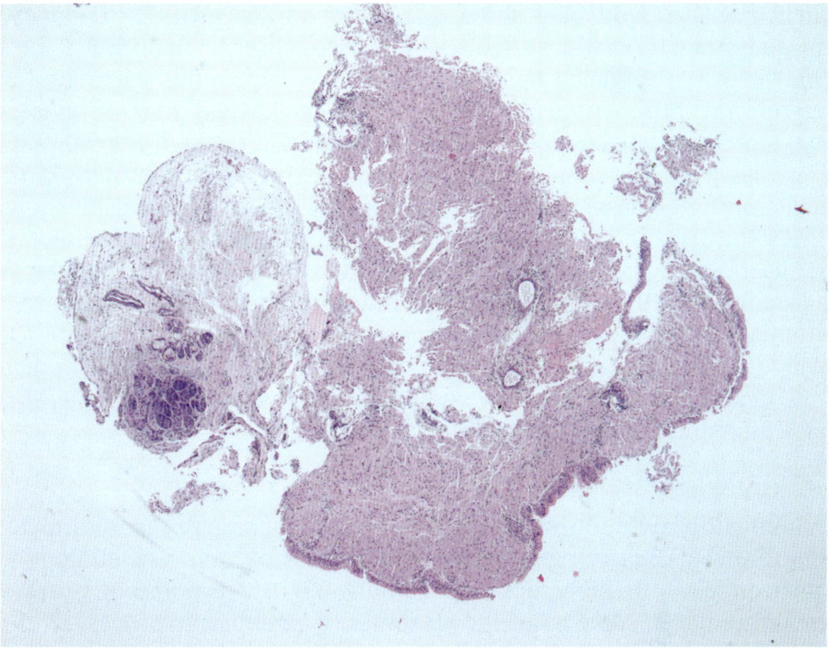

A

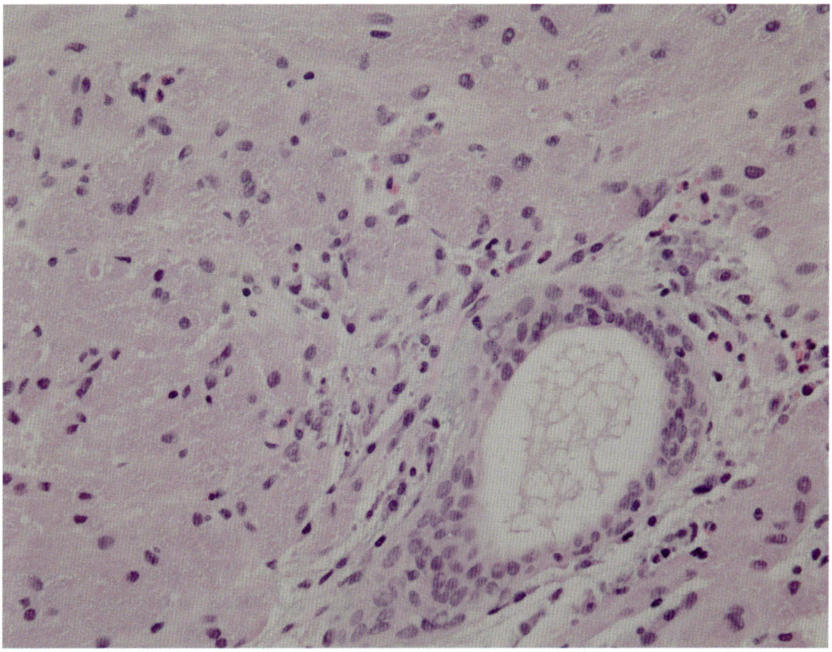

B

FIGURE 14.15 **A:** Endoscopic biopsy of granular cell tumor of the bronchus shows replacement of the submucosa by sheets of large cells with abundant eosinophilic cytoplasm. **B:** Higher magnification shows large cells with small, centrally placed nuclei containing abundant granular eosinophilic cytoplasm.

unencapsulated and may show infiltrative borders, with a tendency to entrap normal bronchial structures in its path as well as small nerve trunks. The overlying bronchial epithelium may show squamous metaplasia and can ulcerate. In rare cases, these tumors can display marked cytologic atypia, mitotic activity, and necrosis heralding a process of transformation to malignancy. The tumor cells consistently express S-100 protein in their nuclei and cytoplasm, and the cytoplasmic granules react positively with PAS stain. The tumors do not react with epithelial, muscle, neuroendocrine, or melanocyte-specific markers such as HMB45 or Melan-A. The diagnosis is usually straightforward on endoscopic biopsies. The only significant differential diagnosis is with an oncocytic carcinoid tumor of the bronchus (well-differentiated neuroendocrine carcinoma), which will be characterized, in addition to the abundant granular cytoplasm, by larger nuclei showing a "salt and pepper" chromatin pattern.

Inflammatory Pseudotumor

Inflammatory pseudotumor, also known as inflammatory myofibroblastic tumor and plasma cell granuloma, is a process of unknown etiology that has been felt to possibly represent an inflammatory response to a previous injury but has in some cases the attributes of a neoplastic process with the capability for infiltration and destruction of lung parenchyma and invasion of adjacent structures. The fact that some of these lesions can recur and progress to a fully malignant tumor has also been cited as evidence of their neoplastic nature. Cytogenetic features have been more recently identified that have also argued in favor of a neoplastic process.[46] The tumors are rare and have a predilection for children and young adults and may have either a central or a peripheral location. Tumors in peripheral locations can often extend into the pleura and involve extrapulmonary structures. Tumors in central locations show a tendency to grow in a polypoid fashion into the bronchial lumen causing symptoms of obstruction. Two patterns can be observed histologically: fibrohistiocytic spindle cell type and plasma cell type. The fibrohistiocytic type is characterized by fascicles of spindle cells with focal storiform pattern admixed with inflammatory cells (Fig. 14.16A). The spindle cells show elongated nuclei with inconspicuous nucleoli surrounded by a rim of amphophilic-to-eosinophilic cytoplasm and are generally devoid of cytologic atypia or mitotic activity. Foamy macrophages can be frequently seen admixed with the spindle cells. The plasma cell type is characterized by a predominance of mature plasma cells admixed with a lesser component of fibroblastic spindle cells (Fig. 14.16B). The plasma cell population will type as polyclonal by the immunoperoxidase or other techniques. The spindle cells will show positivity for SMA and vimentin. About one-third of cases have been shown to harbor the anaplastic lymphoma kinase (ALK) rearrangement, which can be detected by FISH or by immunohistochemistry using the ALK antibody-1 (ALK-1).[47] ALK-1 positivity, however, has been observed mostly in children, and absence of this stain does not rule out the diagnosis. It

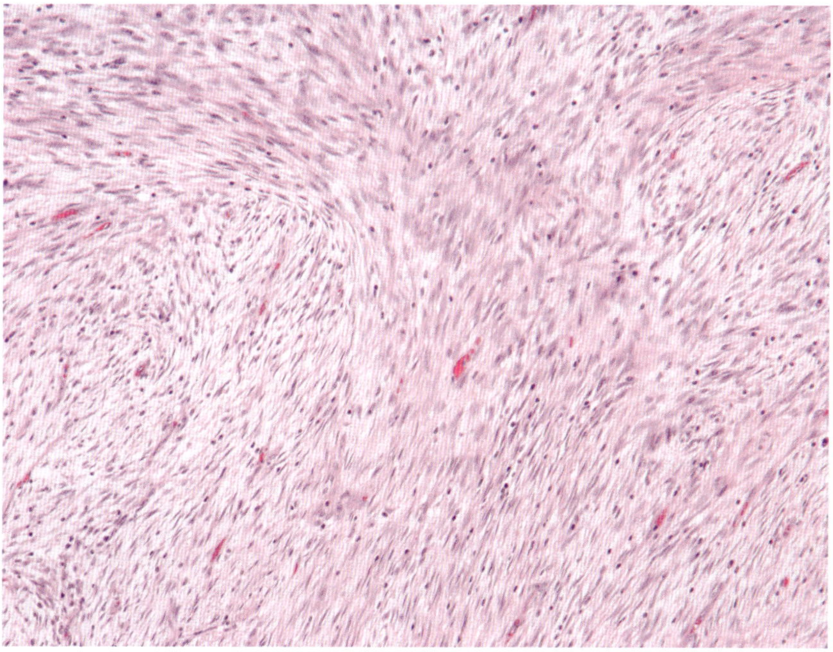

A

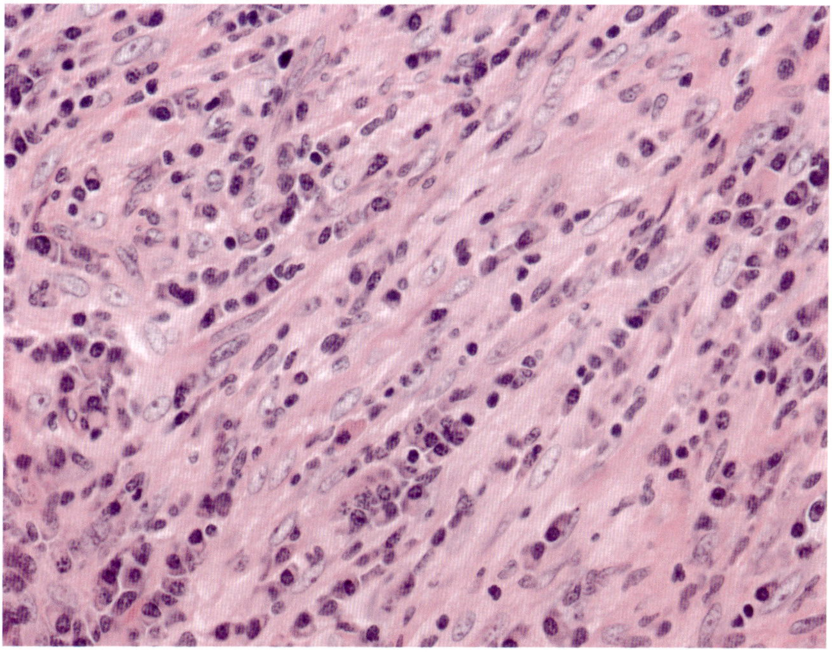

B

FIGURE 14.16 **A:** Inflammatory pseudotumor of lung, fibrohistiocytic type, shows bland-appearing fascicular spindle cell proliferation with minor inflammatory component. **B:** Inflammatory pseudotumor, plasma cell type, shows fibroblastic spindle cell proliferation accompanied by numerous mature plasma cells.

may be difficult in some cases to draw the line between an inflammatory pseudotumor and a spindle cell sarcoma. The presence of marked cytologic atypia, nuclear pleomorphism, mitotic activity, and tumor cell necrosis favors a diagnosis of sarcoma over that of inflammatory pseudotumor.

OTHER BENIGN TUMORS AND TUMOR-LIKE CONDITIONS

A number of other benign tumors and tumor-like conditions can occur in the lung that may be amenable to sampling through endoscopy or by core biopsies.

Alveolar Adenoma

Alveolar adenoma is a rare benign tumor that usually presents as a small coin lesion within pulmonary parenchyma and is characterized by multiple large cystic spaces filled with eosinophilic proteinaceous material that superficially resemble dilated lymphatics. The cystic spaces are lined by cuboidal cells with hobnail appearance resembling alveolar type II pneumocytes (Fig. 14.17A, B). The interstitium separating the cystic spaces shows collagenous stroma containing scattered bland-appearing spindle cells. The epithelial cells lining the dilated cystic spaces are type II alveolar pneumocytes and stain for keratin, CEA, surfactant apoprotein, and TTF-1. The stromal spindle cells stain for SMA and vimentin.[48] The lesion, thus, appears to represent a mixed proliferation of alveolar pneumocytes and septal mesenchyme. Cytogenetic studies have supported a neoplastic genotype. The main differential diagnosis is with lymphangioma and sclerosing hemangioma. The presence of hobnail cells lining the cystic spaces and cytokeratin/TTF-1 positivity will help distinguish the lesion from lymphangioma. The absence of sheets of monotonous TTF-1+ clear cells in the interstitium surrounding the cystic spaces, and the absence of pools of blood in the lumen of the cystic spaces will serve to distinguish it from sclerosing hemangioma.

Mucous Gland Adenoma

Mucous gland adenoma is a rare benign tumor that originates from submucosal seromucinous glands of the proximal airways leading to bronchial obstruction, mostly in adult patients. They usually appear on endoscopic examination as polypoid endobronchial tumors obstructing the lumen. The tumors are usually well circumscribed, with a mucoid consistency and multicystic appearance. Histologically, the tumors are characterized by a proliferation of dilated seromucinous glands as well as nondilated glands and tubules in the submucosa. A distinctive feature of these tumors is the fact that the process is restricted to the submucosa up to the cartilaginous plate and never extends beyond the cartilaginous plate.[49] On higher magnification, the dilated glandular structures are mainly lined by mucinous epithelium, although bland columnar,

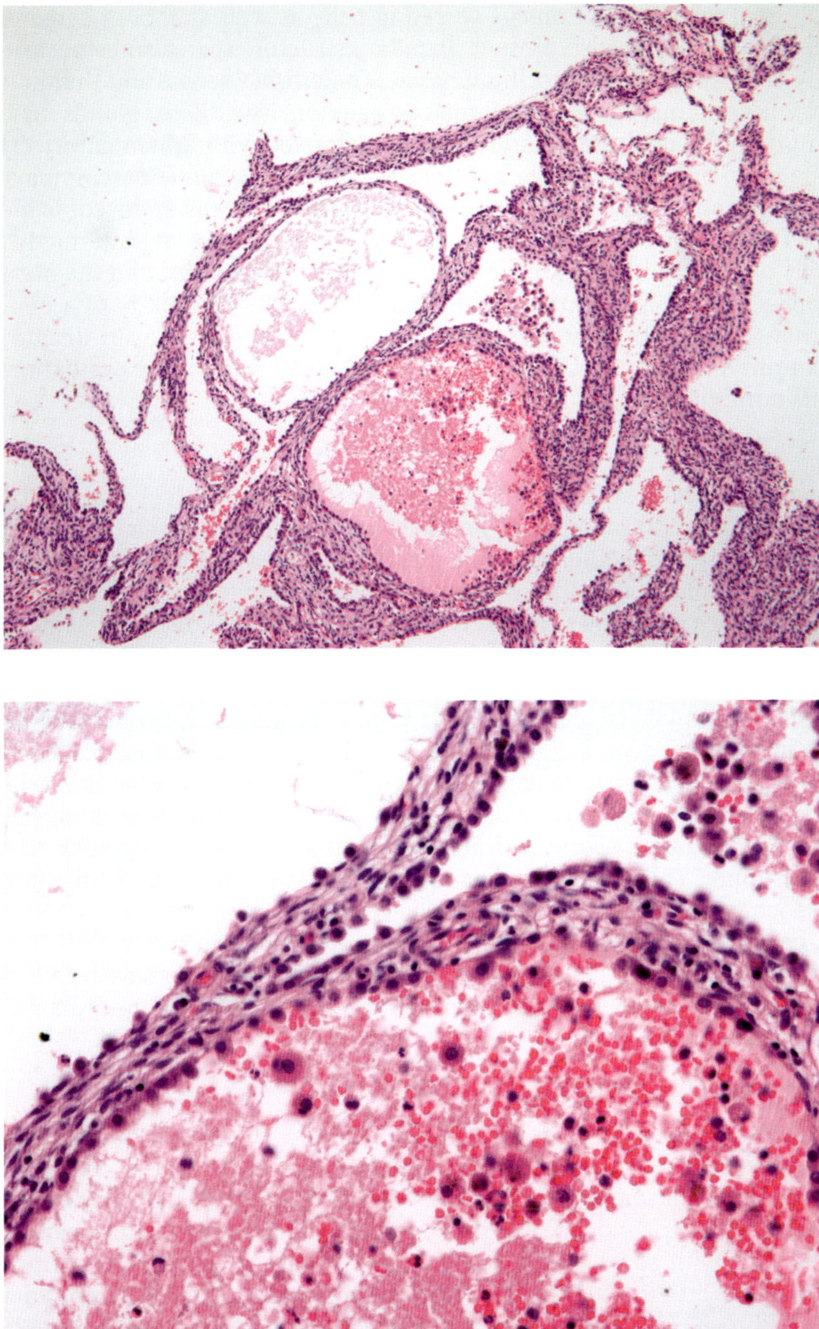

A

B

FIGURE 14.17 **A:** Endobronchial biopsy of alveolar adenoma shows dilated spaces filled with proteinaceous fluid simulating distended lymphatics. **B:** Higher magnification shows lining of the cystic spaces by hobnailed type II pneumocytes. Notice primitive fibroblastic spindle cell proliferation in the septal stroma.

cuboidal, or flattened mucus-secreting cells as well as foci of squamous metaplasia may be also present. Papillary structures can also be occasionally seen protruding into the lumens. The stroma separating the dilated glands contains a dense inflammatory reaction. The dilated glands may be empty or filled with mucinous material admixed with inflammatory cells. The main differential diagnosis is with a mucoepidermoid carcinoma and the distinction can be challenging, especially on a small endoscopic biopsy. The complete absence of cytologic atypia, absence of "intermediate" cells or squamoid foci admixed with scattered mucocytes, and the normal appearance of the dilated glands should raise the possibility of a benign process. Mucous gland adenoma is a hematoxylin and eosin diagnosis; immunohistochemical stains play a very limited role for the evaluation of this condition.

Alveolar Proteinosis

Alveolar proteinosis is a diffuse process of unknown etiology that has been observed in association with immunosuppression and hematologic malignancies.[50] The condition affects patients of all ages and may manifest with cough, dyspnea, and diffuse reticulonodular infiltrates in both lung fields. Coalescence of nodules can lead to areas of consolidation. The hallmark of the process is filling of the alveoli by acellular proteinaceous eosinophilic material that characteristically stains brightly with PAS (Fig. 14.18). The eosinophilic material tends to show prominent granularity, reminiscent of the frothy exudates seen in *Pneumocystis carinii* pneumonia. Electron microscopy has demonstrated lamellar osmiophilic bodies, annular inclusions, and dense granules in the exudate. The underlying pulmonary architecture is preserved, with absence of fibrosis or other significant alteration in the interstitium. The differential diagnosis is with *P. carinii* pneumonia; simple histochemical stains can be of assistance for separating the two. PAS stain is positive in alveolar proteinosis but will not stain the frothy infiltrates in *P. carinii* pneumonia; conversely, Gomori methenamine silver stain will highlight the organisms in *P. carinii* pneumonia and will be negative in alveolar proteinosis.

Placental Transmogrification

Placental transmogrification refers to a rare condition characterized by extensive replacement of lung parenchyma by structures resembling edematous placental villi. The lesions have been described mainly in young adults in association with congenital giant bullous emphysema and in adults with severe emphysema related to smoking. The alveoli in this condition develop a peculiar villous configuration resulting from edema and fibrosis of residual strands of alveolar tissue in lungs affected by severe emphysema, resulting in the development of grape-like structures and softening of lung parenchyma. The villous-like structures are usually lined on their outer surface by a single layer of cuboidal epithelium (Fig. 14.19). The cores of the papillary-like structures are filled with edema

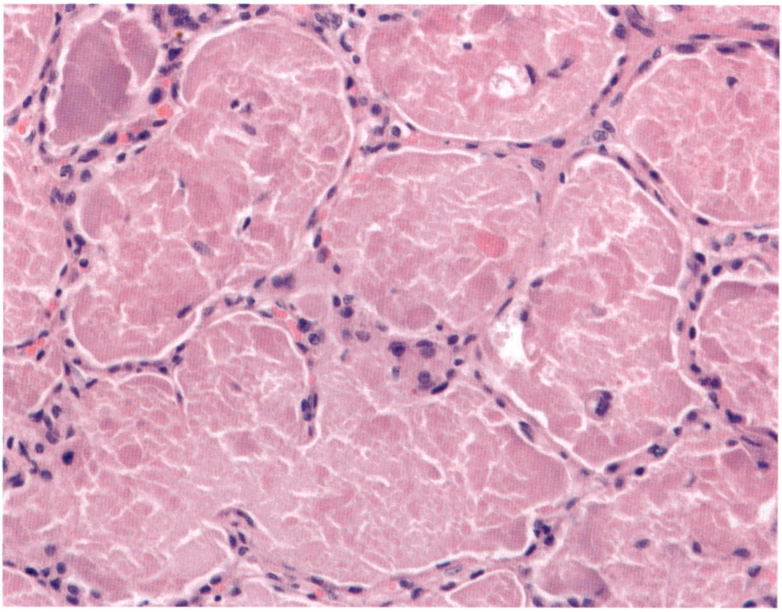

FIGURE 14.18 Alveolar proteinosis is characterized by distention of alveolar spaces with proteinaceous granular eosinophilic material. Notice the absence of inflammation or fibrosis in the alveolar walls, a clue to its noninfectious etiology.

fluid or may show myxoid stroma with scattered small vessels. Some cases may display mature adipose tissue or focal smooth muscle proliferation in the cores. Cases with prominent mature adipose tissue have been interpreted as examples of pulmonary lipomatosis. The striking resemblance to edematous chorionic villi is quite distinctive and greatly facilitates the diagnosis.

Lymphangioleiomyomatosis

Lymphangioleiomyomatosis (LAM) is an unusual disorder of unknown etiology that predominantly occurs in premenopausal women and is associated in some cases with tuberous sclerosis, with which it shares an alteration in the tumor suppressor gene *TSC2* at chromosomal locus 16p13. Patients present clinically with recurrent bouts of pneumothorax and show the characteristic imaging findings of multiple bilateral nodular and cystic changes of lung parenchyma with a honeycomb appearance on computerized tomography scans. Although open lung biopsies are the preferred method for establishing a tissue diagnosis, transbronchial biopsies have also been utilized with good results.[51,52] Histologic examination shows cystic dilatation of airspaces, some of which are at least partially lined by a discrete spindle cell proliferation attached to the walls of the cysts (Fig. 14.20A, B). The spindle cells in these areas resemble smooth

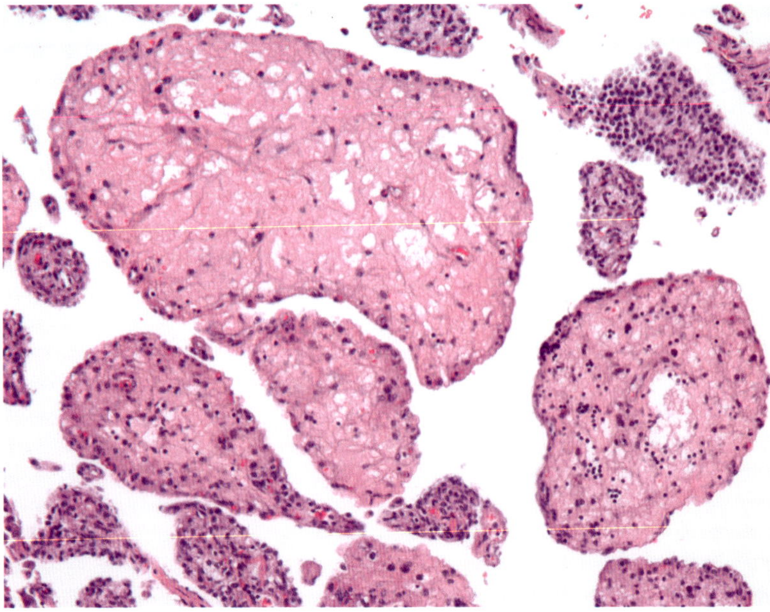

FIGURE 14.19 Transbronchial biopsy in placental transmogrification of the lung shows distended villus-like structures lined by single layer of small cuboidal cells in the surface and containing small vessels admixed with myxoid material in their cores. The structures resemble chorionic villi.

muscle and contain elongated nuclei surrounded by lightly eosinophilic-to-amphophilic fibrillary cytoplasm. The spindle cells may adopt a more epithelioid appearance focally and display abundant clear cytoplasm (Fig. 14.20C). The spindle cell proliferation is not associated with cytologic atypia or mitotic activity. The spindle cell proliferation can be extremely subtle and easily missed on initial examination. Attention to the presence of cystically dilated spaces with focal areas of thickening of the walls should prompt closer examination to identify the smooth muscle proliferation. The spindle cells in LAM have a dual phenotype and coexpress SMA and HMB45; they, thus, also belong in the family of myomelanocytic proliferations related to PECs. The spindle cells can also stain positive for estrogen and progesterone receptors. The lesions can hardly be confused for any other condition; the differential diagnosis is, thus, quite limited. The most important consideration is simply not missing the lesion, which can occur quite often when a proper clinical history has not been provided or attention is not paid to the subtle thickening of the cystic spaces and the focal spindle cell proliferation. Use of immunohistochemical stains, in particular SMA and HMB45, is helpful in highlighting such foci in suspicious cases or in cases with a positive history and typical radiographic findings.

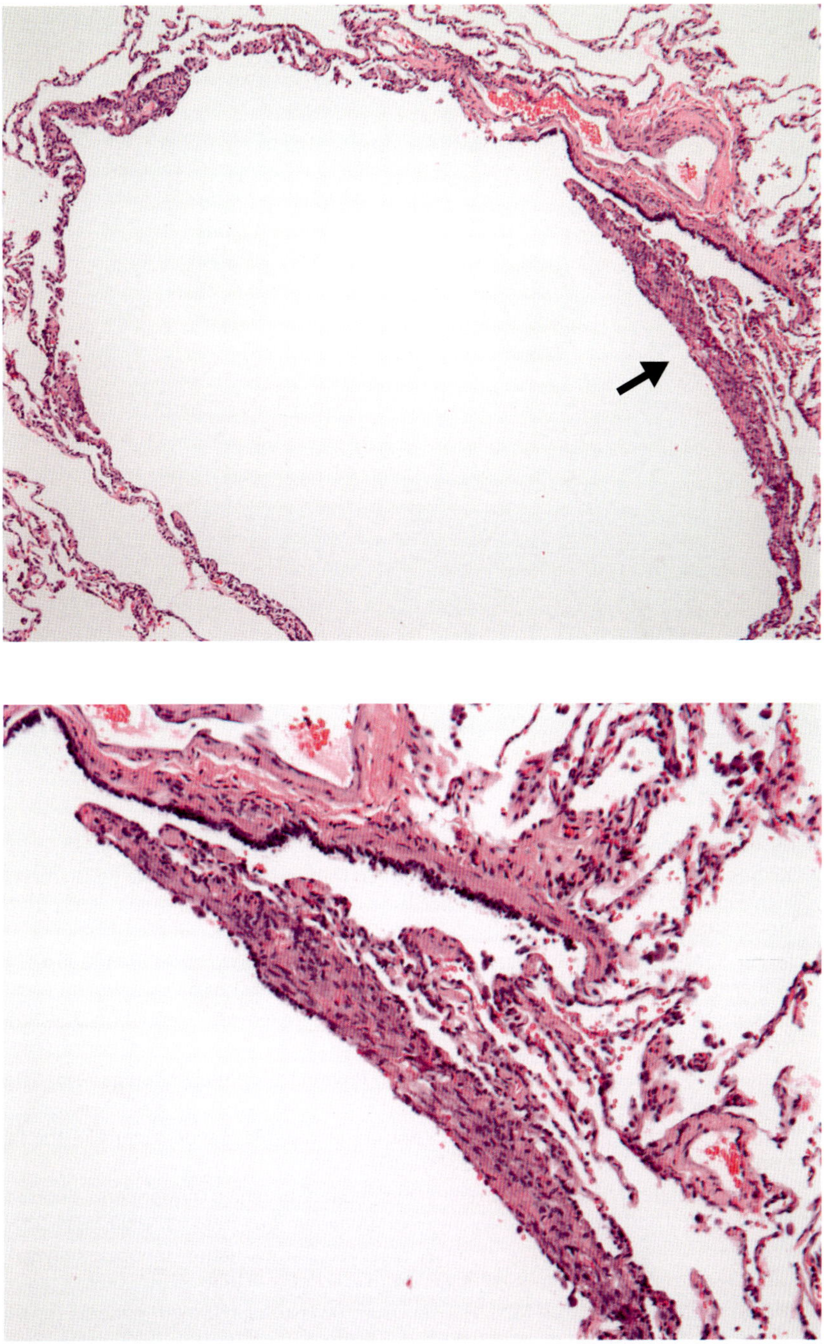

A

B

FIGURE 14.20 Changes seen in endoscopic lung biopsies in LAM: **A:** Cystic dilatation of airspace shows very subtle and focal thickening of the wall (arrow). **B:** Higher magnification from same field shows subtle proliferation of spindle cells beneath the lining mucosa; such case may be very difficult to diagnose in the absence of clinical information suggestive of LAM. *(continued)*

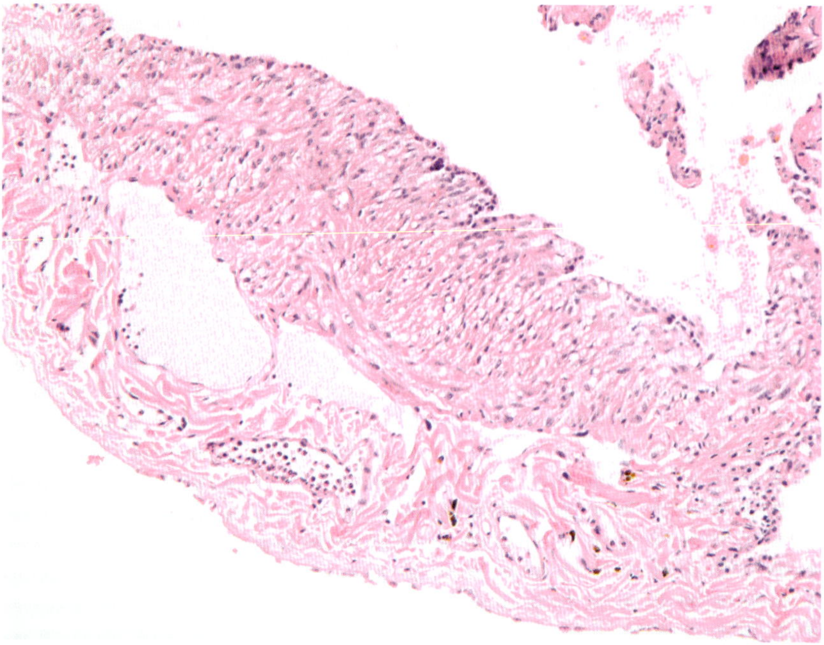

C

FIGURE 14.20 *(continued)* **C:** Another area showing more characteristic spindle cell proliferation with clearing of the cytoplasm. The cells in these areas were positive for actin and HMB45.

REREFENCES

1. Suster S. Primary sarcomas of the lung. *Semin Diagn Pathol.* 1995;12:140–157.
2. Xiao S, Lux ML, Reeves R, et al. HMGI(Y) activation by chromosome 6p21 rearrangements in multilineage mesenchymal cells from pulmonary hamartoma. *Am J Pathol.* 1997;150:901–910.
3. Suster S, Moran CA. Pulmonary adenofibroma: report of two cases of an unusual type of hamartomatous lesion of the lung. *Histopathology.* 1993;23:547–551.
4. Moran CA, Suster S, Koss MN. Endobrionchial lipomas: a clinicopathologic study of four cases. *Mod Pathol.* 1994;7:212–214.
5. Marcheix B, Brouchet L, Lamarche Y, et al. Pulmonary angiomyolipoma. *Ann Thorac Surg.* 2006;82:1504–1506.
6. Yellin A, Rosenman Y, Lieberman Y. Review of smooth muscle tumors of the lower respiratory tract. *Br J Dis Chest.* 1984;78:337–351.
7. Bosch X, Ramirez J, Font J, et al. Primary intrapulmonary benign schwannoma. A case with ultrastructural and immunohistochemical confirmation. *Eur Respir J.* 1990;3:234–237.
8. Yousem SA, Flynn SD. Intrapulmonary localized fibrous tumor: intraparenchymal so-called localized fibrous mesothelioma. *Am J Clin Pathol.* 1988;89:365–369.
9. Moran CA, Suster S, Koss MN. The spectrum of histologic growth patterns in benign and malignant fibrous tumors of the pleura. *Semin Diagn Pathol.* 1992;9:169–180.
10. Rao A, Falconieri G, Moran CA, et al.. Intrapulmonary solitary fibrous tumor. Clinicopathologic and immunohistochemical study of 24 cases. Med.Pathol.2011;24:422A..
11. Moran CA, Suster S, Abbondanzo SL, et al. Primary leiomyosarcomas of the lung: a clinicopathologic and immunohistochemical study of 18 cases. *Mod Pathol.* 1997;10:121–128.

12. Zeren H, Moran CA, Suster S, et al. Primary pulmonary sarcomas with features of monophasic synovial sarcoma: a clinicopathological, immunohistochemical, and ultrastructural study of 25 cases. *Hum Pathol.* 1995;26:474–480.
13. Suster S, Fisher C, Moran CA. The spectrum of bcl-2 oncoprotein reactivity in benign and malignant spindle cell tumors of soft tissue, skin, serosal surfaces, and gastrointestinal tract. An immunohistochemical study of 380 cases. *Am J Surg Pathol.* 1998;22:863–872.
14. Kaplan MA, Goodman MD, Satish J, et al. Primary pulmonary sarcoma with morphologic features of monophasic synovial sarcoma and chromosome translocation t(X;18). *Am J Clin Pathol.* 1996;105:195–199.
15. Yousem SA, Hochholzer L. Malignant fibrous histiocytoma of the lung. *Cancer.* 1987;60:2532–2541.
16. Weiss SW, Ishak KG, Dail DH, et al. Epithelioid hemangioendothelioma and related lesions. *Semin Diagn Pathol.* 1986;3:259–287.
17. Kitaichi M, Nagai S, Nishimura K, et al. Pulmonary epithelioid hemangioendothelioma in 21 patients, including three with partial spontaneous regression. *Eur Respir J.* 1998;12:89–96.
18. Meduri GU, Stover DE, Lee M, et al. Pulmonary Kaposi's sarcoma in the acquired immune deficiency syndrome. Clinical, radiographic and pathologic manifestations. *Am J Med.* 1986;81:11–18.
19. Howard M, Brink N, Miller R, et al. Association of human herpes virus with pulmonary Kaposi's sarcoma. *Lancet.* 1995;346:712.
20. Nash G, Fligiel S. Kaposi's sarcoma presenting as pulmonary disease in the acquired immunodeficiency syndrome: diagnosis by lung biopsy. *Hum Pathol.* 1984;15:999–1001.
21. Yousem SA. Angiosarcoma presenting in the lung. *Arch Pathol Lab Med.* 1986;110:112–115.
22. Spragg RG, Wolf PL, Haghighi P, et al. Angiosarcoma of the lung with fatal pulmonary hemorrhage. *Am J Med.* 1983;74:1072–1076.
23. Wagenvoort CA, Beetstra A, Spijker J. Capillary hemangiomatosis of the lungs. *Histopathology.* 1989;14:212–214.
24. Lantuejoul S, Sheppard MN, Corrin B, et al. Pulmonary veno-occlusive disease and pulmonary capillary hemangiomatosis: a clinicopathologic study of 35 cases. *Am J Surg Pathol.* 2006;30:850–857.
25. Wilson RW, Moran CA. Primary melanoma of the lung: a clinicopathologic and immunohistochemical study of eight cases. *Am J Surg Pathol.* 1997;21:1196–1202.
26. Littman CD. Metastatic melanoma mimicking primary bronchial melanoma. *Histopathology.* 1991;18:561–563.
27. Moran CA, Hochholzer L, Rush W, et al. Primary intrapulmonary meningiomas: a clinicopathologic and immunohistochemical study of ten cases. *Cancer.* 1996;78:2328–2333.
28. Kodama K, Doi O, Higashiyama M, et al. Primary and metastatic meningioma. *Cancer.* 1991;67:1412–1417.
29. Gaffey MJ, Mills SE, Askin FB. Minute pulmonary meningothelial-like nodules: a clinicopathologic study of so-called minute pulmonary chemodectoma. *Am J Surg Pathol.* 1988;12:167–175.
30. Suster S, Moran CA. Diffuse pulmonary meningotheliomatosis. *Am J Surg Pathol.* 2007;31:624–631.
31. Moran CA, Suster S, Fishback NF, et al. Primary intrapulmonary thymoma: a clinicopathologic and immunohistochemical study of eight cases. *Am J Surg Pathol.* 1995;19:304–312.
32. Suster S, Moran CA. Histologic classification of thymoma: the World Health Organization and beyond. *Hematol Oncol Clin North Am.* 2008;22:381–392.
33. Folpe AL, Fanburg-Smith JC, Miettinen M, et al. Atypical and malignant glomus tumors: analysis of 52 cases, with a proposal for the reclassification of glomus tumors. *Am J Surg Pathol.* 2001;25:1–12.

34. Tang CK, Toker C, Foris NP, et al. Glomangioma of the lung. *Am J Surg Pathol.* 1978;2:103–109.
35. Koss MN, Hochholzer L, Moran CA. Primary pulmonary glomus tumor: a clinicopathologic and immunohistochemical study of two cases. *Mod Pathol.* 1998;11:253–258.
36. Cai C, Zeng Y, Chen H, et al. Fibrobronchoscopic evidence of endobronchial hairs in intrapulmonary teratoma with hemoptysis but without trichoptysis. *Am J Med Sci.* 2008;336:441–444.
37. Moran CA, Travis WD, Carter D, et al. Metastatic mature teratomas in lung following testicular embryonal carcinoma and teratocarcinoma. *Arch Pathol Lab Med.* 1993;117:641–644.
38. Katzenstein AL, Gmelich JT, Carrington CB. Sclerosing hemangioma of the lung: a clinicopathologic study of 51 cases. *Am J Surg Pathol.* 1980;4:343–356.
39. Devouassoux-Shiosheboran M, de la Fouchardiere A, Thivolet-Bejui F, et al. Endobronchial variant of sclerosing hemangioma of the lung: histologic and cytological features of endobronchial material. *Mod Pathol.* 2004;17:252–257.
40. Devouassoux-Shisheboran M, Hayashi T, Linnoila RI, et al. A clinicopathologic study of 100 cases of pulmonary sclerosing hemangioma with immunohistochemical studies: TTF-1 is expressed in both round and surface cells, suggesting an origin from primitive respiratory epithelium. *Am J Surg Pathol.* 2000;24:906–916.
41. Satoh Y, Tsuchiya E, Weng SY, et al. Pulmonary sclerosing hemangioma of the lung. A type II pneumocytoma by immunohistochemical and immunoelectron microscopic studies. *Cancer.* 1989;64:1310–1317.
42. Gaffey MJ, Mills SE, Zarbo RJ, et al. Clear cell tumor of the lung. Immunohistochemical and ultrastructural evidence of melanogenesis. *Am J Surg Pathol.* 1991;15:644–653.
43. Fetsch PA, Fetsch JF, Marincola FM, et al. Comparison of melanoma antigen recognized by T-cells (MART-1) to HMB-45: additional evidence to support a common lineage for angiomyolipoma, lymphangiomyomatosis, and clear cell sugar tumor. *Mod Pathol.* 1998;11:699–703.
44. Deavers M, Guinee D, Koss MN, et al. Granular cell tumors of the lung: clinicopathologic study of 20 cases. *Am J Surg Pathol.* 1995;19:627–635.
45. Van der Maten J, Blaauwgeers JL, Sutedja TG, et al. Granular cell tumors of the tracheobronchial tree. *J Thorac Cardiovasc Surg.* 2003;126:740–743.
46. Su LD, Atayde-Perez A, Sheldon S, et al. Inflammatory myofibroblastic tumor: cytogenetic evidence supporting clonal origin. *Mod Pathol.* 1998;11:364–368.
47. Coffin CM, Patel A, Perkins S, et al. ALK1 and p80 expression and chromosomal rearrangements involving 2p23 in inflammatory myofibroblastic tumor. *Mod Pathol.* 2001;14:569–576.
48. Burke LM, Rush WI, Khoor A, et al. Alveolar adenoma: a histochemical, immunohistochemical, and ultrastructural analysis of 17 cases. *Hum Pathol.* 1999;30:156–167.
49. England DM, Hochholzer L. Truly benign "bronchial adenoma": report of 10 cases of mucous gland adenoma with immunohistochemical and ultrastructural findings. *Am J Surg Pathol.* 1995;19:887–899.
50. Bedrossian CW, Luna MA, Conklin RH, et al. Alveolar proteinosis as a consequence of immunosuppression. A hypothesis based on clinical and pathologic observations. *Hum Pathol.* 1980;11:527–535.
51. Bonetti F, Chiodera PL, Pea M, et al. Transbronchial biopsy in lymphangioleiomyomatosis of the lung. HMB45 for diagnosis. *Am J Surg Pathol.* 1993;17:1092–1102.
52. Guinee DG Jr, Feuerstein I, Koss MN, et al. Pulmonary lymphangioleiomyomatosis. Diagnosis based on results of transbronchial biopsy and immunohistochemical studies and correlation with high-resolution computed tomography findings. *Arch Pathol Lab Med.* 1994;118:846–849.

15

METASTATIC TUMORS TO THE LUNG

The lung is one of the commonest visceral sites of metastases for malignancies arising from internal organs. Metastases can reach the lungs through lymphatic or hematogenous routes. The classical presentation of metastatic tumors to the lungs is in the form of multiple bilateral subpleural nodules.[1] Isolated metastases (i.e., "coin" lesion) have also been observed in up to 9% of cases.[2,3] Distinguishing a primary from metastatic lesion in a lung biopsy may be quite difficult in the absence of a proper clinical history as the morphology of many of the tumors that are capable of metastasizing to the lung can show significant overlap with different primary lung tumors. A multidisciplinary approach that includes clinical and pathologic correlation, results of imaging studies, and comparison of the lesion with previous pathologic material will be critical for accurate diagnosis. Several other factors may also play a role in obscuring the proper identification of metastases in the lungs, including late metastases from low-grade tumors that take place many years after the initial recognition of the primary lesion, changes in morphologic appearance of the metastatic deposits in the lung as compared with the original lesion, unusual mode of spread or distribution of the metastatic deposits in the lung, and unusual or peculiar morphologic appearances of metastatic deposits that may lead to the mistaken assumption of a new or separate, unrelated primary tumor.[4] In addition, a small number of metastases to the lung may correspond to the hematogenous spread of tumors that are deemed by convention to be benign and incapable of metastases; the latter have been categorized as "benign metastasizing" tumors.[1]

METASTASES TO THE LUNGS FROM MALIGNANT EPITHELIAL NEOPLASMS

Because the terminal pulmonary bed is one of the most frequent visceral sites involved in the arrest of circulating tumor cells from internal malignancies, the lung is often one of the first organs, other than the lymph nodes, to be involved by metastatic spread of carcinoma. Metastases of carcinoma to the lungs may occur through hematogenous route, through lymphatics, or by retrograde spread from involved mediastinal or hilar lymph nodes. Most metastases from carcinomas are multiple, sharply circumscribed from the surrounding parenchyma, and show rapid growth. The sharp circumscription of the metastatic deposits is a helpful clue on imaging studies to separate them from primary lung cancer that tends to be spiculated on chest X-rays. Solitary metastases from epithelial neoplasms to the lung may be easily mistaken for a primary lung tumor in the absence of a proper clinical history or when the primary tumor remains clinically occult. Clinicopathologic correlation is, thus, indispensable for a correct diagnosis.

Metastases of carcinoma may occasionally adopt a pattern of growth that can closely mimic a primary lung cancer, such as the lepidic (bronchioloalveolar) growth pattern (Fig. 15.1); the latter tends to occur particularly with tumors from the colon, breast, pancreas, stomach, and kidney.[4,5] Another unusual presentation for metastases from carcinomas coming from other organs is an endobronchial location; such tumors will present as a polypoid intrabronchial mass leading to symptoms of obstruction that can closely resemble a primary bronchogenic tumor.[6] A common presentation of carcinoma metastases to the lungs is massive lymphangitic spread, particularly from stomach, prostate, breast, or pancreatic cancer, which may lead to the phenomenon described as "lymphangitis carcinomatosa" characterized by plugging of the peribronchial, septal, and pleural lymphatics by tumor

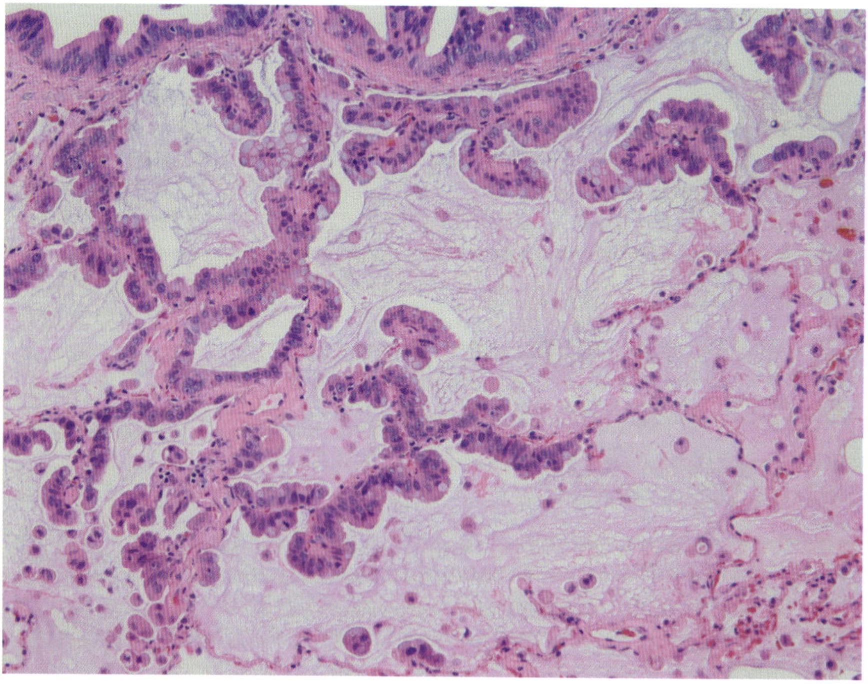

FIGURE 15.1 Metastasis from carcinoma of pancreas showing lepidic growth along preexisting alveolar septa simulating a mucinous primary bronchioloalveolar carcinoma of lung.

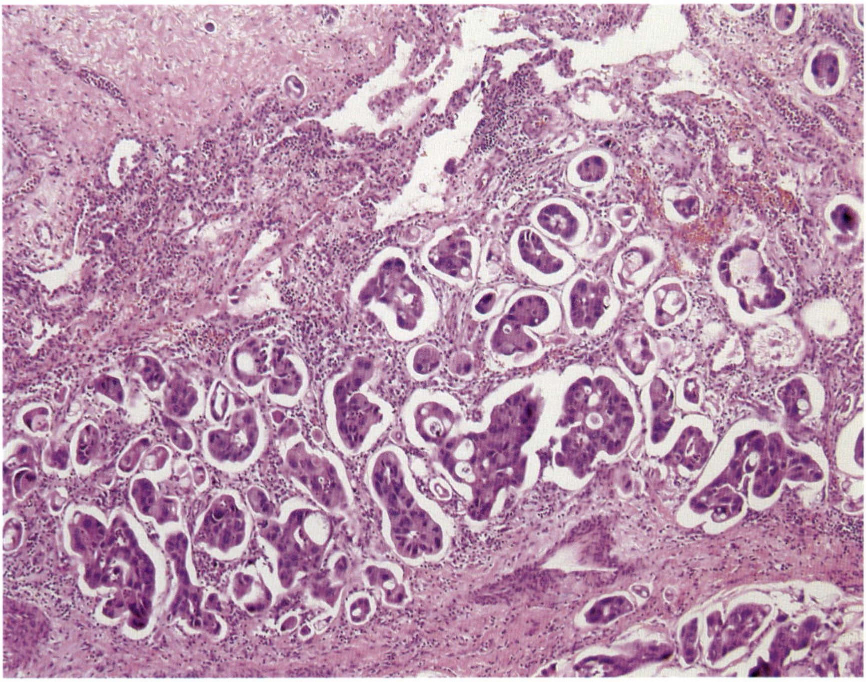

FIGURE 15.2 Metastasis from papillary serous carcinoma of ovary showing extensive lymphangitic spread throughout septal and bronchial lymphatics ("lymphangitis carcinomatosa").

emboli (Fig. 15.2). The diagnosis of metastatic carcinoma to the lung requires communication with the clinician and obtaining a thorough clinical history. Application of immunohistochemical stains or other ancillary techniques may be required in many instances to confirm the lineage of the tumor; review of previous biopsies or resection material will also be necessary to compare with the current lesions, either to confirm the resemblance to the original tumor or to document progression or regression of the malignancy at the metastatic sites.

Metastases from Head and Neck Cancer

Approximately 25% of head and neck cancers metastasize to the lungs.[7] The most common metastatic cancers from the head and neck to the lung originate from the larynx and the oral cavity.[8] The most frequent histologic types are squamous cell carcinoma and basaloid squamous cell carcinoma. The latter, in particular, can be easily confused for the small cell variant of primary squamous cell carcinoma of the lung or for small cell cancer on small endoscopic biopsies (Fig. 15.3). Proper clinical history is, therefore, indispensable for adequate identification of the lesion as a metastasis. Salivary gland tumors can also metastasize to the lungs, particularly adenoid cystic carcinoma and acinic cell carcinoma.[9,10] A detailed

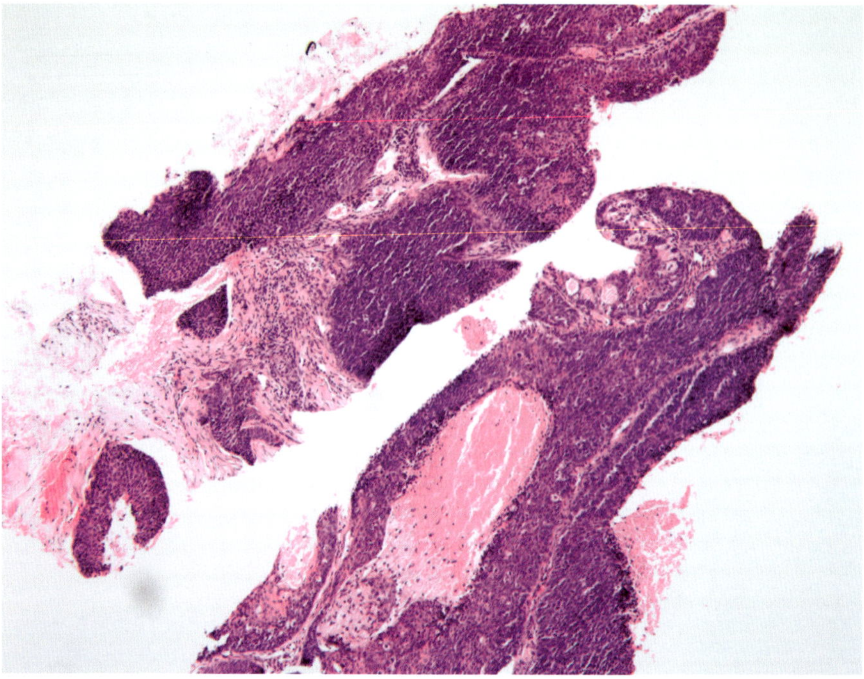

FIGURE 15.3 Pulmonary metastasis of basaloid-squamous carcinoma of the tongue shows islands of tightly packed, uniform small cells with peripheral palisading. In the absence of a proper history, these tumors can be mistaken for a primary squamous cell carcinoma of bronchus of the small cell variant or for basaloid or neuroendocrine carcinoma of the lung.

clinical history is required because salivary gland tumors can often metastasize after a long period of latency and may be easily mistaken for primary salivary gland-type tumors of the lung. Carcinoma of the thyroid, in particular papillary thyroid carcinoma, also metastasizes to the lungs. The clear nuclear features of papillary thyroid carcinoma can sometimes also be observed in some primary lung tumors, such as bronchioloalveolar cell carcinoma (adenocarcinoma with lepidic growth pattern) and in some cribriform-papillary adenocarcinomas.[11] Metastases from papillary thyroid carcinoma can also adopt a bronchioloalveolar pattern of growth closely simulating a primary adenocarcinoma[4]; use of immunohistochemical stains for thyroglobulin is indicated in such instances (Fig. 15.4).

Metastases from the Gastrointestinal Tract

Carcinomas arising from the whole length of the gastrointestinal tract can metastasize to the lungs, in particular colon, pancreas, and stomach. Colonic metastases have a tendency to display a wreath-like pattern of growth with cribriform structures along the periphery and extensive areas of necrosis. The cells are usually tall columnar, may be mucin secreting, and may contain interspersed goblet cells (Fig. 15.5). Unlike primary

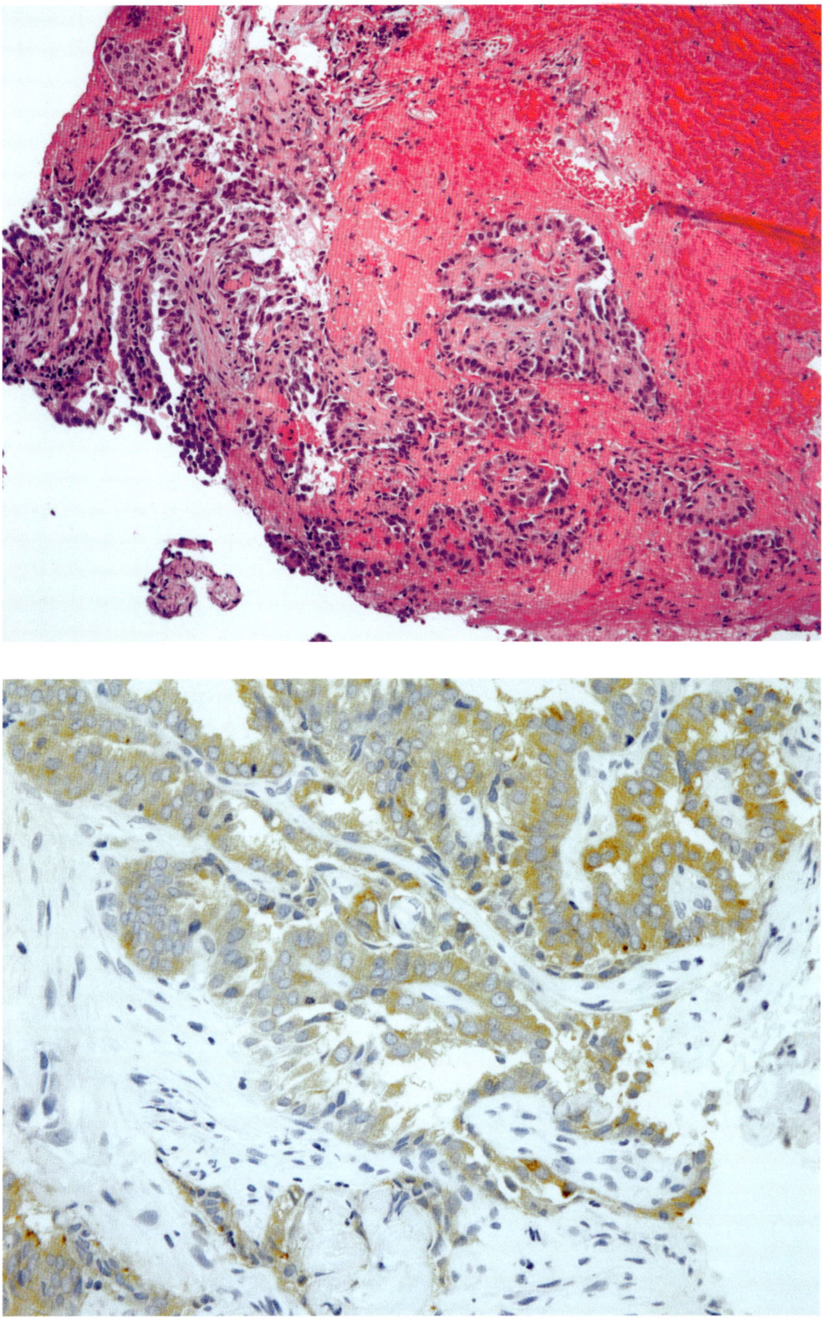

A

B

FIGURE 15.4 **A:** Endobronchial biopsy with metastasis of papillary thyroid carcinoma. The tumor can be easily mistaken for a primary papillary carcinoma of lung on routine microscopy. **B:** Immunohistochemical stain for thyroglobulin shows positivity in the tumor cells supporting thyroid origin.

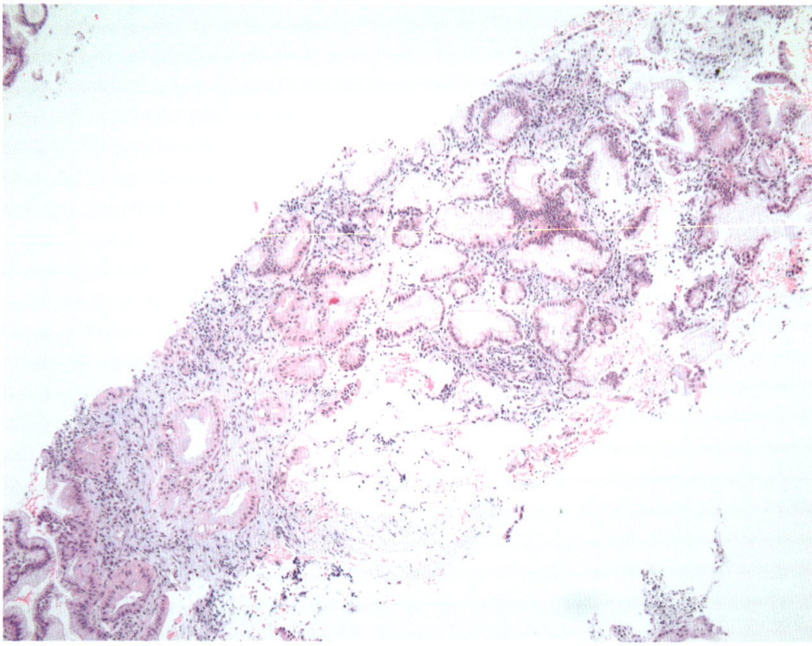

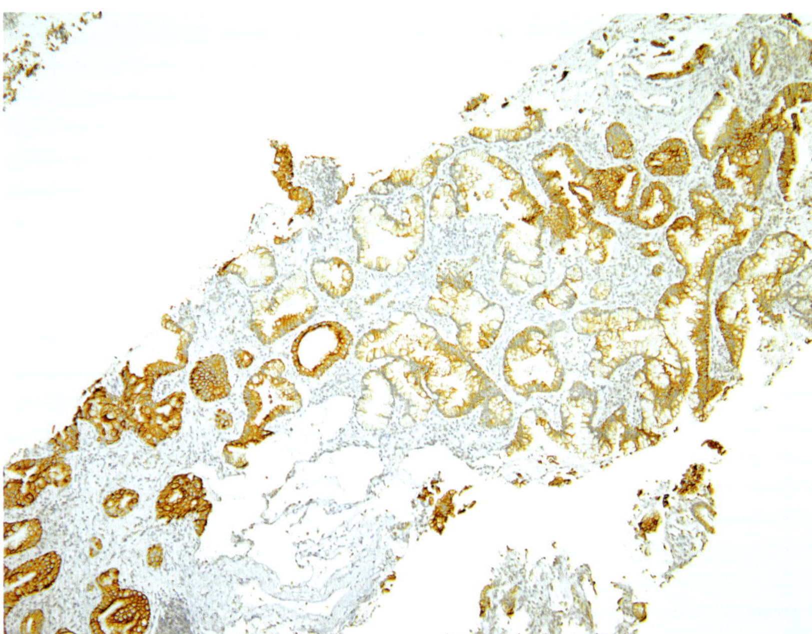

FIGURE 15.5 **A:** Core biopsy of metastatic adenocarcinoma of colon to the lung shows glands lined by tall columnar cells containing cytoplasmic mucin. **B:** The tumor cells were negative for TTF-1 and CK7 and showed strong positivity for CK20 (shown) and CDX2.

mucinous carcinomas of the lung, colonic metastases usually display marked cytologic atypia with prominent mitotic activity (eFigs. 15.1 to 15.3). Immunohistochemical stains may be of limited value in this setting because primary intestinal-type adenocarcinomas of the lung can display an enteric phenotype (CK20+/CDX2+ and CK7–/TTF–1–) or a lung phenotype (CK7+/TTF–1+ and CK20–/CDX2–).[12–14] Strict clinicopathologic correlation and thorough imaging and endoscopic studies may be needed before a definitive diagnosis can be rendered. It is also important to make this distinction because primary lung adenocarcinoma may also adopt a striking cribriform pattern of growth that can be easily confused for a metastasis from the colon or other organs in the gastrointestinal tract.[11] Primary mucin-secreting carcinoma of the lung may also adopt certain other unusual morphologic features that can lead to an erroneous diagnosis of metastases when the tumor is, indeed, a primary lung neoplasm, including production of abundant extracellular mucin (so-called colloid carcinoma) and tumors with signet-ring cell features.[15,16] Because such tumors can exhibit either an intestinal or a primary lung immunophenotype, careful clinicopathologic correlation is indicated to establish the correct diagnosis.

Metastases from primary tumors of the gastrointestinal tract, in particular pancreatic carcinoma, can sometimes adopt a striking lepidic growth pattern that can closely simulate a primary mucinous carcinoma of the lung with bronchioloalveolar pattern. It is important to keep this fact in mind because pulmonary metastases may occasionally represent the initial manifestation of pancreatic carcinoma, with radiographic and clinical features that are indistinguishable from those of a primary lung cancer (eFigs. 15.4 and 15.5).[17] Liver cell carcinoma can also metastasize to the lungs in early and late stages and can present as a solitary nodule (Fig. 15.6). The tumors must be distinguished from different lung primary tumors and other types of metastasis comprising cells with abundant eosinophilic cytoplasm. Immunohistochemical staining for HEP-Par1 and demonstration of a canalicular bile duct pattern of staining with carcinoembryonic antigen (CEA) will be of aid in making this distinction.

Metastases from the Genitourinary Tract

The most common metastases in the lung to originate from the genitourinary tract are from renal cell carcinoma (eFigs. 15.6 to 15.8). Renal cell carcinoma metastases are often multiple but can also present as a solitary lesion; they may precede the clinical detection of the primary tumor or develop several years (<10 years) after detection of the primary tumor in the kidney.[18] Metastatic renal cell carcinoma to the lung can also occur as an endobronchial lesion adopting a polypoid endobronchial configuration, thus clinically simulating a bronchogenic neoplasm.[19] Proper identification of a renal cell carcinoma metastasis to the lung may be of clinical significance because survival following metastasectomy can be

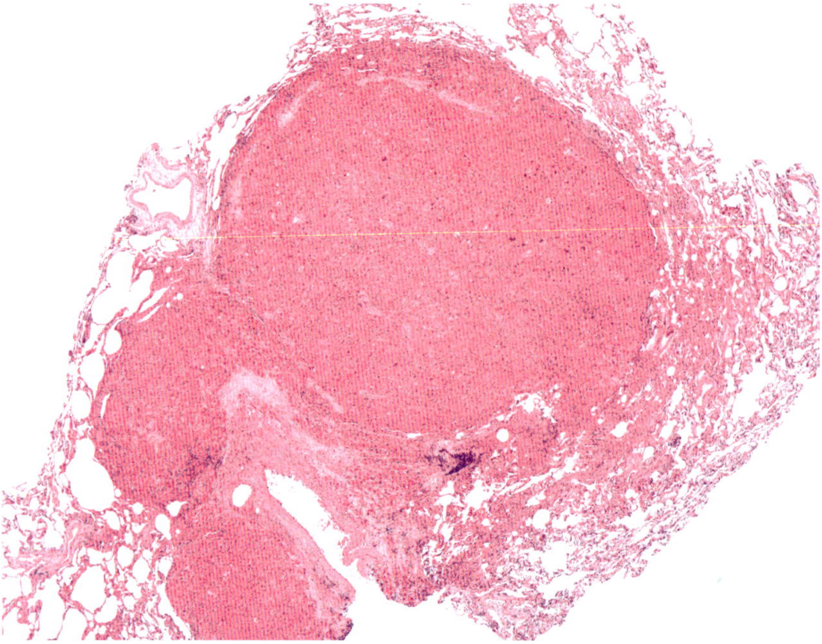

A

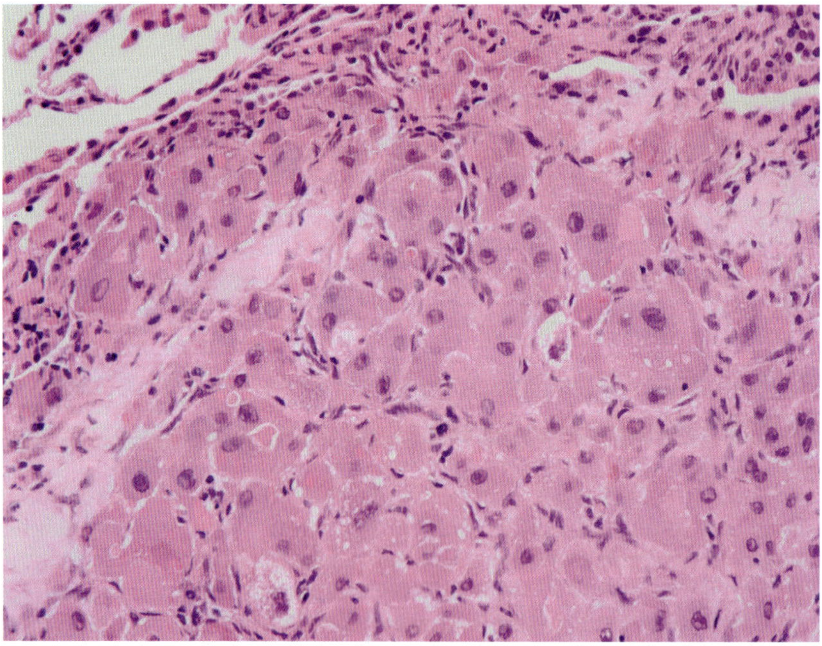

B

FIGURE 15.6 **A:** Metastasis of hepatocellular carcinoma, fibrolamellar type, shows a well-circumscribed pulmonary nodule sharply separated from the surrounding parenchyma. **B:** Higher magnification shows large cells with abundant densely eosinophilic cytoplasm and round nuclei with prominent nucleoli.

quite significant. The majority of renal cell carcinoma metastases to the lung will show the classical clear cell morphology characteristic of these tumors (Fig. 15.7); however, unusual variants can also be observed, such as tumors with abundant eosinophilic granular cytoplasm, tumors with a sarcomatoid appearance, and tumors with a prominent hemangiopericytic growth pattern (Fig. 15.8A, B).[4] Immunohistochemical stains play an important role in the diagnosis of these tumors. All renal cell carcinoma metastases (including the sarcomatoid variant) are strongly positive for cytokeratin antibodies, in particular low-molecular weight cytokeratins, and coexpress vimentin intermediate filaments. The tumors are negative for thyroid transcription factor-1 (TTF-1), p63, and surfactant apoprotein but can be positive for Napsin A. Other helpful markers associated with renal cell carcinoma include CD10, renal cell carcinoma antigen (although the latter has not been very helpful in our hands for metastatic renal cell carcinoma), PAX8, and carbonic anhydrase (CA) IX (Fig. 15.8 C). A potential pitfall for diagnosis occurs with metastases from the papillary variant of renal cell carcinoma. Such tumors may display a prominent papillary growth pattern that can be confused for papillary adenocarcinoma of the lung and other metastatic tumors; moreover, they strongly express CK7, thus overlapping with the immunophenotype of primary lung adenocarcinoma. A helpful marker that can serve to distinguish metastases to the lung from papillary renal cell carcinoma is α-methyl CoA

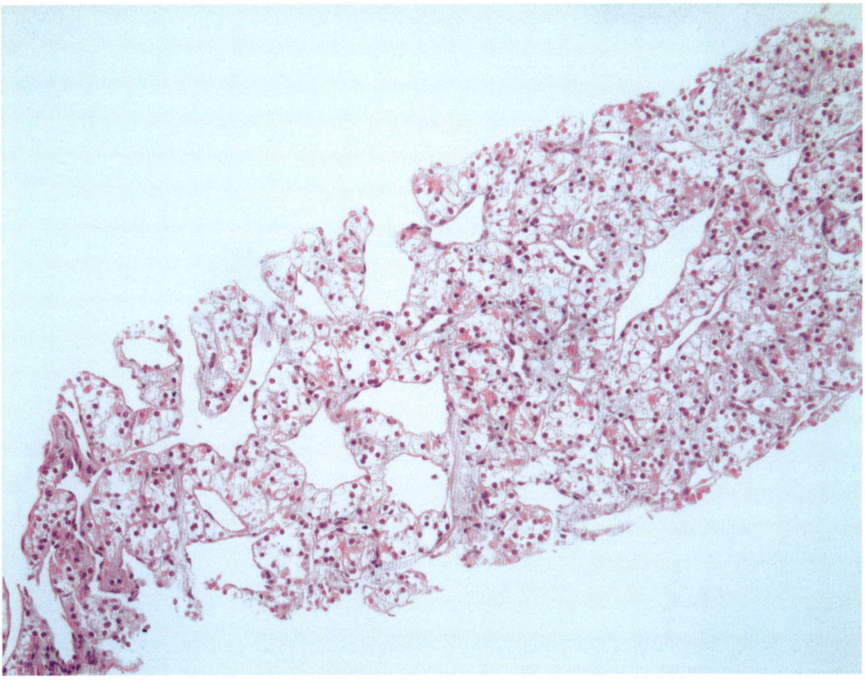

FIGURE 15.7 Core biopsy shows metastasis of clear cell renal cell carcinoma in the lung.

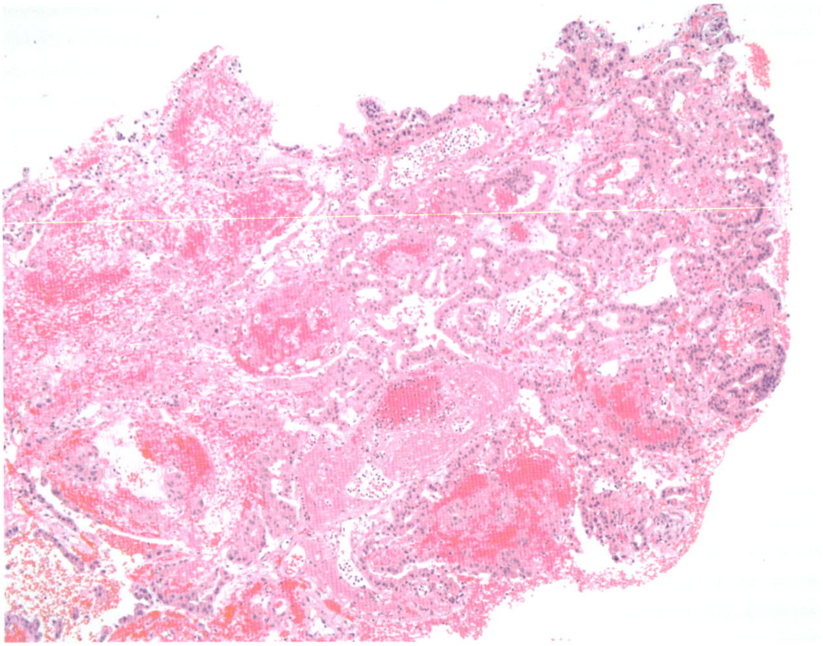

A

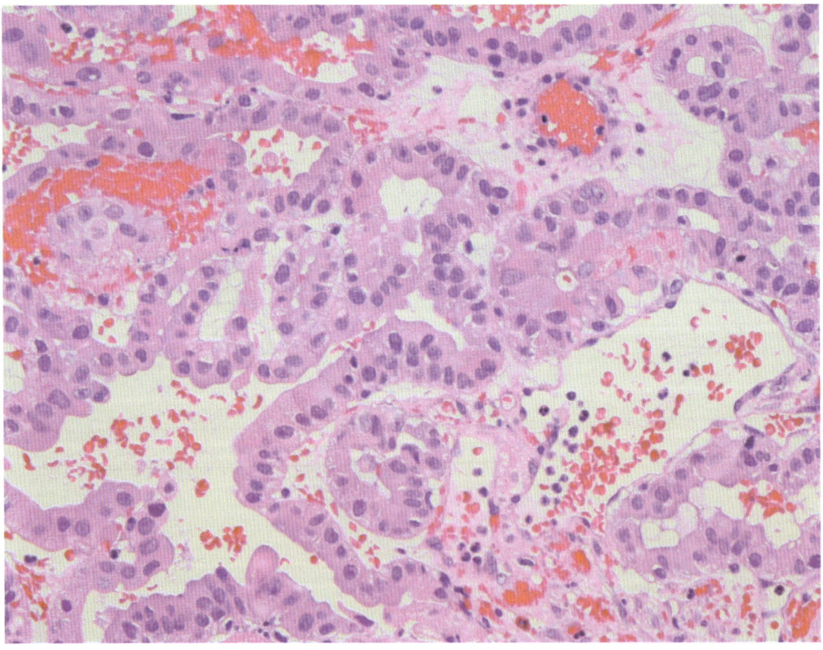

B

FIGURE 15.8 **A:** Endobronchial biopsy shows metastasis of renal cell carcinoma with abundant oncocytic cytoplasm. The tumor adopts a glandular configuration that can simulate other types of epithelial malignancies. **B:** Higher magnification shows glandular structures lined by large cells with abundant eosinophilic cytoplasm.

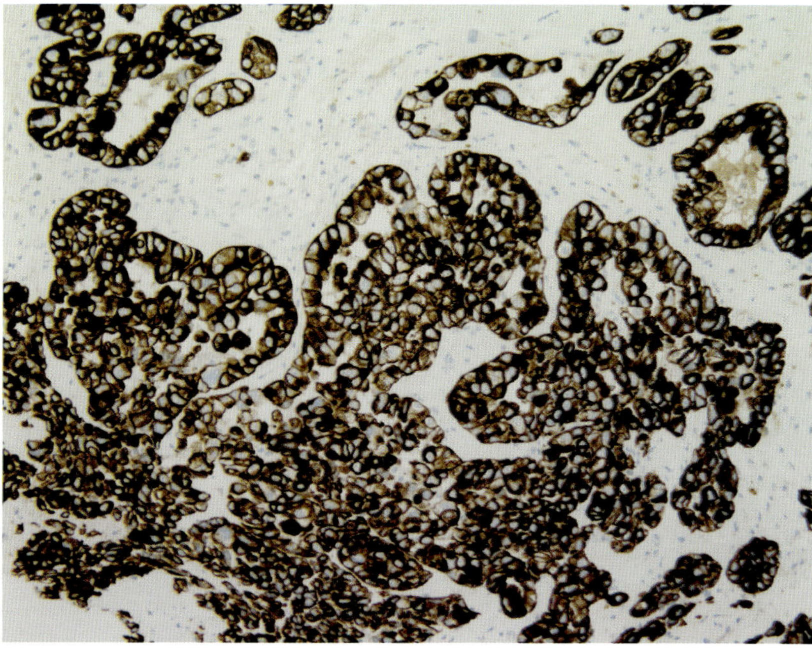

C

FIGURE 15.8 (*continued*) **C:** Immunohistochemical stain for CD10 shows striking cytoplasmic and membranous positivity of the tumor cells.

racemase, which is strongly and preferentially expressed in the papillary variant of renal cell carcinoma.[20] Metastases to the lung characterized by clear cell morphology can also occur in patients with adrenal cortical carcinoma; the lesions may be impossible to distinguish from a clear cell renal cell carcinoma by routine histology. Immunohistochemical stains will be required for proper diagnosis; adrenal carcinoma is most often negative for cytokeratin but will stain strongly with inhibin, whereas renal cell cancer will display the opposite pattern of staining.

Metastases from urothelial carcinoma of the bladder and renal pelvis and from prostate adenocarcinoma can also occur in the lung, particularly in the more advanced stages of the disease. Metastases of urothelial carcinoma are usually disseminated and multiple and will show the characteristic histology of these tumors. Carcinoma of the prostate, although usually presenting first with bony and regional lymph node metastases, can rarely also present initially with metastases to the lungs with no obvious involvement of lymph nodes or bone.[22] Metastases to the lung from prostate cancer often show a marked cribriform pattern (Fig. 15.9); identification of this pattern of growth should prompt ordering stains for prostate-specific antigen and prostate-specific acid phosphatase to rule out prostate cancer.[23] Metastases to the lungs from testicular cancer occurs with frequency, particularly with malignant germ cell tumors.[23,24] Embryonal

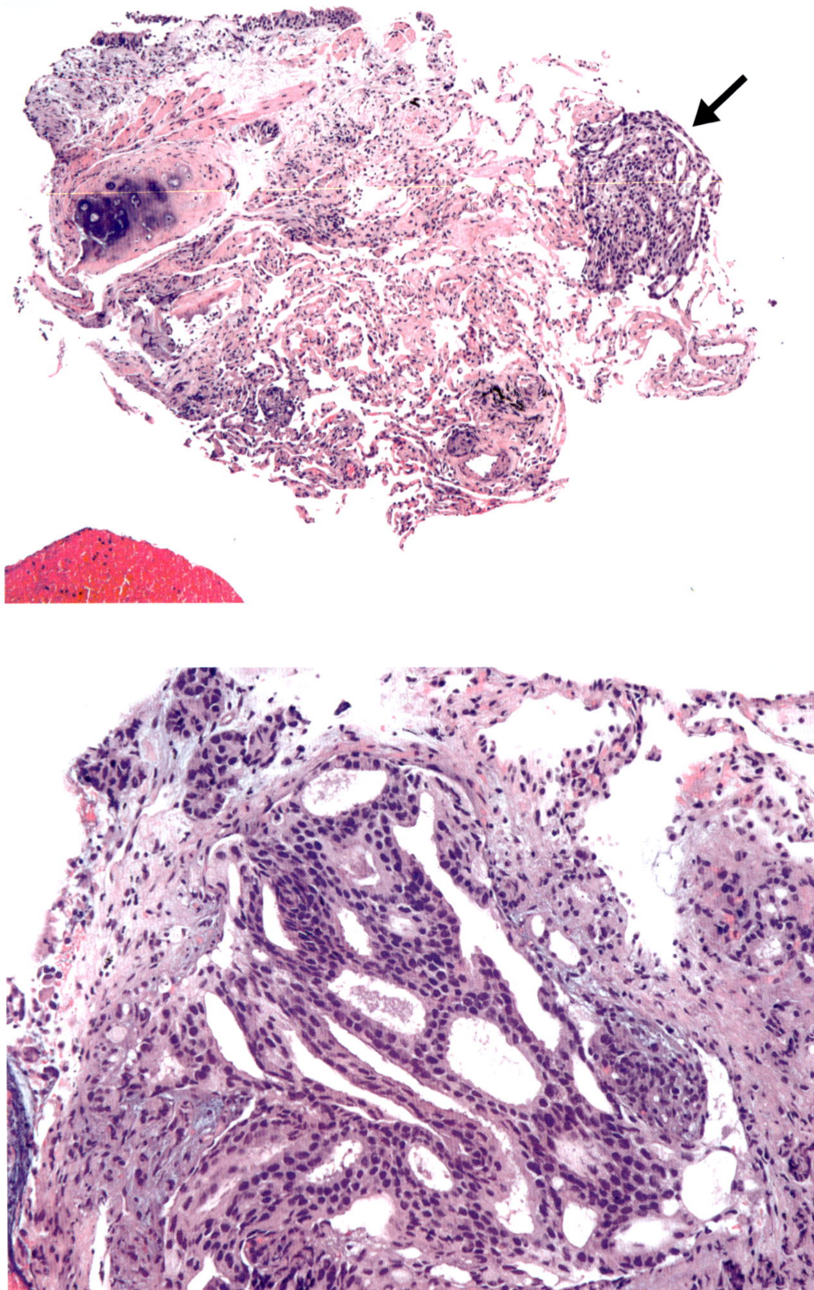

A

B

FIGURE 15.9 **A:** Transbronchial biopsy showing normal bronchial mucosa and cartilaginous plate and a minute focus of adenocarcinoma within alveolated parenchyma (arrow). **B:** Higher magnification shows cribriform glandular spaces lined by atypical cells with hyperchromatic nuclei characteristic of prostate carcinoma.

carcinoma and teratocarcinoma may metastasize as either a synchronous or a metachronous solitary lung nodule. A peculiar phenomenon observed in these tumors at the metastatic site is maturation of the tumor, whereby the metastatic deposits will contain only mature teratomatous elements (Fig. 15.10).[25] The lung is also a favored site of metastasis for testicular and uterine choriocarcinoma characterized by large, hemorrhagic tumor masses, although disseminated disease may also occur. The lesions will usually show bizarre nuclear pleomorphism owing to the syncytiotrophoblastic component, with prominent interstitial hemorrhage; less frequently only the cytotrophoblastic component may be evident. The tumors need to be distinguished from anaplastic large cell carcinoma, pleomorphic sarcomas, and large cell carcinoma of the lung that can occasionally contain a trophoblastic giant cell component. The latter tumors will display focal positivity for β-HCG, making the use of this stain of limited value for separating the two. Clinicopathologic correlations, and a detailed clinical history is indispensable for diagnosis under those circumstances.

Tumors of the female reproductive tract can also be a common source of metastases to the lungs, mainly from carcinoma of the uterus and cervix.[26] Metastases of endometrioid adenocarcinoma of the uterus and ovary can show a back-to-back cribriform arrangement of glands that

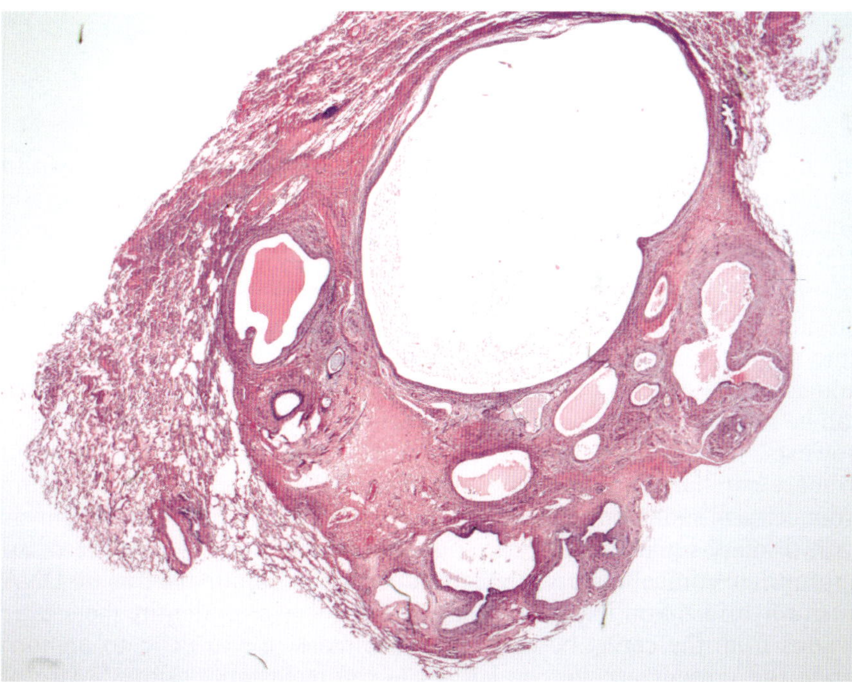

FIGURE 15.10 Lung metastasis from testicular teratocarcinoma shows "maturation" phenomenon, whereby only mature teratomatous elements are present at the metastatic site.

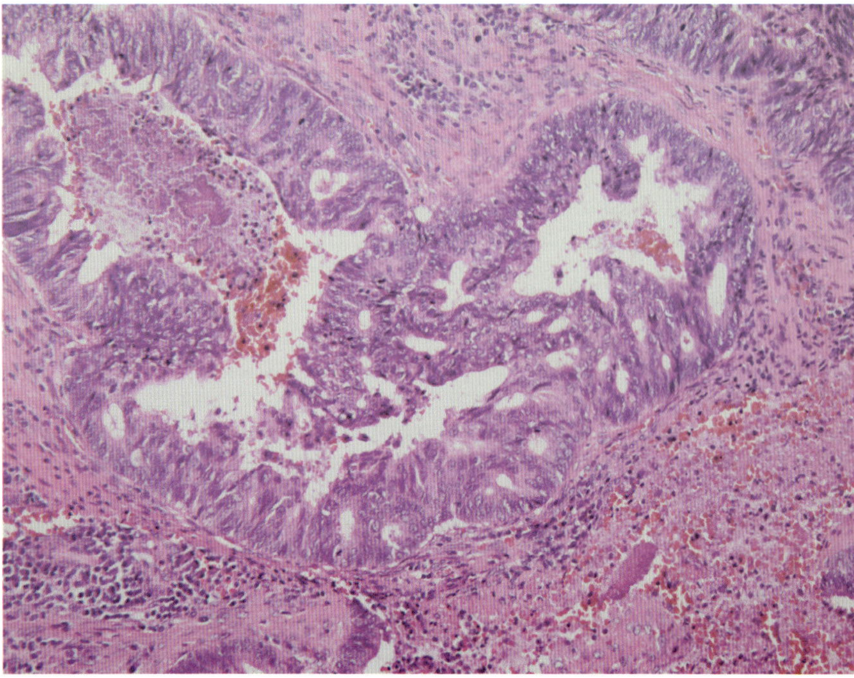

FIGURE 15.11 Metastasis to the lung from endometrioid adenocarcinoma shows back-to-back cribriform arrangement of glands.

can display prominent subnuclear vacuolization; the latter will be helpful for distinguishing it from primary lung adenocarcinoma (Fig. 15.11). The tumors must be distinguished, however, from the fetal-type adenocarcinoma of the lung, which can closely resemble a metastatic endometrioid adenocarcinoma. Fetal-type lung adenocarcinoma will show positivity of the tumor cells for TTF-1 and β-catenin, unlike endometrioid adenocarcinoma that is usually negative for those markers. Papillary serous carcinomas of the ovary or uterus also metastasize distally to the lung. They can be recognized by their high-grade cytology and papillary architecture; however, clinical correlation is always indicated to separate them from primary papillary carcinoma of lung (Fig. 15.12). Metastases to the lung from cervical squamous cell carcinoma can cause difficulties for diagnosis with primary squamous cell carcinoma of the lung in the absence of an appropriate clinical history. Detection of human papillomavirus by DNA in situ hybridization has been utilized with success to identify metastatic lesions from the cervix by reverse transcriptase in situ PCR, to demonstrate the presence of the viral RNA in the metastatic lesions.[27] Use of antibodies to p16 can also be utilized to accomplish similar results, given that squamous cell carcinoma of the lung displays loss of expression of p16.[28]

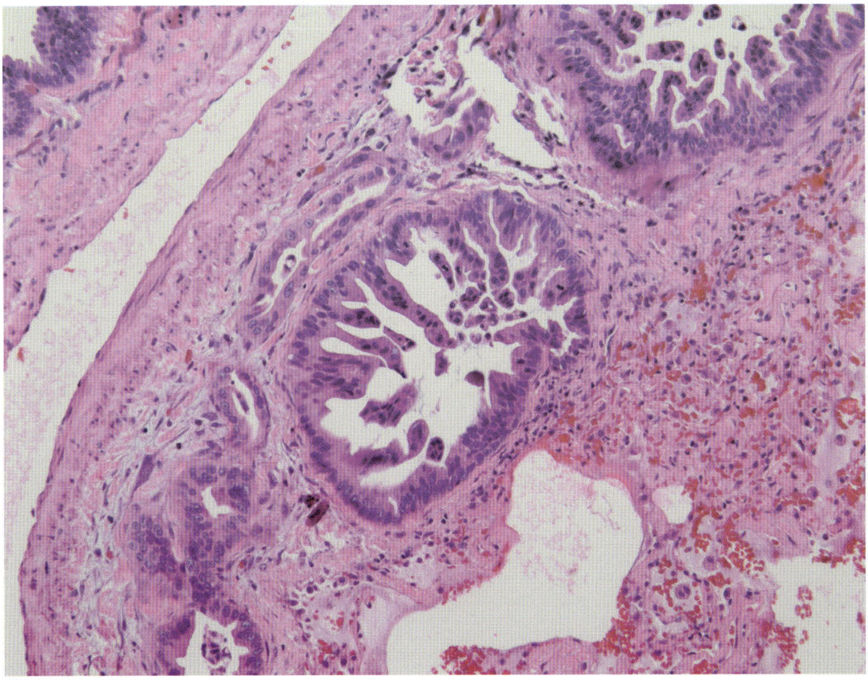

FIGURE 15.12 Metastasis of papillary serous carcinoma of ovary to the lung shows plugging of lymphatics by tumor.

Metastases from Other Epithelial Malignancies

Breast carcinoma is a common source of lung metastases and the lung can be a frequent site of initial relapse for these tumors. Distinction from a second primary lung cancer can be problematic, especially if a long latency period has supervened since the removal of the primary tumor. Moreover, up to 23% of lung metastases from breast cancer can be solitary.[29] Breast cancer metastases to the lung can show a prominent lymphangitic pattern of spread along lymphatics (Fig. 15.13); it can adopt a miliary pattern of distribution with diffusely scattered microscopic nodules; it can show a tubular pattern of spread extending within the airspaces; or it can adopt a lepidic pattern of growth resembling bronchioloalveolar carcinoma (Fig. 15.14) (eFigs. 15.9 and 15.10).[30] They can also display a variety of morphologic appearances that can mimic other primary and metastatic lung tumors. Metastatic ductal carcinomas of the breast to the lung can display an acinar growth pattern, a single-file configuration reminiscent of metastatic anaplastic carcinoma of stomach or invasive lobular carcinoma of breast (Fig. 15.15), a cribriform architecture that recapitulates ductal carcinoma in situ of the breast (Fig. 15.16), or it can grow as sheets of poorly differentiated tumor cells without any specific architecture (Fig. 15.17). Without a proper clinical history, it may be impossible to recognize the tumor as coming from the breast. Lung metastases from

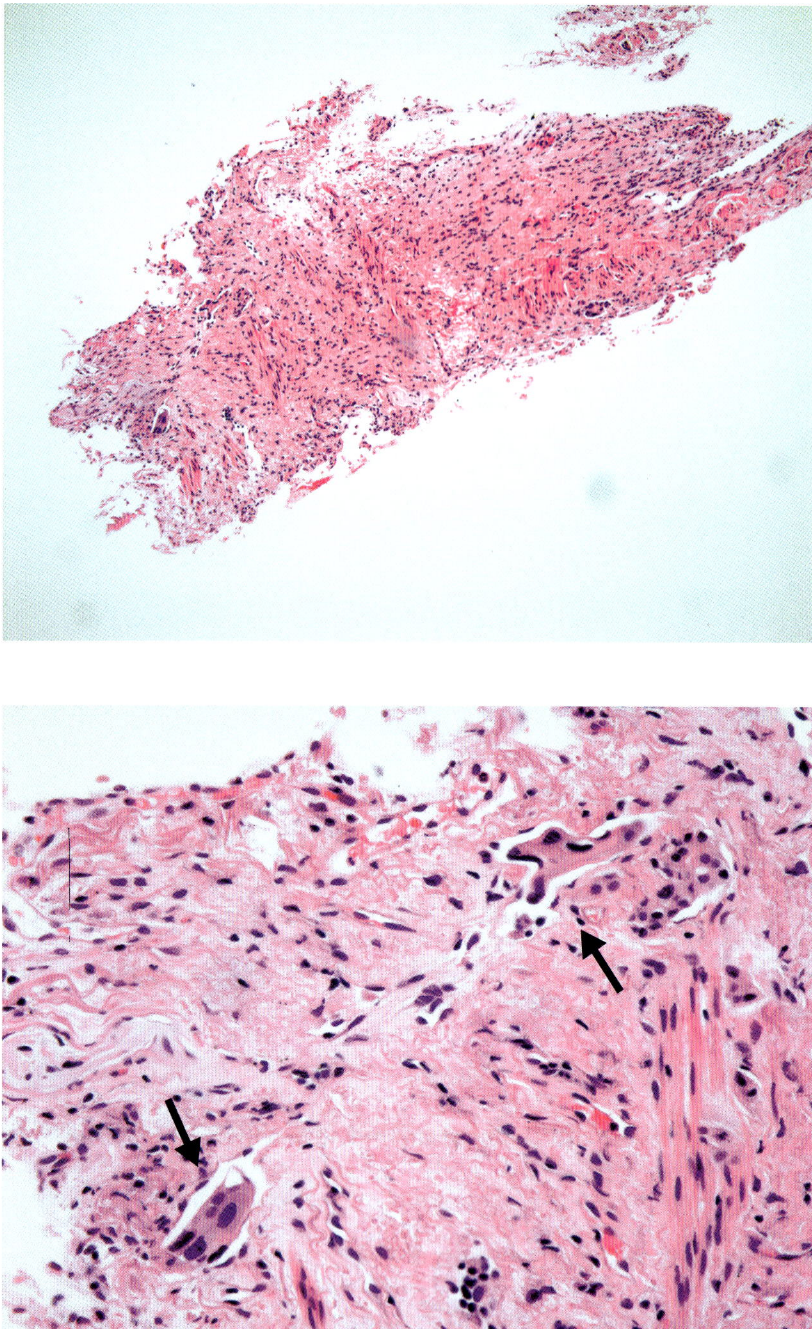

A

B

FIGURE 15.13 **A:** Endobronchial biopsy in patient with history of breast cancer and diffuse reticulonodular lung infiltrates shows deceptively bland appearance with minimal changes. **B:** Higher magnification, however, shows microscopic tumor emboli plugging small lymphatic vessels (arrows).

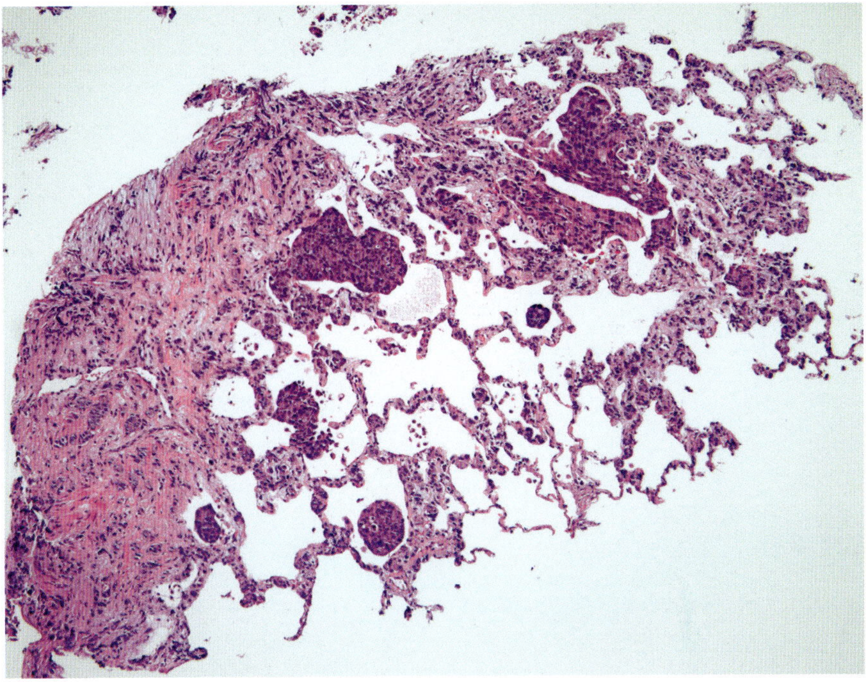

FIGURE 15.14 Transbronchial biopsy shows metastatic breast carcinoma spreading through the airspaces. Tumor plugs are seen within the alveolar lumens.

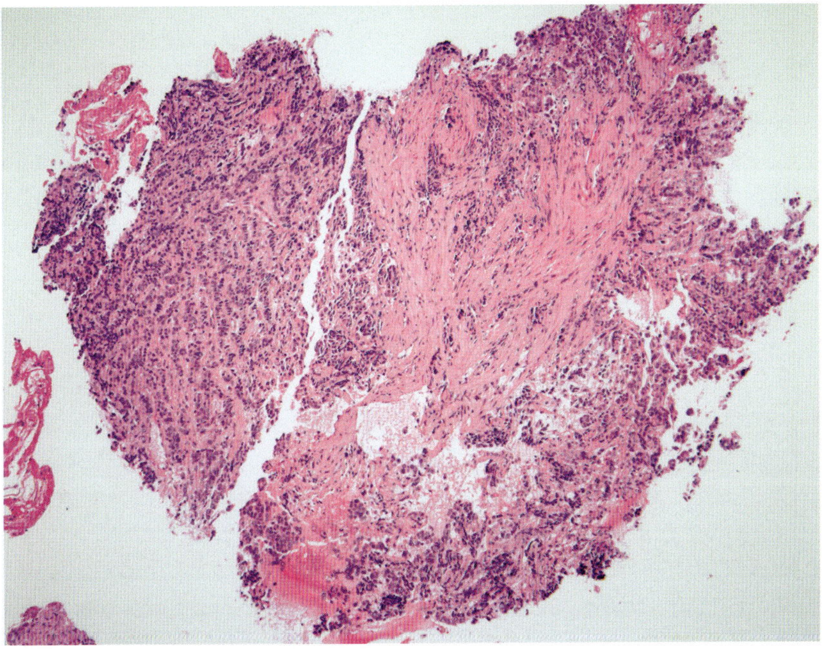

A

FIGURE 15.15 **A:** Endobronchial biopsy in patient with metastasis of breast carcinoma shows replacement of the lung by invasive tumor. *(continued)*

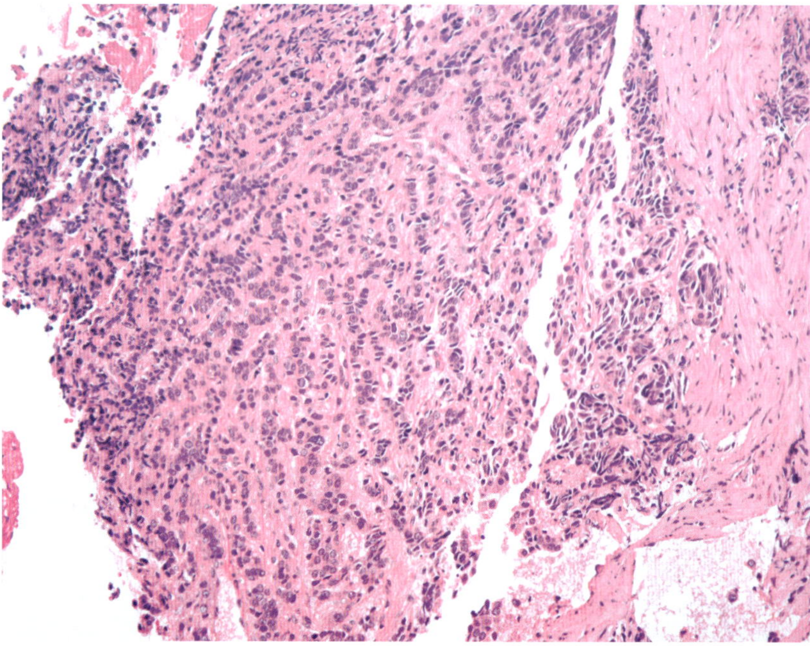

B

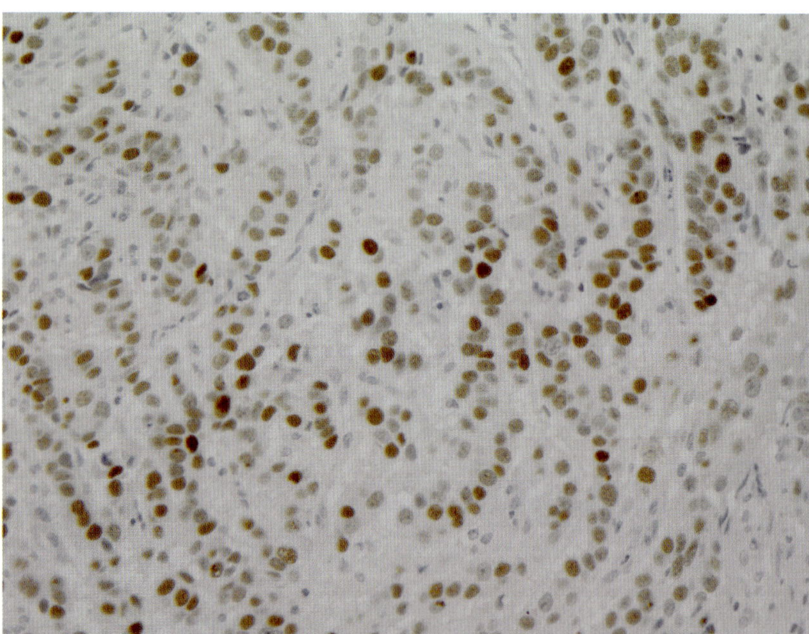

C

FIGURE 15.15 (*continued*) **B:** Higher magnification shows atypical tumor cells infiltrating connective tissue in a single-file arrangement. **C:** Immunohistochemical stain for estrogen receptor shows positive nuclear staining of the tumor cells.

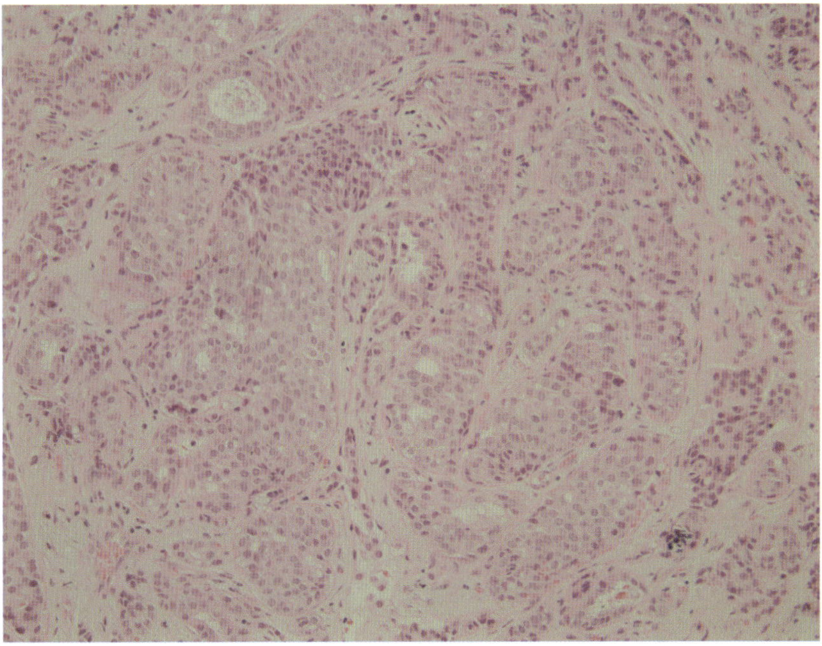

FIGURE 15.16 Metastasis to the lung from invasive ductal carcinoma of the breast shows islands of tumor cells with cribriform architecture resembling breast ductal carcinoma in situ.

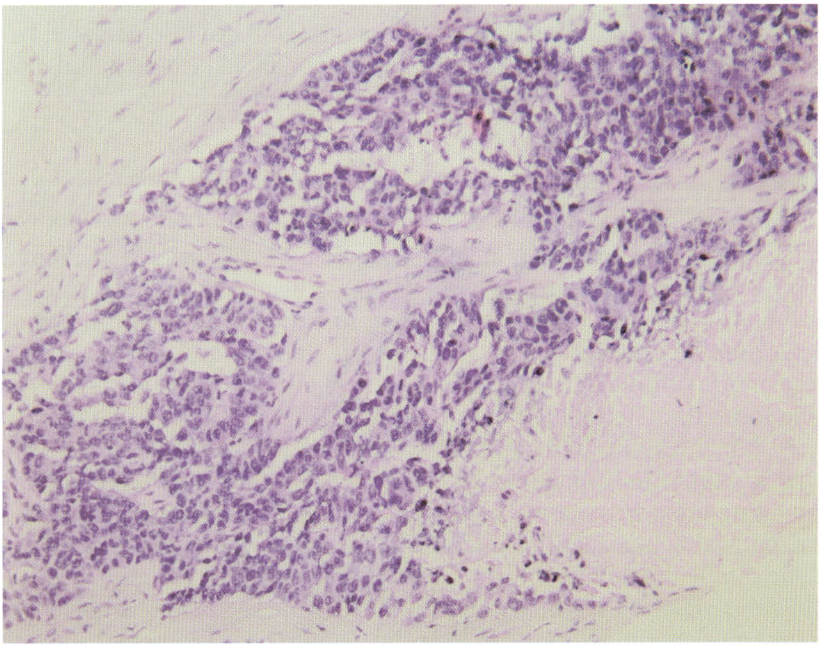

FIGURE 15.17 Metastasis to the lung of invasive ductal carcinoma of breast shows sheets of poorly differentiated tumor cells without any particular architecture.

breast ductal carcinoma usually stain positive for CK5/6, estrogen and progesterone receptors, E-cadherin, GCDFP-15, and mammaglobin, and they are negative for CK7, TTF-1, napsin A, and p63.

Other epithelial neoplasms that can in rare instances metastasize to the lungs include adnexal carcinomas of the skin (squamous cell carcinoma, basal cell carcinoma, basosquamous carcinoma, and other malignant adnexal tumors) and thymomas. Adnexal carcinomas are almost universally positive for p63; care must be taken not to mistake them on small biopsies for squamous cell carcinoma of the lung. As with all other metastases to the lung, an adequate clinical history will be indispensable for proper interpretation.

METASTASES FROM BONE AND SOFT TISSUE SARCOMAS

Bone and soft tissue sarcomas are a frequent source of metastases to the lungs; the lung is, in fact, the most common site of metastases for malignant bone tumors and soft tissue sarcoma. Histologic distinction between a primary and a secondary tumor is not possible based on histologic examination alone; clinicopathologic correlation is required to make this determination. It must be remembered that metastases of sarcoma to the lung significantly outnumber primary mesenchymal tumors of the lung. Establishing a correct diagnosis of metastatic sarcoma to the lung is of clinical importance because resection of the metastatic lesions has been associated with improved survival.[24,31] Metastases to the lung from sarcomas are most often peripheral and subpleural and well demarcated from the surrounding lung parenchyma. Endobronchial metastases simulating a bronchogenic neoplasm, however, have also been described.[32]

Metastases from Bone Tumors

Osteogenic sarcoma is the commonest malignant bone tumor to metastasize to the lungs. Although, in the past, lungs were the first site of relapse for patients with osteosarcoma, the incidence of isolated pulmonary metastases from osteosarcoma has been reduced significantly since the introduction of some of the newer chemotherapy protocols for this tumor. Metastases from osteosarcoma occurring in children and young adults are most often multiple and peripheral but may also be single and more centrally located.[33] Metastatic deposits of osteosarcoma in the lung generally show similar features to the primary lesions (Fig. 15.18); however, they may show a maturation phenomenon with massive chondroid differentiation simulating chondrosarcoma or with massive collagenization leaving only minimal viable malignant elements. The malignant components may, thus, not be sampled in limited biopsy material precluding an accurate diagnosis. Clinical correlation is, thus, indispensable under such circumstances. The second most common bone tumor in the pediatric age group to metastasize to the lungs is Ewing sarcoma (Fig. 15.19). The tumor can be confused histologically for other small round blue cell tumors in this age group, such

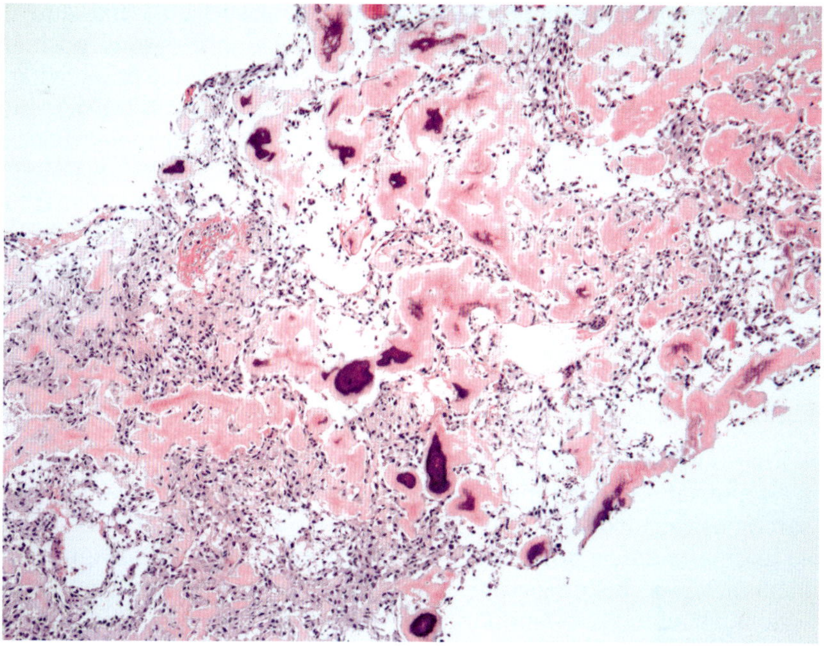

FIGURE 15.18 Core biopsy of peripheral lung nodule with metastatic osteosarcoma shows abundant osteoid flanked by an atypical spindle cell proliferation.

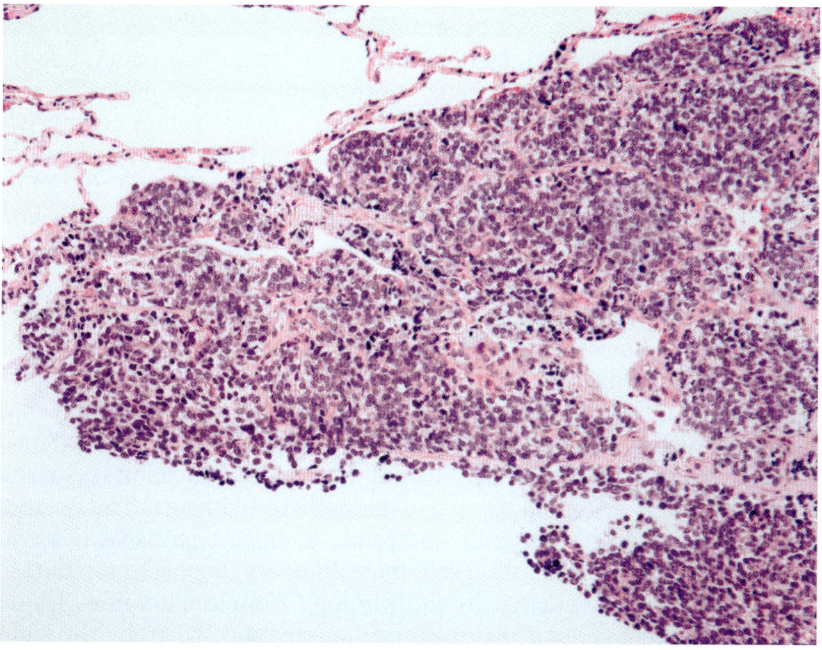

FIGURE 15.19 Lung metastasis of Ewing sarcoma shows sheets of small round blue cells; the tumor cells were strongly positive for CD99 and negative for other differentiation markers.

as rhabdomyosarcoma, neuroblastoma, lymphoblastic leukemia, and the polyphenotypical desmoplastic small round cell tumor; strong positivity for CD99, to the exclusion of other markers, will be of value for arriving at the correct diagnosis. An additional tool in equivocal cases is the detection of the EWS/FLI-1 translocation on chromosome 22q12 by molecular testing or by use of the monoclonal antibody to Friend leukemia integration-1 (FLI-1) by immunohistochemistry. However, it should be remembered that cases of acute lymphoblastic leukemia can also be positive for CD99 and FLI-1.[34] Evaluation of pediatric small round blue cell tumors should, thus, be carried out using a panel of immunohistochemical stains that include CD99, FLI-1, CD3, CD10, CD20, CD43, TdT, cytokeratins, neuroendocrine, and myogenic markers (desmin, myogenin, etc.).

Metastases from Soft Tissue Sarcomas

The lung is a favored site of metastases for soft tissue sarcomas. Virtually any type of sarcoma can metastasize to the lung. Because a large variety of sarcomas can also arise as primary tumors in the lung, it may be impossible to differentiate a primary from a metastatic lesion without supportive clinical data. The histologic differential diagnosis for sarcomas metastatic to the lung includes pulmonary carcinosarcoma, sarcomatoid (spindle cell) carcinoma, and biphasic pulmonary blastoma. Making this distinction on a small biopsy may be impossible unless very distinctive or clearly diagnostic areas for these tumors are present in the sample. In many instances, the best diagnosis that can be offered will be that of "spindle cell malignant neoplasm, not otherwise specified (NOS)" or "high-grade sarcoma, NOS." In general, metastases from soft tissue sarcomas can predominantly comprise spindle cells, epithelioid cells, pleomorphic cells, or an admixture in varying proportions of the above. Tumors comprising predominantly or exclusively of spindle cells include synovial sarcoma, fibrosarcoma (malignant solitary fibrous tumor), malignant peripheral nerve sheath tumor, leiomyosarcoma, and myofibroblastic sarcomas (Fig. 15.20). Tumors comprising epithelioid cells include epithelioid sarcoma, alveolar soft parts sarcoma, malignant peripheral nerve sheath tumor, epithelioid fibrosarcoma, and others (Fig. 15.21). Tumors characterized by pleomorphic tumor cells include pleomorphic liposarcoma and pleomorphic high-grade sarcoma ("malignant fibrous histiocytoma"). Virtually any of these lesions can display areas exhibiting "rhabdoid" morphology in high-grade tumors; that is, tumor cells with globular, densely eosinophilic cytoplasmic inclusions that displace the nuclei to the periphery and comprise accumulations of intermediate filaments. The presence of "rhabdoid" features generally portends a more aggressive behavior. A peculiar phenomenon observed in pulmonary metastases from soft tissue sarcomas is a change in morphology from the original lesion.[4] Some tumors may show a maturation phenomenon, whereby the tumor cells adopt a better differentiated morphology or undergo cartilaginous, smooth muscle, or other types of differentiation; others may undergo a

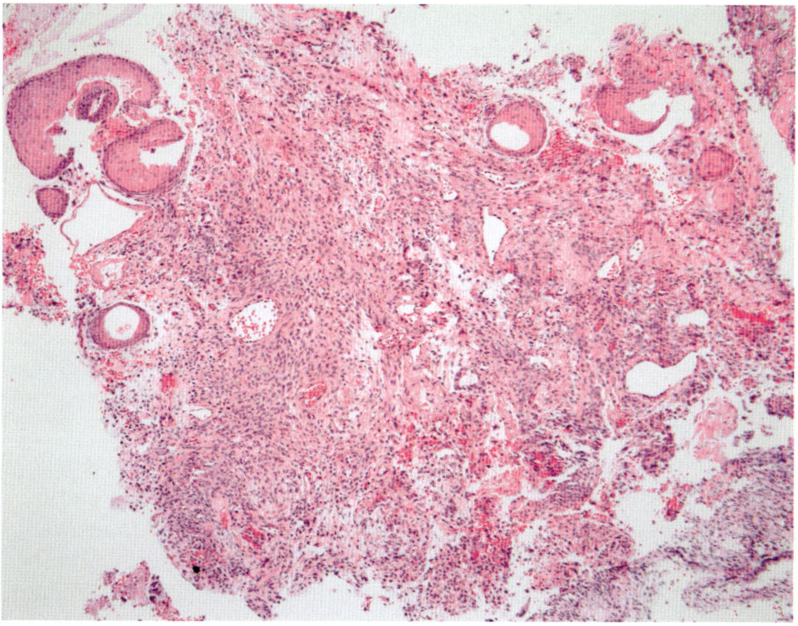

FIGURE 15.20 Endobronchial metastasis of synovial sarcoma shows monotonous population of spindle cells entrapping bronchial glands. The patient had a known history of synovial sarcoma of the ankle.

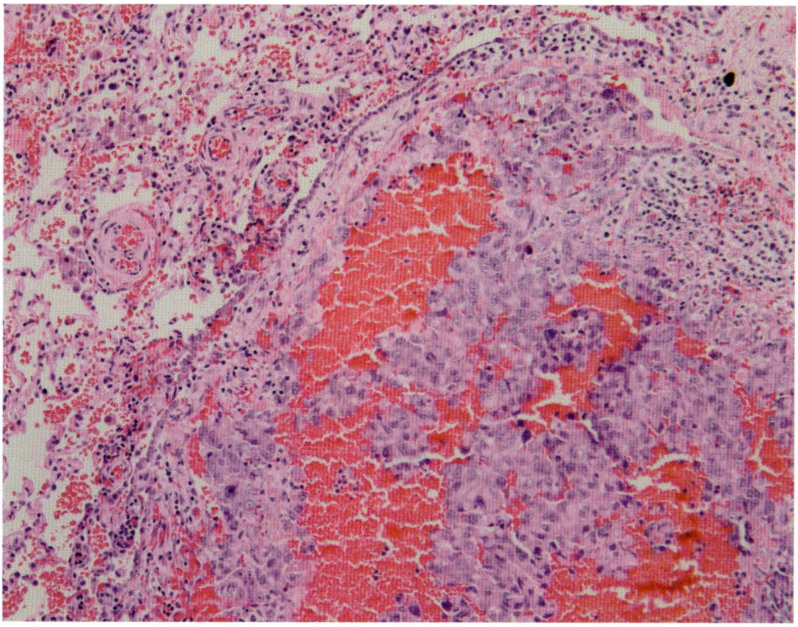

FIGURE 15.21 Metastasis to the lung from epithelioid sarcoma of hand; notice the cluster of round, epithelioid cells with abundant cytoplasm. Some of the cells display homogeneous eosinophilic "rhabdoid" inclusions in the cytoplasm.

regressive process in which they will revert to a more primitive phenotype, reminiscent of a malignant fibrous histiocytoma. Another feature of metastases of soft tissue sarcoma to the lungs is the tendency for the tumor to entrap normal airspaces in the advancing border of the lesions at the periphery simulating a biphasic neoplasm, a pitfall that can be averted by noticing the normal, benign appearance of the epithelial structures and by demonstration of TTF-1 or napsin A positivity in those cells.

Immunohistochemistry and molecular pathology can play a major role in identifying the specific type of sarcoma (Table 15.1); however, strict clinicopathologic correlation will be indispensable to establish whether the lesion represents a primary or metastatic tumor.

Sarcomas of the Female Genital Tract

Uterine leiomyosarcoma is the commonest type of sarcoma of the female genital tract to metastasize to the lungs. Metastases to the lung from uterine leiomyosarcoma are generally a late event, and the metastases may appear very well differentiated and of low-grade histology leading to confusion with a benign smooth muscle proliferation.[35] Metastatic leiomyosarcoma shows immunoreactivity with smooth muscle-associated markers, including SMA, SMMS, and H-caldesmon, but use of these markers will not permit a distinction between a tumor originating in the lung, uterus, and soft tissue. A helpful adjunct for diagnosis in such cases is the use of bcl-2, an oncofetal protein involved in the regulation of apoptosis that is strongly expressed in Mullerian-derived (female genital) smooth muscle but not in smooth muscle tumors arising from extragenital soft tissue.[36] Strong positivity of the tumor cells for bcl-2 will strongly point in the direction of a metastasis from the female genital tract. Metastases of high-grade uterine leiomyosarcoma may occur synchronously with the primary tumor and will show a bizarre morphology reminiscent of a pleomorphic high-grade sarcoma (malignant fibrous histiocytoma).

Endometrial stromal sarcoma is another uterine tumor that shows a propensity to metastasize to the lungs, particularly in late stages of low-grade lesions. A solitary lung metastasis may occasionally be the first manifestation of the tumor.[37] Metastases of endometrial stromal sarcoma can be easily mistaken for a variety of other mesenchymal neoplasms and usually present as a monotonous proliferation of uniform small round or oval cells that may adopt a striking hemangiopericytomatous growth pattern. A distinctive feature that should bring to mind the possibility of endometrial stromal sarcoma is the identification of small spiral arterioles scattered in the stroma (Fig. 15.22A). Immunohistochemical stains will also play a role in the diagnosis because the tumors are strongly positive for CD10, a marker that is not commonly expressed in other tumors bearing similar morphologic features (Fig. 15.22B). The tumors are also characterized by positivity for estrogen and progesterone receptors. More recently, a specific molecular genetic abnormality has been demonstrated in these tumors that is characterized by a (7;17) translocation with involvement of

TABLE 15.1 Translocations, Gene Fusion Products, and Immunoprofile in Soft Tissue Sarcomas

Tumor Type	Genetic Abnormality	Gene Fusion Product	Immunoprofile
Synovial sarcoma	t(X;18)	SYT–SSX	Keratin, epithelial membrane antigen (EMA), bcl-2, CD99, calponin, TLE-1, S100 protein
Low-grade fibromyxoid sarcoma	t(7;16)	TLS–CREB3C2	Vimentin
Well-differentiated liposarcoma and dedifferentiated liposarcoma	Supernumerary ring and giant marker chromosomes	Amplification of 12q14–15, including MDM2 and CDK4	S-100 protein, MDM2, CDK4
Myxoid/round cell liposarcoma	t(12;16) t(12;22)	TLS–CHOP EWS–CHOP	S-100 protein
Clear cell sarcoma of tendons and aponeuroses	t(12;22)	EWS–ATF1	S-100 protein, HMB45, melan-A, vimentin
Extraskeletal myxoid chondrosarcoma	t(9;22) t(9;17) t(9;15)	EWS–CHN TAF2N–CHN TCF12–CHN	Vimentin, CD99
Alveolar soft parts sarcoma	der(17)(X;17)	ASPC–TFE3	TFE3
Extrarenal rhabdoid tumor	Inactivation of 22q11.2	hSNF5/INI1	INI1
Ewing sarcoma/PNET	t(11;22) t(21;22)	EWS–FLI1 EWS–ERE	CD99
Desmoplastic small round cell tumor	t(11;22)	EWS–WT1	Keratin, desmin, chromogranin, synaptophysin, vimentin

(Continued)

TABLE 15.1 *(Continued)*

Tumor Type	Genetic Abnormality	Gene Fusion Product	Immunoprofile
Alveolar rhabdomyosarcoma	t(2;13) t(1;13)	PAX3–FKHR PAX7–FKHR	Desmin, myoglobin, myogenin, myo-D1
Leiomyosarcoma	Complex karyotype with numerous gains and losses, but no consistent recurrent aberration at the chromosomal level	None	SMA, SMMS, desmin, calponin, H-caldesmon
Endometrial stromal sarcoma	t(7;17)	JAZF1–JJAZ1	Vimentin, desmin, CD10, ER/PR
Epithelioid sarcoma	None	None	Keratin, vimentin, CD34
Fibrosarcoma (malignant solitary fibrous tumor)	None	None	Vimentin, CD34, bcl-2, CD99

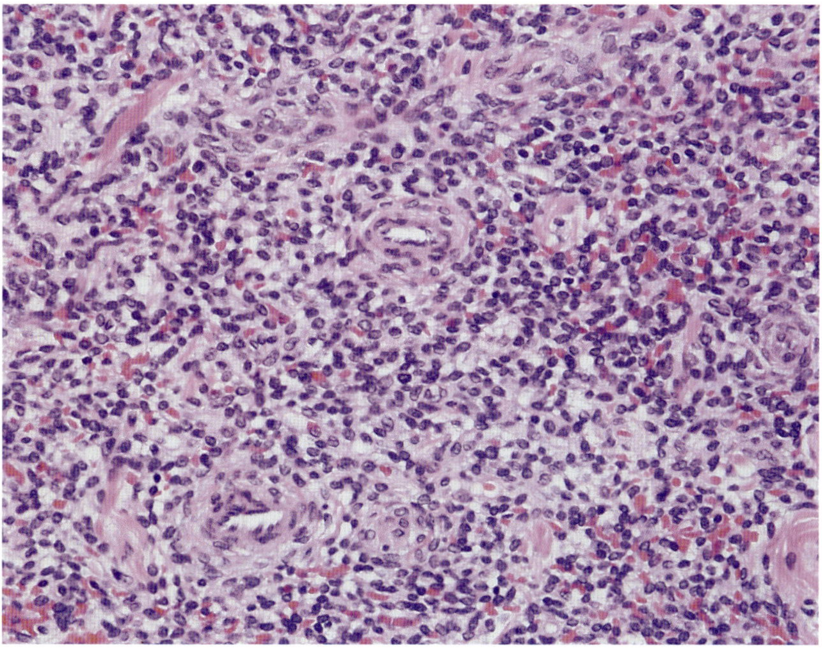

A

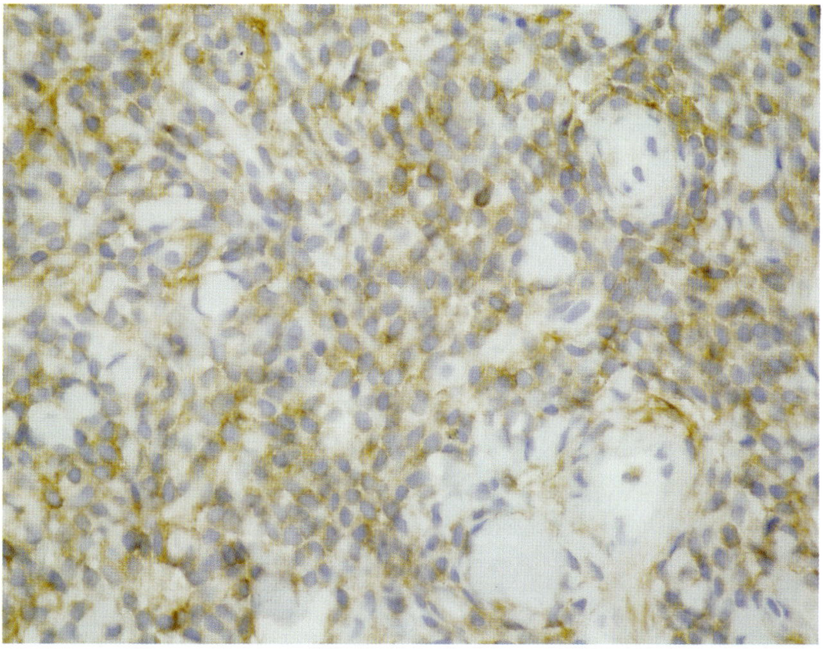

B

FIGURE 15.22 **A:** Pulmonary metastasis from endometrial stromal sarcoma shows monotonous population of small-to-oval cells containing a few spiral arterioles in the stroma. **B:** Immunohistochemical staining for CD10 is seen in endometrial stromal sarcoma metastasis.

chromosome arms 6p and 7p resulting in a fusion protein, *JAZF1/JJAZ1*, which can be identified in paraffin sections by FISH.[38] There needs to be a high level of suspicion, however, for the proper recognition of this tumor at metastatic sites. Confirmation of the existence of a previous uterine endometrial stromal sarcoma through a proper clinical history will be helpful for definitive diagnosis.

METASTASES FROM MALIGNANT MELANOMA

The lung is the second most frequent site of metastases from malignant melanoma and the first site of relapse for the disease. In a large autopsy series, the lungs were involved with metastases of melanoma in less than 70% of cases, second only to lymph nodes.[39] The presence of lung metastases in melanoma generally portends a poor prognosis. Metastases of malignant melanoma are most often multiple and bilateral; however, solitary metastases may also occur. Endobronchial metastases of malignant melanoma present with symptoms of bronchial obstruction owing to an endobronchial polypoid mass. Because malignant melanoma can have a protean morphologic appearance, metastases of melanoma can be difficult to diagnose and may simulate a large number of other tumors. Identification of melanin pigment in the tumor cells facilitates greatly the diagnosis (Fig. 15.23); however, several pulmonary metastases from

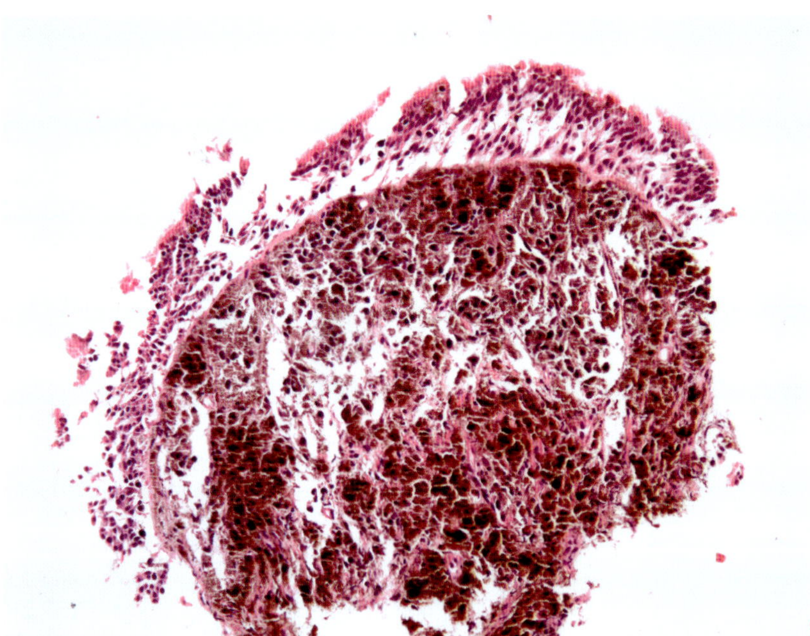

FIGURE 15.23 Endobronchial biopsy in patient with metastatic malignant melanoma shows heavily pigmented atypical cell population underlying the bronchial mucosa.

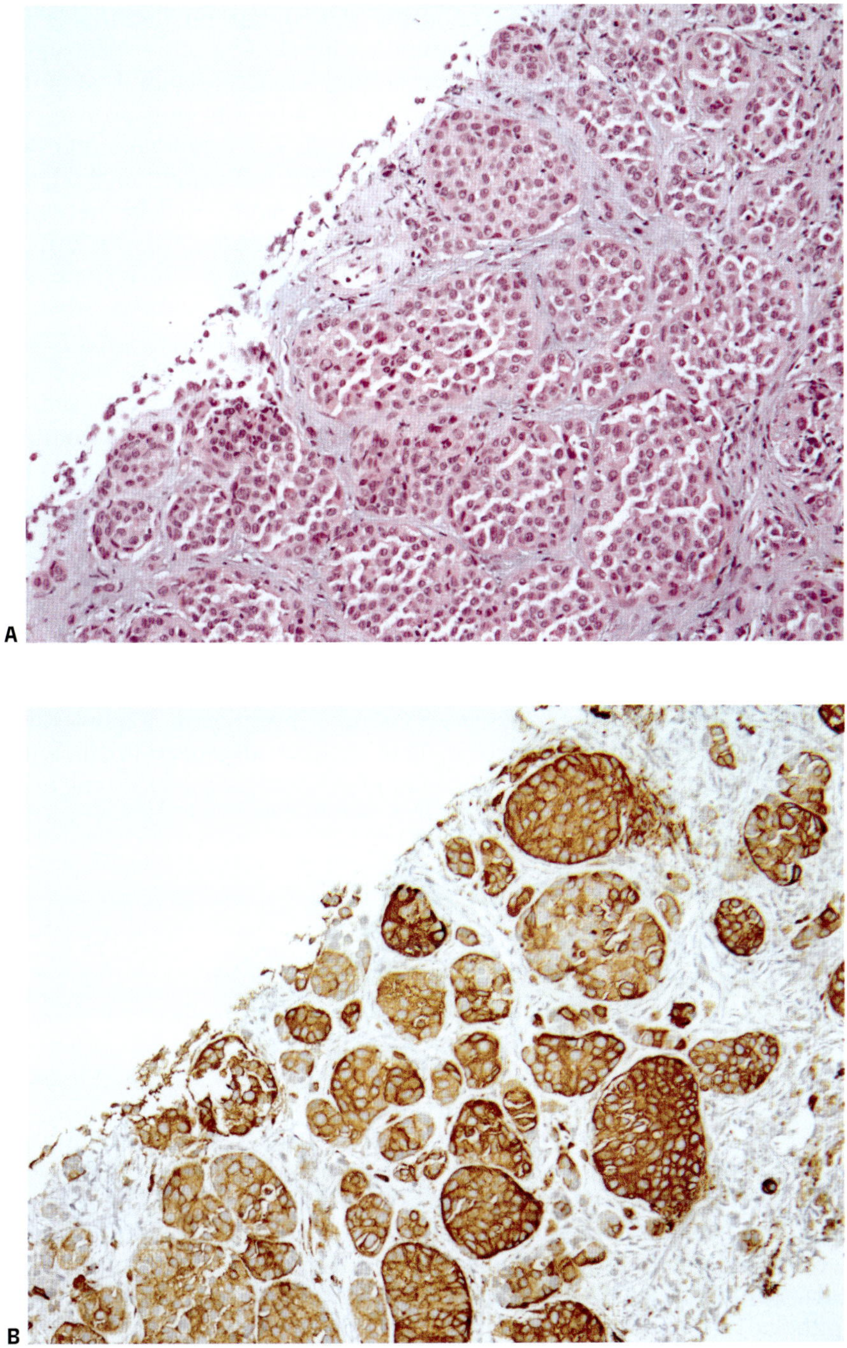

FIGURE 15.24 **A:** Core biopsy of peripheral lung nodule in patient with history of malignant melanoma shows nests of epithelioid tumor cells devoid of melanin pigment. **B:** Immunohistochemical stain with HMB45 shows cytoplasmic staining of the tumor cells supporting the diagnosis of metastatic malignant melanoma.

malignant melanoma are amelanotic and will contain no identifiable pigment (Fig. 15.24). Malignant melanomas can show a wide spectrum of cytologic appearances, including epithelioid, spindle, balloon, granular, signet-ring, rhabdoid, small lymphocyte-like, granular, and bizarre anaplastic tumor cells. In addition, the tumor cells can adopt varied growth patterns, including fascicular, nested, sheet-like, trabecular, myxoid, and sclerosing.[4] The use of immunohistochemical stains will be necessary for arriving at a definitive diagnosis in many instances. The majority of metastatic malignant melanomas stain positive for S-100 protein and will react with one or more melanocyte-associated markers, such as HMB45, melan-A, and tyrosinase. Rare cases (>5%) may lose their reactivity for S-100 protein or for some of the other melanocyte-associated markers. Moreover, a few melanoma metastases will express epithelium-associated markers, such as CEA and epithelial membrane antigen (EMA), introducing a major pitfall for diagnosis in these tumors. The use of a panel of antibodies that includes epithelial and melanocytic markers is, therefore, recommended in the evaluation of poorly differentiated tumors suspected of being malignant melanoma. Comparison of the pulmonary lesion with prior biopsies from the primary tumor may also be of assistance in defining whether the two lesions correspond to the same neoplasm. It should be kept in mind, however, that malignant melanoma may also show a tendency to undergo changes in morphologic appearances at metastatic sites.[4] Likewise, changes in antigenic expression of markers in metastatic lesions of melanoma have also been documented that can introduce difficulties when comparing metastases with the original lesion.[40]

METASTASES FROM "BENIGN" TUMORS

Metastases to the lungs from tumors that are generally regarded as benign ("benign metastasizing tumors") have been recorded in a number of instances. The commonest example is the condition known as "benign metastasizing leiomyoma."

Benign Metastasizing Leiomyoma

This term is used to describe single or multiple lung nodules comprising benign-appearing smooth muscle occurring in women of reproductive age or older with a history of prior or concurrent benign uterine leiomyomas. Another term used for the condition is leiomyomatous hamartoma, because of the tendency for the lesions to entrap normal respiratory glandular epithelium at their periphery creating the impression of a biphasic epithelial–mesenchymal neoplasm. The lesions appear to be hormonally dependent and contain estrogen and progesterone receptors. The exact nature of these lesions is still debatable; some believe them to be hamartomatous, whereas others contend that they represent actual metastases from low-grade, well-differentiated uterine leiomyosarcomas.[35]Recent study using a micro-RNA (i.e., miRNA) assay in these tumors found that the lesions did not express these translational inhibitors in any of the 10 cases studied, compared with high expression in all cases of leiomyosarcoma tested.[41] The authors concluded that benign metastasizing leiomyoma is, indeed, a benign process. Another distinguishing feature was the strong expression of bcl-2, which helps to separate them from primary smooth muscle tumors of the lung that are negative for this marker. Because of their small size and peripheral location, the lesions are seldom biopsied and are most often examined in resection specimens or removed by wedge biopsy.

Other "Benign" Metastases to the Lung

Some of the other tumors that can show metastatic deposits in the lung after a considerable latency period include intracranial meningioma and giant cell tumor of bone.

Benign metastasizing meningioma is a term that refers to a benign-appearing pulmonary nodule with features of meningioma that develops after a long latency period in a patient with a history of benign-appearing intracranial meningioma.[42] The lesions are well circumscribed and show the characteristic features of meningioma, with spindle or oval cells devoid of nuclear atypia or mitotic activity that tend to adopt a whorling configuration. The main differential diagnosis is with minute meningothelial nodules, which are generally microscopic, usually seen as an incidental finding in patients whose lungs were resected for other causes, and do not arise in the background of a patient with a prior history of meningioma.

Benign metastasizing giant cell tumor of bone refers to an analogous situation in which a pulmonary metastasis showing the features of a conventional giant cell tumor of bone develops in a patient with a prior history of benign giant cell tumor of bone.[43] Histologically, the lesions are identical to conventional giant cell tumor of bone.

REFERENCES

1. Suster S. Pulmonary metastases of extrapulmonary tumors. In: Saldana M. ed. *Pathology of Pulmonary Disease*. Philadelphia, PA: J.B. Lippincot; 1994:701–710.
2. Davis EW, Peabody JW, Katz S. The solitary pulmonary nodule. A ten year study based on 215 cases. *J Thorac Surg*. 1956;32:728–771.
3. Toomes H, Delphendahl A, Manke H-G, et al. The coin lesion of the lung. A review of 995 resected coin lesions. *Cancer*. 1983;51:534–537.
4. Suster S, Moran CA. Unusual manifestations of metastatic tumors to the lungs. *Semin Diagn Pathol*. 1995;12:193–206.
5. Rosenblatt MB, Lisa JR, Collier F. Primary and metastatic bronchioloalveolar carcinoma. *Dis Chest*. 1967;52:147–153.
6. Sheperd MP. Endobronchial metastatic disease. *Thorax*. 1982;37:362–369.
7. Viadora E, Brass IDJ, Pickren JW. Cascade spread of blood-borne metastases in solid

and non-solid cancers of humans. In: Weiss L, Gilbert HA, eds. *Pulmonary Metastases*. Boston: GK Hall; 1978.
8. Papac RJ. Distant metastases from head and neck tumors. *Cancer*. 1984;53:342–346.
9. Spiro RH, Huvos AG, Strong EW. Adenoid cystic carcinoma of salivary origin. A clinicopathologic study of 242 cases. *Am J Surg*. 1974;128:512–518.
10. Sidhu GS, Forrester EM. Acinic cell carcinoma: long-term survival after pulmonary metastases. *Cancer*. 1977;40:756–759.
11. Luevano A, Rao N, Mackinnon A, et al. *Cribriform Adenocarcinoma of the Lung. Clinicopathologic, Immunohistochemical and Molecular Study of 15 Cases*. Med. Pathol 2012;25:483A..
12. Yousem SA. Pulmonary intestinal-type adenocarcinoma does not show enteric differentiation by immunohistochemical study. *Mod Pathol*. 2005;18:816–821.
13. Inamura K, Satoh Y, Okumura S, et al. Pulmonary adenocarcinomas with enteric differentiation: histologic and immunohistochemical characteristics compared with metastatic colorectal cancers and usual pulmonary adenocarcinomas. *Am J Surg Pathol*. 2005;29:660–665.
14. Canney A, Sheahan K, Keegan D, et al. Synchronous lung tumors in a patient with metachronous colorectal carcinoma and a germline MSH2 mutation. *J Clin Pathol*. 2009;62:471–473.
15. Moran CA, Hochholzer L, Fishback NL, et al. Mucinous (so-called "colloid") adenocarcinoma of the lung. *Mod Pathol*. 1992;5:634–638.
16. Castro CY, Moran CA, Flieder DG, et al. Primary signet-ring cell adenocarcinoma of the lung: a clinicopathologic study of 15 cases. *Histopathology*. 2001;39:397–401.
17. Cassiere SG, McLain DA, Emory WB, et al. Metastatic carcinoma of the pancreas simulating primary bronchogenic carcinomas. *Cancer*. 1980;46:2319–2321.
18. Katzenstein A-L, Purvi R Jr., Gmelich J, et al. Pulmonary resection for metastatic renal adenocarcinomas. Pathologic findings and therapeutic value. *Cancer*. 1978;41:712–723.
19. Trinidad S, Lisa JR, Rosenblatt MB. Bronchogenic carcinoma simulated by metastatic tumors. *Cancer*. 1963;16:1521–1529.
20. Eichelberg C, Minner S, Isbarn H, et al. Prognostic value of alpha-methyl CoA racemase (AMACR) expression in renal cell carcinoma. *World J Urol*. (Epub ahead of print, Oct. 19, 2011).
21. Gentile PS, Carlon HW, Huang T-Y, et al. Disseminated prostatic carcinoma simulating primary lung cancer. Indications for immunodiagnostic studies. *Cancer*. 1998;62:711–715.
22. Copeland JN, Amin MB, Humphrey PA, et al. The morphologic spectrum of metastatic prostatic adenocarcinoma to the lung: special emphasis on histologic features overlapping with other pulmonary neoplasms. *Am J Clin Pathol*. 2002;117:552–557.
23. Morrow CE, Vassilopolous PP, Grage TB. Surgical resection for metastatic neoplasms of the lung: experience at the university of Minnesota Hospitals. *Cancer*. 1980;45:2981–2992.
24. Mountain CF, McMurtrey MJ, Hermes KE. Surgery for pulmonary metastases: a 20-year experience. Ann Thorac Surg 1984;38:323–327.
25. Moran CA, Travis WD, Carter D, et al. Metastatic mature teratomas in lung following testicular embryonal carcinoma and teratocarcinoma. *Arch Pathol Lab Med*. 1993;117:641–644.
26. Mountain CF, Khalil KG, Hermes KE, et al. The contribution of surgery to the management of carcinomatous pulmonary metastases. *Cancer*. 1978;41:833–841.
27. Plaza JA, Ramirez N, Nuovo GJ. Utility of HPV analysis for evaluation of possible metastatic disease in women with cervical cancer. *Int J Gynecol Pathol*. 2004;23:7–12.
28. Sterlacci W, Tzankov A, Veits L, et al. A comprehensive analysis of p16 expression, gene status, and promoter hypermethylation in surgically resected non-small cell lung carcinomas. *J Thorac Oncol*. 2011;6:1649–1657.

29. Schlappack OK, Baur M, Steger G, et al. The clinical course of lung metastases from breast cancer. *Klin Wochensch.* 1988;66:790–795.
30. Rossman P, Vortel V. Pulmonary metastases imitating alveolar cell carcinoma. *J Pathol Bacteriol.* 1961;81:313–317.
31. Predina JD, Puc MM, Bergey MR, et al. Improved survival after pulmonary metastasectomy for soft tissue sarcoma. *J Thorac Oncol.* 2011;6:913–919.
32. Udelsman R, Roth JA, Lees D, et al. Endobronchial metastases from soft tissue sarcomas. *J Thorac Cardiovasc Surg.* 1984;87:260–269.
33. Rasalkar DD, Chu WC, Lee V, et al. Pulmonary metastases in children with osteosarcoma: characteristics and impact on patient survival. *Pediatr Radiol.* 2011;41:227–236.
34. Lin O, Fillipa DA, Teruya-Feldstein J. Immunohistochemical evaluation of FLI-1 in acute lymphoblastic lymphoma (ALL): a potential diagnostic pitfall. *Appl Immunohistochem Mol Morphol.* 2009;17:409–412.
35. Wolff M, Kaye G, Silva F. Pulmonary metastases (with admixed epithelial elements) from smooth muscle neoplasms. Report of nine cases, including three males. *Am J Surg Pathol.* 1979;3:325–331.
36. Suster S, Fisher C, Moran CA. The spectrum of bcl-2 oncoprotein reactivity in benign and malignant spindle cell tumors of soft tissue, skin, serosal surfaces, and gastrointestinal tract. An immunohistochemical study of 380 cases. *Am J Surg Pathol.* 1998;22:863–872.
37. Abrams J, Talcott J, Corson JM. Pulmonary metastases in patients with low-grade endometrial stromal sarcoma. Clinicopathologic findings and immunohistochemical characterization. *Am J Surg Pathol.* 1989;13:133–139.
38. Micci F, Walter CU, Texeira MR, et al. Cytogenetic and molecular genetic analyses of endometrial stromal sarcoma: nonrandom involvement of chromosome arms 6p and 7p and confirmation of JAZF1/JJAZ1 gene fusion in t(7;17). *Cancer Genet Cytogenet.* 2003;144:119–124.
39. Patel JK, Didolkar MS, Pickren JW, et al. Metastatic patterns of malignant melanoma. A study of 216 autopsy cases. *Am J Surg.* 1978;135:807–812.
40. Plaza JA, Suster D, Perez-Montiel D. Expression of immunohistochemical markers in primary and metastatic malignant melanoma: a comparative study in 70 patients using a tissue microarray technique. *Appl Immunohistochem Mol Morphol.* 2007;15:421–425.
41. Nuovo GJ, Schmittgen TD. Benign metastasizing leiomyoma of the lung: clinicopathologic, immunohistochemical and micro-RNA analysis. *Diagn Mol Pathol.* 2008;17:145–150.
42. Miller DC, Ojemann RG, Proppe KH, et al. Benign metastasizing meningioma. *J Neurosurg.* 1985;62:763–769.
43. Bertoni F, Present D, Sudanese A, et al. Giant cell tumor of bone with pulmonary metastases. Six case reports and review of the literature. *Clin Orthop Rel Res.* 1988;237:275–282.

INDEX

Note: Page numbers followed by *f* indicate figures; those followed by *t* indicate tables respectively.

R